WHAT PARENTS AND HEA
SAY ABOUT T

MW00682756

"A well organized book that is very easy to read, understand. I like the tip boxes as they summarize key points in each section, and the information is very thorough and informative, and the questions asked are common and realistic concerns of parents."
- *Wan Lu (Registered Dietitian, Master of Applied Nutrition)*

"A full understanding of important topics, offers practical aspects of feeding and nutrition, and answers the most frequently asked parent questions. It also allows parents to have a better understanding of feeding and nutrition for their babies and toddlers and allows them to formulate their own questions so that they know what to ask their health care provider."
- *Dr. Diane Sacks (Former President of Canadian Pediatric Society; Staff Pediatrician at North York General Hospital)*

"It covers absolutely everything - from making the choice of feeding style and maternal diet to full meals and related nutritional issues until the age of 5 years. It covers the most important details that every parent asks their health practitioner, and, in many cases, answers to questions we didn't even know to ask! I, as a parent, feel empowered that I am in control and am educated about my children's nutritional status and I know I'm providing my children with the best possible start to life!"
- *Ariella Azogui (Parent)*

"Very informative and super-practical with thorough key information and organization without the extra useless information found in most books. The best gift to any parent who cares about providing their child with the best care early in life. It is definitely a wonderful book that every parent should have."
- *Ariel Nahmias (Parent)*

"This book allows parents to feel in control about their child's feeding and nutrition and saves their time by providing thorough notes that are screened and directly to the point (there is no extra jargon). It is great for the new mother and/or new baby as it provides a wealth of practical information."
- *Dr. Rebecca Bodok (Family Practice)*

"Dr. Levy's book is most informative, practical and down-to-earth. It will be a big help to me as I talk to parents regarding many day-to-day issues in the care of their children."
- *Dr. John Hsuen (Staff Pediatrician at North York General Hospital & Hospital for Sick Children)*

"I would recommend that each mother read and educate herself on these sensitive issues of nutrition and various related topics. It is easy to read and to understand, as it is written in simple English. It is of major help to me to have this information readily available. Great job!"
- *Ella Vinick (Parent)*

"This book is amazingly full of important information for all mothers. It is very detailed and puts your mind at ease."
- *Anna Livshe (Parent)*

BABY & TODDLER
FEEDING and NUTRITIONAL HEALTH
A Complete Practical Guide

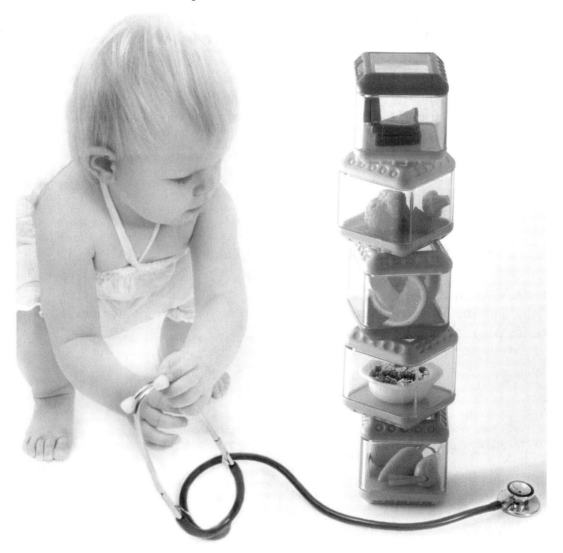

Dr. Maurice Levy, M.D, M.Sc., F.A.A.P, F.R.C.P(C)

White Knight Books

Ordering information CANADA: White Knight Books c/o Georgetwon Terminal Warehouses 34 Armstrong Avenue, Georgetown, ON, L7G 4R9, T:1-866-485-5556 F: 1-866-485-6665 and UNITED STATES APG Distributors (Associated Publishers' Group) 1501 County Hospital Road, Nashville, TN 37218 USA T: 1-888-725-2606, F: 1-800-510-3650

First Printing: 2008

Library and Archives Canada Cataloguing in Publication

Levy, Maurice, 1951-
Baby and Toddler: a complete, practical guide for feeding and nutritional health/ Maurice Levy.

Includes bibliographical references and index.
ISBN: 978-1-897456-00-2

1. Infant-Nutrition. 2. Toddlers-Nutrition. 3. Infants-Health and hygiene.
4. Toddlers-Health and hygiene. I. Title. RJ216.L49 2007 649'.3 C2007-904825-0

Produced by: Book Coach Press
Edited by: Karen Opas-Lanouette
Cover Designed by: Donald Lanouette

Printed and Bound in Canada

For more information visit
www.babyandtoddlerhealth.com

Dedication

~

In Loving Memory & Dedication to my parents, Jacob & Heftzibah Levy
This book would not have been possible without the encouragement, love,
support, understanding, and patience of my beautiful wife, Brigitte,
who has always been supportive of me in my professional life.

Dedicated with love and gratitude to my four children, Lital, Liran,
Roy, and Jonathan for their support, understanding, and patience
during the writing of this book.

A special thanks and dedication to my eldest daughter, Lital,
for her tireless efforts to transform my ramblings into the beautiful book
you have before you, and for her invaluable support and encouragement.

~

Introduction

Welcome

I have been a doctor specializing in pediatrics for over 25 years. The most common issues that parents bring to me revolve around the proper feeding and nutrition of their children. And they are right to have these concerns! Feeding your baby and toddler the proper foods in the proper amount at the proper developmental stage gives your baby life long advantages.

The developmental period in babies and toddlers is the most important stage of a child's life. It is a time of rapid brain growth, during which nerve connections are made, the brain differentiates and develops higher functions, and the body's systems also grow and begin maturing. It is greatly dependent upon appropriate feeding and nutrition.

Parents are responsible for providing healthy and proper nutrition to their babies and toddlers so that they are able to grow and develop optimally. Parents are often either dangerously misinformed or simply lack the information to properly feed their babies and toddlers.

Parents will do the right thing for their child, if they only know what the right thing is. For that, parents need solid nutritional knowledge. It can be difficult to find a comprehensive source of infant and toddler nutritional information.

This book is written using the most recent research and nutritional information, and is based on research, training, and professional experience. It is current and provides sound scientific evidence, to the best of my knowledge. This book will become an invaluable resource and reference for parents.

Intention & Purpose

This book is intended for parents of babies and toddlers and is definitely useful for health professionals (e.g., pediatricians, family doctors, dieticians, nutritionists, etc.). It will help parents by providing information on the optimal feeding and nutrition for babies and toddlers, and will ease concerns over a variety of related issues.

Nutritional and feeding aspects are covered from a medical perspective, from the time the baby is born until toddler age (and even older), in a practical, simple, and easy to read manner.

It is important for parents to educate themselves about their child's feeding and nutrition, as the responsibility is on them; parents are the child's primary caregivers and are responsible for what, when, and how the child eats, and the effects of inappropriate feeding and nutrition.

Although the information provided in this book equally applies to children of either sex, "he" and "she" alternate through the book to prevent the awkward use of he/she. If a particular problem is related to one sex more than the other, it will be stated; otherwise it is equal to both sexes without the intent to give offense.

How this Book is Different

The following characteristics distinguish this book from other reference books:

The entire book is focused on the feeding and nutrition of babies and toddlers in a detailed, simple, step-by-step organized plan for mothers and fathers, as well as health professionals.

It is written by a pediatrician (previously the family medical columnist for the women's weekly magazine *Laisha*), who has listened to and answered many of the same questions (although each baby is unique) that were posed by parents over the last 25 years of medical practice.

Each topic in the book is discussed in specific and practical detail, covering various questions and parental concerns, with case descriptions and added tips in each chapter that answer other, related concerns.

The main message is clearly stated and each chapter presents the main points a parent should know to provide the best feeding and nutrition for their babies and toddlers. In contrast to other books, this provides a point-by-point description. Parents do not have to read between the lines or "look" for the answer in a long story—it is given to them directly and clearly.

Parents will save lots of time reading this book, because it is written in brief, direct points and sentences that are easy to find and understand.

Recipes and menus are included as a guide to set the parents on the right track when preparing foods for their baby. Also included are general home food preparation and sample instructions for each age group (newborn to toddler), which gives the parents a basic understanding of the best feeding and nutrition for their child.

Parents will greatly appreciate the fact that not only does this book discuss problems and issues that arise with feeding and nutrition, it also discusses the role of prevention.

The book is updated with the feeding changes and recommendations that occurred as recently as 2007.

It includes unique chapters that are not included in any other books, such as the picky eater, hiccups, burping, warming the bottle, spices, tastes and flavoring, spoon and cup use, dairy products, nutrition and oral health, pacifier and its effects on feeding, stool characteristics, infant obesity, vitamins and minerals, water and fluid intake, and more.

How to Use This Book

The book contains eight sections with various chapters contained within each section related to the main topic (sub-headings are organized in a logical manner; e.g., when to introduce, what to introduce, how much, etc.). It is designed according to the developmental ability and the feeding stage of your baby and toddler.

Use the table of contents or the index to quickly find specific information on any nutritional concern.

Each chapter begins with general introductory notes to allow the reader to understand what will be discussed in the chapter and gives an overview of why it is important.

Common parental concerns are emphasized in a question and answer format that addresses the most usual questions asked of pediatricians. Each chapter contains tips relevant to that particular topic and stresses aspects of clinical significance.

Case descriptions of issues that occur most frequently in clinical practice are provided to help readers understand what is being discussed.

There are basic recipes and sample menus for the new parents that will provide tasty, age appropriate, and healthy food experiences for your baby and toddler. Various tables throughout the chapters summarize important information for parents.

Disclaimer

Despite the fact that the best effort has been made to ensure that this book is detailed and very practical, and in most cases, will fit your child's case, you must always work in concert with your pediatrician. This is because your doctor knows your child's unique needs and, over time, recommendations may change or differ according to individual consideration and geographical variation.

The contents of this book are not intended and should not be taken as a substitute for your doctor's advice. It is meant purely for informational purposes. Anything contained in this book should not be considered as specific medical advice with respect to any specific condition and/or person. It is meant to ease your concerns and give you knowledge that complements the information your pediatrician or health professional provides.

Thus, the author respectfully and specifically disclaims any liability, risk (personal or otherwise) that may be incurred as a consequence (directly or indirectly) from the use or application of any of the information provided in this book.

Furthermore, this book contains various names of companies and corporations used for the sole purpose of providing parents with clear examples of what is meant: the use of such names is not intended and should not be understood as, endorsing, prohibiting, or advertising any of the companies mentioned or omitted.

Acknowledgements

I wish to acknowledge and offer my sincere thanks to all those who have commented on this book. To begin, I thank my colleagues who have provided valuable suggestions and comments in response to various chapters. These include:

Dr. Diane Sacks: Former president of the Canadian Pediatric Society and pediatrician, North York General Hospital

Dr. Joe Telch: Pediatrician, North York General Hospital and nutritionist

Dr. Kurt Andre: Pediatrician, York Central Hospital

Dr. David Meisels: Family Dentistry

Dr. Susan Kovacs: Pediatric gastroenterologist, North York General Hospital

Dr. Steven Moss: Pediatrician, North York General Hospital

Dr. John Hsuen: Pediatrician, North York General Hospital

Dr. Jay Govan: Pediatrician and neonatologist, North York General Hospital

Dr. Jin Edward: Pediatrician, North York General Hospital

Dr. Stephen Comay: Pediatrician and hematologist, North York General Hospital

Dr. Phyllis Spier: Pediatric and adolescent medicine, North York General Hospital

Elizabeth Zemelman: Registered dietitian in private practice

Wan Lu: Registered dietitian, master of applied nutrition

Janice Newman: lactation specialist, North York General Hospital

Various pediatricians from North York General Hospital and York Central Hospital

Special Thanks

Dr. Sasson Lavi: Pediatric allergist, Hospital for Sick Children

Nancy Girvan: Registered nurse,
International Board Certified Lactation consultant

Karen Balko: Registered dietitian, pediatric department,
North York General Hospital

I would like to thank my patients and others who were generous enough to supplement this book with pictures and comments, in addition to the generous support of these individuals:

Librarians at North York General Hospital; Maureen Pakosh, Gaby Fernandes, Aleine Bernstein
Sofia Abramoviche, Secretarial Help

A special thanks to all my family, friends and colleagues
who supported the production of this book.

I would like to express a sincere thanks to Book Coach Press, particularly Serena Williamson, President of Book Coach Press; Karen Opas-Lanouette, Editor-in-Chief and Donald Lanouette, Book Designer for their support and tremendous amount of work on the production of the book along with their goodwill, patience, and great professional skills to produce an excellent final product. Thank you.

LET'S START WITH THE REAL STUFF!

TABLE OF CONTENTS

Section 1: Breastfeeding

Section 2:
Bottle-feeding

Cup Use

Cow's Milk

Eggs

Section 5:
Issues Related to Feeding & Nutrition

Burping

Stool Characteristics of Babies & Toddlers in Health & Diseases

Constipation

Crying & Fussing In Relation to Feeding & Nutrition

Section 6:
Food Allergy & Food Safety

Feeding & Food Allergy

Section 7:
Growth Characteristics & Assessment

Section 8:
Specific Feeding & Nutrition Issues

Iron & Iron Deficiency

Section 1: Breastfeeding

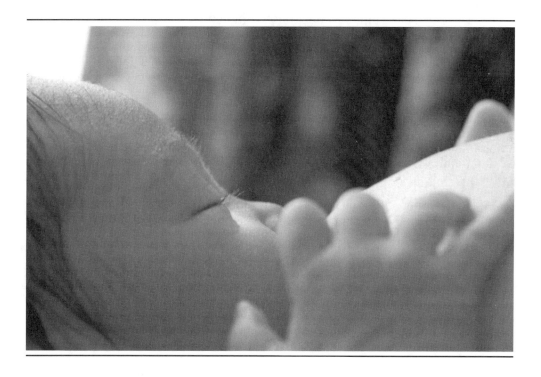

Introduction to Breastfeeding

General

Breastfeeding may be defined as feeding your baby breast milk, either directly from the breast or expressed for feedings using other methods such as the bottle, cup, etc. World health organizations, including the American Academy of Pediatrics, agree that breast milk is the best source of nutrition for at least the first 6 months of your baby's life (including premature and sick newborns). Solid foods should start as a complementary addition to breast milk at around 6 months of age.

Breast milk has a unique nutritional value and will always be considered better for your child than infant formulas. This is due to a difference in composition (that changes to match your baby's changing nutritional needs as he grows) of proteins, cholesterol, fatty acids, carbohydrates, digestive enzymes, infection fighting factors (not found in formula), minerals, vitamins, etc., all of which makes breast milk a better food choice than formula or cow's milk.

Artificial formulas will never be able to fully replicate the nature of breast milk. Its unique composition promotes the development of the brain and protects against various illnesses. In addition, mothers feel an extended physical and emotional bond with their infants, as they are able to nourish, comfort, and meet the emotional need of their babies.

While breastfeeding is a natural function, it does not necessarily mean it is a natural instinct. Many mothers require education, support, and assistance to enjoy breastfeeding their babies. While most first-time mothers may be apprehensive about being able to breastfeed, many feel it is definitely worth the effort, depending upon expectations, attitudes, and concerns.

Ultimately, breastfeeding is a personal decision on the mother's part as she balances her baby's optimal health and development with the demands of her own life. A woman must carefully consider all the facts and options available to her and to her partner, to make an informed and responsible decision.

Tip: Breastfeeding and Intellectual Development

Some studies suggest that formula-fed babies are more prone to learning disorders, overfeeding and obesity, and lower levels of intellectual functioning than breastfed infants (Huggins, 2005).

The Decision to Breastfeed

The following set of questions may be helpful for mothers when deciding whether or not to breastfeed:

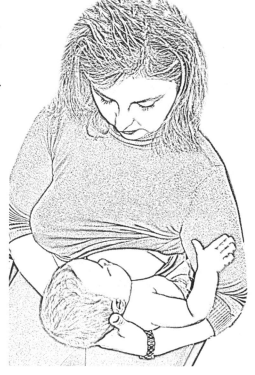

- What are the benefits of breastfeeding my baby compared to the bottle?

- Do I want to breastfeed my baby?

- What do I expect the breastfeeding experience to be like?

- Will I feel incompetent or unable to provide for my baby if the baby and/or I are unable to breastfeed?

- Can I change my mind about breastfeeding after I have already begun?

- Will breastfeeding affect my relationship with my family (spouse or other children)?

- Can I handle my baby's dependence on me for food?

- Are there any difficulties associated with breastfeeding?

Tip: Breastfeeding Problems and Solutions

Much of the physical discomfort (usually of short duration) associated with breastfeeding can be solved with appropriate help and management.

Making the Decision Before Delivery

- While some mothers have made the decision to breastfeed before the delivery, many others are hesitant to make the decision.

- Each mother has her own set of beliefs in various feeding methods with justifications for each one. Educational, cultural beliefs, parental experiences (e.g., breastfeeding mother, grandmother's experiences, etc.), and previous experiences will affect the mother's decision to breastfeed.

- It is best to decide whether or not you will be breastfeeding before giving birth to your baby.

- Consult with your doctor in a relaxed environment and discuss questions and concerns you may have about which feeding method is best suited for you and your family's emotional and physical needs.
- Typically, the individual decision to breastfeed is made during pregnancy, and sometimes even before that.
- Education and support are important for successful feeding, including spousal support, in either feeding methods.

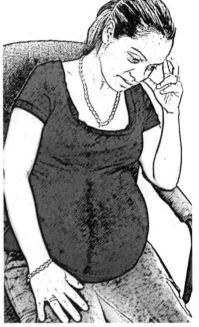

Tip: *Cultural Notes*

Many Asian cultures view breastfeeding in public as an embarrassing display.

The people of Kenya and many Africans view breastfeeding as a natural process and feed their babies on demand (anywhere and at any time).

The Japanese culture views breastfeeding as a necessary requirement for healthy children.

Making the Decision After Delivery

- The first question put to a mother after the delivery of her baby (if she has not decided beforehand) is whether or not she will be breastfeeding.
- It is not recommended that you make this decision during the delivery period, since it is a very tiring and emotional day.
- It is also not recommended to make the decision to breastfeed after you have already begun to bottle feed, since your breast milk production may diminish after birth if no breastfeeding is done and there is a risk of nipple confusion (preference). However, you may combine breast and bottle, as any amount of breast milk is better than none.

Tip: **Why Is the Choice Important?**

The majority of your baby's weight gain during the first year of life is based on the milk your baby receives, whether it is breast, formula, or both. Much of the time spent with your baby is when feeding him. This close contact enhances bonding and love, and can be relaxing for the mother.

Difficulties & Success with Breastfeeding

Initial Difficulties

- There are various obstacles and difficulties when initiating and continuing to successfully breastfeed and these include:

  ❖ Lack of family and societal support, encouragement, and/or guidance.

  ❖ Absence of internal decision (mother is unsure of full importance and need to breastfeed).

  ❖ Insufficient prenatal education or misinformation about breastfeeding.

  ❖ Media influence on commercial promotion of infant formula (distribution upon hospital discharge).

  ❖ Latching difficulties, nipple problems (e.g., sore and cracked nipples, etc.).

  ❖ Baby's refusal to feed from the breast.

  ❖ Insufficient breast milk supply (whether a false impression or truly insufficient milk).

  ❖ Sleepy baby after birth from maternal medications.

  ❖ Post-partum depression.

  ❖ Abnormal maternal diet.

  ❖ Emotional and physical tiredness (anxiety on the mother's part).

  ❖ Maternal employment.

TIP: Reason for Stopping Breastfeeding

Reasons why mothers stop breastfeeding include a perception of not enough milk, sore nipples, etc. The more support a mother has for breastfeeding, the more likely she will continue.

Successful Breastfeeding

The following suggestions are helpful when trying to succeed in breastfeeding your baby:

- Your baby should begin feeding from the breast immediately after birth since early skin-to-skin contact has been shown to have positive effects on successful breastfeeding (unless there is a medical problem).

- You and your baby should room together at all times to provide a better chance of successful breastfeeding. You will be able to immediately feed your baby when he is hungry or anytime he shows interest (24-hour rooming is considered to be ideal).

- Breastfeeding should take place in a relaxed, quiet, and comfortable environment.

- Do not give your baby any bottles when trying to quiet him. Your baby will be reluctant to struggle with your nipple after a few encounters with the bottle's easy artificial nipple.

- Do not give supplemental bottles of formula in the first few days of life if your baby is not gaining weight, unless recommended to do so by your doctor or lactation specialist. There are other alternatives to help initially until breastfeeding is established (e.g., cup feeding, lactation aids, etc.).

- Proper latching technique is crucial to the success of breastfeeding.

- Pacifiers and formula feedings interfere with nursing your baby, so avoid or minimize their use and use them appropriately (after breastfeeding has been established).

- Feed your baby on demand when he is hungry, and not by a schedule. In most cases, you will have to initiate feedings since your baby will be more sleepy than hungry in the first few weeks of life. Initially, you may have to wake your sleepy baby to feed him.

- Breastfeed your baby 8-12 times a day at first; keeping him happy and satisfied while stimulating the hormone (prolactin) responsible for milk production.

- Watch for suckling versus sucking; *suckling* is when your baby extracts milk from your breast; *sucking* is gumming on your breast with no results. Watch your baby for a strong, steady suckle and swallow feeding pattern.

- It is important for you to maintain strong support from your family, friends, breastfeeding specialist, etc.

- Be persistent and determined when you breastfeed your baby—do not give up easily.

Tip: Taking Care of Your Nipples

Do not wash your nipples frequently in soap, as this causes dryness.

Use olive oil or breast milk to protect your nipples from dryness and lesions.

Let your nipple air dry after each feeding.

Keep your nipples dry between feedings by using an absorbing pad.

How Long to Breastfeed

- The American Academy of Pediatrics (AAP) and other health organizations suggest that your child should be exclusively breastfed for the first six months of life, with partial breastfeeding continued (if possible) until the age of one year or longer.

- The Canadian Pediatric Society (CPS) states the following about breastfeeding duration: "Exclusive breastfeeding is recommended for the first six months of life for healthy term infants, as breast milk is the best food for optimal growth. Infants should be introduced to nutrient-rich, solid foods with particular attention to iron at six months with continued breastfeeding for up to two years and beyond."

- The general point is that a mother should continue breastfeeding for as long as she would like to, or as mutually desired by both mother and child.

- The longer the baby is breastfed and receives human milk, the greater the benefits are.

Tip: Breastfeeding Duration

A recent study (Pediatrics 113: 283, 2004) showed that by the time babies reached 12 weeks of age, only 53% of the participating mothers were exclusively breastfeeding. Discontinuation of exclusive breastfeeding was attributed to difficulties with latching or sucking techniques, and formula supplementation, due to various reasons.

Parent Concerns

Does the size of the breast affect the ability to breastfeed?

- No, there is little correlation between breast size and the capacity to produce milk. Only a small number of women with insufficient breast tissue will be unable to breastfeed.

- Difficulties in milk production may be related to breast surgery (e.g., breast reduction), however this is not always the case.

- Minimal changes in the breast during pregnancy and failure of post-partum engorgement may be early signs of difficulties with breast milk production.

- Consult your health profession or lactation specialist to help you assess the situation.

Are there any health benefits to breastfeeding past the age of six months?

- Yes, there are various health benefits to breastfeeding past six months of age.

- Breastfeeding should continue for as long as mutually desired by both mother and baby, since the longer you breastfeed, the greater the benefits to your child.
- Even for older infants and toddlers, breast milk provides energy, protein, essential fatty acids, and antibodies which protect against illnesses.
- Furthermore, the Society of Obstetricians and Gynecologists of Canada show new evidence indicating that extended breastfeeding reduces pre-menopausal breast cancer in you and obesity in your child.

Is it possible to switch to breastfeeding after bottle-feeding?
- If a woman is unsure about whether or not she wants to breastfeed, she can try it for a few weeks and then switch to the bottle if she changes her mind. However, it is very difficult to switch to the breast after bottle-feeding has been given (see *Re-lactation*).

Tip: Breastfeeding Insight
If you plan to breastfeed, you should learn as much as possible about it before the baby is born.

Can I keep breastfeeding when I have a cold?
- Yes, you can continue to breastfeed when you have a cold.
- It is important to continue breastfeeding to provide your baby with the benefits of breast milk (factors that fight infection; especially as antibodies to the cold virus you have developed will be transferred to the baby and lessen his chances of catching it or decrease the severity if he does catch it).
- Use hygienic measures to protect you and your baby, including hand washing, covering your mouth (a mask to cover transmission of virus to your baby), etc.
- Despite hygienic measures, you may still transfer the virus to your baby, even before clear symptoms of a cold are present.

My breast milk is clear. Is this the reason why my baby is not gaining weight? Is there any way to test breast milk?
- Breast milk that comes out clear does not necessarily mean anything.
- Milk testing is not done, as it is impractical for a variety of reasons.
- Difficulties with weight gain in your baby can be due to various factors, which must be discussed with your doctor.

Does a cesarean section delivery affect successful breastfeeding?
- With a cesarean section, there may be a delay in milk production for the first few days after delivery. The mother may also be more tired after the operation, and the baby is sleepier and less interested in feeding. As such, he may not be able to start breastfeeding as early as a vaginal delivery baby.

> **Tip: First Doctor Office Visit**
>
> A pediatrician or other knowledgeable experienced health care professional should see all breastfeeding newborns at about three days of age (within 48 hours after discharge) to assess infant feeding and hydration, as well as to evaluate other conditions. The earlier you visit, the easier it is to solve any problems.

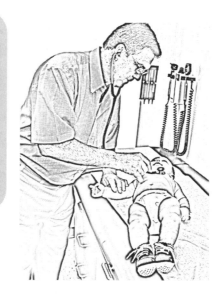

Will I have to breastfeed in public?
- You may have to breastfeed in public if your baby is hungry and needs a feeding.

- However, breastfeeding in public should be done appropriately and comfortably in a specific setting (see *Breastfeeding in Public*).

When can I start dieting, if I am breastfeeding?
- Dieting is not recommended, especially in the early weeks of breastfeeding, until your breastfeeding is established and your baby is gaining weight well.

- In the first few months, you should lose weight slowly to return to your pre-pregnancy weight.

- Remember that you are eating for two and dieting, especially incorrectly, may affect you and your baby.

- Make sure you are eating a healthy, well-balanced diet.

Can breastfeeding ruin the shape of the breast?
- Typically, breastfeeding does not ruin the shape of your breast.

- Most women's breasts return to the size and shape they had before nursing.

When should I start breastfeeding—right after the delivery?

- Start breastfeeding as early as possible, even immediately after the delivery (provided you and your baby have no medical problems, or if you feel physically able). The earlier you start breastfeeding (skin-to-skin contact), the better it is for milk production and future breastfeeding maintenance.

Will breastfeeding a toddler make him more dependent?

- Many experts but not all believe that a toddler who is breastfed will generally become independent, confident, and secure, as he has received comfort from the breast.

Should my spouse play a role in the feeding decision?

- Both parents should discuss feeding options and review the appropriate information for both breast and bottle-feeding. The decision should be one that is informed and responsible. Studies show that spouses have a major influence on the initiation and maintenance of breastfeeding.

I heard that you are given free formula upon discharging from the hospital. What does this mean?

- Formula companies supply the hospital with formulas as an endorsement for bottle-feeding and the hope that formula will be used. This does not mean that bottle-feeding is superior to breastfeeding; it is simply a promotion of a commercial product.

What are some feeding cues?

- Feeding cues can include rooting, suckling motions, motion activity (hands to mouth flexing arms, moving legs like riding a bike), posture effects, tense and clenched fists, crying, etc. (see *Feeding By Schedule or On Demand*).

What are the causes for feeding resistance after a few weeks or months with no problems?

- Sometimes, babies develop feeding resistance after a while of having no problems. Among other possibilities, you should consider whether your breast milk taste has changed due to new foods in your diet, new medicine, strenuous exercise, a new pregnancy, mastitis, illness of your baby, etc.

Resources for Help & Information

There are various resources you can go to for information and help with breastfeeding, including the following:

- Healthcare professionals (physicians, dietitians, nurses, etc.).
- La Leche League International (800-LA-LECHE www.lalecheleague.org).
- Lactation consultants and counselors.
- Doctor or health professional in your area.

Tip: The Decision To Breastfeed

Breastfeeding mothers were asked what made them decide to breastfeed. Some of the answers include:

Because breast milk has all sorts of health benefits for my baby that formula doesn't.

My baby is more important to me than my comfort.

There was no question as to whether to breastfeed; it is a matter of physical and emotional readiness.

It is part of my culture to breastfeed.

I want a special bond with my baby.

Conclusion

- There is no real substitute for breast milk.
- It is the best source of nutrition for your baby, as it contains immunological and anti-inflammatory cells and antibodies that formula can't provide.
- The American Academy of Pediatrics and Canadian Pediatrics Society recommends exclusive breastfeeding for the first six months of life (this may not always be possible, due to various reasons).
- Feeding your child in the early years of life helps determine his physical and mental future health (*Medical Post*, March 14, 2006).
- No one should make you feel guilty or incompetent if you are unable to breastfeed, for whatever reasons.
- The decision is yours and depends on personal choice, cultural beliefs, and previous experiences. As long as you have been presented with the appropriate information for both feeding methods, you are making an informed, responsible decision that can only be made by you.

Breast Milk & Its Benefits

General

Whether you are eagerly awaiting the birth of your baby, or are already experiencing the joys and challenges of a new baby, you made an important decision when you chose to breastfeed your baby. The health, cost, and psychological benefits of breastfeeding make it a great choice.

Breast milk is natural and uniquely produced—each mother makes a "customized" milk for her own baby. It has the right amount and quality of nutrients to suit the baby's first food needs. The composition of breast milk changes within the same day and as breastfeeding progresses to meet the baby's changing needs. The ratio of carbohydrates, fats, and minerals vary at different ages (e.g., 8 days, 9-12 days, 12-24 days, 2 months, etc.).

Convenience is a great factor in breastfeeding—it is always ready and at the right temperature.

The Canadian Pediatric Society and the American Academy of Pediatrics recommend exclusive breastfeeding for the first six months of life. The baby is then ready for complementary foods, but breastfeeding continues to provide many health benefits for as long as the mother is nursing and beyond. Most babies wean at about two years of age on average. Some mothers wish to stop sooner than that and others prefer to nurse longer.

Breast Milk

Colostrum

- Colostrum is the first milk produced at the end of pregnancy and during the first few days after delivery.
- It is yellow in color, thick, creamy, and contains a high amount of minerals, proteins, and antibodies to protect the baby from germs (it contains white blood cells to fight infections). It is low in fat, and easy to digest.
- Colostrum helps babies pass the first stools (meconium, a dark-green, almost black stool) more easily and acts as a laxative. It stimulates the baby's bowel movement and helps eliminate bilirubin (a chemical excreted by the liver which causes yellow skin coloration/jaundice).

- Colostrum coats the lining of the baby's immature digestive system, protecting it against bacterial infection and allergies.

- It is low in volume, but usually just the right amount for a newborn baby (his stomach is about the size of a chickpea at birth). The volume will increase daily, as the baby nurses more and his stomach expands. Around day three there is a big jump in volume when production of more mature milk starts.

- For a period of two to three weeks there is "transitional milk." The amount of colostrum decreases and the mature milk increases. The yellow color will gradually disappear.

Mature Breast Milk
- By about the third day, the milk changes and contains more water (the breast is fuller).

- By about the tenth day your milk changes into mature milk, which has two components:

  ❖ *Foremilk* is milk the baby receives at the beginning of any feeding, It is high in water, which satisfies thirst and supplies water soluble vitamins and lactose sugar. It is bluish-white in color and has a thinner consistency.

  ❖ *Hindmilk* is milk the baby receives as the feeding session progresses; it is high in protein, fat, and calories. This milk is thicker and whiter in color.

- To ensure the infant receives the calorically dense hindmilk, you should keep breastfeeding until your baby pulls away or falls asleep

- Inadequate weight gain and a frequent need for feeding may indicate that your baby is not getting enough hindmilk. This usually happens when a mother switches her baby to the other breast before he is finished feeding on the first breast.

- Mature milk is suited to a baby at any age—milk matures as the baby grows and it is easier to digest than formula or cow's milk.

- Breast milk has a relatively low percentage of protein, making it easy on the baby's immature kidneys.

- The concentration of cholesterol found in breast milk is just right for the needs of your baby's developing brain.

- There is a better absorption and use of important elements such as calcium, iron, and zinc with breast milk than with formula or cow's milk.

Breast Milk Benefits for the Baby

Breast Milk Protects Against Illness

- Breastfeeding protects against ear infections due to a factor in the milk that fights the infection. Also, breastfed babies are fed in an upright position, so they are less likely to experience milk backing up through the Eustachian Tube.

- Breastfed infants experience fewer colds, urinary tract infections, and allergies. The baby is protected by his mother's antibodies, so that he gets less digestive and respiratory infections. The immune components in breast milk protect babies, especially in their first months of life, from allergies and asthma until their immune system has matured (at around six months of age).

- When there is family history of eczema, asthma, hay fever, or other allergies, it is especially important to breastfeed in order to reduce the risk of developing allergic symptoms (the longer you nurse, the better).

- If and when infections do occur, they are usually less severe in a breastfed infant.

- Breast milk also protects against diarrhea by promoting helpful bacteria in digestion.

- It protects against Pneumonia, Meningitis (brain infection), and Urinary Tract Infection.

- Breast feeding is one of the factors found to reduce the risk of Sudden Infant Death Syndrome (SIDS).

- There are fewer problems with food reflux, as milk is emptied twice as fast from the stomachs of breastfed babies than from those of formula fed babies.

- Breast milk lowers the risk of heart disease and juvenile diabetes. A child who breastfeeds for more than 12 months may be 76% less likely to develop diabetes as a teen (*Archives of Pediatric & Adolescent Medicine*, July 2002).

- Breast milk also offers fewer risks of chronic diseases, Hodgkin disease, rheumatoid arthritis, celiac disease, childhood cancer, dental caries, and liver disease.

- Breastfed babies have a better chance of survival than formula-fed babies in places where there is no clean water, and pre-mixed formula is too expensive for the family's budget.

Tip: Immune Constituents of Breast Milk

The following are constituents in breast milk that help fight against infections:

Live cells (e.g., lymphocytes, neutrophils, etc.) attack bacteria and produce antibodies.

Immunoglobulin antibodies (most important antibody secreted is immunoglobulin A).

Lysozyme breaks down bacterial cell walls.

Lactoferrin is a protein that binds iron so it is not available for the growth of bacteria or yeast, which require it to survive. It kills certain kinds of bacteria, viruses, and fungi.

Bifidus Factor promotes growth of beneficial bacteria.

Antistaphylococcal factor acts against staphylococci bacteria.

Overfeeding & Digestion

- When breastfeeding, there is less chance of overfeeding your baby, as he controls the amount he needs by the sucking intensity and duration.

- Breast milk digests easily and produces loose bowel movements. As such, constipation is rare in breastfed infants.

- A British study discovered that bad LDL cholesterol was lower in adults who were breastfed as infants, due to efficient digestion (*Pediatrics*, Sept. 2002).

Tip: Breast Milk Properties and Infection

Maternal milk is a live food, sometimes referred to as "white blood" because of its immune properties and ability to destroy bacteria. Iron in breast milk is low, as it is meant to be, but it is nearly completely absorbed by the baby, versus a 10% absorption rate from formula.

During infectious diarrhea or colds, continue breastfeeding your baby. Your body produces antibodies in your breast milk to help protect your baby, even before you know that you are ill. This does not mean that he won't get sick, but if he does he will be less ill than if you give him formula. Hand washing is important, especially when you are ill.

Developmental Benefits
- There is optimal development of a baby's jaw and mouth when breastfed.
- The sucking effort of breastfeeding is stronger than that of the bottle, leading to better muscle development of the jaws, muscles, and teeth, and better speech development.
- It is less likely that a breastfed baby will need dental work, as the sucking motion involves face and tongue muscles (well shaped jaw and straight teeth).
- Breast milk contains all the necessary elements for the development of nerve cells in the brain. Long non-saturated fatty acids are also contained in breast milk and necessary for the optimal visual development and function of the brain.
- Some studies have shown that breast milk increases intellectual function, by increasing the child's IQ by 8.3 points, on average.
- Other studies have shown that breastfed children average slightly better in academics than formula-fed children. It has been proven that the longer children were breastfed, the better they did academically. These advantages have been shown to persist well beyond childhood.

> **Tip: Enhanced Security & Warmth**
>
> Bonding between mother and baby is facilitated by endorphins in the breast milk that promote relaxation and satisfaction. This provides the baby with an enhanced feeling of security and warmth.
>
> Breastfed babies respond better to vaccines.

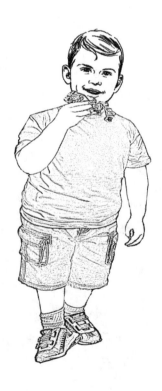

Obesity
- There is probably less of a chance of obesity in breastfed infants than in bottle-fed babies, because the baby will stop feeding when full, while the bottle-fed baby may continue sucking until the bottle is empty.
- There are contradictory studies on the relationship between breastfeeding and long term obesity in the child and adolescent. Some studies suggest that

breastfeeding reduces obesity; others suggest it makes no difference, whether you breastfeed for a short or long period of time, nor if you delay food introduction (Hillard Burdette, *American Journal of Clinical Nutrition*, March 2006).

- The key factors in childhood obesity are inadequate diets and low levels of physical activity. However, genetic aspects should also be considered (Hallal, *International Journal of Obesity*, March 2006).

Breast Milk Benefits for the Mother

- Returns the uterus to its normal state and lessens the risk of bleeding.
  - ❖ Oxytocin is a hormone that causes the "milk ejection reflex" during breastfeeding.
  - ❖ The same hormone causes contraction of the uterus and as such, speeds the return of the uterus to its normal size.
  - ❖ Decreases the risk of postpartum uterine bleeding.

- Breastfeeding is convenient and always ready to serve!
  - ❖ There is no need to prepare utensils and formula before feeding.
  - ❖ Baby's food is always ready for feedings at any place, and it is fresh, clean, and at the right temperature.
  - ❖ Saves energy and time in food preparation; no errors will be made in preparation, either.
  - ❖ There are no worries when traveling about having enough formula or clean water.

- There are financial savings associated with breastfeeding.
  - ❖ Breastfeeding can be absolutely free. All you needs are your breasts and your baby.
  - ❖ It costs more than $1200 per year for formula-fed babies, but only an estimated $400 (with increased food for the mother and extra supplies she may want to buy) for the first year of breastfeeding.

- You are able to return to your pre-pregnancy weight much quicker.
  - ❖ The fat that accumulates during pregnancy is now used to produce breast milk.
  - ❖ Breastfeeding uses extra calories, which helps the mother to lose weight.
  - ❖ When your body is making breast milk, it burns about 500 more calories per day.

- Breastfeeding promotes bonding and intimacy between you and your baby. The mother feels a sense of fulfillment and joy in being able to feed her child. Your newborn also benefits from the physical closeness of nursing. The baby feels loved and protected and understands that you are there for him.

- Switching from breastfeeding to formula can always be done, however it is more difficult to relactate if you decide to breastfeed after formula feeding for a week or so.

- Depending on breastfeeding as a method of birth control is risky. A woman must be exclusively breastfeeding, using no formula supplements, have no vaginal bleeding after post partum bleeding has stopped, and her baby is younger than six months.

Tip: Long-Term Effects for the Mother

There is evidence that breastfeeding decreases risks of breast cancer, ovarian, uterine, and cervical cancer, and prevents hip fracture later in life. The greater the total number of months of breastfeeding, the lower the risk of developing breast cancer.

The mother who breastfeeds for longer than three months has a lower risk of pre-or-post menopausal breast cancer (26-31% less risk).

Short-term effect of breastfeeding is associated with less risk of post-partum depression.

Benefits to Society & the Environment

- There is a decreased cost in the health care system as breastfed babies are healthier, less hospitalized, less infections, etc. (Cattanea et al., *Pediatrics 95*: 540-546, 2006).

- There is less cost to the welfare system since breastfeeding is not as expensive as formula-fed babies.

- There is no garbage, as there is from the packaging used for formula.

- Breastfeeding eliminates the water and fuel energy used in preparing and sterilizing the equipment needed for bottle-feeding.

Latching & Positioning

General

Some mothers have no problems with positioning and latching their babies onto the breast. They experience no nipple pain and their babies gain weight beautifully. Mothers in this category wonder why there should be a big fuss about breastfeeding. The majority of mothers do have some difficulty. By learning about proper positioning and latching before your baby arrives, you can avoid getting sore nipples and ensure that your baby is feeding properly.

Once your baby has arrived, you will have time to practice the things that you have been reading about or have learned in prenatal classes. Coordinating positioning and latching with a real baby is different than using a doll (like you did in prenatal sessions). You may have some challenges but, with practice, you will improve.

Ask for help, both in the birthing room and afterwards during your hospital stay, if you require it. The midwife, doula, delivery room nurse, post partum nurse, or lactation consultant should all be able to assist you.

There are several nursing positions that you may want to learn in the first few days so that you can choose the position that is the most comfortable for you and your baby.

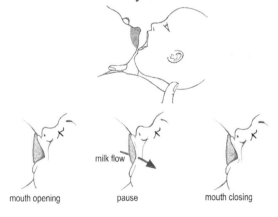

mouth opening   milk flow   pause   mouth closing

Many breastfeeding problems (e.g., sore and cracked nipples, insufficient milk supply, etc.) can be resolved by improving basic techniques.

Tip: Areola Definition

The areola on the breast is the darker pigmented skin area surrounding the nipple.

Establishing a Successful Beginning

- In order to have a successful and established breastfeeding technique, you require:

1) A good start or beginning.
2) Proper positioning so that the baby will latch onto the breast properly.

- In order to have the best start in successfully establishing the breastfeeding technique, you will need to do the following:

  ❖ Place the baby at the breast immediately after birth. Usually, a mother requires help in the beginning and should patiently wait for the breastfeeding to be initiated by the baby. Do not hurry or push your baby aggressively to latch onto the breast, as this may lead to resistance. Simply allow your baby to self-attach (skin-to-skin contact) so that the process happens naturally. When given the chance, the baby will crawl up to your breast from the abdomen, latch on, and start breastfeeding (drugs given to the mother, during labour may interfere with the baby's ability to crawl, seek the mother's breast and breastfeeding behaviour).

  ❖ Both mother and baby should be staying in the same room together.

  ❖ Do not give your baby artificial nipples as he may prefer the rapid flow of the bottle's nipple. It is difficult to know in advance which babies will have problems.

- Refrain from offering any supplements of water, sugar, or formula. If supplements are required, they should only be given with a lactation aid such as a cup, finger, bottle, or syringe. You will need to be instructed in the use of these aids. If you do not wish to use these aids and request a bottle, it certainly is your right to do so, but be aware that you may be removing your option to breastfeed at a later time.

- Do not place any restrictions on the duration (length) or frequency of breastfeeding.

- In order to establish a successful breastfeeding position, you need to do the following (discussed in further detail later in this chapter):

  ❖ Position yourself properly and comfortably.

  ❖ Position your baby properly and comfortably.

  ❖ Present your breast.

  ❖ Ensure proper latching of the breast.

  ❖ Make adjustments for your baby's breathing.

  ❖ Support your breast when breastfeeding.

  ❖ Know how to break a breastfeeding session.

Positioning Mother & Baby

General Guidelines

- It is important to remember that every breast is a little different, even in the same mother. Sometimes, babies prefer one breast over another. Mothers may use more than one position when nursing (e.g., cradle hold for one breast and then switch to the football hold for the other breast).

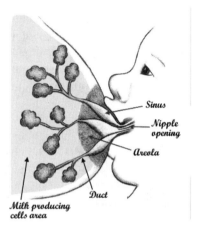

Sinus

Nipple opening

Areola

Duct

Milk producing cells area

- The use of extra pillows will help to give you good support when positioning your baby. Prenatal instructors usually advise you to bring three pillows to the hospital with you to use when you are breastfeeding. Special breastfeeding pillows are good, but they need to be large enough to fit around you properly. Many on the market are too small and are useless, unless you are quite tiny.

- Comfortable nursing positions require the correct positioning of your baby at the breast. In any position, you should follow these guidelines:

  ❖ Make sure you are comfortable, whether it be sitting up in your bed, a rocking chair, or armchair (if you are sitting in a chair, use a footstool, books or anything that will support your feet).

  ❖ You may also lie on your side in bed, facing your baby with a pillow to support your head, back, and upper leg (place a pillow behind your back, on your lap and under the arm for increased support).

  ❖ Have your baby positioned so that his nose is in line with your nipple in any of the positions you try. The goal is to have your baby grasp more of the lower areola (where his chin is) and less of the upper areola (where his nose is). When your baby tries to latch onto your breast he will naturally tilt his head back so his chin comes in closer to the breast. If your baby's mouth is in line with the nipple he will grasp too close to the nipple when he tilts his head.

❖ Your baby's body and head should be facing you with his head, neck, and back in a straight line.

❖ Be careful that your breast is not blocking your baby's nose (press your breast down with your free hand to give your baby clear breathing space).

❖ Place a pillow between your back and under your baby to support his body and prevent getting shoulder and neck aches during a seated feeding.

❖ Avoid slouching, and bring the baby up to you rather than bending over.

Nursing Positions

Position
Cradle Hold (tummy to tummy)
Steps to Follow

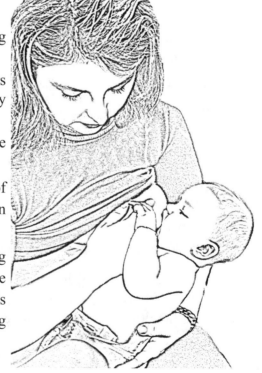

- Sit upright in an armchair, rocking chair or bed.

- Make sure that your back, shoulders and knees are well supported (may need to use pillows).

- Ensure that you are in a comfortable and relaxed position.

- Place your baby's head in the bend of your elbow while your hand holds on to his bottom.

- The baby's tummy should be facing your stomach and his head should be at the level of your breast with his arms on either side of the nursing breast.

- You may continue to support your baby's arms and body with pillows to make the process more comfortable.

- Support your breast with the opposite hand.

- Remember, your baby's head, back, and legs should all be in a straight line.

- If you feel that your nipple begins to hurt you halfway through the feeding, check to see if your baby slipped off the breast.

- *"C" Hold*: Make a "C" with your thumb and fingers. Cup your breast and hold it with your fingers well back from the areola with your thumb resting lightly on top. This is a good hold for using with the football and cross cradle position.

  ❖ *This position is the most common and comfortable position used by mothers when breastfeeding and it may be used for the entire duration of the feeding.*

Position
Cross Cradle (LT Breast)
Steps to Follow

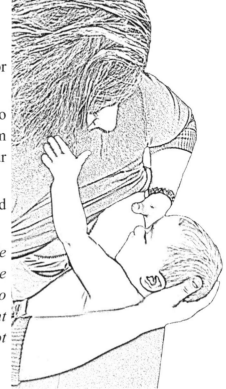

- Hold your baby the same way you did for the above cradle hold position.

- The difference between these two positions is that you use the opposite arm to support the baby's neck and use your forearm to support his body.

- The breast is supported and held by the arm that is on the same side.

  ❖ *When considering the cross cradle position on your left side, follow the same guidelines except switch arms to hold your baby with your right arm, supported by your forearm (not your hands or fingers).*

Position
Football Hold (clutch hold)
Steps to Follow

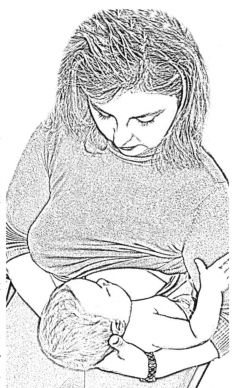

- Sit upright in a chair or bed. Put two pillows lengthways behind your back (but not where your baby's feet will go). One or two pillows should be placed close by your side to support your arm and bring your baby to the level of your breast. Using pillows in this way will allow your baby to be moved closer to the breast without doubling up his legs.

- Support your baby's neck and base of his head in one hand with your forearm supporting his upper body against your side. Your elbow should be bent.

- Move him back so that his nose is in line with your nipple. His legs and feet will be stretched out on the pillow under your arm.

- Support your breast with your other hand using a "C" hold (fingers below and thumb above).

- Tickle your baby's lip lightly with your nipple. Wait for a wide open mouth; bring him in quickly so that he grasps the underside of the areola first. Your nipple should be drawn back into his throat and his upper lip should cover a little of the areola. His chin should be close to your breast and his nose tilted away from your breast.

- You can also do this position using your left hand, if you wish.

    ❖ *This position allows you to control the baby's head and ensure a good position for latching properly (however, it may still be difficult to ensure proper latching). This technique is best and most commonly used when:*

❖ You require a good view of your baby breastfeeding to ensure that the technique is correct and your baby is feeding properly.

❖ Your baby is small, or premature, or you had a cesarean section and you need to keep the baby's weight off the incision and stitches.

❖ Your baby's mouth tends to slide off the areola and grasps only the nipple.

❖ You have a large breast or flat/inverted nipple (since the mother can see both her nipple and the baby's mouth, she can easily control the baby's head).

❖ Your baby tends to fall asleep while breastfeeding (it is easier to compress your breast with your free hand in this position.

❖ To nurse twins, as each baby can nurse on each side.

❖ *Remember to keep your hand low at the base of your baby's head. This will prevent his nose from burying into the breast. He will incline his head, thereby keeping his chin in close to the breast and his nose will be clear for easy breathing.*

Position
Side-Lying Hold

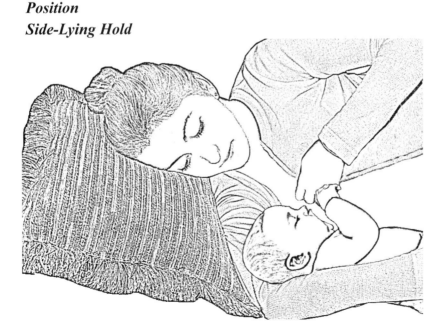

Steps to Follow

- Lie on your side with one pillow under your head, one pillow behind your back for support, and a small towel between your knees for comfort.

- Lay your baby facing you, tummy-to-tummy, nose in line with your nipple.

- If your baby is small, he may lay on your arm (much like in the cradle hold). Use your upper hand to hold your breast. Tickle the baby's lips. When he opens wide draw him onto the breast. Your baby remains on your arm.

- If your baby is large, or you wish to use a different hold, you can support your breast with the hand closest to the bed, and use your upper hand to move the baby by the shoulders in towards the breast.

- Place a pillow or a rolled towel behind your baby from the neck down to support his body. His head should be well supported by the bed. He needs to be able to tilt his head back so his chin touches the breast and his nose is not buried into the breast.

  ❖ *This position is great for feeding a newborn or for a mother right after a cesarean section. It is also great for bedtime or nighttime feedings, when you are tired (e.g., the day following the birth of your baby). It enables both the mother and baby to rest during a nursing session.*

  ❖ *Often a mother will require some help getting her baby to latch in this position for the first few feedings because she can't see what she is doing as well. A lot will depend on her baby's cooperation (interest).*

  ❖ *For safety reasons, when feeding in bed make sure that the baby is not close to the edge of the bed.*

- In any of the above nursing positions, the baby should be aligned so that you are able to draw a straight line that connects the baby's ear, shoulders, and hips on either side of the baby's body.

- Have the baby's nose in line with the nipple as a starting point to ensure a better latch.

- In most cases (other than the reclining position), it will be necessary to support your breast (at least in the early days of breastfeeding) in order for your baby to attach properly. This is especially true as milk production increases your breast size and weight.

Presenting the Breast

- Look at what direction your baby's mouth lies in relation to your breast. Is it horizontal or vertical? By compressing your breast between your fingers and thumb you can shape your breast so that it is easier for your baby to grasp.

- A "C" shape is usually easier when using a football hold or side lying position. Using your free hand, place your fingers under the breast and your thumb on top to present the nipple to your baby ("C" hold position).

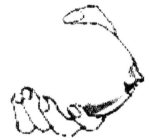

"C" hold position

- For the Cross Cradle hold a "U" hold (cupping the breast from underneath with the fingers towards the inner side and thumb on the outer side of your breast) will give a better shape for the baby to grasp the breast

- For the Cradle hold, a "C" hold may or may not work. Some mothers find an inverted "U," holding a shape from the top of the breast works better. Experiment!

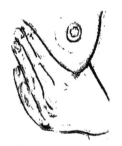

"U" hold position

- Make sure your fingers are behind the areola when holding your breast, so that your baby can latch deeply onto the underside.

- With the breast supported, tickle your baby's lips lightly with your nipple to encourage a wide-open mouth.

- When your baby opens his mouth wide, pull him towards you onto the breast gently but quickly (do not push your breast into his mouth).

- Both of your baby's lips should be turned out. If there is no pain the latch is good. If you are experiencing pain, gently pull down on your baby's lower chin. If the pain does not resolve, break suction by placing a clean finger between your baby's gums and slip your nipple out.

- Do not let your baby suckle if pain continues for more than 30 seconds.

- Your baby's tongue should be extended over his gums and should be curved under your breast (it should feel like a pulling, not biting, sensation).

- If your baby is a little sleepy, compress your breast with your free hand. This will speed up the flow. Do not do compressions if he is actively drinking.

- Make adjustments for your baby's breathing. If your baby's nose seems to be blocked, pull his bottom closer to you and slightly change the angle of his position. A small cloth rolled and placed underneath a very large breast will lift it up.

- Some mothers use their thumb to press on their breast to uncover their baby's nose. Be careful if you are doing this. If you push on the breast tissue too much, there is pulling in two opposing directions (you are pushing back away from the baby's nose and he is tugging towards his mouth). This can cause cracking of the skin at the edge of the nipple/areola. It is painful! If your baby does not manage to latch on properly the first time, gently detach him from the breast and keep practicing the latch until you and your baby master it.

Tip: Pain During Latching

If pain persists throughout nursing, detach the baby by inserting your finger in the corner of his mouth to break the suction and re-latch him. Make sure that his mouth is open wide before latching.

Latching

Proper Latching

The following are signs of proper latching:

- The baby's mouth should cover as much of the areola as possible, with the lower lip covering more of the areola than his upper lip (some areola is seen above the upper lip).

- Your baby's mouth should be open wide with lips rolled outward (curled out).

- The baby's chin (and not necessarily his nose) should be touching your breast.

- You should be experieincing no pain after the initial latching and first few suckles (see *Parent Concerns*).

> ### *Tip: Successful Latching*
> The key to successful latching involves taking enough of the breast into the mouth so that the nipple is drawn to the back of the baby's mouth and his gums and tongue are compressing the areola. If you do not wait until your baby opens his mouth wide before pulling him to the breast, the baby may suck on the nipple only, limiting the amount of milk received and leading to sore nipples.

Improper Latching
The following are signs of an improper latch. Check to see if you are making any of the following mistakes:

- Your baby should be lying on his side rather than on his back, since this position allows him to latch onto the breast comfortably.

- Make sure that your baby's head is not positioned too far over on your left side. Your baby should be positioned so that his mouth is right at the nipple or slightly to the right of it (aimed towards the top of his mouth).

- Do not place your baby onto the breast until he opens his mouth wide.

- Try to place the breast into your baby's mouth instead of moving him onto the breast. Push only your baby's head toward your breast while you use your hand instead of your whole forearm to move the baby. Make sure that your baby's legs are tucked into your side with your elbow.

- Other signs of incorrect/ineffective nursing include:

  ❖ The baby is sucking with the nipple only instead of suckling on the areola.

  ❖ The baby is suckling in a light, quick and fluttery manner, rather than taking deep, regular suckles.

- While written instructions may be helpful, person-to-person help is often required to fix a painful latch since you need to ensure that it is done properly (the earlier, the better). The mother is shown how to help the baby latch on.

Signs of Effective Feeding
The following are signs that your baby is receiving enough milk once he is latched onto the breast correctly:

- Your baby should be feeding with a suckle-pause-swallow rhythm.

- Your baby may suckle quickly at first to bring the milk out of the nipple.

- A definite pause (movement of his chin as he opens his mouth to the maximum while suckling) occurs when your baby receives milk in substantial quantities since this means that his mouth is filling up with milk.

- Your baby opens his mouth wide, keeps it open for a few seconds, and closes it again just before opening it once more.

- A baby who is not receiving enough milk will present a fast sucking pattern without any of the above wide-open pauses (he simply opens and closes his mouth).

Supporting Your Breast

- After your baby has properly latched onto your breast, hold your breast throughout the feeding session so that its weight does not tire your newborn's mouth.

- Supporting your breast will become less necessary as your baby gets older (you will have a full hand available during most of the feeding).

- If your breast is large and hard to support, use a rolled-up hand towel and place it under your breast to help support its weight.

Parent Concerns

How can I tell whether my baby is latching and sucking efficiently?

- It is not easy for you to recognize inappropriate latching, so if you do have any concerns, consult your doctor or lactation specialist.

- Refer to the above sections on proper and improper latching.

- Remember, sore nipples are an indication of improper latching. But pain-free latching does not necessarily mean that the latch is good.

- If your baby is only making small suckling motions and not doing the "open mouth wide-pause-close mouth" type of suckling, he is probably not latching onto the breast well.

- Also, babies who seem frustrated or dissatisfied after a feeding (especially for long durations) may not be receiving enough milk, due to an improper latch.

The following points are important in ensuring a proper latch:
- Ensure that both you and your baby are calm and relaxed.
- Support the breast in a "C" or "U" hold position ("U" hold fits better in the baby's mouth).
- Brush your baby's lips with your nipple.
- Aim the nipple towards the roof of the baby's mouth.
- Bring your baby quickly and deeply onto the breast.
- Maintain infant and breast support.
- Ensure that your baby's mouth is wide open, lips are rolled back, most of the areola is covered, and that the baby's chin is touching the breast.

Why is skin-to-skin contact important?
- Other than the fact that skin-to-skin contact provides comfort and security to your baby, it also helps build your milk supply.
- Studies show that skin-to-skin contact helps in continuing to breastfeed for a long duration.

What is the best way to end a breastfeeding session?

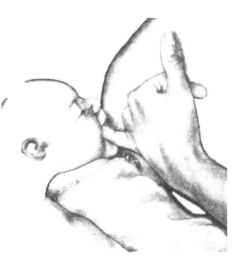

- The best way to end the feeding session is to wait until your baby lets go of the nipple.
- If your baby does not let go of the nipple, end the feeding when rhythmic suck-swallow slows down, or place your finger at the corner of his mouth and slowly allow him to let go.

How is breast milk produced?
- Breast milk works on a supply and demand system. The more often you nurse your baby, the more milk your breasts will produce.

- Only a small number of mothers do not have enough milk for their babies (due to breast reduction surgery, hormonal problems, thyroid problems, illness, etc.). For the best milk production, breastfeed as early as possible and as often as possible.

How do I breastfeed twins?

- You can breastfeed both babies and, if there are any difficulties with exclusive breastfeeding, you may use supplements at the breast rather than using bottles.

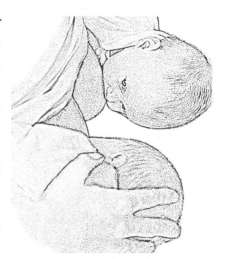

- You may need to express breast milk as well as breastfeed if both babies were born prematurely and require special care until they adjust to breastfeeding and are gaining weight well.

- You can breastfeed your babies simultaneously or separately; there are advantages and disadvantages with each method.

- It is better to nurse each baby one at a time, but it will take up more of your time each day.

- Try practicing various breastfeeding positions (many mothers have found the football hold to be most successful with twins).

- You may try the cross cradle position with your babies facing each other and have the legs of one twin tucked under the other twin.

- Try the parallel position as well, with both babies facing the same way. Basically, one baby is in the football hold and the other is in the cradle hold position.

- Alternate breasts rather than always nursing the same baby on the same breast as this gives both babies extra visual stimulation and improves visual coordination.

- Accept help when it is offered from family, friends, support network, etc.

When should breast compression be done?

- The purpose of breast compression is to stimulate the let-down reflex and to continue the flow of milk to the baby once he no longer drinks (open-pause-closed type of suck). Thus, breast compression keeps him drinking milk, especially the milk received at the end of the feeding (hindmilk that is high in fat); finish the first side before offering the second.

- It works especially well in the first few days to help babies get more colostrum.

- Breast compression is useful when:

    ❖ A baby has poor weight gain.

    ❖ Colic is present in a breastfed baby.

    ❖ A baby requires frequent feedings and/or long feedings.

    ❖ The mother has sore nipples.

    ❖ The mother has recurrent engorgement and mastitis.

    ❖ Encouraging a sleepy baby to continue feeding.

- It is not necessary if all is going well (see other details in this chapter, if there is not enough milk).

Do I need to feed from both breasts or just one breast at every feeding?

- It is not a good idea to feed the baby on just one side. There is no point in just keeping the baby sucking without getting any milk for long periods of time.

- You should "finish" one side and, if the baby wants more, offer the other.

- Your baby is "finished" on the first side when he is no longer drinking, even with compression. This does not mean you must take your baby off the breast as soon as he doesn't drink at all for a minute or two (you may get another milk ejection reflex or let-down reflex, so give it a little time). If it is obvious that the baby is not drinking, take him off the breast and if he wants more, offer the other side.

- Babies often let go of the breast on their own; it does not necessarily mean that he has "finished" that side. Babies often let go of the breast when the flow of milk slows, or sometimes when the mother gets a milk ejection reflex and the baby, surprised by the sudden, rapid flow, pulls off. Try him again on that side if he wants more, but if the baby is obviously not drinking, even with compression, switch sides.

How long should breastfeeding sessions be?

- It is important to make the distinction between "being on the breast" and "breastfeeding" (or actually drinking milk). When breastfeeding, you need to ensure that your baby is properly suckling the breast.

- There should be no restrictions or time limits on the length and frequency of feedings. Learn your baby's cues as to when he is full or "finished."

- If your baby has been on the breast for hours, it means that the baby is not latching on properly and is not really getting enough milk. He may be at the breast, but not actually breastfeeding. These babies usually use a rapid, fluttering, sucking pattern that may stimulate some milk let-down. They do not do the slow suckling with distinct pauses that indicate a good flow of milk. Once the latching is proper, your baby will no longer spend hours on the breast (see *Low Milk Supply*).

- Some babies get plenty of milk, but enjoy spending time on the breast for comfort and security reasons.

What are some frequent causes of poor weight gain or weight loss?

- Inadequate milk production.
- Infrequent feedings.
- No response to subtle feeding cues.
- Poor latching.
- Poor milk transfer from breast to baby.
- Lethargy or tiredness of the baby.

What are some alternative feeding methods or methods of supplementation?

- Lactation aids, cups, finger, spoon, syringe, medicine dropper, bottle, etc.

Tip: Combining Breast and Bottle Feeding

If you complement breast milk with a bottle, use a method that is close to breastfeeding in which you hold the bottle perpendicular to the baby's face (you will need to burp him more in this position).

- The following section details various methods of supplementation and related comments.

Methods of Supplementation

If you are concerned about your baby's breast milk intake or weight gain, consult with your doctor BEFORE beginning any supplemental feeding methods. If your doctor feels that supplementation is called for, review the various methods with either your physician or a lactation specialist.

Cup Feeding

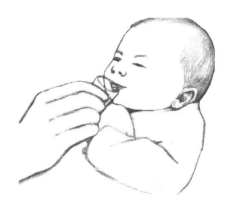

- Cup feeding is useful when the baby is not latching onto the breast and/or when the mother has to be separated from the baby.

- Do not use cup feeding when the baby is latching onto the breast well and simply needs supplementation.

- Cup feeding does not seem to interfere with breastfeeding as much as a bottle does and it is faster than finger feeding. Also, sipping from a cup is different from suckling and as such, nipple confusion is unlikely to occur.

- The technique of cup feeding is simple to learn and safe for use.

- You may use any small cup or one that is made especially and designed for babies (there are special cups designed for premature babies).

Lactation Aids

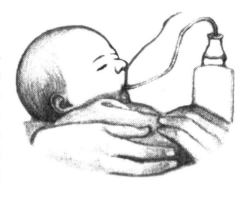

- A lactation aid is a device (usually a feeding bottle with an enlarge nipple hole and long, thin tube attached to the nipple, leading from a container) that allows a breastfeeding mother to supplement her baby with expressed breast milk or formula, without using an artificial nipple.

- The better a baby latches on, the more easy it is for him to get milk, particularly if the mother's milk supply is low.

- The baby may not get enough milk from the breast due to a poor latch, and may require the use of a lactation aid until he learns to breastfeed properly.

- With lactation aids, babies and mothers learn how to breastfeed by breastfeeding, babies continue to receive the mother's milk while being supplemented, and the baby will not reject the breast.

- Use lactation aids only after the baby has nursed on both sides (the baby's suction will make the milk flow).

- As things improve, the mother will introduce the lactation aid later in the feeding until the baby eventually refuses the supplement.

- A lactation specialist should demonstrate the use of the lactation aid to the mother.

Finger Feeding

- Finger feeding is good for the baby who has difficulties latching onto the breast or who is refusing the breast.

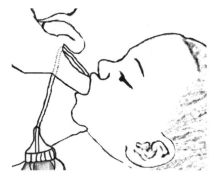

- Use finger feeding as a method of encouragement for your baby to suck in a similar manner to breastfeeding.

- Finger feeding helps your baby latch onto the breast and also wakes up a sleepy baby (especially in the first few days).

- Use this method before a feeding to bring the baby's tongue down (and before everyone is fed up and tired).

- Once finger feeding has calmed your baby and improved his suckling technique, there is a better chance that he will take the breast.

- A disadvantage to finger feeding is that it is quite slow and as the baby gets older, it may take longer and longer.

  As with all methods of feeding, finger feeding can teach the baby to prefer the finger to the breast. It is better to not use any supplementation at all if is unnecessary.

Breastfeeding Problems & Solutions

Red Flags

Breastfeeding Problems & Solutions discuss various problems that may be encountered with breastfeeding for the baby, mother, or both. Most problems and physical discomfort are of short duration and can be solved with appropriate help. In fact, most of these problems can be easily prevented and quickly cured. However, there are times when it is vital to have you and/or your child examined by a health professional.

The following may be considered red flags while you are breastfeeding, requiring discussion with your health professional and/or lactation specialist:

Mother

❖ Mother is having trouble latching the baby onto the breast.

❖ Painful latch.

❖ Severe engorgement (may prevent latching).

❖ Sore and cracked nipples.

❖ Milk has not come in after 5 days.

❖ Mother does not care to feed the baby.

Baby

❖ Loss of about 10% of birth weight in the first few days of life.

❖ Meconium stool on day four.

❖ Concentrated urine and reduced urine (especially in the first few days).

❖ Signs of poor latch (painful latch, sore nipple, etc) in the mother.

❖ Choking and gagging.

❖ Fussing at the breast.

❖ Baby often seems hungry after feedings.

❖ Sleepy newborn (more than four hours at night).

❖ Refusal to breastfeed.

Other red flags are those due to various illnesses of the baby and may include fever, vomiting, irritability, shortness of breath, etc.

Sore & Cracked Nipples

General

Breastfeeding is meant to be an enjoyable experience for both baby and mother.

Many mothers believe that sore and cracked nipples are normal at the beginning of the nursing process, but this is not true. Some mild nipple soreness may occur in the first few days and then disappear, if the baby is latching well.

Sore and cracked nipples can lead to mastitis (if this happens, contact your doctor). Some blood may be swallowed from the bleeding nipple and either vomited or excreted in your baby's stool (this blood will not hurt your baby). Severely cracked and bleeding nipples can be very painful and may require a rest from breastfeeding to allow them to heal before resuming nursing.

Moms who are in this situation should be seen by a breastfeeding specialist either at a breastfeeding clinic (usually covered by your health plan) or with a private visit to the home (fee for service). Milk can be either hand-expressed (if the mother is comfortable doing so), or an electric breast pump can be rented to remove milk from the breast until the nipple is healed.

Mothers do not have to suffer the pain and trauma of sore and cracked nipples. They need immediate help at the first sign of pain to learn how to correctly latch the baby on to the breast. Most post-partum nurses have special training in teaching mothers the correct techniques. Some hospitals have lactation consultants who will teach the technique to mothers. A lactation consultant is helpful to teach and support the mother until painless breastfeeding is accomplished.

Causes

The cause of sore nipples is almost always due to a baby's poor positioning and latching technique. The following may cause nipple pain:

- The baby's body is turned away from mom when trying to latch.
- The baby is positioned too high so he grasps too close to the base of the nipple.

- Holding the baby's head and pushing him into the breast, so that his nose touches the breast but the chin does not.

- Not waiting for a wide open mouth before bringing the baby to the breast.

- Trying to latch a baby onto an engorged breast without softening the areola (see *Breast Engorgement*).

    Other causes include:

    ❖ Trying to pull the baby off the breast without breaking suction.

    ❖ Baby with tongue-tie (frenulum too close to the tip of tongue).

    ❖ Baby with disorganized suckle.

    ❖ Baby with ineffective suckle.

    ❖ Baby with unusual shaped palate.

    ❖ Baby who is teething and bites the breast.

    ❖ Early use of bottle or pacifier which may interfere with a good latch.

    ❖ Eczema of the nipple or other skin conditions.

    ❖ Yeast infection of the breast (thrush/Candida).

    ❖ Nipple (milk) blisters.

    ❖ Raynaud's of the nipple (breast vasospasm).

    ❖ Improper use of a breast pump.

Tip: Proper Positioning and Latching

Your baby's latch may not be good, even though you have pain-free nipples. (Watch for poor weight gain. An improved latch might improve milk intake.)

In the first few days of breastfeeding when milk volume is low, a good latch is vital to maximize colostrum intake.

Long feedings do not cause any damage to the nipple when the latch is done properly.

See *Proper Positioning and Latching* if you are having problems.

Treatment

- The best treatment for your sore and cracked nipples is prevention, which includes getting your baby to latch on well from the beginning (e.g., learning about positioning and latching during pregnancy, or in the first few days after birth).

- Sore nipples should be treated early.

- For minor soreness, expressed breast milk put on nipples after each feeding will help to soothe them. Purified lanolin (Purelan or Lansinoh) is also safe to use and many mothers feel that they have helped with healing.

- For badly cracked nipples see a specialist as soon as possible. While you may try the suggestions included in this chapter, do not delay getting help.

- Nipples will usually heal quickly once the latch is improved. However, if your pain persists after you have made changes to your latch, consult your doctor or lactation specialist.

Ointment for the Nipple

- For bruised and minor blisters or slightly cracked nipples, expressed breast milk or purified lanolin works well for healing. Studies show that a mother's own milk heals as well or better than any cream.

- Be careful of other breast creams, some are not recommended because they have ingredients that the mother or baby may be sensitive to.

- For severely cracked nipples, or those that are not getting better within a week, mothers are encouraged to see a doctor, as they may require a special prescription ointment that accelerates healing (a combination of antibacterial, anti-inflammatory, and antifungal ingredients).

- You may use this ointment after all feedings; once you are pain free you may use the ointment less frequently.

- The following table outlines the ingredients in the ointment:

Antibacterial	Skin bacteria worsening the situation or causing infections. Prevents the risk of mastitis. Bacteria makes the healing process more complex. e.g., Mupirocin, 2% ointment, fucidic acid or Bactroban.
Antifungal	Decreases inflammation. Reduces pain. e.g., Miconazole powder added so that its final content is 2%, Clotrimazole, nystatin, Ketoconazole.

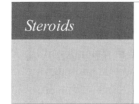 *Steroids*	Decreases inflammation.
	Reduces pain.
	e.g., Betamethasone 0.1% ointment.

- These combinations work well for most cases of sore nipples.
- The baby's body does not absorb much of the ingested ingredients, so they are not considered harmful to him.
- Ointments are more healing than creams.
- Pain medications for sore and cracked nipples may also include acetaminophen and ibuprofen.

Other Helpful Measures
- A baby who is very hungry can sometimes be too aggressive when latching and sucking on the breast. Watch for early feeding cues and feed your baby more frequently.
- If your nipples are more painful and the baby is due to begin a feeding on that side, you may try beginning to feed on the less painful side. Switch the baby to the sore side once the let-down has occurred.
- If your milk is flowing before the baby latches on, he does not need to suck as hard to get the milk flow started. This can reduce discomfort. Encourage a let-down before a feeding by hand-expressing, massaging, and applying heat to your breasts.
- Breast compression often allows the mother to complete a feeding on just one side. As such, it spares the other side that is sore from trauma. If the baby spends less time on this sore breast, the nipple will heal faster. Breast compression is especially important when there is only a small amount of milk available.
- It is better to keep your nipples exposed to air as much as possible. Avoid excessive moisture between feedings and refrain from using plastic-lined nursing pads for the same reason. Lanolin may help you feel more comfortable as you heal.
- If your breasts become engorged, try expressing a little milk first to soften the areola. Engorged breasts make it even more difficult for your baby to latch on.

Parent Concerns

What if I have sore and cracked nipples and have tried all the treatment measures described above, yet nothing works?

- This problem may arise, particularly when appropriate treatment was not started early (day 4). However, your nipples will get better with time.

- You still have the ability to provide expressed milk to your baby, even when the pain of sore nipples is bad.

- You can express milk by hand or pump. There are excellent hospital grade electric pumps that allow a mom to single or double pump their breasts comfortably until the nipples are healed. (See a lactation consultant or breastfeeding specialist about this option.)

- If both nipples are severely cracked, try feeding your baby using other methods, such as cup feeding or finger feeding until you are able to nurse again.

- Maintain your milk supply with frequent expression of milk (pump or hand). In this way, you give time for your nipples to heal.

- Refrain from breastfeeding for a few days or more, so that when your baby returns to the breast it is less painful. Once you restart, you can gradually keep feeding on the breast that is not as sore, while the other heals.

- If you find that you don't have enough milk to satisfy your baby feeding from just one breast, you can express milk from the sore breast and feed it to your baby by means of a lactation aid.

- If the amount in one breast is sufficient, any milk pumped can be frozen for later use. Some moms are able to breastfeed completely on only one breast.

- Formula may be used via the lactation aid if there is not enough milk for the baby while he is feeding only on the one side (in cases where mom cannot express or pump enough to supply the rest of the milk).

Do I need to remove the ointment I put on the nipple before I feed my baby?

- No, you do not need to wash off the ointment since most of the ingredients used in the ointment are not absorbed by the baby's digestive system. There is no need to wipe or wash the area, even when your baby goes on the breast.

- Cleaning (if it has to be done at all) should be done gently. Washing the nipple with a little breast milk would be perfectly acceptable, especially if the baby does not like the taste of the ointment.

- If you do wash your nipple, do not use soap, alcohol, or pre-moistened towlettes. Only use water and do not use any creams that contain alcohol.

My nipple turns white with burning pain after my baby comes off the breast.

- Some mothers may experience pain that (usually) begins after the feeding is over. This pain is associated with the nipple becoming white, as if blood is not getting to the end of the nipples—which is actually the problem.

- The pain may last several minutes or more before the nipple is able to return to its normal color. After this, a new type of pain (often described as throbbing) may begin, lasting anywhere from seconds to minutes.

- All of this is due to spasms and relaxation of the blood vessels in the nipple.

- These spasms of the blood vessels are probably due to injury or hypersensitivity of the blood vessels of the nipple. Treating the cause of the nipple pain during the feeding usually treats the pain due to the spasm.

- Ensure that your baby is latching properly and apply heat (hot washcloth, hot water bottle, hair dryer on low setting etc.) to the nipple immediately after nursing to prevent or decrease the reaction. Dry heat is usually better than wet heat.

- If it is a persistent problem, then discuss it with your doctor and lactation specialist.

Breast Engorgement

Normal Engorgement

Normal engorgement (breast fullness) occurs when your breast milk is changing from colostrum to transitional breast milk. Usually this happens around three to four days after giving birth. Some moms may experience this as early as day two, and a few may have this happen a little later.

When the milk becomes plentiful, your breasts may seem full. This fullness is due to increased congestion, blood flow to the breast, and increased milk production. Engorgement is sometimes painful. Some mothers notice little to moderate fullness, while others become engorged with each of their babies. The feeling of fullness makes the breasts sensitive to touch.

It is important to continue nursing your baby frequently (every 2-3 hours). Removing milk from the breast relieves the congestion and can prevent severe engorgement. Warm showers followed by nursing may also help relieve the fullness. The best solution for engorgement is frequent breastfeeding.

Fullness of the breasts usually subsides within a few days.

Tip: More on Breast Engorgement

Not every woman experiences breast engorgement, and some women hardly notice any pain with it.

Engorgement may cause not only pain; it can also cause problems with breastfeeding, such as difficulties latching, decreased milk production, and progression to abnormal engorgement.

Abnormal Engorgement

- It is not normal for a woman to get severe engorgement.
- Causes of abnormal engorgement may include inadequate emptying of the breast due to ineffective or infrequent suckling by the baby, or failure to express colostrum/milk frequently when baby is not able to breastfeed (e.g., baby is separated from the mother).
- Supplementing babies with formula (if it is perceived by the mother and/or health professional that the baby is not getting enough milk) in the early days is associated with increased risk of engorgement.

- Symptoms of abnormal engorgement include excessive swelling (sometimes extended to the armpit), redness, fullness (congested, warm breast), pain, hardness of breast tissue, low fever, and throbbing or lumpy breasts.
- If your breasts are severely engorged, your baby may not be able to latch on. The nipple becomes flat, injured, and sore, since the baby can only grab the end of it.

The following table outlines some points in helping you differentiate between mastitis and severe engorgement:

Mastitis	Severe Engorgement
• Usually occurs on one breast. • Usually occurs during the first few weeks after the birth, if mom has cracked nipples or unresolved blocked ducts. • High fever. • Requires antibiotics for treatment if due to cracked nipples.	• Usually occurs in both breasts. • Low grade fever can occur. • No antibiotics are required for treatment.

Tip: Preventing Engorgement

The best way to prevent severe engorgement is to feed the baby as frequently as possible from the very first day, and ensuring that he is properly latched onto the breast.

Treatment for Severe Engorgement

General Measures

- Wear a well-fitted and supportive bra, but ensure that it is not too tight.
- Wear loose clothing that does not rub against your breasts.
- Get plenty of rest.
- Do not sleep on your stomach or your breasts, as milk ducts become clogged when the breasts are not emptied.
- Breastfeeding will help soften your breasts, however expect that they will harden again within one to two hours.

- Pain relief medication (e.g., ibuprofen—a combined pain reliever and anti-inflammatory) during the feeding session.

- Ensure that the latching technique is good, so that your baby can extract the milk easily (see *Positioning & Latching*).

- You can massage your breasts at the beginning of a feeding session to encourage milk flow.

- To get the milk flowing, you may have to compress the breasts. Once the milk flows, pressure and tension in the breasts improve. Expression of milk will also help lessen the engorgement and pain.

- Some moms like to apply heat to the breast before feeding, but if the breast is very swollen cold compresses are better. Cold reduces swelling and allows the milk to flow, whereas heat increases congestion.

- Sometimes, the baby refuses to take the breast and/or cannot latch because of the flattening of the nipple and areola, as well as hardness of the breast. In this case, remove some milk to relieve fullness by hand-expressing milk. Once the nipple and areola are soft and less flat, the baby will be able to latch on well and feed.

- If your baby is still not able to take the breast, use alternative methods to feed the baby your expressed milk (via cup feeding, finger feeding, syringe, etc.).

- Remember that engorgement lasts only a few days, with the worst being in the first 36 hours.

- Sometimes the breast is swollen mainly in one part, so you may change feeding positions (have the baby's chin pointing towards this area) to ensure that all milk ducts are being emptied.

- Enabling the baby to latch on effectively will help soften the breasts and eventually eliminates the problem.

Between Feeding Sessions

- Ice packs or cold compresses (wrapped in a towel) can be used between feeding sessions to reduce swelling. A bag of frozen peas works well for this purpose because it fits the contours of the breast.

- Green cabbage leaves seem to have a beneficial effect on engorgement. It is not clear how they work.

❖ Wash the leaves well, dry, and keep in the refrigerator until you are ready to use them.

❖ Use a rolling pin to break the veins of the cabbage leaves so they will contour easily around the breast. Apply the leaves directly on your breasts, inside your bra.

❖ You may re-apply cabbage leaves between feedings until your breasts feel comfortable (about 3-4 times per day).

❖ Do not use leaves for longer than that, in order to avoid affecting your milk supply.

❖ Some recommend leaving the cabbage leaves on your breasts until they wilt, or leaving them on for about 20 minutes each time (maybe after each feeding).

❖ You may use cabbage leaves until the swelling and pain subsides.

Tip: Engorgement and Expressing Milk

Do not worry that expressing milk in small amounts will lead to a decrease in your milk supply. Expressing milk helps you decrease the engorgement and pain.

Engorgement When Choosing Not to Breastfeed

- Use green cabbage to relieve severe discomfort and when you are unable to breastfeed. Cabbage leaves may be wrapped around the breast and left for about 20 minutes on the breast, 2-4 times per day.
- Relieve breast pain with pain medications and ice packs.
- Use moist, cool compresses.
- Do not pump or express the milk.
- When weaning your baby, do it gradually and not "cold turkey."

Parent Concerns

Is engorgement a reason to stop breastfeeding?

- No, engorgement is not a reason to stop breastfeeding.
- You can and you should continue breastfeeding, since unrelieved engorgement may lead to mastitis (infection of the breast) and decreased milk production.

My baby feeds from one breast and then he is full, meanwhile my other breast is engorged. What should I do?

- You need to ensure that your baby is gaining weight properly while feeding from only one breast.

- Alternate breasts at each feeding. If he seems to fall asleep, stimulate him to continue feeding.

- You can pump or manually express milk for a few minutes (about 1oz/30g) from the engorged breast for comfort. You can store the milk for later use.

- You may also use pain medications occasionally for some relief.

- Breasts may also be engorged in the morning, if you have not expressed milk or breastfed during the night.

What is the difference between breast fullness and breast engorgement?

- *Breast fullness* is a gradual build-up of milk in the breast that could be an indication of early lactation. It is a transitory phenomenon where breast tissue remains compressible. It usually does not cause difficulties with breastfeeding and rarely lasts longer than 24-36 hours. Fullness disappears on its own with the increase of breast milk. Mothers will feel well, contrary to breast engorgement.

- *Breast engorgement* can cause difficulties with breastfeeding due to mismanagement of the state of transient fullness because of a delay or restriction in duration and frequency of breastfeeding and because many mothers receive IV fluid. Numbness and tingling may occur with severe engorgement, due to pressure on the nerve in the armpit. Fever is also a sign of engorgement and pain is generalized (there is a feeling of general tiredness).

- Both conditions can occur in both breasts simultaneously, with an overall swelling of the breasts.

Mastitis

General

Mastitis is an inflammation of the breast and is a common problem for breastfeeding mothers. *Infective mastitis* is caused by bacteria entering through a cracked nipple, while *obstructive mastitis* is caused by a blocked duct. It typically develops only in one breast.

A mother who has infective mastitis usually develops it early in her breastfeeding experience, whereas obstructive mastitis may happen at any time that milk is blocked and not removed from the breast. Mothers who do not breastfeed may also get obstructive mastitis if their breasts are engorged.

Some mothers may develop mastitis more than once during the course of lactation. Prevention, therefore, is important.

> ### Tip: Mastitis and Milk Supply
>
> Mothers who experience mastitis may experience decreased or low milk supply in the affected breast. The sodium content is higher in the affected breast, which may lead the baby to refuse the breast. If the baby will not nurse, pumping will help to maintain the supply by emptying the breast. Milk from the affected breast is good, and will not harm the baby.

Possible Trigger Factors

The following could trigger the occurrence of mastitis:

- Cracked or sore nipples may allow bacteria to enter the breast by way of the baby's saliva (infective).

- Fatigue, stress, or malnutrition can cause a decreased resistance to illness (infective).

- An overabundant milk supply, breast engorgement, or breast trauma (obstructive).

- Plugged ducts (obstructive).

- A tight, constricting bra, under-wire bras, or incorrect sleep positions (obstructive).

- Abrupt change in frequency of feedings or missed feeding (obstructive).
- Milk plug on the nipple, causing blocked ducts (obstructive).

Tip: Cracked Nipples and Mastitis

Most women with cracked nipples do not get infective mastitis and women without soreness in the nipples may get obstructive mastitis.

Symptoms

Symptoms associated with mastitis include the following:

- Local swelling, hardness, and redness (usually starts with a small, reddened area that spreads quickly if not attended to promptly).
- Hot and tender breasts.
- Breast pain.
- Fever and chills.
- Fatigue, malaise, flu-like symptoms, and generalized aching; you may feel very ill with no strength or energy.

The following is a table to help you distinguish between mastitis and blocked ducts.

Mastitis	Blocked Ducts
Skin is redder and hotter. More of a fever (may occur without a fever).	Painful, swollen, and less red; lumps are usually associated with plugged ducts.
Pain is more intense.	Absence of fever (may occur, though).
More general symptoms associated with fever.	Pain is less intense.
Complications may include abscess if not resolved.	Does not soften with feeding.
	Complications may include mastitis.
Usually requires treatment, especially if mother has a crack in the nipple.	No treatment with antibiotics required (resolves spontaneously in 24-48 hours).

- Prompt and proper treatment of a plugged duct will usually keep mastitis from developing. Infections will also clear up faster if you breastfeed frequently, thus keeping your breast empty.

- Treatment of plugged duct includes the following:

  ❖ Breastfeed often to promote drainage.

  ❖ Apply moist heat to the area several times per day.

  ❖ Massage affected breast before and after feeding to stimulate milk flow.

  ❖ Change position of the baby, so his chin points in the direction of the hardened area of the breast.

  ❖ Avoid constrictive clothing.

- Get help with latching if cracked nipples are not healing.

- If you have a milk blister (plug) on the nipple, it will be very painful to touch and more painful when you are breastfeeding. Wash your hands before trying to open the blister. Sterilize a needle (by the flame of a match or candle), let it cool and gently prick the blister. Then carefully squeeze the plug using a tissue or clean facecloth. Thick white material may come from the underlying duct and milk may start to spray out. If your baby is ready to breastfeed he will probably clear the blockage. Massaging over the hardened area towards the nipple while he is nursing will help to clear it. Use a pump if your baby will not nurse.

Treatment

The following are suggestions for how to treat mastitis:

- Continue breastfeeding unless it is too painful to do so (restart as soon as possible; the sooner, the better).

- If you cannot breastfeed, express your milk from the affected breast manually or with a breast pump to relieve the pressure and drain the breast.

- Increase your fluid intake.

- Get plenty of rest to reduce stress and fatigue (e.g., prioritize tasks more efficiently from most important to least important—write a list). Delegate tasks to others, if possible.

- Heating pads or warm compresses may be placed on the breast's affected area to help the infection.

- Take pain relievers that may also help your fever (e.g., acetaminophen or ibuprofen).

- Open both sides of your bra and allow milk to flow from the breast while you are feeding your baby on the opposite side, so that you can finish the feeding on the infected side with less discomfort.

- When symptoms of mastitis last longer than 24 hours, speak to your doctor about antibiotics. Antibiotics can help decrease the symptoms in about 24-48 hours. Resolution may take three-five days.

- If treatment with antibiotics is effective, you may try to restart breastfeeding in 24 hours (if you had stopped due to pain).

- If your baby will not feed on the infected breast, remove milk from that breast at each feeding manually or by pump.

> ### Tip: Feeding During Mastitis
>
> By continuing to breastfeed, the baby may empty the breast more effectively than by using a pump or hand expressing. Hospital grade pumps can be rented in cases where the baby is not nursing. They are gentle, fast, and most effective, allowing mom to get more rest.

Complications of Mastitis

- Consult with your doctor again if:
  - ❖ Your symptoms do not improve significantly within 5 days after starting antibiotics.
  - ❖ The symptoms worsen within 24-48 hours of treatment.
  - ❖ If you feel a lump in the breast that is very tender when squeezed.

- Mastitis may sometimes lead to breast abscess (a pocket of pus-filled areas/localized infection), especially when treatment is delayed or ineffective for mastitis. Treatment of the abscess may include antibiotics and open drainage of the abscess through surgery or repeated aspiration—sucking and drawing fluid out of a cavity (usually with local anesthesia).

- Breast abscess is treated with incision and drainage. If the incision is made close to the areola, the mother may not be able to breastfeed immediately after the operation, due to pain and/or a dressing placed on the nipple and areola. This incision (if close to the areola) can compromise future milk production.

- It is better to keep breastfeeding from the abscessed breast if possible, to keep better drainage of the area.

- There are alternatives to incision and drainage, such as ultrasound guided needle aspiration or placement of catheter for drainage rather than by incision.

- Lumps in the breasts that do not go away on their own or after treatment need to be seen by a doctor to rule out other causes.

Tip: Mastitis and Treatment

If you start antibiotics, take them for the full course, despite improvements in the first few days. Recurrence of infection can occur if you stop treatment early. Some mothers may develop yeast infection of the breast after taking antibiotics. See your doctor if you develop increased pain or burning sensation when you are breastfeeding.

Parent Concerns

Should I stop nursing if I have mastitis?

- It is important, safe, and actually better, to continue nursing from the infected breast when you have mastitis, or even abscess, if you can. If surgery is required for the abscess, you may continue nursing from the unaffected breast, but you must continue to pump milk from the abscessed breast for a day or two.

- Frequent feeding keeps your milk supply flowing and prevents further blockage or engorgement, which makes the breast more painful.

- Sometimes there is large swelling on the breast tissue, making it difficult for your baby to latch on.

Will mastitis affect my baby?

- Mastitis will not affect your baby, though it may reduce milk supply in the infected breast. Do not worry about passing any germs to your baby, since they probably came from your baby in the first place. Drinking your breast milk will not harm your baby.

Will antibiotics taken for mastitis affect my baby?

- The antibiotics given to mothers to treat mastitis generally do not cause any problems for the nursing infant; however the baby's stools will be looser than usual. The amount of acetaminophen or ibuprofen that the baby receives in breast milk is insignificant.

Are antibiotics always required to treat mastitis?

- Mild cases of mastitis may require only rest, frequent nursing, warm compresses, or draining of the breast to relieve pain. These cases may improve spontaneously within 48 hours with no antibiotics. However, if symptoms of mastitis should worsen (more pain, increased redness and hardening of the area, and fever), antibiotics are required. If you develop abscess, antibiotics are needed, along with surgical drainage or the previously suggested treatments for abscess.

Flat or Inverted Nipples

General

Breast nipples come in various shapes and sizes. Some nipples make the breastfeeding process more challenging, while others seem to ease the process. In order for the baby to suckle effectively, he will need to draw your nipple far back into his mouth where it is protected. His jaws move on the areola and the tongue strokes the underside of the areola, stripping the milk from the ducts and sending it to the back of the throat so the baby can swallow it.

A mother's nipple is normally stretched to twice its original length during breastfeeding. Flat and inverted nipples can be a challenge because they do not stretch as far back into the throat and may be difficult for a baby to grasp. A mother may have one flat or inverted nipple or have a nipple that protrudes more than the other. There are changes in elasticity of the nipple/areola in the third trimester of pregnancy and in the first few weeks after delivery. Despite recommendations to begin treatment during the last trimester of your pregnancy, studies have shown that prenatal preparation does not really make any difference over post-delivery treatment. Pregnant women should be reassured that almost all nipple shapes and sizes are compatible with effective breastfeeding, once postioning and attachement is correct.

Some babies have little trouble with flat or inverted nipples because they are eager, vigorous feeders. Talk to your doctor or lactation specialist if you have any concerns about breastfeeding.

Identification & Types of Nipples

A Pinch Test is the best way to tell if a nipple is truly flat or inverted

- To do a Pinch Test:

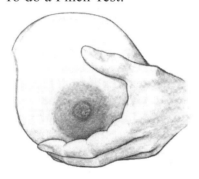
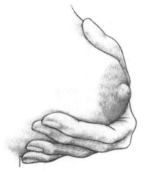

❖ Hold your breast between your thumb and index finger near the base of the nipple.

❖ Press gently and firmly behind your nipple (about 1 inch/2.7 cm). You should be able to feel where the larger mass of the breast tissue ends and the nipple begins.

❖ If your nipples protrudes, then you should not experience problems when latching.

❖ If your nipple does not protrude nor retract inside the breast, it is a flat nipple.

❖ Inverted nipples retract inward, towards the breast, instead of protruding when the areola is gently squeezed. The degree of retraction varies from minimal to severe.

❖ If your nipple disappears, then it is an inverted nipple.

- A truly inverted nipple is caused by adhesion at the base of the nipple that binds the skin to the underlying tissue.

Tip: Nipple Confusion

Avoid the use of any artificial nipples, because the baby who is learning how to nurse, especially when his mother's nipple is flat or inverted, may have more difficulty with latching.

Flat Nipples

- Flat nipples usually cause fewer problems than inverted nipples.
- A good latching technique is usually all that is necessary.
- You may try to gently compress the areola to make the nipple as erect as possible before you nurse your baby.
- Nurse as soon as possible after birth and frequently thereafter to avoid breast engorgement (See *Breast Engorgement*).

Inverted Nipples

- Inverted nipples can create a problem during the breastfeeding process by making it more difficult for your baby to latch onto the breast. In some cases, when the baby starts to breastfeed the breast tissue shrinks back so that your baby has difficulty grasping it. If he does grasp the nipple he may bite down on it if he cannot draw it back into his throat. This will cause sore or cracked nipples.

- Many inverted nipples become less inverted or protrude normally as the baby starts to latch on. Over time, the suckling of a baby who is latching on will make the nipple protrude and he will be able to draw it further back into his mouth to nurse.

Improving the Feeding Process

The following are suggestions of what can be done to improve the feeding process when you have flat or inverted nipples:

- Stimulating your nipple is helpful in making it protrude before nursing. You may try to grasp the nipple and "roll" it in-between two fingers (thumb and index fingers) for approximately 30 seconds.

- If your nipple is severely inside your breast, squeeze it with your two fingers to expose it so that your baby will be able to latch onto your breast.(It may just pop back in when the baby comes to the breast again).

- Breast pumps help draw out the nipple right before a feeding session and sometimes your baby may latch on after a few minutes of pumping. They also help stimulate your production of milk. Any milk pumped can be given to your baby by cup, syringe or finger feeding until your baby is breastfeeding.

- You can help the baby get a better grip during nursing by taking the outside part of the areola between your thumb and forefinger and compressing the entire area for sucking (shaping the breast). Make sure your fingers are not too close to the nipple.

- In most cases, only one nipple is inverted and the other breast is easier for your baby to latch onto. You may feed on the one that is easier to grasp and pump the more challenging one until that nipple is more pliable.

- Continue breastfeeding your baby if you are not experiencing any pain and your baby is gaining weight well (able to take the milk properly). With time, the problem of flat or inverted nipples will correct itself.

- Try various positions when breastfeeding your baby to help your baby grasp the breast (e.g., football hold, cross-cradle, or lying down).

- Avoid the use of artificial nipples since the baby may become nipple confused, especially when your own nipple does not protrude.

- Consult a lactation specialist for further assistance and advice.

Tip: Nipple Soreness and Baby Comfort

Some mothers with flat or inverted nipples experience nipple soreness or pain (see *Sore & Cracked Nipples*).

Stop and comfort your baby if feeding sessions becomes stressful rather than relaxed. You may try rocking your baby, offering your finger for him to suck, walking around with him, etc., until your baby has calmed down.

It is good to have some milk pumped ahead. If either you or the baby get upset, feed your milk by an alternative method, pump your breast, and try again next time.

Tip: Improper Latching

If your baby is unable to latch on well, this may lead to decreased milk supply unless you pump your breast. If this problem persists for more than a few days, talk to your doctor or lactation specialist about breast shells and other solutions.

Extra Tips on Pumps & Flat or Inverted Nipples

- Pumps help pull out the center of the nipple rather than compress the areola (helps to break adhesions).

- When soreness of the nipples lasts longer than a week you have to keep up your milk supply, which requires the use of a high quality pump (e.g., Symphony, Lactina, Pump in Style, or Hollister pump). Speak to a lactation consultant about the best kind of pump for your particular situation.

- When your both nipples are severely inverted, double pumping (every 2 to 3 hours) may be necessary until your nipples protrude.

- Pumping to draw out inverted nipples may last only a few days while others have to pump for weeks, or even months (depends on degree of inversion and your baby's sucking patterns).

- If the nipple inverts again during pauses in the baby's feeding, you may need to stop and pump again for a few minutes and then put the baby back on the breast.

Comments on the Use of Breast Shells & Nipple Shields

The difference between breast shells and nipple shields can be a little confusing.

- *Breast shells* have different backs on them (Medela makes soft and silicone made shells whereas Hollister's are hard plastic like the front of the shells). The back with the smaller hole is supposed to put pressure at the base of the nipple to encourage the nipple to come out evert.

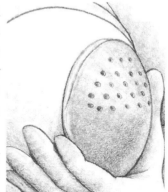

breast shell

- Shells with larger holes are provided for mothers with sore nipples to keep anything away from touching the nipple directly (for quicker healing).

- Breast shells are better when they have many holes on the front part for air circulation (mothers who do wear these shells, may have to wear a larger size bra to avoid blocked ducts).

- There is some controversy over the use of breast shells, as they have not been proven to be completely effective.

- Like breast shells, nipple shields can be used for sore nipples.

- *Nipple shields* are made of thin silicone (they look like a Mexican hat). These fit directly over the nipple during a feeding and help the baby latch onto the breast (if the mother has flat or inverted nipples).

- The risk in using nipple shields is that it may be difficult to get your baby to nurse without them. Milk supply can drop about 22%, so mothers are instructed to pump to keep up the supply until the baby is latching directly on the breast.

- They have proven to be beneficial to premature babies. The nipple shield stays deep in the infant's mouth and encourages him to suckle stronger (the lack of fat pads in his cheeks makes it harder for him). He also tires easily. His intake is usually higher using a shield. Nipple shields should not be used as a first resort for moms with flat or inverted nipples.

- If you do decide to use a nipple shield, you should be taught how to use it properly, get the correct size, and track your baby's weight a few times with your health specialist or lactation expert.

Breast Milk Leakage: How to Cope

General

Many new mothers experience leakage of colostrum during the last few weeks of pregnancy. It is normal; usually these mothers have a large volume of colostrum at birth ready to feed their baby. Mothers who do not leak before delivery should not be concerned, because their body will release and produce enough colostrum for their babies in response to the hormonal shift that takes place after the placenta is delivered (estrogen and progesterone go down while prolactin and oxytocin go up).

Some mothers do not experience any breast milk leakage throughout their breastfeeding experience, while others leak a little or a lot. Either is normal.

Some mothers are embarrassed when they leak milk because of its unpredictability and their inability to control it (especially if leaking continues beyond the first several months). The amount of breast milk leakage usually declines over time. If this leakage is bothersome, a mother needs to know how to cope, so that she is not tempted to wean early.

Tip: Leaking Variations

Leaking is normal in the first month while your body is learning how much milk to produce for your baby. Leaking varies among mothers with respect to stimuli, amount of leakage, and duration of leakage. Some mothers leak throughout their breastfeeding experience. This, too, is normal.

Causes

- Breasts usually leak when they are full of milk and when the hormone oxytocin triggers the let-down reflex, causing breast milk leakage.
- Sometimes, the let-down reflex may occur spontaneously due to:
  - ❖ A baby's crying (milk stimulating sounds).
  - ❖ Sitting or being in a chair where you breastfeed.
  - ❖ Picking up your baby.
  - ❖ Thinking of your baby or seeing/smelling his clothes.

❖ Sexual activity.

❖ Engorged breasts.

❖ Over stimulation of the nipple or massaging the breasts.

❖ Over production of milk.

❖ Less storage capacity for milk in the breasts.

❖ Hormone imbalance and medication.

> ### Tip: Sympathetic Let-Down
>
> This occurs when your baby is feeding from one breast and milk leaks out from the other. Placing a towel or cloth to catch the milk flow saves getting your clothes wet. You may wish to catch the milk flow into a cup or bottle and refrigerate it for later use.

Tools for Coping

The following suggestions can help you prevent or cope with breast milk leakage:

- Nurse before your breasts get too full. Avoid missing a feeding.

- Be aware of when you leak the most and plan ahead so that you may be prepared (e.g., in the mornings).

- Wear disposable nursing pads or reusable cotton pads to absorb milk leaks and change them frequently.

- When breastfeeding, leave the flap of your bra open on the other side and have an absorbent diaper or towel under your breast to catch any leakage or hold a clean container under your breast and collect any leaked milk to save for a supplement. Breast milk can be refrigerated or frozen for later use.

- Avoid nursing pads that have plastic backings, since these retain moisture and may cause nipple soreness. Products such as these should be used only on rare occasions when you can not afford a leak (e.g., during a wedding, you are a member of the wedding party, are wearing a solid top and cannot go to feed your baby or pump your breasts).

- If you do seem to leak through your clothes, wear patterned or printed shirts to camouflage leaks. Carry an extra shirt and bra pads with you when you go out. If your baby is not with you take a hand pump in case you need to pump.

- To stop the leaking, push on your nipple with the palm of your hand or apply some pressure against your breasts. Gentle pressure for a few seconds on a leaking breast is usually sufficient to cue it to retain milk for a brief time. When the mother feels that her milk is letting-down, crossing both arms over the chest and pressing gently for 5-10 seconds usually stops the leaking.

- Feed the baby before lovemaking to avoid "milk showers" (Some couples do not mind this, while others do). Putting a large towel across the top of the bed will also prevent bedding from getting wet. Some women wear a bra, if leaking during intimacy bothers them or their partner.

Parent Concerns

How long does breast milk leakage last?

- It usually lasts for up to the 10 weeks after giving birth and then completely stops. However, breast milk leakage varies in duration and amount with each mother and may continue throughout your breastfeeding experience.

I do not leak any milk—does this mean that I do not produce enough milk for my baby?

- Many women never leak any milk at all and this is also natural. If you have leaked milk before and it has stopped, it is not an indication that the supply has dwindled. It simply means that you and your baby are in sync with one another, especially if the baby is healthy, gaining weight, and content.

Are leaking breasts helpful for my baby at all?

- It is helpful for a baby who is sleepy or hesitant to take the breast as the leaking breasts provide your child with sensory input. He will see the leaking milk and he may smell it or taste it, causing him to want a feeding.

- Breast milk leakage helps you as well, since it relieves pressure and reminds you that it is time to feed your baby.

- Perhaps leaking is helpful for the new baby who is still learning how to nurse efficiently. Also, it may act as a safety valve to prevent mastitis (infection of the breast).

Is it normal to leak from the breast if I am not breastfeeding?

- This is normal. If you do not start breastfeeding in the first few days after giving birth your body will naturally adjust within a week. When your breasts become engorged and you do not empty your breasts, your body gets the signal that milk is not needed, prolactin receptors shut down, you stop producing milk and any milk in the breasts is reabsorbed and disappears. Avoid taking drugs to "dry up milk." They can have serious side effects. Do not bind your breasts (it leads to mastitis).

- Wear a well-fitted bra and apply ice packs or green cabbage to dry up the milk.

- This may prove to be painful and uncomfortable. Take comfort knowing it does not last long.

- If you have been breastfeeding for several days and then decide to stop, wean slowly, by dropping one feeding and then waiting a few days to drop another. Stopping "cold turkey" may lead to blocked ducts and then mastitis.

- Mothers can often express a few drops of milk from their breasts several months after weaning. This is normal.

I returned to work and I leak sometimes when I am asked or am thinking about my baby. Is this normal?

- Various stimuli may cause milk leakage. Leaking breasts are usually not a problem by the time your baby is older. You can wear good absorbent breast pads and change them frequently.

- You may also try to press against your breast with your arms folded across your chest (heels of your hands pushing on your nipples) to prevent leaking, as pressure applied directly against the nipples will keep milk from leaking.

- You can wear patterned clothes to help you disguise your leaks.

- Try expressing or pumping your milk before you get full and notice the sensations (e.g., full or hardening breasts) that may signal a leakage occurrence.

- Most mothers need to pump their breasts two or three times when they are back to work. It is suggested to pump 10 minutes at break time and 15 minutes at lunch time.

Overabundant Milk Supply

General

Some mothers produce a lot more milk than their babies need. Mothers who have an overabundant supply of milk usually have an overactive let-down, characterized by milk streaming out of the breast, especially during the first few minutes of nursing. Mothers have multiple letdowns during one feeding, but they are usually more manageable than the first one.

The fast flow of milk may cause the baby to struggle and choke when he is trying to nurse. He may pull off the breast and cry. He may refuse to nurse because he is afraid that it may happen again. Some babies bite down on the nipple to stop the flood of milk until they catch their breath and then resume nursing.

When a baby is allowed to set the pattern in regards to length of time on a breast, he will get both the foremilk (the watery milk that is high in sugar) and the hind milk (the thicker milk that is high in fat) in the right balance. When a mother switches her baby before he has finished on the first breast just to relieve the second breast, he may get too much foremilk, which can cause him to be very irritable. Mothers with an overabundant supply often only need to feed from one breast per feeding.

Usually, overabundant milk supply issues will resolve as the mother's supply adjusts to the baby's needs. Remember that this, too, shall pass. However, if the problem persists, discuss the issue with your lactation specialist, doctor, etc.

Tip: The Let-Down Process

When your baby suckles, there are a two hormones that begin to work together to lead to milk production and the release of milk for feedings:

The suckling movement stimulates nerve fibers in the nipple.

These nerves carry the request for milk to the pituitary gland in your brain via the spinal column.

continued

This gland responds to this message by releasing the hormones prolactin (from the anterior pituitary gland) and oxytocin (from the posterior pituitary gland).

Prolactin stimulates the production of milk in the alveoli (grapelike structures) within the breast.

Oxytocin stimulates contractions of tiny muscle cells (myoepithelial cells) around the alveoli, squeezing them and forcing milk into the milk ducts. When these cells contract at the same time, a let-down occurs.

- Inhibitions of the let-down reflex can occur because of stress, pain, fatigue, anxiety, nicotine, alcohol, and certain medications.
- Stimulation of the let-down reflex can occur after hearing your baby cry, thinking about your baby, massaging the breasts, smelling the baby's clothes, etc.

Symptoms in Mother & Baby of Overabundant Milk Supply

Mother

Some mothers can experience pain when milk ejection reflex occurs.
- The mother's breasts feel full and tender between feedings, even after several weeks of breastfeeding.
- There is frequent spraying of milk from one or both breasts and excessive leaking.
- Engorged breasts and repeated mastitis may occur due to blocked ducts.

Baby
- The baby may swallow air, gulp, spit, hiccup, gag, or choke and struggle when feeding, due to an overactive let-down.
- The baby may pull away frequently to break the suction to catch his breath, or he may bite down on the nipple to stop the flow, and then resume nursing.
- The baby may cry and refuse to latch again because he is afraid of a repeat performance.
- Babies who fill up on the watery foremilk (due to mother switching to the second breast too soon) may have laxative effects from large quantities of the lactose sugar. They may get stomach pain, fussiness, and gas. Stools may be frequent, explosive, and watery green in colour.

- Babies may have normal or excessive weight gain, but may also experience slow weight gain.

Coping with Overabundant Milk Supply

In coping with overabundant milk, the goals are to reduce milk production, provide a more relaxed feeding session with less forceful let-down, and have a contented baby. The following suggestions may help.

- Offer one breast at each feeding by allowing your baby to nurse as long as he wants on that one side. If he has nursed less than 15-20 minutes on that one breast and wants to nurse again in less than an hour or two, put him back on the same breast.

- If your baby gets a little squirmy during the feeding, take him off the breast, burp him and offer the same breast again. If your baby seems to like a faster flow, do some breast compressions during the remainder of the feeding to get more hind milk into the baby. He will be more satisfied and sleep longer.

- Many mothers with an overabundant milk supply only need to offer one breast per feeding.

- If the other breast gets uncomfortably full before the next feeding, express just enough milk to relieve the discomfort (not to empty it completely).

- If you have an overactive let-down you can start the flow of milk by hand expressing, allow the foremilk to stream from your breast onto a towel until it slows down to a manageable rate before offering the breast to your baby. The second let-down is usually less forceful.

- Since gravity can help slow down the flow of milk, you may try various breastfeeding positions. Have a towel ready to catch the leakage as the excess milk may dribble out of your baby's mouth. Try the side lying position or lying on your back with the baby on top of the breast. You may also lean back slightly when sitting up, so your baby is suckling uphill against gravity. When your flow slows down, resume an upright position.

- Babies who gulp and choke when the mother has a forceful let-down will often swallow air, so you may need to burp your baby often.

- Avoid pumping or expressing milk as it will lead to more milk production. Pump or express your milk only if you need to relieve the fullness of your breast (about 1 oz/30g).

- Generally, you will notice a decrease in your milk supply in about a week, as it adjusts to meet your baby's demands without over producing.

- Cold cabbage leaves are used as a comfort measure for breast engorgement and can be helpful until milk supply is more balanced (see *Breast Engorgement).*

Parent Concerns

I have a lot of milk and my baby gasps for air, gags, and fusses when I start to feed him. What do I do?

- Babies whose mothers have too much milk will often exhibit symptoms such as choking, fussiness, pulling off the breast, crying, gassiness, spitting up, and hiccups.

- They may gain weight quicker than the average baby, or may gain weight more slowly.

- Try to follow the previous recommendations until the problem is gradually settled or is better tolerated by your baby.

Can I pump breast milk if I have an overactive let-down reflex and overabundant milk?

It is not recommended to pump during an oversupply of milk. Continuing to pump breast milk will increase your milk supply, making matters worse. You can express a small amount just for comfort or right before a feeding session to decrease the forceful milk flow.

My baby gets upset when the flow slows down. What should I do?

- A baby who is used to a fast flow of milk may get frustrated when the flow slows down. However, it is important that the baby stays on the first breast until it is soft (to ensure he receives the fat in the hind milk).

- You can compress the breast with your fingers and thumb and continue to do so to keep your baby interested in breastfeeding. This will also eliminate his frustration and increase the amount of fat he receives in a feeding.

Insufficient (Low) Milk Supply

General

Many mothers are concerned about their babies receiving enough milk. These concerns sometimes lead parents to offer formula supplementation or even wean their baby too early. Most mothers produce an adequate amount of milk; the problem is usually that the baby is not getting enough milk.

When discussing milk supply, one should consider two factors:

1) Mother has good milk supply, but the baby is not feeding effectively.

2) Mother has low milk supply.

It is important to have your baby assessed by a doctor within 72 hours after the hospital discharge. Visiting the doctor in the first 2-3 weeks of your baby's life is important to ensure good weight gain and successful breastfeeding. It also ensures that there are no signs of dehydration and weight loss.

Weight gain is the most important indicator of proper nutrition in your child.

The time the baby spends on the breast is not an indicator of successful feeding. Even when the amount of milk is sufficient, the baby must latch onto the breast properly in order to get enough milk.

In general, if your baby has a good latch and you have abundant milk, he will probably have good weight gain, whether his feedings are short or long and infrequent. If you have abundant milk but your baby's latch is poor, there may be slow or no weight gain (and you may have sore nipples). If your baby has a good latch and you have an average milk supply, then your baby will probably have good weight gain, whether the feedings are short and frequent or long and infrequent.

False Alarms of Low Milk Supply (Perceived Lack of Supply)

- Some mothers think that they do not have enough milk, when there are actually no problems with their milk supply. It is a frequent reason for premature cessation of breastfeeding.

- Most symptoms that mothers worry about are normal patterns in breast feeding and do not always mean that milk supply is low or has decreased.

- False alarms of low milk supply may occur within the first few days after delivery or may occur later (after breastfeeding has already been established).

Immediate Period After Birth
- During the first 48 hours after the birth (when a mother's perception of insufficient milk supply may begin), only a small volume of colostrum is normally available for and required by the newborn baby.
- The newborn's stomach capacity is very limited at birth.
- Babies feed frequently in the first several days of life (usually 12 or more times in the first 24 hours).
- Initially, the more frequent and effective the baby's feeding becomes, the more milk the breast will produce (supply and demand).
- Attempting to pump the breast at this time will only yield very small amounts of colostrum, which is normal.
- Unnecessary formula supplementation during this time period (in the first several days of life), can lead to low milk supply, engorgement, and nipple confusion.
- If breastfeeding is painful, then consult your lactation specialist immediately to receive proper help and advice.

Later Time Period
- Some concerns or perceived alarms of low milk supply are false; these concerns include:
  - ❖ *Softer or Less Engorged Breasts*: This occurs as your milk production adjusts to your baby's demands and the initial fullness or engorgement subsides.
  - ❖ *Feeding More Frequently & Longer Durations*: Your baby wanting to feed more frequently does not necessarily mean that your baby is hungry. Many babies have a strong need to suck and enjoy continuous contact with their mother. Frequent nursing assures that your baby is getting enough milk.
  - ❖ *Fussy Baby*: Some babies are fussy all the time or experience fussy periods. Fussiness can be due to various reasons and as such, you should consult with your doctor to ensure that your baby is gaining weight properly and that there are no other reasons for this fussiness.

❖ *Breast Leakage:* Leaking often stops after your milk supply becomes established and is regulated to your baby's needs. Thus, little to no leaking does not mean that your milk supply has decreased.

❖ *Let-Down Reflex Sensation:* If you do not feel the let-down reflex as strongly as you used to, it does not always mean that your milk supply is low. Some mothers do not even feel the let-down reflex sensation at all.

Feeding Frequency

Frequencies of feedings are not a very useful indicator of determining how much milk the baby is actually receiving.

- A baby who breastfeeds well will wake up when he is hungry.

- If your baby is on the breast more frequently, it does not mean that he is receiving more milk than if he is on the breast less frequently (the same is true for babies who are on the breast for longer periods).

- Some babies feed infrequently, because they are being kept on a schedule rather than on demand. At some point, the baby will give up crying, even when he is hungry. Some will give up crying and simply return to sleep. If the baby is latching onto the breast well, more frequent feedings are a solution.

- Babies also experience occasional growth spurts (frequently around 2-3 weeks, 6 weeks, and 3 months). During this time, babies nurse more often than usual to bring in more milk for their expanding needs. Also, babies will gain weight normally or even more than usual, compared to when you have low milk supply.

- Sometimes, a baby decreases the amount of time spent on the breast. He simply may be able to extract milk more quickly now as he is more experienced. If his weight gain is good, then there should be no concerns.

Tip: Variations in Nursing, Sleeping and Weight Gain

Do not compare your baby to other babies in terms of nursing habits, sleeping patterns, and weight gain. Each baby is a unique individual and there is a wide variation in nursing routines.

Causes of True Low Milk Supply

When it seems as though your milk supply is not meeting your baby's needs (your baby is not gaining weight appropriately despite effective latching) as observed by health professionals, try determining the interfering factors in your milk production. The following are causes or contributing factors to lessened milk supply (alone or in combination):

Bottle Supplementation

- Bottle supplementation (even occasional) of formula, juice, or water can interfere with your milk supply.

- Supplementation fills up your baby and causes him to wait longer for the next feeding, thereby decreasing milk production and breast sucking.

- Frequent bottle supplementation will teach your baby poor latching techniques at a time when he expects rapid flow (even when milk supply is already established).

- When there is a slow flow of milk the baby may pull away from the breast, causing a decreased milk supply.

- Your baby may become confused with the use of an artificial nipple, as it requires a different type of sucking. If your baby is not sucking properly, then he will not be able to stimulate your breast for milk production.

Pacifiers

- Some babies are willing to meet their sucking needs with a pacifier, which may significantly reduce their sucking time at the breast.

Scheduled (Stretching) Feedings

- Delaying a baby's feeding until the clock dictates that a certain amount of time has passed (i.e. limiting the number of feedings) can interfere with milk supply and demand.

- Cutting back in the length of your baby's feedings will also decrease your milk supply, so allow your baby to come off the breast on his own when he feels full. Taking your baby off the breast not only prevents your milk supply from increasing, but also decreases the valuable milk fat content that he could obtain if you allow him to nurse longer.

- Follow your baby's cues instead, and offer the breast when your baby shows signs of hunger.

Offering One Breast

- Offering only one breast per feeding may interfere with your milk supply. If you are working to increase your milk supply, use both breasts and do not limit breastfeeding to only one breast.

Pills & Medications

- Some women take birth control pills while they are breastfeeding and, while progesterone pills are better, these may still decrease your milk supply. Medications such as antihistamines may also decrease your milk supply.

Pregnancy & Illness

- Being pregnant or being ill (e.g., mastitis) may decrease your milk supply.

Fatigue, Tension & Emotional Shock

- Mothers who are doing too much and breastfeeding must take care of themselves in order to provide an adequate milk supply for their babies.
- Fatigue and tension can interfere with your let-down reflex and contribute to inadequate milk supply, so take the time to relax.

Excessive Dieting & Smoking

- Both excessive dieting and/or smoking will have detrimental effects on your milk supply.

Breast Surgery or Hypoplasia

- Some women are unable to produce an adequate supply of milk due to breast surgery or breast hypoplasia (decreased breast tissue).

Placid/Sleepy Baby

- Some babies sleep most of the time and nurse infrequently or for short periods of time.
- If your baby only has a few wet diapers and is not gaining weight, then you should awaken him regularly and encourage him to nurse until he wakes by himself to feed.

Late Onset of Low Milk Supply

For no obvious reasons, some women have a low milk supply around 2-4 months of the baby's life. Possible explanations for late onset of low milk supply may include:

❖ Baby returns to poor latching technique.

❖ Baby has not nursed well from the beginning (yet gained weight normally due to abundant milk supply).

❖ An older baby discontent with the milk flow.

Increasing Milk Supply

Try the following suggestions when trying to increase your milk supply:

• Drink plenty of fluids and eat a well balanced diet.

• Make sure that you are rested and relaxed.

• Feed in a quiet and relaxed place that is free of any distractions.

• Compress your breasts to increase the amount of milk your baby receives at the breast. You may start compressing once the baby is no longer drinking (to keep him actively sucking for a longer time).

❖ Do not do anything if your baby is actively breastfeeding.

❖ To compress your breasts, hold your breast with one hand (thumb on one side and fingers on the other) and watch your baby

❖ Squeeze your breast firmly and keep it compressed (do not release the pressure; keep squeezing while the baby nurses and then release). The faster milk flow should cause your baby to start nursing actively again.

❖ Wait until your baby stops nursing to compress your breast again. If your baby does not stop nursing, rotate your fingers slightly around the breast and squeeze again.

❖ Repeat as needed in different areas of the breast until your compression technique no longer keeps him active, and then switch to the other breast.

- Nursing on both breasts at each feeding ensures that your baby receives all the milk available, as well as allowing both breasts to be stimulated frequently.

- Another way to increase milk supply is to do "switch nursing." When your baby is no longer actively nursing switch to the opposite breast. Do this a few times. When the baby is nursing on one breast, milk is let-down on the opposite breast, so baby will have a faster flow on that breast. This works well for a sleepy baby.

- Nurse frequently for as long as your baby wants to nurse. A sleepy baby may need to be encouraged to nurse more frequently. If your baby wants to be at the breast for a longer period of time, feed him lying down.

- Herbs (e.g., fenugreek and blessed thistle) may help in increasing your milk supply.

- Avoid bottles and pacifiers, as these interfere with nursing.

- It is not always easy to decide if your baby requires supplementation. If your baby does not drink well or is not gaining weight, supplementation may become necessary. If temporary supplements are necessary, they can be given with a nursing supplement while your baby nurses (e.g., spoon, cup, etc.).

- It is sometimes difficult to differentiate between true low milk supply and your baby not receiving enough milk. It is important to have your baby regularly checked for weight gain and examination. In order to rule out the possibility of inappropriate feeding technique before concluding true low milk supply, a lactation specialist or doctor must do observation of feedings.

- If all of the above suggestions do not improve your milk supply fairly quickly, a medication that stimulates breast milk production such as domperidone is a possibility.

Tip: Low Milk Supply and Introduction of Solid Food

When experiencing low milk supply and when your baby is older than 4 months, extra calories can be offered from solid foods. Solids should be given after breastfeeding; otherwise the baby may become full on the solids and take less breast milk. Milk volume may drop because of less breastfeeding. Breast milk should still be a significant part of the baby's diet, if possible.

How To Know: Is My Baby Getting Enough Milk?

Signs of adequate milk supply include the following:

Weight Gain

- Weight gain is the best indicator of whether your child is receiving enough milk.

- Your baby will lose weight in the first few days of life before actually beginning to gain weight. He should start gaining weight by the fourth or fifth day of life. If your baby is breastfeeding well, he should be back to his birth weight by day 7-14.

- With a poor start it may take a few days longer, so follow your baby's weight closely with your doctor or lactation specialist.

- Babies should be plotted appropriately for their age on the WHO (World Health Organization) growth standard charts.

Weight Gain Averages:

- ❖ On average, your baby should be gaining 5-7oz/150-210 g per week, within the first 3 months, or about 1.5-2 lbs/680-908 g per month.

- ❖ The average weight gain in a 4-6 month old baby is 4-5 oz/113-142 g per week.

- ❖ The average weight gain for a 6-12 month old baby is 2-4 oz/57-113 g per week.

Tip: Growth and Breastfeeding Technique

See *Growth Chart*. Note that growth charts available for babies who are formula-fed are different than for those who are exclusively breastfed. Slow or no weight gain can be improved when the breastfeeding technique is improved.

Nursing Characteristics

- See *Positioning & Latching*.

- Open, pause, close type of suckling. The longer the pause, the greater the volume taken.

- Once milk volume increases by day 3 or 4, you may hear or see your baby gulping or swallowing.

Appropriate Output—Urine & Stool

The following are only suggested guidelines for the number of wet and dirty diapers a baby should have. Although it seems important, especially in the first few days, I cannot say it is a good indicator of milk intake for parents to rely on absolutely.

- Once the baby is examined, and despite the doctor having an idea of the number of wet and dirty diapers as told by the parents, the baby is still going to be weighed by the doctor.

- In the first several days of life, the risk of dehydration and possible associated consequences means that it is crucial to ensure that the baby is gaining weight.

- Because it is difficult for parents to estimate the number of wet and dirty diapers their baby has, and because it is difficult for the doctor to accurately assess for signs of dehydration, weighing is important, as are the previously mentioned signs of poor milk intake and dehydration.

- Some parents may report "little" stool of variable frequency, while other report normal looking size with a certain frequency. Some may say the stool was "watery" and may have been mixed with urine. Disposable diapers are very absorbent and, for the first few days, it may be difficult to tell if your baby is wet (you can put a piece of Kleenex inside the diaper for the first few days if you are having difficulties with knowing if your baby is wet).

- The following can be considered to be some guidelines for watching for *dirty diapers*:

  ❖ Day 1: At least one meconium bowel movement (black and sticky).

  ❖ Day 2: At least two meconium bowel movements turning greenish in color and not as sticky.

  ❖ Day 3: At least two or three loose greenish bowel movements.

  ❖ Day 4-6: at least two or three yellow stools per day.

  ❖ Day 6 to 4-6 Weeks of Age: three or four soft stools that are usually golden-yellow to brown, and are runny or seedy.

  ❖ After 4-6 weeks: Some babies may go several days without having any bowel movements, which is not a cause for concern as long as they are healthy and gaining weight appropriately.

- Consult your doctor if you have any concerns.

- The following are considered to be some guidelines for *wet diapers*:

  ❖ The first three days, the diaper will not be heavy. This is the time when the baby is taking smaller volumes. He is getting colostrum. A heavy wet diaper is equal to about three tablespoons of water in the stool.

  ❖ Day 1: 1 wet diaper in the first 24 hours.

  ❖ Day 2: two wet diapers in the second 24 hours.

  ❖ Day 3: three wet diapers in the third 24 hours.

  ❖ Day 4: four wet, heavier diapers in the fourth 24 hours.

  ❖ Day 5: five wet heavy diapers.

  ❖ Day 6 and after: six to eight wet and heavy diapers.

> ### Tip: Red Stain on Baby's Diapers
>
> You may notice urate crystals (a staining on the diaper that is orangy-red in colour). It can be normal in the newborn period and should not be an indication of dehydration or poor milk intake, although it may have some significance in the first few days. Many babies who are growing well from the beginning may also have these red-orangy colors with no significant importance. When milk volume has increased and your baby is drinking more, the urate crystals will disappear.

- Although the above are guidelines and are important, especially in the first few days, I do not find it to be a very good indicator of a baby's milk intake, since different parents report stool and urine differently.

- The following signs may indicate poor milk intake and dehydration that requires medical attention: decreased urine and stool output, lethargy, listlessness, weak cries, dry mouth, skin that loses its resilience (when pressed, it stays pressed), worsening jaundice, etc. These are not always easy to detect on your own (or even for your doctor) and that is why it is important to follow up with your doctor and check your baby's weight.

Parent Concerns

The soft spot (fontanel) on my baby's head is sunken. Does this mean he is dehydrated?

It is very difficult to assess dehydration simply from your baby's fontanel in the first few months of life, even by an experienced pediatrician. It is not a reliable measurement of dehydration unless severe (see *Water, Fluids & Drinks*).

Breastfeeding in Public

General

A breastfeeding mother has the right to nurse her baby anywhere and at any time. Many mothers breastfeed in public. Others are hesitant or uncomfortable to do so. This may be due to shyness or fear of the reaction of those around them. There are ways to breastfeed discreetly which may make you feel more comfortable when you are nursing in public.

Society has mixed emotions when it comes to breastfeeding in public. Some people are uncomfortable just knowing that a woman is breastfeeding in their presence, even if her breast is not showing. The same people often have no qualms about seeing a scantily dressed woman walking around in public. Many people in the North American culture see breasts as sexual but have difficulty with them being functional.

Others are very supportive of mothers nursing in public, perhaps because they come from a breastfeeding friendly culture, have breastfed in public themselves, and have a very supportive family. These people see breastfeeding for what it is; a normal part of everyday life. Babies need to be fed when they are hungry and breast is best.

Nursing your baby is a natural and beautiful experience and, with time, you will be more comfortable nursing in public. Be proud that you are able to nurse your baby and never be ashamed of this fact.

How to Breastfeed in Public

The following are tips and suggestions of how to nurse your baby in public discreetly:

- Plan ahead so that you may have some idea where you will be when your baby wants to nurse. How long are you going to be away from home?

- Breastfeeding your baby right before you go out will give you more time before he is hungry again (you might even be back home by then).

- You may buy special nursing tops that provide easy access to the breast. Many of these clothes have small openings that reveal just enough for your baby to be able to breastfeed. If you are wearing a t-shirt or sweater, you can lift it up for easy access to the breast. Your baby covers your midriff while nursing. If you are wearing a buttoned top, undo the lower buttons only.

- If you are in a mall or store, ask if it is possible to nurse in a fitting room. Somelarger malls have special baby care rooms with chairs where you may nurse your baby. If you are in a restaurant, ask for a booth so that you may have more privacy.

- Some of the baby slings like "Heart to Heart" or Over the Shoulder" are very useful when nursing in public. Your baby is in close and you can even nurse "hands free" if you wish.

- Never breastfeed in a bathroom, since no one enjoys eating where the toilets are.

- Feed your baby before he gets too hungry and draws more attention to you. This will allow your baby to feed in a calm and relaxed manner.

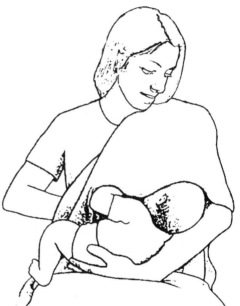

- Distract your baby's hands away from your shirt, so that he does not lift it while you are nursing. Carry a soft toy for your baby to hold during a feeding session.

- Never cover yourself with a blanket since this only draws more attention to the fact that you are nursing. It may also be uncomfortable for your baby.

- Many new mothers who wish to try public nursing but are uncomfortable may want to practice by standing in front of a mirror when they are nursing to see just how much others actually see. If they wish, a light blanket or shawl draped over the shoulder can be used to cover any exposed areas.

- Mothers, who choose not to breastfeed publicly, can take some expressed breast milk with them and bottle-feed it to their baby. (This is not advised until your baby has established solid breastfeeding habits.)

Breast Preference

General

It is not unusual for a newborn baby to latch and nurse well on one breast, but then refuse the other (probably because the first breast is easier to grasp). Breast preference may also occur in the later stages of breastfeeding. It is important for your baby to try to feed from both breasts, so that you do not lose your milk supply in the unused breast.

Some mothers are concerned that nursing from one breast only will alter the unused breast's shape or size. The breast that is not nursed on or pumped will gradually dry up and remain smaller than the breast the baby is nursing from. Women typically have one larger breast, even before pregnancy or breastfeeding. Many mothers can breastfeed totally (meeting all the baby's nutritional needs) from only one breast.

Causes

There are various reasons why babies prefer one breast to the other.

- Your baby may notice a difference in the nipple shape or size. Babies usually will latch on easier if the nipple protrudes, whereas they may have more difficulty latching on a breast that has a flat or inverted nipple (see *Flat and Inverted Nipples*).

- Your baby may not be able to properly latch on to one of the breasts (poor latching technique, probably). This may be due to your comfort in holding your baby. Are you right or left-handed? Do you have an I.V. in your preferred hand (in hospital)?

- Breast engorgement in a particular breast may cause your baby to refuse that breast because it is more difficult for him to latch on to the engorged breast.

- There may be low milk supply in one of the breasts, causing your baby to suck harder for the milk (it is important to rule this out as a cause).

- Your baby may be sick with an ear infection or have a blocked nostril, causing him to prefer one breast to the other.

- A fracture of one side of the collarbone or trauma at birth may predispose your baby to prefer one side of the breast.

> ### Tip: Breast Refusal
>
> When your baby refuses one breast, you must pump that breast regularly in order to continue producing milk. In time, your baby will probably feed from both breasts.

How to Overcome Breast Preference

The following suggestions may help in getting your baby to begin feeding from the refused breast:

- Gently encourage your baby to nurse from the refused breast.

- Pump the refused breast if the baby does not nurse on that side. In the case of a flat or inverted nipple, pumping may draw out the nipple so that it is easier for the baby to latch. The nipple needs to be drawn back into the baby's mouth to keep him from slipping off it while he is nursing.

- Try pumping for a few minutes before latching on your baby. Always offer the refused breast first when your baby is just starting to wake up.

- Offer the rejected breast when your baby is tired or sleepy. Again, pump it a little before trying to latch. Keep your baby in skin-to-skin contact when trying.

- Try using different positions when breastfeeding to encourage the refused breast (e.g., Football hold on the rejected side). Mothers usually feel more comfortable holding their baby with their dominant hand. Therefore using a Football hold on the right side and a Cross Cradle hold on the left side often works for a right-handed mother. The opposite is true for the left-handed mother.

- If your baby is old enough and your milk is well established already, allow your baby to feed off the one breast as long as you are not experiencing any problems and he is receiving enough milk and gaining weight. Some older babies can finish feeding in five minutes and gain weight well.

- Mothers and babies often will fall into the pattern of nursing where it is easiest. If milk supply is low on the refused side, pumping may help to build it up (see *Increasing Milk Supply*).

- In cases of birth trauma, keeping the baby's sore side away from the breast usually works best. Try a different position.

- Ask a lactation expert for help and advice if your baby continues to reject one side, or suddenly rejects one breast.

Nursing Strike

General

Occasionally, a baby who was feeding well may suddenly stop taking the breast for no apparent reason, even though he is obviously hungry. This is known as a *nursing strike*. Nursing strikes usually last 2-5 days and not more than two weeks. They usually occur in babies between 3-8 months of age, although this can vary.

Many mothers believe their babies are beginning to naturally wean when they are really on a nursing strike. Beginning to wean during the first months to year of life is rare; it is a gradual process and not a sudden rejection of the breast. Don't mistake nursing strike as a cue to prematurely stop breastfeeding.

Tip: Staying Calm

The mother should not feel frustrated, upset, guilty, or believe that her baby's refusal to nurse means that she has done something wrong. Staying calm is the best for mother and baby.

Baby's Behavior During the Strike

The following behaviors are characteristic of babies on a nursing strike:

- Your baby may cry, scream, and push you away if you try to place him on the breast (the more you try, the more your baby gets upset).

- Typically, your baby does not refuse the breast all the time. He may choose to breastfeed at certain times (e.g., at night, when sleepy, or just starting to arouse). If this is the case, your baby may continue to gain weight appropriately.

- Sometimes the baby on a nursing strike will go to the breast for a very short period of time, just long enough to satisfy his hunger and then pull away.

- Babies may prefer to suck their hands when they are on a nursing strike.

- The nursing strike may stop suddenly (just like it started) or may gradually worsen over a few days.

Causes

The cause of a nursing strike is often unclear.

- Something may have frightened the baby while he was breastfeeding. For example, if the baby bites his mother, her reaction may upset him (see *Biting the Breast*). She may also have an overactive let-down. If her milk comes too fast he may choke on it, pull away, and be reluctant to try it again.

- The baby may have a stuffy nose or ear pain.

- Milk flow may be too slow due to decreased supply, or baby has become used to fast flow of bottles and prefers them over breastfeeding.

- Sometimes, a baby who is ready to wean (usually over a year old) and is eating lots of solid foods and drinking from a cup gradually loses interest in nursing.

> **Tip: Possible reasons for a nursing strike:**
>
> Nursing becomes a stressful time with too many outside interruptions.
>
> Limited and/or rigid feeding schedules instead of allowing the baby to lead the way.
>
> Baby becomes more dependent on a pacifier, thumb, or is given too many bottles.

Nursing Strikes & Decreased Milk Supply

- Some mothers have a drop in milk supply for no apparent reason at approximately 3 months after birth. In this case, the baby wants to nurse but quickly becomes frustrated and cries because he is unable to receive milk adequately. He may yank on the breast trying to make the milk come faster.

- It is important to know if the baby is getting the milk. Watch his behavior. Does he suckle properly (open his mouth wide, pause, close) in a relaxed manner? Can you hear him swallow frequently?

- Some causes of low milk supply include (see *Low Milk Supply*):
  - ❖ Use of birth control pills or pregnancy.
  - ❖ Using the bottle more than usual.
  - ❖ Emotional "shock."

❖ Illness in the mother (e.g., mastitis).

❖ Long time between feedings.

❖ Use of decongestants like Benadryl.

❖ Mother is doing too much (e.g., Supermom).

What To Do

The following are some suggestions of what you can do with a baby on nursing strike:

- Patience and support of your baby are key in helping your baby find his way back to the breast.

- Feed in a quiet place; provide more eye-to-eye contact and skin-to-skin contact without specifically trying to offer the breast (remember that nursing strikes get better spontaneously).

- If your baby becomes upset when you are trying to feed, stop and attempt to calm him before trying again.

- Try nursing your baby when he is falling asleep.

- Watch to make sure that your baby is receiving enough milk (follow his weight gain, etc.).

- Do not try to force the baby to breastfeed, as he will get more upset.

- Try feeding at night in your bed with lots of skin-to-skin contact. This can encourage him to feed.

- Try walking with your baby while he is in a breastfeeding position until he gets a little sleepy; you may then try and place him on the breast.

- It is advisable to pump your milk frequently to keep up your milk supply until your baby resumes nursing well.

- If you are concerned about his milk intake, give him expressed milk by cup or eyedropper, etc. If your baby is eight months of age or older, expressed breast milk can be mixed with other solid foods (usually, strikes do not last long when the baby is older than three months of age).

Parent Concerns

How do I know if my baby is on a nursing strike or the beginning of a weaning process?

- The following will help you differentiate between the two:
  - ❖ Typically, the baby has been nursing well and then suddenly refuses to nurse with no apparent reason (nursing strike).
  - ❖ Your baby seems unhappy during breastfeeding, briefly taking the breast and then beginning to fuss and refuses to take the breast (nursing strike).
  - ❖ If your baby is less than a year old and has not been eating much solid foods or drinking from a cup, it is unlikely that he is ready to give up breastfeeding (nursing strike).
  - ❖ Baby-led weaning during the first year of life is uncommon and more gradual than sudden. They wean for the following reasons; milk supply is down, use of bottles, or both, one often causes the other to come into play.
  - ❖ When your baby is naturally weaning himself, he is most likely not to be distressed with the change.

What can happen with a nursing strike?

- Nursing strikes usually last two to four days and usually do not result in permanent weaning.
- In order to maintain breast milk supply and prevent engorgement or mastitis during a nursing strike, express the milk as often as the baby was nursing prior to the strike.
- If you must offer expressed milk, do so with an alternate feeding device such as a cup, spoon, syringe, dropper, etc., rather than a bottle.

How do I deal with my baby's nursing strike?

- Do not interpret the strike as an effort to "self wean."
- If a nursing strike happens and there are other symptoms or illness present, consult your doctor.

- Continue to try to breastfeed your baby and try not to use substitute formula in a bottle. Instead, use the alternative methods of feeding mentioned above, slow down on solid foods, be patient, and follow the suggestions made in this section.
- Contact La Leche League for support, if necessary.

What are the causes of breast refusal and how do I deal with it?
There are various reasons why a baby may refuse the breast and they may include:

- Difficult or long birth (vigorous suctioning of baby after birth).
- Baby is forced onto the breast (especially while crying or not ready to latch).
- Nipple confusion or preference.
- Breast engorgement, inverted nipples, or poor positioning.
- Baby is experiencing pain or has tongue tie.
- Medications the mother is taking or medical complications (jaundice, dehydration, etc.).

What suggestions do you have for dealing with breast refusal?
- Offer lots of skin-to-skin contact.
- Be alert to your baby's feeding cues (e.g., crying, hand movements, head movements, etc.,) and place him on the breast when these cues are noticed.
- Do not force your baby on the breast; handle him gently.
- Proper positioning and latching techniques should be learned with the help of a lactation consultant.
- Try alternate feeding methods if your baby is not latching properly at a feeding (e.g., pump your breasts, cup or spoon feeding, finger feeding).

Tip: Support of Mother During Breast Refusal

Sometimes, mothers require support or someone to talk to when dealing with breast refusal. The La Leche League is great for helping you deal with difficulties (both physical and emotional) you may have when breastfeeding.

Tip: Additional Comment on Breast Refusal

Often babies are mucousy within the first 24 hours of birth. This can lead to breast refusal. When they attempt to latch onto the nipple, they gag, and then throw up mucous. Allow your baby to rest a bit (it seems to help) with lots of skin-to-skin contact to comfort his distress. Also, when a baby lacks interest or is having difficulty latching, the side-laying position seems to work best for him. Have him lie facing you, nose in line with the nipple. He will tilt his head back when you stroke his upper lip with the nipple. By moving him by the shoulders a little, he will first grasp lots of the underside of the areola, then draw the nipple into his mouth and, finally, the upper lip will cover a smaller amount of the areola. A good number of babies latch by themselves with very little assistance in this position, because they are not handled as much.

It sometimes takes several weeks before a baby will breastfeed properly. Rental of an electric breast pump allows the mother to provide her own milk to her baby.

Biting the Breast

General

It is hard to relax and enjoy breastfeeding when your baby has bitten you. You will probably be afraid that it will happen again. While some breastfed babies occasionally bite, it is a fairly simple problem to deal with and should not threaten the success of breastfeeding.

When your baby is latching on correctly and nursing actively, the nipple is far back in your baby's mouth, his tongue is over his lower gum, and he cannot bite. In order to bite the breast, your baby has to adjust his tongue by bringing it behind his lower gum, pushing the nipple to the front of his mouth.

The best way to prevent biting involves anticipating the behavior and stopping it before it happens. This may require persistence on your part, as the baby may not stop biting immediately. Remember that this, too, shall pass!

Causes

- The most common reason for biting the breast is sore gums due to teething.
- Sometimes, your baby will bite when he is almost finished nursing and is startled by something, or just wants to play.
- If milk flow is slow, biting or yanking the breast usually occurs quite early in feeding session.
- If milk flow is too fast, some babies may clamp down on the nipple to stop the spray, catch their breath, and then resume nursing.
- Physical illness (e.g., cold, ear infection, etc.) may make it difficult for your baby to swallow while breastfeeding. For example, if his nose is blocked (babies are nose breathers in the first year of life), he will probably bite.
- Some babies bite the breast to get mother's attention, while some bite due to stress.

How to Stop Breast Biting

- A mother should be prepared to intervene when the baby bites the breast.

Notice your baby's biting pattern (e.g., time it occurs—early or late in the feeding—the baby's level of interest when feeding, during physical illness, teething, etc.).

- Some babies are very fast feeders when they are older. They may only nurse for 5 to 7 minutes and get all the milk they need. If your baby is a biter, slip your finger into the corner of his mouth to release your nipple whenever he starts to pull away from the breast. Pulling the baby straight off without breaking suction may cause sore nipples.

- The following are some steps you can take to help stop your baby stop breast biting:

  ❖ Keep your finger close to your baby's mouth so that you can unlatch him from the breast quickly.

  ❖ Remove your baby from the breast gently and react in the following manner:

    1) Say "No biting."

    2) Put him down gently or give him to someone else.

    3) Wait a few minutes before you start nursing again.

  These actions will teach your baby that biting is "not acceptable" and that the milk goes away when he bites. Sensitive babies may cry at these actions, so calm your baby (e.g., rocking, walking, singing, etc.) and resume feeding.

  ❖ Repeat these steps until your baby understands to stop biting.

  ❖ Be sure not to yell or scream at your baby, as time and attitude do convey the meaning. Too much anger or amusement may interest the baby enough to make him want to repeat the experiment again, rather than making him stop.

  ❖ If the baby bites early during a feeding session due to frustration while trying to get your milk to let-down, do some breast compressions to speed up the flow.

  ❖ If you have an overactive let-down, take your baby off the breast and allow some of the milk to spray onto a towel until it seems manageable, and then relatch him. You may also try to lean backwards so that he is suckling against gravity until the initial flow has slowed down.

  ❖ If your baby bites near the end of a feeding session, unlatch him from the breast.

❖ If your baby is very young and still learning to nurse properly, try various positions and repositioning until he gets the latching technique right. Some babies may require suck training if they are persistent in keeping the tongue behind the lower gum.

❖ If your baby is teething and bites your breast after a short period of breastfeeding take him off for a few minutes, then relatch. You may offer something else for him to chew on before nursing and in-between feedings. Teething rings are good substitutes; however some experts do not recommend this, as it may reinforce the unwanted behavior. A cold, wet facecloth may help to soothe sore gums.

❖ A baby is less likely to bite to get attention if his mother gives him lots of eye contact and touches and talks softly to him while he is feeding.

Tip: Response to Breast Biting

React firmly but calmly when he bites, since screaming or pushing your baby away may be frightening to him. He may cry and refuse to nurse.

Sometimes older babies with teeth leave marks after a breastfeeding session. Generally, this is not painful and is caused by the teeth resting on your breast during breastfeeding.

Saying "No biting" does not work with all babies. Some can be frightened and go on a nursing strike (see *Nursing Strike*). Others enjoy the reaction and want to continue the game.

Tongue Tie & Breastfeeding

General

Tongue tie is a term used for a condition in which a baby is born with a tight or shortened frenulum (a whitish, vertical membrane which attaches the tongue to the floor of the mouth).

Both breastfed and formula-fed babies may have difficulties feeding if they have a tight frenulum, leading to complications in the baby and mother. If the frenulum is too short or tight, the breastfed baby will not be able to latch onto the breast or extract milk from the mother's breast properly and the mother may end up supplementing milk by the bottle. The bottle-fed baby with tongue tie will have less difficulty, as some formula does drip into his mouth, even without active sucking.

Often, there is a family history of tongue tie.

Symptoms of Tongue Tie

Symptoms of tongue tie and associated problems may vary widely and may result in the following:

❖ Poor weight gain or weight loss in the baby.

❖ Frustration: The baby cannot get the milk easily from the breast and may give up on breastfeeding (fatigue early on when beginning to nurse).

❖ Crying and fussiness in the baby.

❖ A mother will often have cracked nipples and experience painful breastfeeding (if the mother persists in breastfeeding, her milk supply may drop due to inadequate emptying of the breast).

❖ Mastitis (infective) may also develop because of cracked nipples.

❖ Addition of other factors such as poor positioning, early bottle introduction, etc., combined with moderate tongue tie may lead to an inability to take the breast and untimely weaning.

> **Tip: Tongue Tie and Feeding Problem**
>
> Consult your doctor or lactation specialist sooner rather than later.

Treatment of Tongue Tie

Treatment for tongue tie is usually best decided on a case-by-case basis.

- Clipping the frenulum:

  ❖ Clipping the frenulum is quick, simple, safe, and is usually a painless procedure that can be done in the doctor's office. It is a simple "snip" with a blunt ended scissor. Bleeding is very minimal with this procedure and it is not dangerous or complicated (less traumatic than ear piercing and less invasive than circumcision).

  ❖ It is worth trying to clip the tongue tie, particularly if there are symptoms in the baby (e.g., not gaining weight properly, etc.) or mother (e.g., pain with nursing, etc.).

  ❖ Clipping of the frenulum should be done within the first few weeks after birth, if it is interfering with breastfeeding to ensure good milk production and comfort for the mother. However, if the problem persists after clipping the frenulum, you should be re-assessed by your doctor or lactation specialist for other contributing factors to pain, etc., in the mother and baby.

If there are no symptoms of feeding difficulties (or there is "mild to moderate" tongue tie), then treatment is usually decided on a case-by-case basis by your doctor.

Parent Concerns

What are indicators of tongue tie requiring treatment?

- Indicators of tongue tie snipping include the following:

  ❖ Latch on is painful and uncomfortable for the mother and/or baby (symptoms as stated above).

  ❖ When the baby cries, the tongue should curl upward and form a trough. With tongue tie, the tongue curls under.

  ❖ The tip of the tongue does not protrude past the lower gum or past the lips.

❖ The tongue cannot touch the roof of the mouth and cannot be moved sideways.

❖ When extended, the tip of the tongue looks flat and square, instead of pointy.

Remember that successful feeding depends on the severity of the tongue tie and that clipping is usually quick, with no complications.

At what age should the tongue tie be cut?

- Tongue tie may be cut at any age, when problems related to feeding or speech difficulties are noted.

- Some cases may resolve spontaneously or the affected person learns to compensate with it, while others may benefit from the treatment.

- If the tongue tie was not cut in infancy, watch to see if it becomes looser (in these cases, the tongue protrudes past the lower lip) and if your child shows speech difficulties; if so, treatment may be required.

Conclusion

- Tongue tie can be an obstacle to breastfeeding, so intervene quickly in symptomatic cases.

- Tongue tie may cause breast soreness and cracked and bleeding nipples in the mother, while the infant may struggle with nursing effectively and have associated poor weight gain or weight loss.

- Many mothers report that after clipping is done, effective breastfeeding is able to resume immediately, without any difficulty.

- Do not resist or ignore the pain simply to continue breastfeeding, as many mothers do. It is in no way beneficial to you or your baby to force the natural process of breastfeeding.

- Speak to your doctor or lactation specialist about breastfeeding difficulties.

- Remember that tongue tie is a possible cause for feeding difficulties.

Breastfeeding & Jaundice

General

Jaundice is a yellow pigmentation of the eye/skin caused by an accumulation of a chemical component in the blood called bilirubin (an orange/yellow pigment) in the tissue.

Newborn babies often become jaundiced, commonly due to the following reasons:

Normal full term newborns naturally have higher numbers of red blood cells than adults (to get enough oxygen in the womb from the mother's blood). When the baby is out of the womb and the lungs supply plenty of oxygen, these extra red blood cells are broken down, leading to increased bilirubin. This makes jaundice more common in newborn babies.

Liver enzymes, which metabolize the bilirubin, are relatively immature in some newborns (this is more pronounced in a premature baby). If the build-up is faster than the newborn's liver can handle, the excess of bilirubin accumulates in the tissues and gives a yellow discoloration to the eyes and skin.

The bilirubin formed does not usually cause jaundice, as the liver metabolizes it and receives aid from the intestine/gut, since bilirubin is excreted in the baby's stool. Some of the bilirubin that gets to the intestine is re-absorbed by the body, especially if the baby does not have many bowel movements or is not taking in enough breast milk or formula. This bilirubin re-absorption (called enterohepatic circulation) makes the baby become more jaundiced.

Various factors may cause increased production of bilirubin. For example, Hemolysis is the destruction of red blood cells caused by a blood group incompatibility between mother and baby (which occurs after birth). If your baby has bruises, or hematomas (this may occur during delivery), these damaged extra red blood cells are available to produce more bilirubin as they breakdown.

Tip: Direct & Indirect Bilirubin

Once bilirubin is produced, the liver adds something to it to make it water-soluble and it is excreted in the urine or passed through the intestine in the stool.

continued

Water-soluble bilirubin is called direct bilirubin or conjugated bilirubin. It is filtered through the kidney and excreted in the urine.

The fat-soluble bilirubin is called indirect bilirubin or unconjugated bilirubin.

Causes & Types of Jaundice

Normal or Physiologic Jaundice

- This type of jaundice affects nearly all newborns to some degree and it is usually harmless.

- In healthy, full-term babies, normal jaundice begins on the second to fourth day after birth, peaks on the third to fifth day, and then begins to decline steadily to normal levels through the first two weeks.

- There is an accumulation of bilirubin (indirect) due to inability of the immature liver enzymes to handle increased breakdown of red cells.

- It requires no intervention in the majority of infants, as it usually resolves on its own. However, other risk factors (e.g., babies who are premature or low birth weight, those who are not feeding enough or not producing enough stool, or those who are dehydrated or have bruises/hematoma, etc.) may develop high bilirubin levels, requiring phototherapy (light treatment).

- In a baby with normal or physiologic jaundice, breastfeeding should continue or even be increased.

Breast Milk Jaundice

- Breast milk jaundice occurs in approximately 2% of breastfed, thriving babies.

- The cause of breast milk jaundice is unknown; it may sometimes increase baby's physiologic jaundice; however this condition is usually harmless.

- This type of jaundice usually develops in the second week of life and peaks at 10-21 days of life (indirect bilirubin levels).

- Breast milk jaundice can last up to two to three months.

- Jaundice (bilirubin) levels may be from low (mildly yellow baby) to quite yellow for a longer time.

- You may sometimes be asked by your doctor to stop breastfeeding for a day to see if bilirubin levels are decreasing. If you do this, use a good quality electric breast pump to express your breast milk, so that it doesn't dry up. Although this practice has been done more in the past, there really is no reason to stop breastfeeding or start a formula supplement. Experts agree that it is not in the best interest of mother and baby to stop nursing, even for one day.

- Bilirubin levels do drop rapidly if other milk is provided along with, or as a temporary substitution for, the mother's milk.

- Abnormal (pathological) causes of jaundice are excluded (see below).

- In most cases, jaundice requires no intervention.

Abnormal (Pathological) Jaundice

- Abnormal and pathological jaundice may aggravate and/or simulate previous types of jaundice. Your doctor may check for these if they have any concerns.

- Examples of causes of abnormal jaundice include:

  ❖ Blood group incompatibilities (most common).

  ❖ Under-functioning of the thyroid.

  ❖ Liver diseases.

  ❖ Infection (e.g., urine infection).

  ❖ Metabolic/genetic disease (e.g., Galactosemia), etc.

Diagnosis

- Jaundice is typically visible on the baby's face including the white part of the eye. The yellowing in the eyes is the first to appear as bilirubin levels reach a certain point and they are the last to disappear as bilirubin levels decrease.

- Yellowing of the skin starts with the baby's head and works its way down towards the toes.

- If bilirubin levels increase, the jaundice (yellowness) moves from the face and becomes more apparent in the trunk and extremities.

- The following infant characteristics are taken into consideration:

- ❖ *Race/Ethnic* grouping may have a varied effect on jaundice (e.g., Japanese have an increased risk).

- ❖ *Birth weight*: A lower birth weight is related to a likelihood of higher bilirubin levels (partly because of the less mature liver enzymes).

- ❖ *Stool pattern*: Infrequent bowel movements will cause an increase in jaundice as bilirubin is reabsorbed into the body (enterohepatic circulation).

- ❖ *Type of feeding*: Jaundice is seen more in breastfeeding babies and is worse if feedings are not effective and the baby does not have frequent bowel movements.

- ❖ *Supplemental Feeding*: Delay in establishing breast milk supply may contribute to increase bilirubin. Water supplementation may also interfere with lactation.

- The following aspects should be considered when assessing the relationship of breastfeeding and jaundice:

  - ❖ What is the frequency and duration of breastfeeding? He should be nursing at least 8-12 times over 24 hours in the first few days.

  - ❖ Is the baby suckling well when he is put to the breast? Can you hear the baby gulping?

  - ❖ Is he actively nursing or does he keep falling asleep?

  - ❖ Does he wake up to feed frequently or do you have to wake him up?

  - ❖ Baby stool frequency and colour of stools: The more frequent the better!

  - ❖ Changing color from meconium/black stools to green and then yellow is a good sign.

  - ❖ Are any additional/complimentary/supplementary feeds being given? Why?

  - ❖ Is the baby being fed at night? Babies usually feed at least 3 times during the night for the first few weeks.

- Laboratory tests of bilirubin levels, including parameters such as baby's birth weight/prematurity, age, clinical condition, blood group types, etc., will help your doctor determine whether your baby needs a simple follow-up (with or without a blood test for bilirubin levels) or phototherapy treatment.

- If the baby has an abnormally high level of bilirubin or if the levels are rising rapidly, the bilirubin test may be repeated as dictated by your doctor in order to monitor the changes in bilirubin levels.

> ### Tip: Jaundice and Urgent Doctor Visit
>
> If your baby has prolonged jaundice and white or pale stool, notify your doctor immediately (the earlier the diagnosis, the better) as it may be due to a congenital abnormality of the liver requiring surgery.
>
> The more yellowness in the skin is noted from top to bottom (eye, face, upper trunk, complete trunk, extremities, palm and sole) the higher the level of jaundice (usually).

Treatment

- Decisions about treatment depend on the age of the baby, birth weight, speed of increasing bilirubin levels, and other associated health issues.
- Frequent breastfeeding while under phototherapy is important to help avoid dehydration.
- *Do not stop breastfeeding.* Ensure that the baby is breastfeeding well or, if you cannot breastfeed, express milk for your baby. Colostrum in particular has a laxative effect which will help your baby have lots of bowel movements. This will decrease the level of jaundice.
- Avoid water supplements which fill up your baby so that he does not nurse well.
- *Phototherapy treatment* alters the bilirubin, helping the baby get rid of jaundice.
  - ❖ It prevents bilirubin from reaching high levels or from accumulating and causing brain damage.
  - ❖ During treatment, the baby is naked with eyes closed and only a diaper on. The baby should have extra fluids to prevent dehydration due to water loss through the skin. This can be done by frequent nursing or using a lactation aid on the breast to give supplements (of expressed milk with sugar water). In some cases formula may be necessary (e.g., a delay in milk production).

❖ Bilirubin levels are then followed and the baby is discharged when levels are within normal range.

❖ Your doctor requires close follow-ups during phototherapy treatment to make sure your baby's bilirubin levels are not increasing to a point of being a concern.

- Rarely, in extreme cases, babies may be given exchange blood transfusions (some of the jaundiced blood is removed and exchanged for new blood), as it is the fastest way to bring bilirubin levels down.

Parent Concerns

Why is there such great medical concern over jaundice when it seems to be a harmless condition that in most cases resolves itself?

- Jaundice is a harmless condition which does, in most cases, resolve itself. However, in rare situations the Bilirubin levels can get high and cause brain damage.

Why is it important to know all three types of jaundice: physiologic, breast milk, and abnormal jaundice?

- Each type of jaundice has a different cause and different outcomes. It is important for doctors to rule out certain types of jaundice, because they need to know what additional tests and evaluations to conduct, or in case urgent treatment is required.

Do frequent stools help lower bilirubin levels in my baby?

- Frequent stools do help lower bilirubin levels since bilirubin is excreted through the stool. The more the better! When it is not excreted, it re-circulates in your baby's system, the bilirubin levels increase, and he may become more jaundiced.

When is phototherapy treatment appropriate?

- Phototherapy treatment is usually done when your baby's bilirubin levels are rapidly increasing to a level of medical concern. Phototherapy breaks down the bilirubin until it is within the recommended range. The baby is referred to the hospital for phototherapy if bilirubin levels are high for the suggested age and weight of your baby (dependent on your baby's blood group, birth weight, and associated issues, etc.).

After phototherapy, will my baby's bilirubin levels stay low or will they increase again?

- Typically, after a day or two of phototherapy treatment bilirubin levels drop significantly and, once the levels begin to decline, they usually continue to decrease. However, there may sometimes be a sudden increase of bilirubin once phototherapy has been stopped. If you notice your baby is very yellow, consult your doctor.

Tip: Jaundice, Skin Colour and Light Exposure

Skin color may look different in different light exposures.

Am I able to know whether or not my child needs phototherapy just by his color?

- If your baby shows intense color all over his body, high bilirubin levels may be suspected and your child may need phototherapy. However, the final decision depends on the bilirubin level in the blood and the age of your baby.

- Even an experienced pediatrician may not always be able to estimate bilirubin levels by eye, as the intensity of color may vary according to the baby's skin color, which is why a blood test is required.

Should I put my jaundiced baby close to the window for sun?

- Your baby should not be placed close to the window and should not be directly exposed to sunlight, since his skin is sensitive and may burn. It is not an effective way to decrease high bilirubin levels which require phototherapy. Simply place him in a room that has a lot of light. More information is available from www.caringforkids.cps.ca.

Breastfeeding & Drugs

General

Most drug medications are safe to use when you are breastfeeding, since a very small amount passes through your breast milk to your baby. However, there are some drugs that are not safe to use when you are nursing.

If you must take drugs when you are breastfeeding, consult with your doctor or call the appropriate health service for information available and advice (e.g., "Motherisk" at Toronto's Sick Kids Hospital 416-813-6780).

It is important to remember that stopping breastfeeding while on drugs may result in low milk production and, subsequently, your baby may refuse to breastfeed. The decision to stop breastfeeding should be based on medical advice, with a proper scientific base. Check with your doctor about any drugs you may take while breastfeeding, including those that do not require a prescription.

Tip: Breast Implant and Breast Feeding

Although some doctors believe that women with silicone breast implants should not breastfeed, there is no evidence showing that babies are harmed by implants. In any case, you should discuss concerns with your doctor.

Drugs Considered Safe

Guidelines for safety include (upon consultation with your doctor):

- Drugs that are either not excreted into the milk or are excreted in small amounts.
- Drugs that are not absorbed by the digestive system.
- Medications applied to the skin or eyes are almost always safe.
- Inhaled medications (e.g., those used for asthma) are usually safe.
- Drugs for local or regional anesthesia that are not absorbed through the baby's digestive system.
- Drugs for general anesthesia usually get into your breast milk in very small amounts. They are unlikely to cause any effects on your baby and disappear from your body very quickly. You can breastfeed after consulting with your doctor.

- There is no need to stop breastfeeding because of x-rays and most scans (CT, MRI, etc.).
- Common drugs which are safe to use during breastfeeding include: acetaminophen (Tylenol, Tempra), prednisone, thyroxin, omeprazole, metronidazole, penicillin, nix, kwellade, etc.

Tip: Safe and Non-Safe Medication

If the baby can take the same medication as you, it is probably safe for you to take it.

Example of drugs that are not safe during breastfeeding are bromocriptine, cocaine, codeine, cyclophosphamide, cyclosporine, doxorubicin, ergotamine, lithium, methotrexate, etc.

Drugs with Possible Effects on the Baby or Breast Milk

The following drugs have an effect on your breast milk and/or baby:
- Most antibiotics are safe and usually do not cause any problems for the mother or baby. However, they may occasionally cause diarrhea and allergic reactions.
- Drugs (diuretics) causing excessive urination or increased urination may cause decreased breast milk production.
- Hormonal pills (birth control) can cause decreased breast milk production.
- Laxatives are known to have an effect on your baby's stool.
- Sedatives or drugs for sedation (sleeping pills) may affect your baby's behavior and his responses.
- Anti-cancer drugs may be harmful during breastfeeding, along with lithium and beta blockers.
- Migraine drugs (ergot) may suppress your ability to lactate efficiently.
- Some medications may be dangerous and cause respiratory arrest (e.g., drugs that contain codeine, such as Tylenol 3, etc.).

Tip: Herbal Remedy Caution

Some herbal remedies can be toxic to your baby.

Considerations Before Taking a Drug

- When considering the use of drugs during breastfeeding, one must consider the benefits of using and the risks of the mother not taking the drugs.

- It is also important to consider the benefits and risks this poses to both mother and baby, if the mother does not take the specific medication.

- Further aspects to consider are the following:

  ❖ Alternatives (that may have less side effects on the baby), or where more information is available.

  ❖ Low dosage use.

  ❖ Various effects on milk production.

  ❖ Duration of drug use.

  ❖ Is it necessary to temporarily stop breastfeeding?

  ❖ The illness itself should be discussed with your doctor (e.g., herpes, chicken pox, etc.).

Tip: Stopping Breastfeeding—What You Need To Do

Be sure that this is the only option for you.

Express your milk in advance, if possible.

How long do you need to take the medication?

Can you "pump & dump" your breast milk, to keep up your milk supply until breastfeeding can resume?

Know that you run the risk of breast engorgement if you do not pump.

With some medications, you may not be able to return to breastfeeding at all (long term treatment).

Increasing Baby Safety

The following are some suggestions of how to increase your baby's safety when you are taking drugs during breastfeeding:

- Find the most reliable and up to date information on the medication you are taking, especially if it is not commonly used.

- If possible, take the medication after the last breastfeeding session or before you go to sleep. Speak to your doctor about taking the medications in a way that will decrease the amount passed to your baby.

- Adjust the drug treatment to meet breastfeeding habits.

- Consider any allergic reactions or effect it may have on your baby (kidney function has to be normal for drugs that are excreted by the kidneys).

- Be aware of your baby's reactions and responses, and consult with your health professional.

Tip: Breastfeeding During Illness

Wash your hands before handling your baby or before a feeding session.

Drink many extra fluids (especially water).

Eat a healthy and well-balanced diet.

Talk to your doctor about extra precautionary measures.

Further Aspects to Consider

When Not to Breastfeed

- If your baby has a rare (1:85,000) condition known as Galactosemia, you should not breastfeed. Babies with this condition are unable to metabolize the sugar in breast milk and should be fed lactose free formula.

- A mother who has HIV or AIDS should not breastfeed.

- Do not breastfeed if you have active tuberculosis.

- Do not breastfeed if you are using illegal drugs (see *Recreational Drugs*).

- Mothers who are undergoing radiation therapy or when radioisotopes are used for diagnosis may not breastfeed for a period of time. The mother may express the milk until the period of radioactivity has passed.

- Do not breastfeed if you have leukemia (especially T-cell virus type I leukemia,) herpes, pertussis, hepatitis, etc. Discuss your disease and the associated risks of breastfeeding with your doctor.

Tip: Breastfeeding & Radioactive Scanning

When a mother receives radioactive material, it depends which material is used. For example, if it is with Technetium, then all of it disappears after 30 hours. The mother can then nurse her baby without any risks of radiation. Although she may be able to breastfeed earlier (since about 75% of it disappears after 12-15 hours). Discuss this with your doctor.

In respect to thyroid scans, it is definitely a concern, as the radioactive material will concentrate in the baby's thyroid and stay there for a long time.

The question is whether a scan is really needed and if another radioactive material can be used.

Use of iodinated and gadolinium in lactation (Jaw, Webb et al., *EUR Radiology* 15, Dec. 2004) suggest that breastfeeding may continue when iodinated agents are given to the mother. You need to discuss this with your doctor

Breastfeeding: Birth Control & Menstruation

- You are able to continue breastfeeding when you have your period (menstruating).

- Menstruation usually begins after you wean from breastfeeding; however, it sometimes occurs during the breastfeeding period.

- Menstruation is sometimes associated with hormonal changes in your body, leading to a temporary reduction in breast milk.

- Some women who take the pill may find that their milk supply decreases, especially with estrogen pills. It is preferred (upon discussion with your doctor) that you use progestin only pills without any estrogen (Yet it may still cause a decrease in your milk supply). If it is possible, avoid or at least wait to take birth control pills until your baby is taking other foods at four to six months of age.

Smoking & Breastfeeding

- When one is a heavy smoker (more than 1 pack per day) and breastfeeding, there is a decrease in milk production.

- Smoking also exposes your baby to nicotine and makes your baby irritable, difficult for him to sleep, and in some cases, the baby vomits or has diarrhea.

- The toxic substances in tobacco reach the maternal milk and are passed on to your baby.

- It is therefore recommended to decrease or stop smoking altogether, if you would like to continue breastfeeding.

- Breastfeed before having a cigarette, so that nicotine levels will be lower.

- Remember that second hand smoke is especially dangerous for your baby (increased risk of SIDS).

Tip: Street Drugs Dangers

Studies show that the active ingredients in street drugs like marijuana, cocaine, heroin, meth (crystal, crank, or speed), etc., are transmitted to your baby through breast milk if you use them. Heroin in breast milk, for instance, can fatally stop your baby's breathing. Alcohol is also passed in breast milk, so it's certainly not a good idea to drink heavily when you are breastfeeding (see *Maternal Diet & Breastfeeding*). Just how much or how little alcohol, street drug or nicotine use is safe for your baby is very unclear, so the best thing for your baby's health is to abstain from these products while breastfeeding.

Recreational Drugs

- Studies show that many of the active chemicals in recreational drugs do make their way into breast milk. Some of them, in extreme cases, kill your baby (e.g., heroin, codeine).

- At any rate, no matter what your personal choices are, do you really want to be giving your baby the active ingredients in cocaine, marijuana, speed, crystal, mushrooms, heroin, etc.?

- In no cases are recreational drugs advisable for the breastfeeding mother, since their effects on infants may be harmful, lasting, and, at the very least, highly unpredictable. Studies show that SIDS (Sudden Infant Death Syndrome) is more likely to occur among infants with parents who indulge in recreational drugs.

- The whole issue of breastfeeding, or even the mother's ability to care for the baby, needs to be re-evaluated in such cases, as the mother and baby need to be followed carefully if drug abuse is present, etc.

Maternal Diet & Breastfeeding

General

There are many reasons to believe that what you eat will have either positive or negative effects on your baby's future eating and taste habits. Typically, a breastfeeding mother does not have to worry about her diet; if she eats normally and maintains a well balanced diet throughout the day, both mother and baby will get the nutrition they need.

Even with an inadequate diet, many women continue to produce an adequate supply of milk.

Certain foods affect the taste, odor, and quality of the milk you produce. With round-the-clock infant care, it is not always easy to pay attention to your own needs.

There are no foods that you need to avoid when you are breastfeeding. However, if you find that a particular food causes fussiness or pain in your baby each time you eat it, discuss it with your doctor (especially when there is family history of severe food allergy). The need to avoid particular foods may be necessary to see what happens. Retry the food in a few weeks to see if it causes the same reaction. If you stop for longer periods of time, look for nutrient replacements. If there is a particular food you do not like, there are other substitutes (e.g., cheese and yogurt are good substitutes for milk; eggs are a good alternative for meat and fish, as are a combination of whole grains, nuts, dried peas, beans, lentils and brown rice, etc.).

Tip: Food Use Priority

Fresh foods are usually better than frozen, and frozen foods are preferable to canned.

Breastfeeding Mothers that Require Special Attention

To ensure a healthy, well-balanced diet, the following women must be carefully monitored:

- Women with limited foods or who are vegetarians.

- Thin women (sometimes decrease caloric intake or have unhealthy eating habits).
- Young mothers who tend to eat irregularly.
- Obese mothers (sometimes decrease caloric intake too quickly).
- Women drinking alcohol in excess.
- Heavy smokers.
- Those with chronic illness on medications (may have decreased appetite).
- Women with breast surgery (severed ducts may not rejoin, therefore decreasing milk supply).

There are no rules, but mothers need to eat and drink to satisfy their hunger and thirst. Follow the Food Groups. There is also a special food guide for vegetarians.

Tip: Pregnancy and Diet

Do not attempt to restrict your weight during pregnancy or follow restrictive diets in the pre-conceptual period.

Maternal Diet & Effects on Baby

Maternal Diet & Baby Growth

Milk volume can be decreased by an insufficient diet or lack of enough fluids. A healthy, well-balanced diet is advisable for the health of the mother. In cases of malnutrition, breast milk will be made from maternal stores; however, it will be at the mother's expense. Some of the effects of a maternal diet on breast milk or your baby may include the following:

- Some babies may be sensitive to certain foods taken in the mother's diet and as a result, the baby may experience the following:
  - ❖ Abdominal pain and gassiness.
  - ❖ Colic—the most frequent offender is cow's milk in a mothers' diet.
  - ❖ Skin rash (especially to cow's milk, citrus, egg, nuts and wheat; rashes sometimes appear after the mother has eaten red peppers), hives, or eczema.
  - ❖ Alternating vomiting and diarrhea (often with bloody stool, etc.). If you notice any of these symptoms, speak to your doctor.

- Breast milk color may change to a pink-orange color, when the mother drinks orange soda; green breast milk results when kelp, seaweed, or other natural vitamins are taken. The color change does not affect the baby.

- Studies have shown that babies often drink more breast milk when the mother has eaten garlic. They seem to like the flavor!

- All foods eaten affect the flavor of breast milk. This is how babies are exposed to cultural foods that they will be eating later.

Tip: Calcium Sources and Allergies

Yogurt, hard cheese (cheddar, Swiss, and parmesan), and cottage cheese are good sources of calcium. Many people with milk allergies can tolerate at least a small amount of these. Other sources of calcium include calcium-enriched tofu, soy bean products, bok choy, collard & kale, sesame seeds, and fish (canned sardines and canned sockeye salmon).

Maternal Non-alcoholic Drinks & Effects on Baby

- You should drink normally to satisfy your thirst and ensure a good milk supply, which means at least 8 daily glasses of water, milk, or other fluids (soups, vegetable juice, etc.).

- Drinking excessively (anything but water) may cause decreased milk production.

- Avoid or cut back on alcohol, caffeine, herbs, and other chemicals.

Alcohol

- Limit your alcohol consumption while you are breastfeeding.

- Heavy drinking may cause your baby to be sleepy, sluggish, unresponsive, and nurse poorly. Drinking may also cause breathing problems in your baby.

- Drinking affects you in that it impairs your functioning and causes you to be unable to protect, care for, or feed your baby. It also makes you susceptible to depression and/or fatigue.

- If you decide to take the occasional drink, then it is not a problem if it is in moderation. Try to take it right after you nurse (or even during nursing) rather than before. This allows a couple of hours to metabolize the alcohol before the next feeding (the body rids itself of the alcohol).

Tip: Beer and Milk Production

There are no conclusive studies that show the correlation between drinking beer and stimulating milk production. Drinking beer should not be counted on for successful breastfeeding.

Caffeine
- Moderation seems to be acceptable; one or two cups a day.
- Increased amounts of caffeinated beverages are popularly thought to cause you and your baby to be jittery and irritable. However, most studies do not support this reasoning, as the amount of caffeine found in a healthy infant is usually very small to, in other cases, undetectable.
- Caffeine is found in some over-the-counter medication as well as colas, tea, and coffee.
- If your baby seems sensitive to caffeine, try eliminating it for a week to see if there is a difference in your baby's behavior.
- Babies born prematurely are slower to eliminate caffeine, suggesting that their mothers' caffeine intake may affect the premature baby more than the full term baby.

Herbs
- The effects of some herbs on your baby are unclear, so it is better to discuss the issue with your doctor before drinking infused herbs whose active ingredients may end up in your breast milk. Your baby's system is much more delicate than yours.
- You may drink teas such as peppermint, raspberry, rose lip, red bush (rooibus), and orange spice.
- Blessed thistle and fenugreek have been used to increase milk supply (there is no scientifically documented proof).

Tip: Chemicals

Chemicals added to food are not good for you or your baby.

Avoid them if possible.

Foods in their natural state are healthier.

Parent Concerns & Tips

Do flavored or spicy foods affect the breastfed baby?

- In general, breastfeeding mothers can eat any spicy and strong flavored foods. The flavor appears in breast milk about 5 hours after ingestion.

- Garlic and spices (or any food, for that matter) do not need to be avoided, unless your baby reacts negatively to them (e.g., fussy, irritable, rash, hives, etc.).

- There is no evidence that spicy or flavored foods cause babies to be more gassy or colicky, since many cultures consume spicy and flavored foods.

- Breastfed infants enjoy tastes and flavors already in the womb.

- Breastfeeding may expose them to many flavors they will encounter later in life and may ease the flavor's acceptance.

How does dieting affect breastfeeding?

- Dieting is not suggested when breastfeeding, at least in the first few months of life.

- It is better to eat well (a healthy, balanced diet) and exercise regularly while you breastfeed.

- Vegetarian or vegan mothers may need additional supplements when breastfeeding (almost like dieting).

- The breastfeeding process makes use of the fat cells stored in the body during pregnancy. Remember that you burn extra calories to ensure adequate milk production.

- Severe diet, weight loss, drugs, and liquid diets can negatively affect your milk supply.

- After your child starts solid foods (after six months of age), you may start to restrict your caloric intake if you find that you need to lose more weight. Remember that lactation seems to metabolize fat accumulated even before pregnancy, but it is important to go slowly.

- Any kind of drastic weight loss carries the risk of low milk supply.

- Overall, moderate exercise during the breastfeeding process is safe and beneficial for most women. It is wise to wear a good support bra and breastfeed before doing any exercise that causes the breast to bounce.

- Very athletic women who exercise to exhaustion will have an increase of lactic acid in their breast milk. The baby may refuse the breast because the milk tastes different. These mothers sometimes pump their milk before exercising, so that they can feed their baby "normal" tasting milk at the next feeding.
- Be careful when performing exercise that involves the chest.
- After exercising clean your breast to clean any salty taste, but do not soap the nipple.
- Consult your doctor about your exercise and diet while breastfeeding.

Should a breastfeeding mother eat and drink more to produce enough milk?

- Some mothers gain weight when they are breastfeeding. This is due to poor food choices, like eating a lot of high calorie junk food or desserts.
- To maintain body weight, 200-500 extra calories more than a mother's non-breastfeeding requirement are usually sufficient.
- Overall, breastfeeding mothers need to eat a healthy, well balanced diet as dictated by their appetite.

Tip: Diet and Food Replacement

If you are on a special diet, you need to figure out how to obtain replacements for you and your baby. If you are a vegetarian, discuss the possibility of vitamin and mineral supplementation with your doctor.

Tip: Foods & Increased Milk Production—Is There a Connection?

Many mothers believe that if they eat certain foods, milk production will increase. There is no documented proof that this is so. Each culture has its own list of recommended foods that are comforting for mother and are believed to be beneficial. As long as mother and baby are happy, that is all that matters.

Breastfeeding & Returning to Work

General

The Canadian Pediatric Society and the American Academy of Pediatrics recommends that, if you can, the best thing for your baby is to feed him only breast milk for his first six months and continue providing breast milk (along with other foods) up until he is two years old. Many women who decide to breastfeed are concerned about how to continue doing so when they return to work.

Going back to work does not mean that you have to stop breastfeeding. You simply have to plan the feeding strategy for the times you will be away from your baby. If you intend to continue breastfeeding, find solutions ahead of time. Discuss your plans with your employer. Similarly, if you intend on returning to school, you need to discuss it ahead of time with your teachers and a guidance counselor.

Coming home after a busy day at work can be very relaxing, when you and your baby share the comforting bond between you as you breastfeed.

Some mothers continue with breastfeeding when they are at home but have formula given to the baby when they are at work. Although breast milk is preferable to formula, some breast milk is always better than none. Mothers who choose this option need to wean the baby for the hours they will be separated from their baby.

Suggestions for Breastfeeding & Working

If you cannot explore the possibility of working from home, try the following suggestions:

- *Return to work part time and gradually increase your hours*. For example, start off by going to work a couple days out of the week and slowly lead up to working an entire week. This allows time for you and your baby to get accustomed to new feeding techniques and schedules.
- *Change your schedule* (if you can) to accommodate nursing (e.g., going home to feed and then returning to work).
- *Plan your schedule* to be able to maximize the amount of time spent

breastfeeding your baby. Some mothers have their baby sitter bring their baby to the work site, if it is not too far away.

- You need to *schedule time to pump* for about 10 minutes at break times and 15 minutes at lunch hour, approximately every 3-4 hours.

- *Plan ahead for storage of expressed breast milk.* Try to pump milk one to two weeks before returning to work and freeze it for future use (e.g., for the first days of returning to work).

What To Do At the Workplace

- You need a private place and regular breaks to pump milk.

- Do not express your milk in an area that lacks privacy or sanitation (e.g., ladies washroom). It is undesirable!

- To maintain your milk supply, it is important to be consistent in expressing breast milk. For example, you can pump everyday to provide milk for the following day while you are at work. Always be at least one day ahead.

- You will require a refrigerator for storing the milk during working hours. Milk can only be kept at room temperature (66-72 F/19-22 C) for four hours.

- If you use a portable cooler with ice packs you can keep the breast milk chilled. (24 hours at 59 F/15 C). Place the milk in the refrigerator or freezer as soon as you return home.

- Use a breast pump that will allow you to express milk from both breasts at the same time, so that you will collect more milk in a shorter amount of time. Many mothers who go back to work very early buy a double pumping electric personal use breast pump (e.g., "Pump in Style" by Medela or "Purely Yours" by Hollister).

- Wear patterned tops in case of leakage and change your breast pads frequently. It would be a good idea to carry an extra top and breast pads with you "just in case."

- Pump a little more than your baby usually drinks during the period that you are separated, in case his appetite increases.

- If you forget to bring an electrical pump with you to work, you can still hand express the milk. You may want to put your cleaned pump in the car to avoid forgetting it.

> **Tip: Care of Breast Milk**
>
> Expressed breast milk may be refrigerated for up to 7 days and frozen for up to 3 to 4 months in the freezer compartment. Once the milk is thawed, it cannot be refrozen. Holding the container under warm running water to thaw breast milk. Gently swirl the milk to mix the layers which separate. Do not shake breast milk or you will destroy some of the milk properties.

Feeding at Home & the Caretaker

- Select a caregiver or a childcare program that can handle and feed your stored breast milk to your baby.

- Do not give your baby a bottle until your milk supply has been established (takes about 4 weeks).

- Start the process of drinking breast milk from a bottle. Your baby may show resistance to the bottle initially, but simply try again at the next feeding (see *Tips & Tricks to Overcome Bottle Rejection*).

- Provide exclusive and additional breastfeeding on the weekends and nurse when the baby shows interest.

- Some babies are happy to increase nighttime feedings to make up for missed feedings during the day.

- Do not use the bottle when you are home all day (weekends, holidays). Have someone else offer the bottle to your baby so that he associates bottle feedings with other people and breastfeeding with you.

- When your baby is close to six months, feed him before going to work, offer expressed milk during lunchtime, and breastfeed when you return from work. In a childcare program, you can give formula or stored, breast milk.

- After six months of age, less pumping may be needed, as the baby will start eating solid foods.

- If your work is close to home, you may want to go home and breastfeed during your breaks.

- Ensure that your babysitter knows how to handle the milk you leave for your baby.

- Explain what to do if no expressed milk is available for your babysitter to feed your baby (e.g., solids, formula).

Parent Concerns

I am supposed to return to work in 5 weeks. Should I start giving the bottle?

- You may start offering the bottle once your milk supply has been well established and your baby is breastfeeding well, to avoid creating a preference for the bottle's nipple.

- Once you know you are returning to work and breastfeeding has been established, start to offer bottled breast milk a few days prior to returning to work.

- In some cases, babies refuse to take the bottle and that is why it is better to offer it several days before going back to work.

- Because a baby's immune system is not totally developed before 6 months, it is better to give only breast milk until that time.

- Remember that if you give formula early, it will interfere with your milk production.

- In case you return to work after your baby is six months old, solid foods may be given to your baby until you return home from work to breastfeed. Your breast milk can be given by a cup or "sippy cup." Continue pumping and expressing milk at work so that your milk production continues. You may have to mix the expressed milk with cereal (given with a spoon) or mix it with other solid foods.

What do I do if my breasts are leaking at work?

- Leaking breasts may occur, especially if you return to work when your baby is still very young.

- Wear good, absorbent breast pads and have spares on hand so that you can change them if you need to.

- Wear patterned tops that make breast milk leakage less noticeable.

- Pump and express your milk frequently to prevent breasts from becoming too full.

- If you feel like you are about to leak milk, fold your arms across your chest, pressing against your breasts for a few minutes. Go and pump as soon as you can. (See *Breast Milk Leakage*).

My milk supply is decreasing since I started pumping at work.

- Once your baby takes expressed milk or formula through a bottle, your milk supply may decrease, as breastfeeding has decreased.

- Stimulation for milk production is a good way of maintaining your milk supply.

- Try pumping more frequently to build up your milk production (even if you see no milk flow, pump for a while longer).

Expressing Breast Milk

General

Expressing breast milk is an effective method of continuing to provide breast milk without actually feeding from the breast. Milk can be expressed by hand, or using a breast pump

There are many different breast pumps on the market; not all are good or effective.

The size of the breast shield is important (the part that fits over the areola/nipple). If the opening on the shield is too tight, it may be both uncomfortable and ineffective at pumping milk.

Expressing breast milk does not stimulate the breast and extract milk as effectively as a baby who is breastfeeding well, but the newer pumps on the market are improving. With all manual and electric pumps, follow the directions carefully. If in doubt, contact a breastfeeding specialist for guidance.

It takes practice to hand express milk. It is a good idea to learn this while in the hospital or from a person who is experienced in doing so (lactation consultant, midwife, nurse, doctor, or family member).

Babies can take expressed breast milk in a cup, by spoon, syringe, bottle, etc.

When & Why

The following are reasons to express milk, whether it is for a brief period of time or a longer duration:

- In the first few days it is good to learn how to hand express colostrum, which can be used to entice a sleepy baby or a reluctant nurser. It is also good to put on your nipples after a feeding, as it is very healing.

- Expression of colostrum by hand is usually more effective than a pump in the first few days. With practice, you can often get a higher volume. Expressing a little milk before latching helps in situations where the areola may be non-pliable (e.g., engorgement).

- Hospital grade pumps are recommended if the baby is unable to breastfeed within 24 hours. This may happen if the baby is in the Special Care Nursery and unable to be put to the breast for a while. Double pumping raises prolactin levels more, and is recommended because it obtains more colostrum/milk for the baby. It is also less tiring for a new mother (she is done in 15 minutes).

- Expressing milk is recommended whenever the baby cannot breastfeed (for whatever reason) to avoid engorgement and blocked ducts, and to keep up the milk supply and provide the best milk for your baby (e.g., back to work, to build up a low milk supply, etc.).

- Illness of the mother or baby, where breastfeeding must temporarily be stopped (very rare).

- You are taking medications that are unsafe for your baby (most are safe). You must check with your doctor or contact your local health department (e.g., "Motherisk" at Sick Children's Hospital in Toronto, Ontario at 416-813-6780).

- If you are pumping to have some milk for storage, the best time is in the morning, when the breast is at its fullest. Nurse your baby first, and then collect the remaining milk for later use.

- Some mothers like to have some milk on hand for dad to feed the baby in the evening (once breastfeeding is established). Many mothers find their supply lower in the evening and welcome the break.

- If you go out in the evening and your baby has been fed while you are away, you may need to pump your breast when you come home to avoid blocked ducts. This milk can be used for a supplement later, as long as it is stored properly.

- If your baby is found to be allergic to formula, you may decide to express milk so that you can relactate. This would require a hospital grade pump (rental).

Tip: More On Breast Milk Expression

Express breast milk manually or with a pump as often as required, depending on your circumstances. If you do express milk, do it after a feeding at the breast and not before, since you want your baby to take as much of your milk as possible. You may use breast compression once the baby stops nursing on his own.

Expressing Milk Manually

The manual method of expressing milk is easy to learn. Follow these steps:

Wash your hands with soap and water.

- To assist the milk ejection reflex, use the flat of your fingers and massage your breast similar to the motion used in breast examination (e.g., circular, clockwise, towards your nipple.) Stroke your breast from the chest wall to the nipple from all directions.

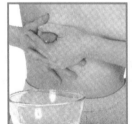

- Place a clean container under your breast so that you are prepared when breast milk is expressed (clean glass or plastic container).

- Do not cup your breast. Form the letter "C" with your hand. (Place your thumb and forefinger on either side of the nipple about 1-1 ½ inches/3-4 cm away from the nipple).

- Push into your chest wall, keeping your fingers together. Gently roll your thumb and first 2 fingers in a rhythmic manner towards the nipple. Work your way around the breast to empty all the ducts. Switch hands as required to reach all areas.

- When the flow of milk slows down, switch to the other breast.

- Remember that hand expression is free and you cannot forget to bring it to work.

Tip: Hand Expressed Milk

❖ While hand expressing milk, you may find milk squirting off to the side from other ducts. Sometimes expressing into a larger container (like a sterile bowl) will make it easier to catch deviant sprays. Then you can transfer the milk into a bottle.

Pumping

- If you are pumping for a premature baby or ill baby, follow the guidelines from the Special Care Nursery for pumping and storage of breast milk. They are different than for full term or healthy babies.

- With practice, the use of pumps will become more comfortable for you to use.

- Pump breast milk in a quiet, relaxed setting and ensure that your hand and the container you use to collect milk are clean.

- Follow the instructions of the manufacturer for cleaning the pump and for pump use.

- A working mother will be looking for a breast pump that offers ease, convenience, and one that is easy to wash. You will need to carry the pump back and forth, and you need to be able to use it quickly and efficiently.

- If you are at home and your baby is with you, the baby suckling will cause the milk to flow. For this reason, some will nurse on one side and pump on the other breast. Others will nurse the baby first and then use the pump.

- If your baby is not with you, you may need to take a few extra steps for the milk to flow easily, such as the following:

  ❖ Apply warm and wet wash cloths to your breasts.

  ❖ Gently massage your breasts (top of the breast to the nipple).

  ❖ Stroke the nipple with the palm of your hand or roll the nipple between your finger and thumb.

  ❖ Sometimes, seeing a picture of your baby or smelling his clothes can start milk flow.

- Each pump is a little different. You want a pump that fits your breast, creating a good but comfortable seal. All nipples are not the same. The standard size breast shield is 24 mm. Many mothers require a larger opening. Some companies (like Medela) have customized shields to fit mothers who have a wide based nipple. They come in 27 mm, 30 mm, and 36 mm. If your nipple is big, check out the pump to see if you can get a larger shield to fit it. A lactation consultant or breastfeeding specialist can advise you regarding a proper fit.

- If pumping your breasts is painful, stop and readjust the pump.

- Common problems that may occur with pumping include sore nipples, obtaining only small amounts of milk per pumping session, erratic or delayed milk ejection reflex, and decreasing milk supply over a long course of pumping. Should any problems arise, discuss them with your lactation specialist or doctor.

Manual Pumps:
- These are hand-operated devices, which need to be worked manually in order to create suction. Some can be used with one hand, while others require both hands.
- Some mothers find these pumps to be hard work. Many mothers prefer them over hand expressing (not as messy).
- Some popular one-handed pumps are: " Harmony," by Medela, "Avent", and "One-Handed breast pump" by Hollister.
- Follow directions on the pump of your choice.
- These are good if you plan to pump only occasionally, or for a short period of time.
- Manual pumps are usually slower than using electric pumps.

Tip: Suction and Pumping Breast Milk

Do not use pumps with a rubber bulb. The suction is too strong and can damage your nipples. A good pump will mimic the baby's sucking (compress and release automatically). Sustained pressure is not good.

Mini-Electric/Battery Pumps
- Mini electric pumps are available, some for single pumping and others for double pumping. Double pumping saves time and increases milk volume! These pumps are good for mothers going back to work who need to pump once or twice a day.
- The warranty on most these pumps is three months.
- Follow the directions on the pump of your choice, since each one is operated differently.
- In regards to battery pumps, the suction is not considered as powerful as electric operated pumps.
- If the pump is painful don't use it. You may require a larger shield.

Retail Electric Pumps
- Retail electric breast pumps are available for mothers who will be pumping a lot. They pump both breasts at a time. The warranty is generally for one year on the motor. They are more expensive, but are better pumps (e.g., "Pump in Style" by Medela," "Purely Yours" by Hollister).

Rental Pumps

- Hospital grade pumps are the best, and are recommended for situations where baby cannot breastfeed (e.g., premature birth), a mother is trying to build up her milk supply, or with a mother who has severely inverted nipples and may need to pump for a longer time before her baby is able to breastfeed.

- Some mothers choose to pump and bottle feed their milk to their baby. A hospital grade (rental pump) will allow her to do this longer.

- You can rent these pumps (e.g., "The Symphony Pump" by Medela, or "Ameda/Egnell" by Hollister).

Tip: More To Know About Pumping

The baby who is nursing well can get much more milk than his mother can pump.

The amount of milk pumped does not accurately tell you how much milk you are able to produce.

Storing Expressed Milk

- Expressed breast milk may be stored for later use.

- Store expressed milk in a small, clean glass or hard plastic containers and make sure that the lids are fitted well. Special freezer bags are also available. Do not use bottle liner bags as they are not strong enough and may break.

- Place the containers in the refrigerator immediately after pumping breast milk.

- Expressed breast milk is safe for 4 hours at room temperature (-2 to -4 F/19 to 22 C); 5-7 days in the refrigerator (32 to 39 F/0 to 4 C); 3-4 months in self-contained freezer compartment; 6-12 months in a deep freezer (-2 F/-19 C).

- Allow the milk to chill for half an hour in the refrigerator before freezing.

- Freeze breast milk in small quantities (2-4 oz/60-120 ml per container or bottle) to minimize waste and allow for easy thawing.

Room Temperature	Refrigerator	Fridge Freezer	Deep Freezer
4 hours	5-7 days	3-4 months	6-12 months

Tip: *Storage and Wasting Breast Milk*

Store in 2-4 oz/60-120 ml portions to prevent wasting any breast milk.

Warming & Administering Expressed Milk

Follow these suggestions in warming and giving expressed milk to your baby:

- To warm expressed milk quickly, place the closed container under warm running water until the milk is body temperature. Drop a few drops on your wrist to check the temperature.

- To thaw frozen expressed breast milk, you can leave it in the refrigerator overnight or you can also put the sealed container in a bowl of warm water for about twenty minutes; you may need to change the water a few times.

- Do **not** shake breast milk! Breast milk is a live food. Shaking it will destroy some of its properties. Gently tilt the bottle back and forth to mix the layers (cream rises to the top).

- Do not thaw breast milk in a microwave or on a stovetop.

- Do not refreeze expressed breast milk once it is thawed.

- Because of possible infection risks, do not offer any breast milk that remains in the bottle or cup from which your baby was feeding at an earlier feeding.

Tip: *Keeping the Nutritional Value of Expressed Breast Milk*

Never thaw expressed milk at room temperature.

Storing Method: up to five days in a refrigerator; up to three to four months in a freezer and, after it has been defrosted, up to 24 hours in the refrigerator.

Freezing Method: make sure to freeze expressed breast milk immediately after expression and in small amounts of 2-3 oz/60-90 ml.

Defrosting Method: this is done with lukewarm water (96.8 F/36 C) and not a microwave or hot water, so that the milk reaches room temperature within 20 minutes.

Nighttime Feedings

General

Many mothers complain that their babies feed more during the night than during the day. This is normal, since babies do not know that nighttime is a time to sleep. It takes babies time to adjust to day and night patterns. Night waking is temporary as children do grow out of this stage.

Being able to sleep through the night is a developmental stage such as toilet training, walking, talking, etc. Babies reach this stage at different times in the first year of life.

Babies usually wake up to feed at night in the first few months of life, unless their stomachs receive and hold enough milk to allow them to sleep through the night.

According to some sleep experts, babies should develop good sleep habits at around 6 months of age. However, they suggest that your baby does need to feed at night after four to six months of age, as this may predispose babies to sleep problems or unhealthy sleeping habits.

Babies are human beings and, each being different from the next, it is impossible to say when your baby will sleep through the night. Some babies sleep through the night at an early age, while some will not. Getting up at night is never a favorite part of parenting, but you can find easy ways of coping, while satisfying your baby's needs. Each family has to see what works out best for them. Waking up to feed is a normal part of parenting in infancy (and even later).

Environment & Sharing Sleep

- Nighttime feedings should include minimum stimulation, fuss and/or communication.

- Change your baby's diapers before feeding him in order to avoid moving him around too much, since this makes him more alert after a feeding.

- Minimize the amount of distractions at night by closing the door, turning off the light, etc.

- Unless your baby is bothered, avoid waking your baby at night to change his diapers or for any other reason—unless suggested by your doctor (to increase weight gain and the need to feed more frequently at night).

g arrangements vary from family to family. Some mothers will nurse the baby in bed whether lying down with him or not, but as soon as the baby stops nursing, the mother will take him to his crib (close or nearby to another room). This plan does not work all the time, since mothers who are feeding the baby in bed lying down can fall asleep while the baby is nursing (in this case, the parents' sleep is less interrupted).

- The following question is raised many times: should I sleep with my baby in the same bed? This is often questioned due to the risk of rolling over your baby and the risk of death. To compare the risk of SIDS (Sudden Infant Death Syndrome), one needs to compare babies who died when they were in bed with the parents, in a crib close to the bed, or in a separate room. Because the cause of SIDS is unknown and due to various other factors, it is hard to definitively assess the risk. You may discuss the recommendations about bed sharing when feeding at night with your doctor.

Tip: SIDS and Sleep

Some studies show that SIDS is more likely to occur among infants who co-sleep with their parents when the parents indulge in recreational drugs or alcohol.

Feeding & Sleeping At Night

- In the early months, it is normal and especially desirable for the baby to nurse during the night as you respond to his needs; it also increases your milk supply, decreases early morning engorgement, and helps your baby with weight gain difficulties.

- Listen to your baby's hunger cues and do not assume that he is not hungry.

- Many mothers find it easy to manage feeding at night if they keep their baby in bed with them or if the baby sleeps in a bassinet or crib right beside the bed.

- The following are suggestions to help your baby develop nighttime sleep patterns (not in the first 3 months):

  ❖ Make the most of your baby's daytime (waking time) hours to help associate daylight hours with play, feedings, and wakefulness.

❖ Try to feed more during the day (depends on your baby) and sleep longer periods during the night.

❖ Feed your child frequently in the evening, closer to the time of sleeping or right before he goes to bed.

❖ Be aware of overtired signs (e.g., quiet, losing interest, fussing, etc.) from your baby.

❖ Allow your baby to fall asleep on your breast, since this is known to be one of the easiest ways for most babies to relax.

❖ When your baby sleeps during the day, use a carriage, cradle, or bassinet. However, when he sleeps at night, place him in a crib to help make the differentiation between daytime and nighttime.

❖ Change sleeping arrangements to find out what works best for your baby. For example, some babies sleep better when they are close to the mother.

❖ Sometimes, sleepy sounds such as lullabies and calming CDs help your baby sleep through the night (especially when played all night). Rocking chairs or swinging motions help the baby fall asleep as well, as this provides your baby with a feeling of comfort and security.

Comment: Ear infections and teething may cause sleeping discomfort at night in your baby. Give pain relievers before bedtime. Also, babies who are ill may have a difficult time sleeping at night, so try different methods of soothing your baby (e.g., massaging, singing, rocking, etc.) and consult your doctor.

Tip: Food on Demand or Schedule

In the end of the first month, you may feed frequently during the day and extend feeding space-time to 3-4 hours at night, but follow your baby's cues and hunger to feed more frequently as needed. There is no schedule and you should feed on demand.

Parent Concerns

I was told that formula-fed babies sleep longer at night—is this true?

• Formula is digested differently than breast milk, and many parents report that the need to feed frequently at night is less in formula-fed babies than in breastfed babies.

- While this may be only partially right, you may try to ensure the following to help your baby sleep for longer periods of time at night:
  - ❖ Baby is latching on well.
  - ❖ Increase the amount taken during the feeding helps him sleep longer.
  - ❖ Use compression to increase the amount of milk the baby receives at the breast.
  - ❖ Finishing the first side before you offer the second breast (allows your baby to receive plenty of high fat milk to allow him to go for a few hours between feedings).
  - ❖ Gradually stretch the hours between feedings so that he eventually sleeps through the night.

Should I feed my baby at night or allow him to sleep through the night when I have to increase his weight gain?

- I usually tell parents to wake up their baby to feed at night if the baby is sleeping for many hours and there seems to be weight gain problems.
- Some babies lose weight because they are left to sleep longer, given pacifiers, suck their thumbs, or feed for only a short period of time during the night.
- "Training" your baby to sleep may lead to inappropriate weight gain, so watch out for:
  - ❖ Your baby's cries.
  - ❖ Hunger cues.
  - ❖ Less frequent feedings at night.
- Let your child stop breastfeeding at night at his own pace.
- There are many tips to encourage your baby to sleep longer while gaining weight well, but many babies continue to feed at night, which is normal human behavior.

  Comment: For a safer sleep see also article in *Paediatrics & Child Health,* May-June 2006, page 313-314 for recommendations to parents.

Dental caries (tooth decay) & nighttime feeding—do I need to wean?

- You need to improve your child's dental hygiene while still continuing to satisfy your child's individual needs through breastfeeding.
- Lactation specialists disagree that milk pooling in the mouth as the baby nurses is a significant cause of dental caries. Rather, they believe that it is due to other factors such as genetics, prenatal diet, and the child's diet.
- Many toddlers who breastfeed at night do not develop caries.

How to Awaken a Sleepy Baby

General

Newborns need to be breastfed about 8-12 times per day (i.e., every 2-3 hours). Your baby should not sleep longer or more frequently than this during the day, otherwise you will need to waken your baby and encourage him to feed. Frequent feedings encourage a good milk supply and help the baby grow and gain weight. Feeding intervals and the length of each feeding session varies depending on the baby's individual needs.

If the newborn falls asleep at the breast very quickly, he may need to be stimulated to breastfeed long enough to ensure adequate milk intake.

Once your milk supply has been well established and your baby is gaining weight well and steadily, you may allow him to set the pace of feedings (on-demand feeding schedule) so that occasional long periods of sleep are fine (whether in the first month of life or later). This usually occurs after three to four weeks. However, if your baby continues to sleep for long periods of time after one month of age and your milk supply is not well established, consult your doctor.

Tip: Sleep

Each baby is unique and there is no exact amount of hours that is appropriate for your baby to sleep between each feed or generally during the day. As long as your baby is healthy and gaining weight, the occasional long nap is fine. If your baby is less than one month of age and sleeps for long periods of time, discuss it with your doctor, since he may be at risk of dehydration and failure to gain weight.

Causes of Sleepy Babies

Some causes that may lead to a sleepy baby include:

- Types of anesthesia or drugs given to mothers during delivery may make your baby sleepy.
- A warm environment or over stimulation (noisy environment or bright lights) may cause some babies to "tune out" by sleeping.

- An inadequate milk intake may cause your baby to become weak and sleepy, rather than demanding to be fed. Weaker babies tire quickly from the work of feeding.

- In the third or fourth day of life, when he starts to lose most of the extra water he was born with.

- Some babies who are circumcised may be more sleepy and uninterested in nursing sessions after the procedure is done.

- Low birth weight and premature babies may fall asleep quickly when beginning to feed, or sleep for longer periods of times. These babies require special attention and their needs should be discussed with your doctor.

- Babies with jaundice may sleep more than other newborns.

Tip: Signs of Illness

If your baby is suddenly becoming lethargic, sleepier, refuses to feed, has different behavior patterns than usual and has or no other associated symptoms (e.g., vomiting, fever, etc.), consult your doctor immediately.

How to Awaken Your Baby

The following table outlines various ways of how to gently awaken or keep awake the sleepy baby in the first few weeks of age. If nothing works, you may have to wait another ½ hour or so and try again.

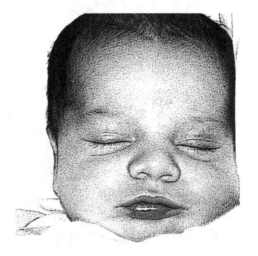

Stimulation

❖ Loosen or remove clothing (do not dress very warm).

❖ Social stimulation (talk, sing, eye contact, etc).

❖ Get skin-to-skin contact with your baby.

❖ Hold him in a sitting or upright position (sitting on your lap, bending him forward at the hips, etc).

❖ Bring him from a horizontal to a vertical position with one hand supporting his head and the other supporting his bottom.

❖ Wipe his face with a cool damp cloth.

❖ Massage parts of his body (work your finger up and down his spine).

❖ Move his legs up and down (bicycling motion).

❖ Stroke the palm of your baby's hands and soles of his feet (rub his feet or blow on them).

❖ Tickle his cheeks and touch the outer part of his ear.

Feeding Related

❖ Stroke his cheek with your nipple.

❖ Switch breasts when milk flow slows down or when he begins to fall asleep.

❖ Burp your baby between sides.

❖ Change feeding positions.

❖ Jiggle the breast in his mouth to dribble milk onto his lips (use breast compression to increase milk flow and keep your baby interested).

Environment

❖ Adjust room lighting (up for stimulation or down for comfort).

❖ Room must not be excessively warm (he will sleep longer).

❖ Undress him or remove his diaper.

Comments

• When your baby has a good latch of the breast, the flow of milk will keep him awake and interested.

• Avoid stimulation that may upset your baby (try anything that works for him).

• Wake your baby when he is in a light sleep (more likely to wake up and feed well).

• If your baby is older than one month and not a premature baby, breast milk and feeding is well established, and the baby is gaining weight well, you may allow your baby to sleep at the breast and occasionally, for longer periods of time than the usual.

• If the baby is tired and hungry and falls asleep at the breast, allow him to sleep, as he will wake up earlier to feed. He may become annoyed if you wake him up earlier and may even bite, refuse the breast, or begin crying.

Issues & Perceptions with Breast and Bottle-Feeding

General

You have the right to choose whether you want to breast or bottle-feed your baby, as it is a personal choice. Do not feel inadequate (especially if you are physically unable to do so), selfish, or inconsiderate (when it does not fit with your lifestyle) if you are not breastfeeding. Women who are not breastfeeding should not be made to feel worse, as they may already feel terrible about it.

There should not be inequality between the father and mother if the mother is breastfeeding, since the father can bond and contribute to his baby's needs in other ways.

Once you have made an informed decision on the type of feeding method you have chosen for your baby, it should be dealt with appropriately and respectfully.

Tip: Switching Breast and Bottle Feeding

It is not difficult to go from breastfeeding to bottle-feeding. It is much more difficult to switch from bottle-feeding to breastfeeding.

Maternal Concerns About Breastfeeding

The following are some maternal concerns regarding breastfeeding when making the decision to breast or bottle-feed. These concerns are short, transient problems that resolve quickly with appropriate care and counseling by a lactation specialist or doctor, when you compare them to the benefits of breast milk.

- Dietary and exercise concerns with weight loss:
  - ❖ Although crash diets and quick weight loss are a bad idea for nursing mothers, moderate exercise during breastfeeding is safe and beneficial for most women. Breastfeeding helps most women lose weight after delivery (at least 500 calories are used with each day of nursing).

- Some concerns about convenience include:
  - ❖ Accommodating the hungry baby.
  - ❖ Having to pump milk when needed.
  - ❖ Returning to work (pumping milk when separated from the baby).
  - ❖ Embarrassment about feeding in public (see *Breastfeeding in Public* for tips on discreet feeding).
  - ❖ Clothing (nursing bras and breast pads).
  - ❖ Commitment time (more frequent feedings with breastfeeding).
- Sore nipples, breast engorgement, leaking breasts, mastitis, overabundant milk supply and inadequate milk supply:
  - ❖ Only in rare situations is the mother unable to produce enough milk—see *Low Milk Supply.*
- Measuring feeding amounts:
  - ❖ Some mothers feel more comfortable with bottle-feeding as they know exactly how much milk the baby is receiving, and there is no need to worry about the maternal diet or medications, etc.
- The effects on the shape and size of the breast after breastfeeding:
  - ❖ It returns to its pre-pregnancy size and shape, depending on weight gain and age.
- Maternal freedom and available help (who can help if I am the only one who can breastfeed?):
  - ❖ Physical freedom increases as your baby gets older. After the first few weeks, feeding will become more regular, giving you predictable times when you do not have to be present for breastfeeding.
  - ❖ If you are bottle-feeding your baby with expressed milk you may feel more flexibility, since everyone in the family can help you and bond with your baby.
- Confusion and lack of experience or support:
  - ❖ The mother feels socially isolated and overwhelmed.
- Reduced sex drive and involuntary milk ejection during sexual stimulation:
  - ❖ Many find this embarrassing; if milk is a problem, nursing the baby before sex and placing a towel underneath the breast can help.

❖ Fathers are sometimes not as supportive of breastfeeding, as the intimacy of a mother-baby relationship can be seen as a threat. The mother may be less interested in her husband after the birth of a new baby, since she now has a new responsibility.

❖ Sexual desire may be decreased during certain phases of breastfeeding and as a result, sex may become less frequent.

Further reasons for decreased sex drive include:
- Mother is tired from caring for the new baby.

- Mother experiences physical changes after pregnancy and birth.

- Nursing her baby may meet all of the mother's intimacy needs.

- Hormones during breastfeeding may cause vaginal lubrication to decrease, causing painful intercourse unless supplemental lubrication is used.

- Mother may be less sensitive to stimulation.

- The interest in sex will gradually increase again as the baby grows.

- Father's bonding with the baby:
  ❖ There are many ways to be a parent besides feeding a baby. Your partner can help with household chores, playing with the baby, rocking the baby to sleep, etc.

  ❖ Also, your partner can offer expressed milk to your baby (see *A Father's Role*).

- Illnesses of the mother (e.g., medications, surgery, radiation, HIV, malnutrition, etc.):
  ❖ It is rare that illness of the mother and/or baby prevents the continuance of breastfeeding, as there are ways to cope with a medical condition while continuing to breastfeed.

- Breast surgery:
  ❖ Previous breast surgery should not stop a mother from nursing her baby (unless otherwise directed by your health professional). With even one breast, you can supply plenty of milk for your baby.

Tip: Bonding

There is a stronger mother and baby bond with breastfeeding than there is with bottle-feeding, since there is more skin-to-skin and eye contact, cuddling opportunities, feelings of security, extra holding, etc.

Baby related concerns for the mother can include:

❖ Premature baby or twins and related difficulties.

❖ Bottle resistance (difficulties when switching at a later stage or weaning).

❖ Baby's illness or disease (physical condition): When the baby is ill, it is not the right time to introduce formula. This is a time when your baby needs your breast milk the most, as it contains active disease fighting components along with its perfect nutritional balance.

❖ Difficulty suckling or latching properly.

❖ Dehydration and breastfeeding jaundice.

❖ An adopted baby.

Tip: Breastfeeding and Antibodies

The baby receives a four to six month supply of antibodies through the maternal blood stream prior to delivery.

A Father's Role

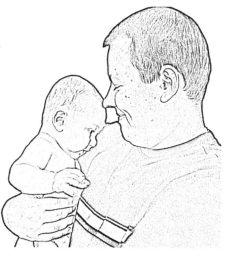

- A mother's perception of the father's attitude towards breastfeeding is one of the greatest factors that influences her decision to breastfeed.

- Sometimes, fathers do not realize how much they can be involved during the breastfeeding period. Studies show that children whose fathers are involved in their lives from birth fare better cognitively, academically, and socially as they grow.

- Fathers have their own concerns including:
  - ❖ Feeling overwhelmed and having concerns about being a new parent.
  - ❖ They may feel excluded at first, while the mother focuses on nursing her new baby.
  - ❖ The issue of sexuality.
  - ❖ Bonding with the baby.
- Feeding a baby is not the only way a parent can bond with a new baby. There are various things a father can do to care for a newborn and create a special father-baby bond such as bathing, sleeping together, rocking the baby, burping, carrying, bottle-feeding, changing diapers, playing, etc.
- Fathers can also help and encourage their wives by:
  - ❖ Helping with household chores.
  - ❖ Providing words of encouragement and support.
  - ❖ Helping in the care of the baby.
  - ❖ Taking time off work to help run the household.
  - ❖ Offering drinks, food, and pillows while the mother is nursing.
  - ❖ Supporting weaning and other decisions.
  - ❖ Boosting the mother's confidence.
  - ❖ Taking care of the baby while the mother naps and gets her rest.

Tip: Breastfeeding and Support

If you are a single mother, you may look for support, help, and encouragement from family and friends.

Doctor's Views & Comments

- Parents are inadequately informed about the risks of formula feeding (artificial milk). Do not accept these risks as normal. They may include unnecessary illnesses such as ear infections, lower respiratory infections, stomach flu, cow's milk allergy, etc. (see *Advantages of Breast Milk*).
- The decision to breast or bottle-feed should be ranked as a first priority and needs to be discussed appropriately.

- Formula-fed babies may have a higher incidence of obesity (because of overfeeding), gastroesophageal reflux, and formula changes.

- Formula will never be able to duplicate the living cells and enzymes and unique properties of breast milk. No one really knows how close formula is to replicating breast milk, as new ingredients and properties are discovered every year in breast milk. Every addition to formula is considered an "abnormal" advance.

- There is more to breastfeeding than just helping your baby grow.

- For bottle-feeding, you need a safe water supply and no errors in its preparation.

- Formula recall and associated consequences are always a concern.

- There is an overall increase in morbidity and mortality in formula-fed infants.

- Although sore nipples, milk leakage, and mastitis can be bothersome, the benefits of breastfeeding far outweigh the temporary inconveniences (most of which can be strategically managed).

- Fathers can bond with their babies by holding them, playing, taking them for walk, giving baths, feeding complementary foods (when age appropriate), etc.

Conclusion

- Human milk is specially designed for the human baby, and the nutritional advantages are certainly numerous. Unless there is a medical problem, there is no real benefit to bottle-feeding.

- It is important to be well informed about the benefits of breastfeeding and associated possible problems, yet be aware of the disadvantages of formula feeding.

- Remember that both types of feeding are possible (breast and bottle) and any amount of breast milk is better than none.

- If you have breastfed and it did not work (with the proper advice), do not feel like you have failed. For successful breastfeeding, you need support at home, at work, from the doctor's office, proper advice, reduced stress and fatigue, etc.

- Hopefully, the breastfeeding section has provided you with more information to help you make an appropriate and informed decision that best fits your lifestyle.

Section 2:
Bottle-feeding

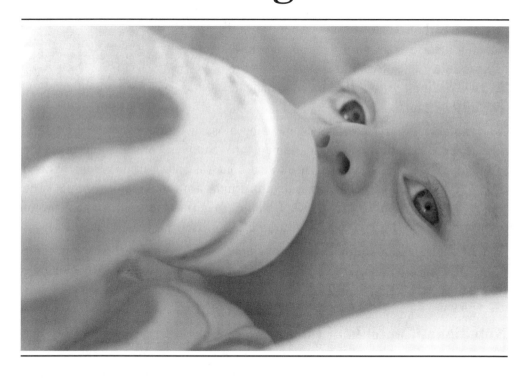

Infant Formulas: Which to Use & How to Choose

General

Formulas are patterned closely after breast milk, the ideal food for a baby's first year. Formula manufacturers start with the basic nutritional elements found in sources such as cow's milk and soybeans. Then they adjust the formula until the proteins, carbohydrates, fats, minerals, and water content are as similar to breast milk as possible. The formula is designed to be easily digested by the baby's delicate intestinal system.

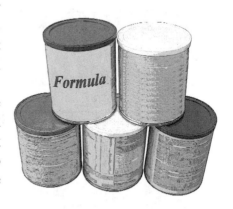

Manufacturers try to make formula as close to human milk as possible, but there are some differences. Human milk changes constantly to meet the growing baby's needs. Human milk also contains living immune factors and digestive enzymes to help your baby, an impossibility for any formula. The frequent changes in formulas are because manufacturers constantly try to improve their product so that the nutrients are closer to breast milk.

While advantages to the baby's development are found in breast milk, the standard formulas are tolerated by most infants. As such, many mothers decide to formula feed.

Nutritional Contents of Formula

Protein

- Protein, an important component of all body cells, is built from amino acids.
- Protein helps in the baby's development by providing new tissue for growth.
- It also helps to control acidity, body fluids and water concentration.
- It has a role in the immune system.
- It can be used for energy if too little fat or carbohydrates are available.
- Protein can be found in meat, poultry, fish, eggs, cheese, dried peas / beans, nuts and peanuts, etc.

- Most formulas have a protein-base derived from cow's milk (casein and/or whey), but some are derived from soybeans.

Carbohydrates
- Carbohydrates (sugars) are an important energy source for the body.
- Foods containing carbohydrates include cereals, flour, bread, rice, potatoes, dried peas and beans, corn, sweet goods, pasta, etc.
- Lactose accounts for most of the carbohydrates in human milk, although small quantities of galactose and fructose are also present.
- Lactose increases (enhances) calcium absorption and is readily metabolized into galactose and glucose.
- The enzyme lactase is necessary to convert lactose into simple sugars that can be easily assimilated by the infant.
- Lactose aids in digestion and promotes normal bowel function.

Fats
- Fats provide a reserve energy source for the body.
- Fats are nutrients which are important for normal body function.
- They help protect your baby's skin and aids in the absorption of vitamins.
- They add taste and texture to various foods and make us feel fuller longer.
- Fats are found in foods such as butter, margarine, some meats, oils, poultry, fish, cream, milk and fried foods.
- Formula contains a mixture of easily digested fats.
- The fat source in formula is a blend of oils; a combination of safflower, sunflower, palm, soy, and coconut oils.

Vitamins
- Vitamins are necessary for growth and development and they are provided in formulas.
- Important vitamins include the following:
  - ❖ *Vitamin A*: good for vision and building body cells.
  - ❖ *Vitamin B*: good for the skin and the nervous system.
  - ❖ *Vitamin C*: good for healthy gums and teeth.
  - ❖ *Vitamin D*: good for strong bones and teeth.
  - ❖ *Vitamin E*: good for proper function of the red blood cells.

Minerals
- Calcium and phosphorus are necessary for proper bone development.
- Iron is also important for healthy red blood cells, etc.

Nucleotides
- Nucleotides are compounds which contain nitrogenous base necessary for energy metabolism, enzyme reaction, growth and maturation of the digestive system and have a role in immune function (e.g., stimulates immunoglobulin production).

Types of Formulas

General

There are a variety of formulas available to meet individual baby needs: formulas for healthy babies, premature babies, babies allergic to cow's milk, those with metabolic conditions (e.g., phenylketonuria), and lactose intolerant babies. There are also hypoallergenic, added rice, follow-up, and organic formulas.

Tip: Phenylketonuria

Phenylketonuria is an inherited disease which causes a buildup of the amino acid phenylalanine in the brain, leading to brain damage. The body does not posses the enzymes necessary to break down phenylalanine. A screening test is usually done at birth for phenylketonuria.

Cow's Milk Based Starter Formula
- Cow's milk based formula is used for children who are able to digest its specific protein and lactose.
- Cow's milk formulas are the most commonly used (if there is family history of allergy, talk to your doctor before starting formula feeding).
- Cow's milk protein contains two protein groups called whey and casein. The protein found in these formulas is hydrolyzed, meaning that it has been partially pre-digested to be less irritating to your baby's digestive tract. More lactose (milk sugar) is added to these formulas to make the concentration closer to breast milk.

- The milk fat is removed and replaced with vegetable fats. In some formulas it is replaced by animal fats that are more easily digestible for infants than cow's milk fats.

- Whole cow's milk is not given before the age of 12 months, as it can cause bleeding in the digestive system and iron deficiency. Talk to your doctor before giving it to your baby.

- High (not low) iron-fortified formula is recommended. This is due to the fact that between four to six months of age, iron stores in your baby are emptying out and additional iron is required for the baby's nutrition. The iron levels in low iron formulas may not be enough to prevent iron deficiency in babies past six months of age.

- These formulas contain Vitamin D and are available as a starter formula to be used between 0-12 months and are used as a follow-up formula from 6-18 months. These come in three convenient forms: concentrated liquid, powder, and ready-to-use.

> ### Tip: Formula
>
> Follow-up formulas usually have more calcium than starter formulas.
> Use formulas that contain omega 3 & 6.
> Use iron-fortified formula (12.0 mg per liter or 0.35 mg per ounce) and do not use those with less iron as they are not a healthy option.
> Note that the name and content of formulas can change with time so always check with your doctor.

Soy Based Starter Formulas
General Information

- Soy is a legume that is rich in protein, vitamins, minerals, and fiber.

- Soy formulas have a modified protein source (i.e. soy protein) as well as a modified carbohydrate source.

- These formulas are different than cow's milk based formulas because of different protein (soy protein) and different carbohydrates (glucose polymer (corn syrup) or sucrose) used in each formula.

- Many parents choose soy based formulas simply because they prefer it over other formulas. Other parents choose to use it because they think their child is allergic to cow's milk based formula.

- The baby will absorb less useable calcium and minerals from soy based formula than from cow's milk formulas.

- Years of use have shown that some babies are better able to tolerate soy based formulas than others.

- Soy based formulas include starter formulas available for 0-12 months and follow-up formulas for 6-24 months.

Tip: Soy Formula Use

Mothers play a greater role than medical personnel in the decision to initiate soy-based formula (Sivan Berger-Achituv et al, JPGN 41:660-666, 2005).

When to Use
- Soy protein based formulas have no advantages over cow's milk formulas.

- Healthy, full-term infants should be given soy formula only when recommended by your doctor for medical reasons. They are not usually recommended as a first choice. However, they do provide nutrients similar to the cow's milk formulas to promote growth and development.

- Soy based formulas should be used when other alternatives (e.g., lactose free, dairy free or hydrolyzed formulas) are unavailable or contraindicated (not to be used) Paediatrics Child Health, 39, 401-405, 2003). Many infants are commonly fed soy protein formulas without good reason.

- Other cases of when soy based formulas should be used include:

When Soy Formula can be Used	Comments
Strict vegetarians	These babies can be offered soy based formulas as they contain no animal products.
Allergy to cow's milk formula	Up to 60% of babies with cow's milk allergy are also allergic to the soy protein formula. An alternative to both cow's milk and soy formulas is hypoallergenic formula.
Unable to digest lactose	Lactose is the most important sugar found in cow's milk based formula. Babies with inherited or congenital lactose intolerance are extremely rare; as such, the use of soy based formulas for this reason is, in most cases, inappropriate. However, lactose intolerance usually occurs after a

Unable to digest lactose	"stomach flu"—called secondary lactose intolerance—and, in this case, one may use soy formula to allow the bowel to rest for a short time, permitting the bowel enzyme that digests the lactose to recover so that lactose can be digested later.
Babies with galactosemia	These babies are unable to digest lactose well.
	They can use soy formulas as the carbohydrates in most of these formulas contain sucrose and/or corn syrup.
	Soy formulas are easily digested and absorbed by these babies.

When Not to Use Soy Formula
- Do not use soy formula for the prevention and/or treatment of colic.
- Soy formulas have no proven value in preventing skin allergic diseases in healthy or high risk babies.
- Many infants with documented cow's milk allergy symptoms (see *Allergies*) can also be sensitive to soy protein formulas and should not be given these formulas. Instead, you may give them hydrolyzed protein formula.
- Also, note that premature babies require more minerals (which are less digestible in soy formulas), so that soy formulas are not considered to be a good choice for premature babies.

Some Concerns with Soy Formulas
- Some children with cow's milk allergy are also allergic to soy formula.
- There is no clear evidence that shows that soy formula decreases the chance of allergies.
- There are questions regarding the effect of vegetable estrogen (phytoestrogen which acts like the estrogen hormone) on the baby's hormonal balance and the risk of both short-term and long-term effects (thyroid problems, reproductive organ functions, and effects on age of puberty).
- Soy based formulas are deficient in some amino acids and these need to be added as they are essential for growth and development.
- These formulas also have more sodium, so they are saltier than the standard formula.
- Lactose is important for calcium absorption and its absorption is decreased with soy formula (which has no lactose). Similarly, phytic acid (a soy plant

vegetable contaminant) can form complexes with various minerals such as calcium and zinc, decreasing mineral absorption. This is the reason why it is not recommended in premature babies (there are reports of rickets and bone mineralization defects). Extra calcium is now added to soy formula to help eliminate this problem.

> ## Tip: Baby Growth On Various Formulas
>
> Despite all the above reasons, experience shows that babies grow well whether they are on cow's milk, soy, or organic formulas.

Cow's Milk & Soy Based Follow-Up Formula

- This type of formula is made for infants six months of age or older.

- They can be based on cow's milk or soy and are iron-fortified.

- Follow-up formulas are considered to be better than straight cow's milk as they contain more calories, iron, protein, and essential fatty acids. They are also easier on the baby's kidneys than cow's milk.

- Follow-up formulas contain slightly higher levels of vitamins, minerals, and protein and slightly lower levels of fat.

- These formulas are enriched with calcium and phosphor to meet the increased needs of the growing infant. The calcium requirement increases by 50% for a baby between the ages of 6-12 months.

- Although follow-up formulas claim to cost 20% less than the standard formulas, you need to assess the amount of formula powder used (in grams) to the amount of ounces diluted that are obtained to make a comparative cost analysis to standard formula.

- Although the companies who make follow-up formulas claim that they contain more benefits than the traditional (starter) formula, this has yet to be proven and parents should continue using the initial starter formula from birth up until 12 months of age.

- The nutrient content of follow-up formulas is adequate; however it is recommended that formulas, regardless of classification, provide no more than 50-65% of the total caloric intake for the infant over 6 months of age. The remainder of calories should come from solid foods.

- Iron in follow-up formulas may be useful if the toddler's diet is deficient in iron (and better for the child than cow's milk).

- Disadvantages of using these formulas are:
  - ❖ The proteins casein and whey ratio in follow-up formulas are different from human milk. Formula may contain variable ratios of the two proteins found in cow's milk (whey and casein). Some follow-up formulas contain ratios of whey/casein that are increased to that of the normal human milk ratio of 60/40 whey to casein. This causes more casein protein group characteristics such as:
    - Casein is less soluble than whey protein.
    - Can take longer to empty from the stomach and the baby may feel satisfied for longer, leading to inadequate nutrional intake.
    - Results in thick curd formation by combining with calcium phosphor, leading to harder stool.
- Some follow-up formulas are sweetened with corn syrup (glucose polymer), which is a good source of calories. They are readily absorbed because they are hydrolyzed by the digestive enzymes (maltase), and impact little on sweetness. Glucose polymer is a frequent addition to infant formulas as it boosts the caloric content in certain difficult feeding situations. However, adding such components as glucose polymer to formula must be done with care, as any additions may cause imbalances of other nutrients (e.g., increased glucose polymer intake may decrease protein intake as a percent of total energy).
- It is essentially better to give your baby a higher amount of the standard formula than follow-up formula. Growing infants require more fluid and all the nutrients (calcium, iron, etc.) can be administered through solid foods at the appropriate age.
- Check with your baby's doctor before using follow-up formula, as some doctors do not recommend them.

Tip: Switching Formula

Do not switch from one formula to another, unless it is recommended by your doctor. If you feel that your baby is not doing well on formula, speak to your doctor first before doing anything.

Specialized Infant Formulas

General

Specialized infant formulas are designed for premature babies and infants who have specific diseases or conditions. These formulas are also used if the baby cannot tolerate the cow's milk protein or the soybean milk protein, and for babies with a history of family allergies. They should be used with the recommendation of your pediatrician.

Hypoallergenic Formulas

Hypoallergenic formulas are used in babies who have allergies to cow's milk and soy based formulas. These babies require a complete degradation (breakdown) of protein.

- Hypoallergenic formulas break down the allergy causing proteins in cow's milk (casein or whey) and soy protein into very small units that are less likely to trigger an allergic reaction.

- The casein hydrolyzed hypoallergenic formulas have a modified carbohydrate source and a modified protein source and can contain medium chain triglyceride (MCT) oil, which is a modified fat.

- These formulas are much more expensive than standard formulas.

- The taste is more bitter and unpalatable in hypoallergenic formulas than in other formulas.

- Hypoallergenic formulas should only be used with a doctor's recommendation for specific medical reasons (e.g., liver disease, children with fat mal-absorption, etc.).

- These formulas do not provide the fatty acids required for the baby's growing brain and they are higher in salts (30-90% more than standard formulas), which is not good for the baby's kidneys.

   ❖ In some hypoallergenic formulas the protein casein has been broken down and can be tolerated in infants with cow's milk allergy. In others the whey protein is broken into smaller incomplete proteins—this is not the best type of formula, as some babies with cow's milk allergy may be intolerant to it.

Hydrolyzed Milk Formulas

These formulas are developed for the extremely sensitive baby.

- Cow's milk protein is large and difficult for the young baby to digest; in hydrolyzed formulas the protein is broken down into smaller, more digestible pieces.

- Some say that using hydrolyzed milk formula from the beginning (if breast milk is not an option) can prevent allergies and many problems such as milk intolerance, intestinal bleeding related to formula feeding, etc. However, there have been reports of allergic reactions to both whey and casein hydrolyzed formulas in highly allergic infants.

- Hydrolyzed milk formulas do not taste as good as other formulas when offered to infants who have tasted other formulas. As such, it is sometimes difficult to switch to hydrolyzed milk formula once you have begun with a different one. Hydrolyzed formulas taste bad due to the presence of sulfated amino acids which tend to impart a sulfur-like flavor. The more complete the hydrolysis, the worse the taste.

- They are more expensive than other formulas and less palatable than soy formula (formula containing partially hydrolyzed whey protein is less expensive than extensively hydrolyzed casein protein formula, yet there can still be an allergy to a hydrolyzed protein formula).

Tip: Colic and Formula

The substitution of cow's milk formula with an extensively hydrolyzed whey formula can help your baby with colic (inconsolable crying of at least 3 hours per day in one week for a period of more than three weeks) occurring in the first three to five months of age (Pediatrics, Dec 2000, 1343-1354).

Lactose Free Formulas

Lactose free formulas are for children who are unable to digest lactose (e.g., babies with bowel disease, lactose intolerance).

- These formulas cannot be used for babies with Galactosemia as they contain residual galactose (sugar).

- They are based on cow's milk, but the lactose (sugar) is removed and replaced with corn syrup.

- Ingredients like corn syrup and sucrose replace lactose.

- Bear in mind that primary lactose intolerance, e.g., congenital (from birth), is actually quite rare.

- The intolerance is usually more common after diarrhea and is called secondary lactose intolerance, in which the bowel temporarily cannot tolerate lactose.

Added Rice Formulas
These formulas are for babies who are spitting up excessively and have weight gain issues.
- Added rice formulas are cow's milk based formulas that also contain rice starch. This helps the formula settle in the baby's stomach.

Formula for Premature Babies
These formulas are designed to meet the special nutritional needs of premature babies.
- They are rich in protein, minerals and vitamins, folic acid, zinc, omega 3 & 6, and iron and provide more calories that standard formulas.

- Premature formulas come in two different categories: premature formulas and follow-up or discharge premature formulas.

Organic Formulas
These are made of milk or soy products that are untouched by pesticides, chemicals, growth hormones, and antibiotics. Therefore, organic foods help minimize the consumption of harmful pesticides, chemicals, antibiotics, and/or hormones.
- While it is commonly believed that organic formulas are more nutritious and/or safer than non-organic formulas, there is no supporting evidence.

- Organic formulas are available in both dairy and soy iron-fortified products that provide the essential nutrients (including omega 3 fatty acids) needed to support your baby's growth and development.

- These formulas meet the nutritional requirements of the Infant Formula Act. They are comparable to others formulas in the market.

- The non-organic formulas carbohydrate sources are processed sugar, corn syrup, or lactose (which may come from cows given antibiotics, bovine growth hormones, and steroids). The certified organic brown rice syrup typically used in organic formulas is an excellent source of naturally occurring carbohydrates and receives minimal processing.

- These formulas can be used to supplement or substitute breast milk and/or can be mixed with cereals for your baby.

- Organic formulas are slightly more expensive than standard non-organic formulas.

Disease Specific Formulas
Disease specific formulas are created to meet the needs of infants' particular health conditions.

- Some of the most common include Portagen for liver disease, and pancreatic insufficiency; Similac PM 6040 for renal or cardiac condition requiring lower minerals, and Phenex-1 or Phenyl-Free for phenylketonuria.

Toddler Formulas
Toddler formulas are made for children in the early years of life, from the age of 1.

- These formulas contain 30 calories per ounce and a complete compilation of vitamins and minerals. They can come with or without fiber.

Choosing a Formula: What You Need to Know

The closest alternative to human milk is an iron-fortified cow's milk based formula (any baby who is not breastfed needs an iron-fortified formula), making it the most appropriate formula first choice for your baby. Use a formula that contains the fatty acids DHA & ARA (found also in breast milk) which helps with brain and retina development—they are more expensive, and there aren't many studies to prove their benefit, but these fatty acids are found in breast milk.

Many parents use soy based formula because of their fear of cow's milk allergy. Only 3% of babies have a true milk allergy and about 15% of these babies will also be allergic to soy. It hasn't been proven, but some parents believe that their babies are less colicky on soy formula. There are some concerns about the effects of soy (which mimics estrogen) formula on hormonal development, fertility, and neurodevelopment. These concerns are theoretical and further study is needed. The best case use for soy formula is if your family is vegetarian, if there is a family history of minor allergies and, of course, for a baby diagnosed with Galactosemia (the inability to digest galactose).

- Babies with severe allergies require specialized formulas. If, for example, your baby is allergic to both cow's milk and soy formula, use hydrolyzed formula.

- If your baby develops symptoms such as blood in their stool, vomiting, diarrhea, or skin rashes, see your doctor immediately, as there may be a formula intolerance.

- When choosing a formula, consider both convenience and cost. For example, is it ready to use, concentrated, or powdered? Choose what is best for you and your baby.

- Never make your own formula or add something to a formula.

The basic point is that you should choose a type of formula that you and your baby are both happy with. Do not constantly switch your baby's formula, as this can upset her digestive system and cause constipation every time there is a dietary change. Your doctor will help you choose the appropriate formula.

Parent Concerns

My baby has diarrhea. Should I switch to soy formula from cow's milk formula?

- If your child has been on the same formula for a few months now and she has the stomach flu, you do not need to change formulas.

- Switching formulas is considered when diarrhea is prolonged. In these situations, babies may not be able to tolerate the lactose well.

- Upon discussion with your doctor, you may use soy or lactose-free formula until your child's bowel is healed.

- In most stomach flu situations, the duration is brief and no formula change is required.

Tip: Vitamins & Formula

You do not need to give your child vitamin supplements when he is formula-fed, as today's commercial formulas are manufactured with all the nutrients that your baby needs.

Can homemade formula be used as an alternative to commercially prepared formula?

- According to Food and Drug Administration (FDA), homemade formula should not be used.

- First, cow's milk cannot be given before your baby is one year of age (see *Cow's Milk*). Second, homemade formula based on cow's milk will not meet your child's nutritional requirements. It will be difficult for your baby to digest it and the high protein and salt contents may place a strain on her immature kidneys.

- Goat's milk is not a good alternative to cow's milk, either, especially if your child has a problem with milk and its protein. Goat's milk is low in vitamin D, B12, iron, and folate, which can lead to anemia in your child.

Is there any one particular formula that is cow's based that is better than other formulas?

- The American Academy of Pediatrics (AAP) and the Canadian Pediatric Society (CPS) does not endorse or recommend using a specific brand of formula. No studies have been done to confirm any one brand is better than another.
- Parents decide on a formula brand for various reasons that include previous experience, formula given in the hospital, and their doctor's recommendation.

Tip: Formula & Age

You can offer formula (toddler formula) as long as you want, but around the age of 3-4 years, your baby may want to make the change on her own. Usually, toddler formula provides some of the necessary nutrients that your child may not be able to consume in solid foods. After the age of 3, you may use milk that is enriched with calcium and iron. Keep in mind that children require milk products for normal growth and development.

When should formula be changed?

- Formula can be changed in the following situations upon discussion with your doctor:
  - ❖ Lactose intolerance.
  - ❖ Milk protein allergy.
  - ❖ Metabolic situations (e.g., Galactosemia, phenylketonuria, etc.).

Tip: Formula Recall

❖ The great majority of formula recalls have been because powdered forms of formula were contaminated with potentially harmful bacteria. The ready-to-feed and concentrate formulas are sterilized, while powder is not.

Do various formulas cause or improve gassiness or colic in my baby?

- A study offering various types of formulas to babies (parents did not know what type of formula was given to their child) did not show any differences in spitting up, gassiness, and crying. The behaviours were the same with all formula groups (Pediatrics 95: 50-54, 1995).

- Different formulas claim to be better than others at preventing gassiness. While it could be true theoretically, it is mostly not true in practice.

- It is important to realize that there may be other causes to fussiness, etc., outside of formula.

Are there kosher formulas?
Yes, there are kosher formulas. Kosher signs include U, D and Pareve. Discuss which to use with your doctor.

Tip: Constipation & Formula

In choosing formulas, use high iron content formulas rather than low iron formulas to prevent your baby developing iron deficiency anemia.

Although studies do not show iron to be a constipating factor, the occasional baby will have bowel movement difficulties (practical experience versus scientific research).

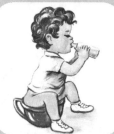

Baby's stool may vary from day to day, depending on the food your baby ingests. Many factors can affect stool color, consistency, and frequency (see *Stool Characteristics & Feeding*).

Tip: Lactose Intolerance

Lactose is a sugar contained in human and cow's milk. It is digested in the intestine by the lactase enzyme into glucose and galactose.

When a baby, child, or adult becomes deficient in this enzyme, they cannot absorb lactose and they develop the following symptoms: bloating, abdominal pain, diarrhea, irritation, and burns around the anus (which is due to lactic acid). Symptoms of lactose intolerance are restricted to the digestive system (there are no hives, chest rashes, etc.). This can be corrected by adding lactase tablets or powder to the diet, replacing the missing enzymes.
Primary lactose intolerance in infants is rare and often over diagnosed. It becomes more common as you get older, when your supply of lactase enzymes determines whether you can tolerate more or less milk products.
1 out of 6500 babies is actually born with no enzymes that break down the sugar lactose.
Many parents mistake their baby's fussiness for lactose intolerance and switch to lactose-free formula. However, in most cases this is not the reason for the fussiness.

continued

There is also a condition called secondary lactose intolerance, which means that the digestive system is injured due to some infection or allergy (e.g., after a stomach flu). Delay the introduction of milk until the lining of the digestive system is healed and more lactose enzyme is available.

- The following tables are only partial examples of formulas and should NOT be considered as being recommended because they are listed here. If you have decided to choose formula feeding over breast milk, discuss the right formula choice for your baby with your doctor. Remember that formula names and content change frequently, so always be sure to confer with your doctor to avoid any possible confusion.

Formula Examples & Tables

The following table contains examples of cow's milk based formulas:

Age	Type	Comments
0 – 12 Months (Starter Formulas)	Enfamil A+	Has omega 3 & 6
	Similac Advance	Has omega 3 & 6
	Good Start	Good Start offers with or without omega 3 & 6
	Enfamil with Iron	Has omega 3 & 6
	Enfamil with Low Iron	
6 – 18 Months & up (Follow-up)	Similac Advance Step 2	
	Good Start 2	Has omega 3 & 6
	Enfapro	With or without omega 3 & 6
	Follow-up Transition	No omega & lactose free

The following table contains examples of soy formulas:

Age	Type	Comments
0 – 12 Months	Isomil 1	Has omega 3 & 6
	Alsoy	Has omega 3 & 6
	Enfamil Soy	
6 – 24 Months	Isomil Step 2	No omega acids
	Alsoy 2	

Lactose Free Formulas Examples
- Examples of lactose free formulas include Enfamil lactose free, Similac lactose free, Nutramigen Hypoallergenic, Pregestimil, Alsoy, and Neocate.

Severe Milk Allergy Formula Examples
- For severe milk allergy, amino acid based formulas are available, but they are extremely costly (e.g., Neocate).

Hypoallergenic Formulas Examples
- In Nutramigen Hypoallergenic formula the protein casein is broken down and can be tolerated in infants with cow's milk allergy.
- In Pregestimil formula the whey protein has been broken into smaller, incomplete proteins. It is still not the best type of formula, as some babies with cow's milk allergy may be intolerant to it.

Hydrolyzed Formula Examples
- Examples of extensively hydrolyzed and hypoallergenic formula are Nutramigen Hypoallergenic and Pregestimil Hypoallergenic.

Added Rice Formula Examples
- An example of this formula includes Enfamil A+ thickened (has rice, starch, and is rich in omega 3 & 6).

Premature Baby Formula Examples
- Enfamil Enfacare A+ and Similac Advance Neosure are examples of formulas for premature babies.

Equipment Used for Formula Preparation & Sterilization

General

There are various items you need to have when you prepare formula. Other equipment to sterilize these items is also necessary. The following is a list of general equipment required:

- Large pot with a lid.
- Bottle/nipple brush.
- Can opener.
- Measuring cup glass.
- Spoon—this is optional for stirring the formula.
- About 6-8 of the following: bottles (full size 8 oz/250 ml; 4 oz/125 ml); nipples; caps (keeps dust away from the sterile nipple); rings (secures the nipple); and discs (placed over the nipple to keep the bottle sealed).
- Plastic funnel (optional; used to pour the made-up formula into the bottle).
- Roll of plastic liners (if using a disposable bottle, you must throw away liners after each use).
- Dishwasher basket and/or drying rack for bottles, nipples, etc.
- Cold packs (1-2) and an insulated container for traveling with homemade bottles.

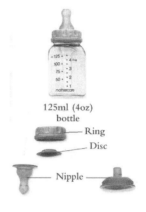

125ml (4oz) bottle

Ring
Disc
Nipple

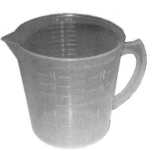

Optional items include a bottle warmer and a warmer in your vehicle that plugs into the lighter opening on your dashboard.

Bottles

Types: Advantages & Disadvantages
There are two basic types of bottles: reusable and disposable.

Reusable	Disposable
Can be filled, sterilized, and refilled (may be used over and over again). Generally made from glass or FDA-approved polycarbonate plastic, both of which are dishwasher safe.	Do not need to be sterilized as they include bags that attach to a plastic holder.

- Whether you opt for reusable or disposable, make sure that the bottle and the bags have clear markings that enable you to measure the correct amount of formula or breast milk for your baby's feedings.

- If you switch between both types of bottles, know that some babies may not like the shape of the nipple (if they sense the difference). If this is the case, then select a brand that offers the same shape nipple on both bottles to avoid nipple confusion.

- Choosing a bottle style and brand depends on your infant as well as your preference.

- There are glass bottles (less popular than they once were) and plastic bottles (also available are bottles for prolonged use).

- The following table outlines the advantages and disadvantages of bottle types:

Bottles	Advantages	Disadvantages
Glass	Easy to keep clean and sterilize. Very durable. May do a better job in retaining nutrients.	Heavy for your baby to hold. Risk of breaking, chipping or cracking so that you can never allow your baby to hold it. Not really portable.
Plastic	Easy to clean and sterilize. Unbreakable and lightweight. Very sturdy (firm).	Usually deteriorates quickly after continuous usage, sterilization and cleaning. Needs to be replaced regularly.
Plastic bottles with Disposable Liners	Easy handling and ideal for cleaning since you throw away plastic liners after use. Comfortable when traveling. Reduces the amount of air the baby swallows (with sucking, the plastic liner bag collapses and so there is a decrease of air entry during feedings). Liners do not need to be sterilized.	Constantly requires that you buy plastic liners. More expensive.

Choosing the Right Bottle

- Parents choose bottles according to affordability and convenience (look at the previous table to help you choose the right bottle for you and your baby).

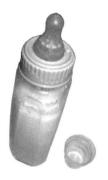

- Many bottles are available these days and each has or claims to have a variety of characteristics.

- No particular bottle or nipple works best for every baby. Some babies are good with any bottle you use. Other babies may have distinct preferences, so you may want to try a few different bottles.

- The bottle and nipple you choose depend on the age and whether your baby is exclusively bottle-fed or breastfed as well (at least part of the time). If you are breastfeeding, choose bottles and nipples that closely resemble the nipple of the breast.

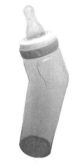

- Bottles come in various sizes. You can choose small bottle volume, if your baby uses small volumes of milk (e.g., if the baby is less than three months of age). Choose a larger bottle of 8-9 oz/240-270 ml when your baby consumes more than the amount of the small volume bottle.

- There are various forms bottles come in to make them easier for your baby to hold. They may be flatter or have a hole in the middle and they may also have a grip or handles on the side. Bottles may also come with removable bottoms to make cleaning easier.

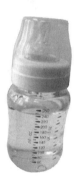

- The following are specific bottles to keep in mind when choosing the right bottle:

  ❖ Bottles with a *wide base* allow for easy filling of formula and cleaning.

  ❖ *Streamlined* bottles are ones the babies can hold onto themselves.

  ❖ *Angled* bottles keep the nipple filled with liquid at all times (e.g., Evenflo's Elite). These are sometimes easier for the baby to hold on his own. Once your baby understands how to hold the bottle, she won't have to tip it as much to get the milk out. Some parents also think that using an angled bottle means less risk of ear infections.

❖ Bottles with *internal vents* prevent air bubbles from forming so that it does not mix with the liquid. This might help in decreasing the amount of spitting up (e.g., Playtex Vent-Air Bottle).

❖ *Wide-necked bottles* are shorter, with a wide base to give added stability and without the interior ridges that encourage germs. These bottles facilitate safe and easy filling and cleaning. *Narrow-necked bottles* may be more difficult to clean and fill. It is important to clean the ridges inside the neck of the bottle, as they act as germ traps.

• There are also bottles with special features such as the *Haberman bottle* that has a nipple with an adjustable flow depending on the position. It is for infants with disorganized sucking patterns. The *"breastfed bottle"* is another bottle that has a short nipple and wide bulb that makes it easier for your baby to suck. Also, the *Adiri bottle* is made of soft rounded silicone, resembling the breast with a straight nipple.

> ### Tip: Testing Bottle Temperature
>
> Never judge the temperature of the liquid by feeling the exterior of the bottle or bag. Take the time to drip a few drops onto your forearm so that you can feel what will be going into your baby's mouth. There are also bottles in the market that are heat sensitive and will alert you when the bottle is too hot.

Replacing Bottles

Bottles and characteristics may change over time. Replace the bottle if you notice the following things:

• *Cracks, chips or breaks*: Your child could cut, pinch or otherwise injure herself (lodging, choking, etc.).

• *Bottles with disposable liners*: Liners should be thrown away after each use.

• *Stickiness, discoloration or swelling of the bottle*: These are signs of nipple and bottle deterioration.

Nipples

General

• The nipple functions as a syringe that allows food to enter the baby's mouth and be swallowed.

• Normally, your baby will learn to suck from any type of nipple given to her, unless there is a medical problem. Keep in mind, however, that it can sometimes take several tries before you find the nipple your baby prefers.

- If your baby has a medical problem (such as cleft lip/palate, etc.), regular nipples can be used once the abnormalities are corrected.

- The best nipple for your baby is the one she feels most comfortable with. If your baby likes the nipple, she will grab onto it quickly and suck vigorously. If she does not like the nipple, she will let go after a few sucks, her body may tense up, and she may begin to fuss or cry.

- No matter what type of nipple you decide to use, be sure to check them regularly for cracks or other signs of deterioration.

- It is also best to use nipples and bottles of the same brand to ensure a proper fit and avoid leaks.

Tip: Nipples and Dental Problems

Dental problems are not related to the type of nipple used; they are related to the duration of use of the same nipple, frequency of bottle use and its content.

Types of Nipples
- There are a variety of nipple shapes. While some nipples will only fit certain types of bottles, many are interchangeable. You may discover that your baby changes her nipple preference as she matures.

- There are three types of nipple material including latex, silicone, and rubber.
  - ❖ *Latex nipples* are golden brown, soft, and a little more flexible than silicone nipples. These are easier for your baby to suck on and good for your baby to start out with. Latex nipples have a distinctive smell, absorb milk fats, and rapidly decompose, creating cracks and tears. Over time, latex nipples will change and do not last as long as silicone nipples.

  - ❖ *Silicone nipples* are clear, heat resistant, and can be cleaned in the dishwasher. These have a sticky texture and are an inert material. They will not change shape nor take on any odors and are less prone to bacteria than latex nipples. Silicone nipples will typically last three to four times longer than latex nipples.

- The following are some nipple shapes for you to choose from:
  - ❖ *Traditional (universal) nipples* are bell shaped with a thin base and tip and are easy to use for most babies. The sucking action with the traditional nipple is unlike that of the breast. It may have 1-3 holes.

There are different rates of milk flow with the universal nipple; flow should be 2-3 drops per second.

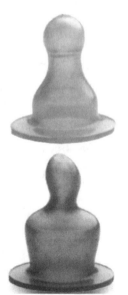

❖ *Naturally shaped nipples* are soft, with a wider base to promote proper latch-on and sucking that helps the baby transition more easily between breastfeeding and bottle-feeding (reinforces the baby's natural reflexes). The longer nipple tip most closely resembles the breast and promotes a suckling action for the baby that is the closest to breastfeeding. The baby's mouth covers the nipple without coming in contact with the plastic nipple-retaining ring. Examples of naturally shaped nipples include the Avent Naturally and Playtex Ventaire.

Tip: Naturally Shaped Nipples

Longer nipples may cause gagging in some babies that are accustomed to their mother's nipple. Nipples must enter your baby's mouth with the holes facing upward so that the milk will spray to the roof of the mouth.

If the nipple has a wide base but short nipple (short shanked nipple), as your baby sucks her lips push against the base and the nipple moves in and out of her mouth. This can be a problem in a baby who is breastfeeding as she may bite, too.

❖ *Nipples for premature babies* are usually given in a hospital setting. It is a smaller and softer nipple than the universal nipple. It has a tinier hole to make the sucking easier until your premature baby gains weight and has more strength.

❖ *Nipples for babies with cleft lip/palate* are designed for babies born with abnormalities of the lip and palate. If the baby has surgical correction early in infancy (especially if the baby only has cleft lip), you can use a regular/universal nipple after the surgery.

❖ *Anti-colic or vented nipples* are soft and naturally shaped, which may help your breastfeeding baby to accept them more easily. There is an anti-vacuum skirt and a one-way valve. These are designed with a tiny hole to let air into the bottle as the baby sucks on the nipple. The hole is meant to prevent the nipple from collapsing and reduces air intake by your baby, as well as ensuring that liquid, and not air, flows through the nipple. The anti-colic feature is built right into the nipple (there are valves in the rims of these nipples).

❖ *Orthodontic nipples* insert further back into the baby's mouth, allowing for a more natural milking action by the tongue. It inconveniently requires a certain way to turn the nipple to accommodate the child's palate and gums. These have a bulb (part of the nipple the baby sucks on) that is flat on one side, which rests on the tongue to resemble the shape of the mother's nipple during breastfeeding. Orthodontic nipples have an irregular shape with an indent in the center. It elongates after repeated sucking to resemble breastfeeding.

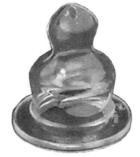

❖ *Multi-flow nipples* can be adjusted to give your baby the right flow of milk, whether it is slow, medium, or fast.

❖ *Slotted multi-flow nipples* are also adjustable, however they feature slots instead of holes. They are good for thickened juices, etc. You can turn the nipple to adjust the flow based on the thickening of the liquid.

Choosing the Right Nipple & Issues to Consider

• Most babies accept whatever nipple you offer them.

• If your baby is bottle-fed, experiment with various types of nipples to see which one works best for your baby.

• If your baby is also breastfed, use a nipple with a wide base and one that resembles the breast.

• When choosing a nipple for your baby, the following issues should be considered:

 ❖ *Flow Rate*: Ensure the flow is right for your baby's age. The speed of formula flow when the bottle is upended with the nipple down should be about one drop per second. As the baby grows, she can probably tolerate a faster speed.

❖ *Hole Size of the Nipple*: If the nipple has a small hole, the baby will suck a lot of air (may require frequent burping) and will use too much effort to get the milk. If the nipple has a big hole, the formula will flow quickly and your baby will not be able to suck effectively, which can lead to gagging or choking. The baby will also stop frequently between sucking until the ingested formula clears the throat. Your baby will let you know if the nipple is too large, as she may gulp or choke; also, milk may drip out of the corners of her mouth.

- There are various sizes when it comes to nipple holes:
  ❖ *Size one* (newborn) is usually labeled for babies up to 6 months of age. The hole is small so as to prevent the baby from taking in too much air at once and gagging. The entire nipple may be smaller than those designed for older babies.

  ❖ *Size two* (nipples for six months and older) are labeled for older babies or as "faster flowing" nipples. These contain a larger hole or, sometimes, there is more than one hole for a quick flow.

  ❖ *Preemie* nipples have tinier holes than others and are softer, so as to make the sucking easier until your premature baby gains weight. They are usually given in the hospital, if you need them.

Tip: Nipples & Gas Problems

Do not look or waste your money on a nipple that claims to make your baby's gas disappear. No nipple has been proven to do this effectively.

If your baby uses a pacifier, she may prefer a nipple shaped like the pacifier nipple. Allow your baby to try one nipple for several days before switching to another (if you need to switch nipples). Trying a wide variety of nipples will probably confuse your baby more, especially if you try few at once or during the same day.

Replacing Nipples

Replace nipples if the following situations arise and check the nipple periodically for signs of wear and tear:

- The formula pours out in a stream when it should drip steadily out of the nipple. If the formula comes rushing out, the hole is too big and you need to replace the nipple.

- Nipple discoloration, stickiness, or swelling indicates deterioration and requires nipple replacement.

- Thinning of the nipple is an early sign that it is weakening. To test the nipple's strength, pull hard on the bulb; it should rebound to its original shape. If it does not, throw the nipple away and replace it with a new one.

- A nipple with any cracks, tears, or rips needs to be tossed out immediately as it is a choking hazard (to avoid choking, follow the manufacturer's advice on the package).

Nipple Care

- Nipples do deteriorate and holes clog up, so make sure to have some spare, sterile nipples.

- Holes that are too small can be enlarged with a needle that has a very fine, sharp point (check the flow regularly when doing this). When enlarging the hole, heat the needle point in a flame until it is hot and then push it into the hole.

Sterilization of Equipment

General

It is very important to sterilize all utensils used in the preparation of infant formula, since bacteria/germs are everywhere and multiply rapidly. Enough germs can cause the baby to develop an illness such as vomiting, diarrhea, etc.

It is recommended that you sterilize everything during the first year of life, especially in the earlier months of life. However, recommendations vary according to your doctor and the water supply of the city in which you live, so discuss this with your doctor. In general, tap water that comes from a municipal system is safe for older babies and children.

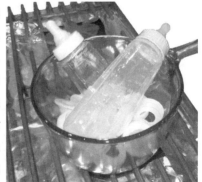

Sterilization Steps
- Wash your hands.
- Using hot, soapy water, wash the bottles, nipples, caps, can opener, and any equipment you may need in preparing the formula. Rinse thoroughly. Wash the bottles thoroughly and remove all milk residues from the bottle and nipple with the brush.
- Place all equipment into a large pot or sterilizer.
- Put water in the pot and cover it.
- Allow it to boil for approximately five to ten minutes.
- Remove the pot from the heat and allow cooling to facilitate the handling and removal of items.
- These items will be placed on a clean paper towel with the open ends of the bottle and nipple facing downward.
- Allow the bottles to dry before feeding.

Improved Steps of Sterilization
Sterilization steps can be improved by doing the following:
- Earlier boiling of the items for 20 minutes, before filling the bottle.
- The water used to mix with formula powder should be boiled for about two minutes.
- Bottles that are filled with formula should be refrigerated and used within 24 hours.
- You can boil water for two minutes and fill a few sterilized bottles with this water. Make sure to keep these bottles at room temperature. You can keep for up to 48 hours. Prior to feeding, add the formula in the appropriate amount, shake well and feed.
- Boiling the bottle with formula in it is not recommended, as this may negatively affect the nutritional quality of the formula.

Tip: Bottle, Nipple and Sterilization

If you are using disposable bottle liners, the only things that need to be sterilized are the nipples, rings, and screw tops of bottles and caps. The liners are sterilized by the manufacturer and should be used only once.

Remember that the nipples that come with these bottles are not disposable and must be carefully cleaned and sterilized before each feeding.

Discuss with your physician at what point it is no longer necessary to sterilize the equipment or water.

Electric Steam & Microwave Sterilization

- There are electric and microwave sterilizers available in the market today, and all you need is access to electricity and a microwave.

- They are a much safer and more consistent means of sterilization than traditional methods.

- Investing in a steam sterilizer makes sense, especially for the working mother. It minimizes the danger of unhygienic sterilization (especially if there are other people helping with sterilization).

- Electric steam sterilization is a quick (8-12 min) and effective method of cleaning equipment. Simply place the equipment that is safe to boil (bottles, nipples, caps, etc.) in the steamer upside down to ensure full sterilization.

- Microwave sterilizers take from five to eight minutes of heating, followed by cooling, to work. Make sure that no metal is placed inside the microwave sterilizer. The best part about microwave sterilizers is that there is no smell or taste involved in the sterilization process and they remain sterile for about 3 hours (as long as the lid is kept on).

- There are also microwave bottles, which can be sterilized in the microwave on their own. Bottles have to be left open during this process. It takes about 90 seconds to sterilize one bottle.

Tip: Microwave and Sterilization

You cannot sterilize in the microwave unless you have the proper microwave sterilizer.

Sterilization Do's & Don'ts

- Bottles, nipples and caps must be sterilized with each feeding.

- Wash your hands thoroughly with soap and water before preparing bottles.

- Utensils used for preparing food must first be washed thoroughly with boiling water.

- Do not touch the inside of the sterilized bottle. Handle the sterilized equipment only from its outside.

- The bottle must be covered with a sterile cap; even during the short time you are burping your baby.

- *Washing bottles with hot boiling water is **NOT** enough to sterilize the bottles.*

Tip: Practicality in Food Preparation

Although these Do's & Don'ts are recommended, in reality not everything suggested is practical, so do your best.

Parent Concerns

How long should I continue sterilizing?

Due to your baby's immature immune system and resulting vulnerability to sickness, you should sterilize your baby's feeding equipment for at least their first year of life. The best practice is to sterilize all equipment until your baby stops using a bottle.

How do I store sterilized bottles?

Once you have sterilized your equipment with the methods previously stated, you can keep it sterilized by keeping it in a sterilized solution. You may leave the bottles and other items in the sterilizing solution until you are ready to use them.

Can I sterilize my equipment in the dishwasher?

You can sterilize the equipment in a dishwasher if you do not want to boil the bottles for sterilization. The equipment (bottles, caps, etc.) must be cleaned of all residues before you use the dishwasher. Place all the equipment in a dishwasher that uses heated water and has a hot drying cycle. The nipples should be boiled separately in a pot.

Formula & Its Preparation

General

Infant formulas come in three forms: powder, ready-to-use, and liquid concentrate. When prepared properly, all formulas have the same nutritional value. Choose your formula based on affordability, a realistic appraisal of your lifestyle, your baby's preference and your doctor's recommendations. Each type of formula has its own set of advantages and disadvantages.

Powder Formulas

Advantages:

- Least expensive.
- Once the can has been opened, it may be stored up to one month before being discarded (tends to go rancid if it is kept more than one month); it does not need to be refrigerated once it has been opened, but must be kept in a cool, dry place (see storage).
- Light weight.
- Easy to transport and use at any time; simply have the sterilized bottle filled with the right amount of formula and add sterile water to it when you need to feed your baby.

Disadvantages:

- Risk of error in measurement of the powder resulting in:
  - ❖ *Too little powder* mixed in the water means that the baby will get too few calories and nutrients, preventing proper weight gain, along with a risk of seizures from water intoxication.
  - ❖ *Too much powder* can lead to dehydration, diarrhea or constipation, stress on the baby's kidneys, and excess calories.
- Risk of powder contamination with germs during formula preparation.

Steps for Preparing Powdered Formula

- These formulas come in cans or packets.
- Formula packets have been measured with a specific amount of formula in them to be added with a set amount of water.

- For preparation of powder formulas, use one spoon (provided in the can of powder) for 2 oz/60 ml of water and then mix thoroughly to ensure that there are no clumps of un-dissolved powder in the bottle.

- When pouring the powder, only use the scoop provided in every can (do not use another spoon or utensil for this—it will have the wrong measurement amount).

- Remember, once the can is open, it should be used within one month. Once open, formula powder should be sealed and stored in a cool, dry place (not in the refrigerator).

- The following are steps for preparing powdered formula:

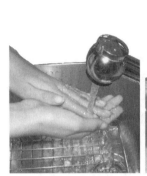 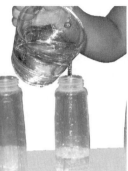 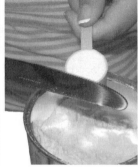 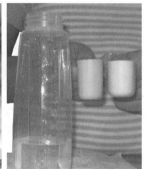

1) Wash your hands with soap.

2) Have all the sterilized items ready.

3) Boil the water for 5 minutes and let it cool to lukewarm water.

4) Check the directions on the can for the correct amount of powder and water needed (e.g., 2 oz/60 ml = 1 scoop; 4 oz/120 ml = 2 scoops; 6 oz/180 ml = 3 scoops, etc.).

5) Pour the water into a clean glass measuring cup.

6) Fill the scoop given in the can with powder and level it with a knife.

7) Add the required number of scoops of powder, according to the amount of water you want to prepare, to the sterilized measuring cup (measure both the formula and water exactly).

8) Mix well.

9) Pour the formula into the bottle(s).

10) Put nipple and caps on the bottle(s).

11) Refrigerate bottles and use them within 24 hours.

12) Warm bottles before use or give at room temperature (either way is good). Make sure to check the temperature by placing a few drops on your forearm before giving it to your child.

13) Discard any remaining formula.

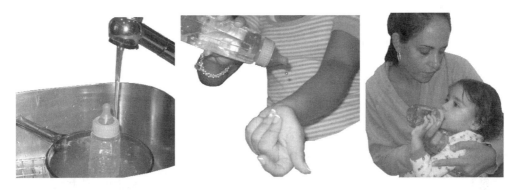

Ready-to-Feed Formulas

Commercially sterile ready-to-feed and liquid-concentrate formulas should be used when available, affordable, and nutritionally appropriate. The powdered form of infant formula should be used when alternative commercially sterile liquid products are not available or affordable. These types of formulas are typically made from cow's milk or a soy base.

Advantages:

- These ready-to-feed formulas provide greater convenience as there is no mixing required. Also, they do not carry the associated health risks of contaminated mixing water or someone mixing the formula incorrectly.

- They are very useful and practical when traveling, or when clean water is not available.

- They can be poured directly into the bottle and refrigerated until needed for use.

- The water/nutrient balance is correct and avoids the possibility of harm to the infant caused by measuring errors during the preparing of powder and liquid concentrate formulas.

- These are better sterilized and thus, more recommended for use if you can afford it (American Dietetic Association).

Disadvantages:

- Most expensive of formulas.
- Once the can is opened, it must be used within 24-48 hours (read the manufacturer's instructions).

Preparation

1) Wash hands with soap.

2) Have sterilized items ready.

3) Rinse the tops of cans with boiled water.

4) Shake the can.

5) Use a sterile can opener.

6) Pour the amount of formula for feeding in the bottle. Do not add water.

7) Put nipple and caps on the bottles.

8) Tightly cover the can if refrigerating the bottles (use within 24 hours) or use right away. It is not safe to leave prepared bottles standing at room temperature for longer than 2 hours.

9) Give it at room temperature or warm (under hot, running tap water) before feeding your baby.

10) Discard any remaining formula.

Liquid Concentrate Formulas

Advantages:

- It is easier to measure and mix than the powder formula.
- It must be diluted with an equal amount of water.
- It is 30-40% more expensive than the powder, but less expensive than the ready-to-use formulas.
- It is poured into a bottle and refrigerated until required for use.

Disadvantages:

- Once the unmixed can is open, it must be used within 48 hours.
- When the formula is mixed with water, it must be used within 24 hours.
- It requires clean boiled water.
- If the water and formula is not properly diluted, it may harm the infant. Too little liquid concentrate of the formula mixed in the water means that the baby will get too few nutrients, preventing proper weight gain along with

other possible risks of seizures from water intoxication. Too much of the liquid concentrate of formula to the appropriate amount of water can lead to dehydration, diarrhea, or constipation, as well as stress on the baby's kidneys and excess calories.

Preparation
1) Wash your hands with soap.

2) Boil the water for 5 minutes and let cool.

3) Have all sterilized items ready.

4) Rinse the top of the can with boiling water.

5) Shake the can well and open it with a sterile can opener.

6) For one bottle preparation, pour an *equal* amount of water and formula (liquid concentrate) into the bottle. To prepare a few bottles, pour the presented amount of concentrated liquid into each sterile bottle and add the presented similar amount of lukewarm water (previously boiled water). For example, 2 oz/60 ml of water for 2 oz/60 ml of can concentrate liquid in the formula preparation.

7) Place all nipples and caps on the bottles.

8) Refrigerate prepared bottles and use within 24 hours.

9) Warm the formula before feeding and shake the bottle when ready to use. Test the temperature before feeding the baby and discard any remaining formula.

Tip: Preparation of a Full Day Supply

You can prepare the necessary bottles for a full day's feeding at one time. As always, all equipment and water must be sterilized. Pour the correct amount of previously boiled water into each bottle. Cap the bottles and keep them in a clean, safe, and protected place. At feeding time, uncap the bottle. Add the measured amount of powder that is appropriate for the amount of water in the bottle, cap the bottle and shake it for 10-15 seconds. You can give it at room temperature or warm it before proceeding to feed.

You can also prepare bottles for liquid concentrate formulas all at the same time and then place them in the refrigerator for the day. Once the formula is prepared, refrigerate the bottles and use within 24 hours. Bottles should be served at warm or room temperature.

continued

Always read the instructions on the label on the can and follow the directions exactly. It will tell you the correct amount of liquid concentrate or powder formula you need to add to each measure of water.

- The nutritional content is the same for all the formulas, if the same one is used.

- The price of powder formulas is cheaper than the prices of liquid concentrate and ready-to-feed formulas.

- In ready-to-feed formulas, the water/nutrient balance is correct and avoids the possibility of harm to the infant caused by measuring errors when preparing powder or liquid concentrate formulas.

Tip: Feeding When Travelling

When traveling, use the ready-to-feed formulas with sterile bottles.

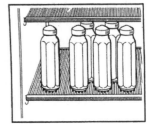

Storage

You must pay attention to how you store your baby's formula and for how long you store it:

- Prepared bottles of formula that are not going to be used immediately should be cooled to room temperature and stored in the refrigerator.

- Keep freshly prepared bottles of formula in the fridge until you are ready to use them for a maximum of 24 hours (including powder formulas).

- Do not keep or re-use left over formula. If your baby always leaves formula in the bottle, put a little less in each bottle next time so that you do not waste formula.

- *Powdered formulas:* Keep the opened can tightly sealed in a cool, dry place (not the refrigerator), and use within one month of opening. Watch the expiry date.

- *Ready-to-use formulas:* Open cans of ready-to-use formulas should be covered, refrigerated, and used within 24 hours.

- *Concentrated formulas:* Open cans of undiluted, concentrated formula should be tightly covered, stored in the refrigerator, and used within 48 hours.

- Do not leave formula in a thermos or bottle warmer.

> ### Tip: Refrigeration Recommendation
>
> Powder Prepared: Store at 35-40 F/2-4 C for no longer than 24 hours.
>
> Concentrate or Ready-to-Feed Prepared: Store at the same temperature as above for a maximum of 48 hours.

Notes on Water in Formula Preparation

- Always use fresh cold tap water to make your baby's formula and boil it only once.
- Do not use the following types of water:
  - ❖ Water that has been repeatedly boiled, or left standing in the kettle.
  - ❖ Water from a tap with a domestic softener attached—the softening ingredients may damage your baby's kidneys.
  - ❖ Water from a tap with a domestic filter attached can trap harmful bacteria and may affect your baby's health.
- The American Academy of Pediatrics agrees that bottled water is okay to use. However, there is no evidence to suggest that bottled water is safer than city water. Bottled water must meet specific FDA requirements for contaminants.
- With mineral water, the sodium and mineral content may be harmful.

Parent Concerns

Do I need to boil the water first when I prepare the formula or boil the prepared formula with water together (e.g., inside the pot)?

- Yes, you need to boil the water first without any formula mixed in. The American Dietetic Association does not recommend preparing formula with boiling hot water due to problems with physical stability of the formula (e.g., clumping or separation) and nutrient degradation.
- When using tap water for preparing formula, use only the cold-water tap. Let it run for about 2 minutes before you use it (lead dissolves in standing water). Using warm tap water may lead to potential lead exposure.

- Most cities use fresh cold-water sources that are quite safe (ask your doctor if your water supply is safe for your baby).

- After you prepare the formula with cold, sterilized water, you may heat the bottle.

Can I switch from ready-to-feed to powder formula?

- There is no harm in switching from one form of formula to another form (while using the same type).

- Most healthy babies are able to accept the change of one form of formula to another.

- Make sure to prepare each formula according to its preparation directions.

Are the different forms of formula the same in terms of nutrition and convenience?

- Nutritionally, all formulas are the same; they vary in terms of convenience and cost.

- Although the most expensive, ready-to-feed formulas provide the greatest convenience of all the formulas.

- Liquid concentrate formulas are reasonably priced and there are fewer mixing errors with this formula compared to powder formula.

- On the other hand, powder formula last up to a month after the can has been opened, making it more convenient for traveling.

How long before a bottle spoils when it is not refrigerated?

- This obviously depends on the temperature in the room and sanitary conditions.

- Generally, formula that has been sitting out and has not yet been given to a baby should be used within 2 hours.

- A bottle that has been partially given to a baby should be used within 1 hour.

Can I use formula beyond its expiration date?

- You cannot use formula beyond its expiration date.

- After formula is expired, vitamin levels change and there are decreased physical properties such as discoloration and separation of fat.

Should infant formula be frozen?
- Infant formula should not be frozen since freezing affects the nutritional quality, sterility, and the physical quality of the formula.

Is it okay to add cereal to my baby's bottle?
- Cereals should not be added to bottles, unless there are medically indicated reasons (e.g., gastroesophageal reflux) and only after consultation with your doctor.
- Adding cereal to the bottle poses risks of choking and excessive weight gain.

My baby is underweight and the doctor advised me to use less water when preparing formula so that she takes relatively more calories. How do I do this?
- Some doctors will advise that you reduce the amount of water in formula preparation to increase caloric intake in your child due to various reasons (e.g., slow weight gain, premature, etc.) for a short period of time while the baby's progress in weight gain is followed.
- For example, if you use powder formula, for every scoop that you usually mix with 2 oz/60 ml of water, use 50 ml of water instead of 60.
- When using ready-to-feed formula, add one scoop of powdered formula to 10 oz/300 ml of ready-to-feed formula.
- In using liquid concentrate, add only 9 oz/270 ml of water to a full can of liquid concentrate for a total of 22 oz/660 ml.
- Increased caloric intake in these cases is usually about 20-24 calories per ounce.
- Your baby's stool may become harder due to formula changes.

How much formula should I be giving my baby?
- You must learn your baby's feeding patterns and know that your baby's eating habits will change as she grow older and is more physically active.
- You know your baby is getting enough formula when she is gaining weight and growing well.
- The following is a general guideline for suggested amounts of formula, however no book can tell you exactly, as it depends on your baby's needs, activity level, genetic tendency, etc. Discuss with your doctor what is appropriate for your baby:

Baby's Age	Formula Amount per Bottle	Number of Bottles
1-2 Weeks	60-90 ml (2-3 oz)	6-10 bottles
3 Weeks – 2 Months	120-150 ml (4-5 oz)	5-8 bottles
2-3 Months	150-180 ml (5-6 oz)	5-6 bottles
3-4 Months	180-210 ml (6-7 oz)	4-5 bottles
5-7 Months	210-240 ml (7-8 oz)	4-5 bottles
8-12 Months	210-240 ml (7-8 oz)	3-4 bottles

Case Description

Sarah is a 3 ½ month old girl who was delivered after a normal pregnancy. She was breastfed and gained weight healthily until the mother stopped breast-feeding and switched to a cow's milk iron-based powdered formula. At this time, Sarah began to be very irritable and ate frequent and larger amounts.

No other associated symptoms such as fever, vomiting, diarrhea, etc., were noticed in Sarah. During a routine examination, Sarah showed normal weight gain for her age, but her urine test showed a low specific gravity (this test indicates how well the kidneys are working). This test is variable, so three follow-up tests were done. All came back low. The doctor asked Sarah's mother to describe how she prepared the formula, and whether she was giving Sarah extra water between feedings.

Sarah's mother explained that she used ½ scoop of powdered formula per 2 oz/60 ml of water, when she was supposed to use one full scoop of powder for 2 oz/60 ml of water.

Tip: Nighttime Bottle Preparation

If you are using powder formula, have the bottle of sterile water ready at room temperature and the formula already pre-measured and in the bottle. This way, all you have to do is pour the water into the bottle, shake it up, and feed.

Have a mini refrigerator in the room and keep a pre-mixed bottle of formula there. When the baby wakes up, take the bottle out of the fridge, shake it well and feed it to your baby at room temperature.

For night use, it is best to use the ready-to-feed formula, since it is the easiest and quickest to serve. Leave the bottle at room temperature and all you have to do is pour in the formula, shake it, and feed the baby.

Warming the Bottle

General

You can give your baby either hot or cold (room temperature) formula. There are no health reasons to warm the formula, nor will room temperature formula result in an upset stomach. Neither temperature is better than the other. However, some babies may refuse cold formula (usually because they are already used to warm formula) while other babies will be happy to take formula at room temperature or slightly cold from the refrigerator.

You save time, especially valuable for those middle-of-the-night feedings, if you accustom your baby to room temperature formula, as you don't have to warm it up each time. This also eliminates the risk of burning your baby with overheated formula.

Babies who are breastfeeding and receive the occasional bottled formula may prefer warm formula, since they are used to breast milk's body temperature. Remember, babies have habits, meaning that they often like things done the same way.

Warming	Not Warming
Advantage Baby preference or comfort.	**Advantage** Less preparation time.
Disadvantage Requires more preparation time. Difficulty when traveling.	Fewer travel concerns. Less concern with leaching of dangerous chemicals from bottle.
If overheated, may leach dangerous chemicals, depending on bottle type.	Nutritional value is not lost through overheating.
Inconvenient for the hungry baby.	Ready to serve for the hungry baby.
Night waking to warm bottle. Risk of burn to baby by overheating formula (especially with microwave's uneven heating).	No microwave risks (uneven heating and burns). No need to warm during the night. No risk of burns.
Overheating of formula can destroy some nutrients.	**Disadvantage** Baby may have room temperature preference.

> ### Tip: Formula Warming
>
> Some experts recommend warming the formula in the first month of life when the baby's ability to regulate body temperature is less effective, as cold formula may cause a drop in the baby's temperature. Warming formula is usually something that is done out of habit.

How to Warm

Warming Formula

Formula can be warmed by:

- Placing the bottled formula in a container of hot (not boiled) water for several minutes, while shaking it occasionally. Lukewarm water is fine.

- Holding the bottle under warm flowing tap water for several minutes.

- Using an electric bottle warmer for a few minutes.

    ❖ Once the bottle is warmed, prevent bacterial growth by using it immediately.

    ❖ After warming the bottle, be sure to shake it well.

    ❖ Check the temperature before feeding your baby. If it is too warm and you need to feed her immediately, cool the bottle under cold tap water. If your baby can wait, allow the bottle to cool on its own to room temperature.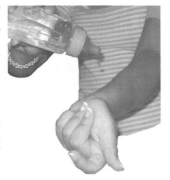

    ❖ Put a few drops of warm formula on the inside of your wrist. It must feel tepid (not hot, not cold) to be suitable for the baby.

Warming Breast Milk

- One should be more careful when warming breast milk in comparison to formula to prevent affecting the milk's composition and hence losing some of its beneficial nutrients and immune factors.

- To warm breast milk, place the bottle in a bowl or pot of warm (not boiling) water.

- Do not shake the bottle; simply move it around a little bit so that it does not lose any of its beneficial nutrients or qualities.

- Do not microwave breast milk since it may kill healthy nutrients, as well as create an uneven distribution of heat.

Microwave Use & Risks

- Do not use a microwave oven to warm your baby's bottle for the following reasons:
    - ❖ It heats the bottle unevenly and it could burn your baby's mouth (e.g., some parts can be cold while others are too hot). You will not be able to detect this by simply feeling the outside of the bottle or using the "wrist test" on the formula.

    - ❖ The bottle or liners may explode after they are taken out of the microwave, especially if the bottle is closed, as the pressure produced inside the bottle may increase and cause an explosion.

    - ❖ Excessive heating may leach chemicals from the bottle or liner into the formula.

    - ❖ Excessive heat in the microwave will damage temperature sensitive proteins and B and C vitamins.

- If, like many parents, you find yourself using the microwave for convenience, follow these steps for safety and nutrient retention:
    - ❖ Help prevent explosions by removing the bottle cap before putting in microwave.

    - ❖ To prevent significantly affecting breast milk's nutritional value, do not heat it past 140 F/60 C.

    - ❖ When you take the bottle out of the microwave, replace the cap and very gently shake the bottle several times, to distribute the heat before giving it the wrist test. Remember, even with these precautions, it is still not a safe practice.

Tip: Reheating Previously Warmed Formula

Do not reheat previously warmed formula. Cold milk (room temperature) may be safer than re-warming. A baby's mouth has germs that can grow in leftover formula and cause infection, especially when reheated.

Parent Concerns

How do I warm the bottle if I am traveling?

- If your baby prefers warm milk and you do not want to serve the bottle at room temperature, bring along a travel bottle warmer or find the means to warm the bottle at your destination. You may also use an insulated container filled with previously boiled water for quick and easy mixing with powder.

> ## Tip: Electric Bottle Warmer
>
> Electric bottle warmers are great for warming bottles at night since they only take about 4-6 minutes to warm the bottle.

There is a concern that plastic bottles made of polycarbonate, could potentially release plastic byproducts when heated. Is this true?

- Scientific evidence supports the safety of plastic bottles, though some results are partly contradictory. In 1999, the FDA released a statement confirming the safety of these plastic polycarbonate bottles (risk concerns include the chemical bisphenol A acting like a female hormone estrogen and interfering with the body's natural process, as well as the risk of cancer, fertility, hormonal effects, male and female reproduction, and altered immune system function). However, some countries are still concerned about these issues and do not favor the use of plastic bottles.

- Given the scientific station of current findings, it is not necessary to stop using baby bottles made of polycarbonate. However, parents who are still uncertain do have the option of changing to glass bottles.

- Bisphenol A in polycarbonate bottles poses no health risk to babies and infants during normal usage. Bisphenol A is a chemical used as the starting material for the production of the polycarbonate plastics. Due to controversy, some suggest replacing the bottle with a glass bottle or replacing these chemicals with safer materials. Overall, many organizations state that, at this point, they are safe for use.

How do I warm refrigerated formula?

- Place it in a container in a pan of warm (not boiling) water on the stove at low heat. Be sure to stir it frequently so that the heat is distributed evenly. For a quick method of warming refrigerated bottles, you may place the bottle under warm, running tap water. If you aren't in a hurry, just leave it out to warm up to room temperature.

In hot weather, should I give cold or warm formula?

- You may feed with either cold or warm formula. In hot weather your baby may enjoy cold formula or chilled expressed breast milk.

Techniques of Bottle-feeding & Related Concerns

General

I f you decide to use the bottle as your feeding technique, do not feel guilty. Each baby is unique and has her own suckling technique. You may need to go through several different styles of bottles and nipples before you find the one that is right for your baby (see *Equipment Used for Formula Preparation & Sterilization*).

As when breastfeeding, make sure you are both relaxed and comfortable. Hold your baby close to give her a feeling of warmth and security, since bottle-feeding is more of a passive action than the process of breastfeeding. Feeding time is a nurturing experience for you and your baby (make sure to keep eye contact and skin-to-skin contact). Let her play with her hands, your fingers, your face, etc.

The first feeding requires some time and patience. While breastfeeding mothers may need an hour or so for the first feedings, bottle-feeding usually takes about 20-30 minutes. Some babies finish quickly when feeding on formula. This is satisfactory as long as you ensure that the nipple hole is not too big (a choking danger).

Techniques of Bottle-Feeding

General Technique

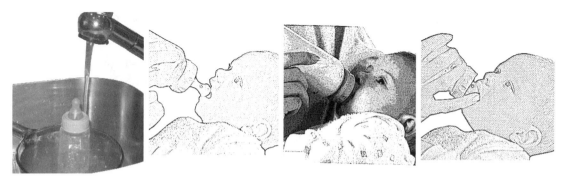

Let your baby know that formula is on its way by stroking her cheek or the tip of her lips with your fingers. This stimulates her *rooting reflex*, prompting her to open her mouth and grasp the nipple

1) Always test the temperature of the milk first.

2) Let a few drops of formula touch the baby's lips.

3) Tilt the bottle so that the formula always fills the nipple completely. Always hold the bottle at the right angle since every bottle system is different (follow instructions).

4) Check the flow of milk (slow or fast):

   ❖ The flow is too fast if the formula drips out of the corner of the baby's mouth (nipple hole is too wide).

   ❖ The flow is too slow if the baby has to work hard and becomes frustrated that hardly anything is coming out (nipple hole is too narrow).

5) Let the baby set the pace for feeding. Allow her to pause to look around or touch the bottle. As the baby get older, she may want to hold the bottle to control its flow.

6) Gently remove the bottle from time to time to let your baby breathe or rest.

7) Learn the signs when your baby has had enough to eat. If your baby is easily distracted after being fed for a while, she is probably finished or almost finished.

8) When the baby is finished feeding, pull the bottle away slowly. Usually, the baby finishes formula feeding in about 10-20 minutes, depending on age, birth weight, etc. When she is finished feeding, slide your finger between the nipple and the corner of her mouth to release the bottle.

9) Do not aggressively encourage the baby to finish the last drops of the bottle. If the baby is drowsing off, do not reawaken her to finish feeding.

10) If the baby is sleeping during a feeding, sit her up with her back upright for a couple of minutes, then offer more formula and see if she takes it.

11) When the feeding is over, throw the remaining formula out. Babies' mouths have germs which can grow in the leftover formula (especially when reheated). Do not use formula that has been out of the refrigerator for more than 2 hours.

12) Make sure your baby is not taking in too much air and that she is not just chewing on the nipple (unable to suck effectively). Suckling technique will change as your baby grows.

13) Never prop up the bottle, as it is may lead to choking, feeding problems, and dental issues.

14) When bottle-feeding in public, try to find a quiet place where you are comfortable. To prevent your baby being distracted, cover your shoulder with a blanket—as though you were breastfeeding.

Tip: Burping

Burping may be done during or after the feeding session (see *Burping: Tips & Tricks*).

Mother's Position

- Make sure your back is properly supported.

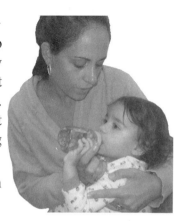

- It is probably more comfortable for you to sit in a chair with an armrest or a pillow underneath the arm so that your arm will not interfere or disturb the baby while she feeds. You can even place your young infant comfortably on a pillow so that she is facing you and you have a free hand to touch her.

- Do not feed your baby if you are lying down flat, because of the risk of choking.

Baby's Position

- Cradle your baby securely in a semi-upright position with support for her head.

- Hold your baby's head higher than the rest of her body to prevent the milk from backing up.

- Holding the baby in your arms is the best way to establish bonding.

- Change sides midway through feeding to promote greater eye stimulation and development.

How to Bottle-Feed a Breastfed Infant

The following are suggestions of how to bottle-feed a breastfed infant:

- Feed on demand rather than on schedule (cues indicate hunger).

- Feed your baby in an upright position so that she does not feed lying down.

- When breastfeeding, you switch sides from one breast to the other. As such, when you are bottle-feeding the breastfed infant, switch from one side to the other side to prevent side preference upon resuming breastfeeding.

- Do not push the nipple of the bottle into your baby's mouth. Rather, let her draw the nipple into her mouth so that she continues to control the feedings. To elicit a rooting response in a wide-open mouth, caress the baby's lips with the nipple of the bottle.

- To mimic the breastfeeding experience, take frequent pauses.

- Use bottles with nipples that are closest in shape to the breast.

Tip: Signals to Stop Feeding

The following are signals that your baby is ready to end the feeding session:

Baby gets sleepy.

Stops sucking.

Turns head away from the bottle.

Closes lips tightly.

Throws the nipple away.

Cries.

Shows their own individual signs that they are finished feeding.

If, by week three or four, your full term baby sucks poorly, feeds slowly, or stops for a long pause, notify your doctor, as this may signal other problems.

Babies with Special Needs

General

- Feeding babies with special needs (e.g., premature babies, low weight for gestational age, specific congenital disease, neuromuscular disease, syndromes, etc.) can be a challenge.

- If your baby was diagnosed at birth with a special need, then you will most likely be shown how to feed your baby or you will have a special team of health professionals to help you.

- A few examples of children with special needs will be discussed later. Situations which are not discussed here can be followed up with your doctor.

Feeding Babies with Cardiac Problems
- Cardiac problems can range from very mild to very serious.

- Despite your hard work and persistence, the baby with serious heart problems may not gain weight well. This is frustrating for many parents.

- Some factors which interfere with your baby's growth in these cases include increased respiratory breathing, poor appetite, greater caloric needs, easy fatigue and decreased food intake, frequent lung infections, and poor nutrient absorption, etc.

- These babies may gain weight slowly, despite taking enough calories from the bottle or breast, due to increased caloric needs.

- It is important to be flexible with feeding methods and schedules for babies with heart problems (both breast and bottle-feeding works well).

- Some babies may require feeding supplements to help with the weight gain, and some even require feeding tubes (breastfeeding supplements can be given via lactation aids—see *Latching & Positioning*).

- Feed more often and on demand as these babies tire quickly. You may need to wake your baby up at night several times until she is able to tolerate a larger volume of milk and feed less often.

- Some of these infants do best with a combination of breast and bottle-feeding. Bottle-feeding may provide more flexibility, particularly if your baby stays in the hospital for treatment after birth.

- The "work" of breastfeeding is actually less than the "work" of bottle-feeding in these cases, since sucking, swallowing, and breathing are easier for a breastfeeding baby to coordinate (your baby's oxygenation remains better when breastfeeding than when bottle-fed).

- If your baby is still not gaining weight well and is unable to tolerate an increased volume of formula, then increasing calories and/or heart surgery may be suggested by your doctor/heart specialist. This will result in a faster growth rate or "catch-up" period.

Feeding Babies with Cleft Lip and/or Palate
- When a baby is born with cleft palate or combined cleft lip and palate, sucking is a more difficult task.

- Typically, a baby needs to position her lips and tongue around the nipple or artificial teat and create both suction and compression during sucking to feed well.

- These babies may have milk escape from the nose during a feeding, especially if the nipple flow is fast. They cough and spit up more often and need to be burped more frequently. They also feed slowly and can show failure to properly gain weight.

- The following table outlines the three types of cleft lip and/or palate and feeding issues:

Cleft Lip	Breastfeeding and/or bottle-feeding is possible (breast tissue fills the gap where the cleft exists and there are no problems with suction or compression since the palate is intact).
Cleft Palate	Most babies cannot generate suction during feeding sessions. Lack of suction makes it difficult to breast or bottle feed efficiently. Feeding is a lengthy and tiring process. Baby may not gain weight well. Presents greater obstacles to breastfeeding; babies feed more effectively with a palatal obturator, a device that fits in the baby's mouth and covers the cleft.
Cleft Lip & Palate	Difficulties compressing the nipple or artificial teat due to an insufficient palate (roof of the mouth) and gums for the tongue to compress the nipple or artificial teat. Compression is important in helping the baby draw the milk out of the breast and/or bottle during sucking.

- *Breastfeeding:*
  - ❖ Babies with cleft lip and/or palate are usually breastfed due to the absence of suction and, in some cases, compression.
  - ❖ Sometimes, babies with a cleft lip or palate are able to extract some milk by compressing the breast between their jaws.
  - ❖ Mothers may also express breast milk into a bottle.

- *Bottle-feeding:*
  - ❖ There are bottles and nipples for babies who cannot generate a suction technique and/or compression during feedings.

Feeding Babies with Neuromuscular Problems

- Due to the baby's weak muscles and depending on the severity of muscle weakness, she may be unable to drink easily from a bottle and may need special feeding techniques or even a tube to feed with until the muscles become stronger.

- Examples of neuromuscular problems include Down's Syndrome, Prader-Willi Syndrome, etc. Babies with these conditions are hypotonic (floppy) at first. They have difficulty latching when breastfeeding and have poor sucking reflexes.

Feeding Low Birth Weight Infants

- These babies have limited stomach capacity and as such, are unable to take very much at each feeding. Feed your baby small frequent feedings and provide concentrated formula (a higher calorie formula than standard formulas) or breast milk to increase caloric intake.

- Feeding is a difficult and tiring challenge, especially if your baby has the associated lung disease of premature babies.

- Babies with gastroesophageal reflux and aspiration, who are gagging and/or coughing after every feeding, require the help of a feeding therapist.

- If you are breastfeeding, place your baby on the breast after let-down has occurred.

- If you are bottle-feeding, make sure the milk flow from the bottle or artificial teat is not too slow or too fast (change hole sizes as needed).

- Some mothers combine breast and formula feeding. Some babies can switch easily from one to the other, while others will have a preference to use the bottle and do not want to take the breast.

- Babies with low birth weight have limited reserves of fat, protein, and other nutrients. As such, breastfeeding may not offer your baby optimal nourishment; in these cases, combined breast milk and formula may be suggested by your doctor.

Discontinuing the Bottle

- Currently, the average age of bottle weaning is about 15 months. Don't stop the bottle until your baby is at least one year old, but don't continue bottle use after 18 months.

- Despite these recommendations, 20% of two year olds and 9% of three year olds still use the bottle.

- Use of a bottle past the age of one year may cause negative effects on their teeth and interfere with consuming important nutrients. The bottle can then become a security object. Keep in mind that the longer children use a bottle, the greater chance they have of being overweight (at risk of obesity). This risk increases by 3% after the age of 15 months.

- As long as the baby takes her liquids from a cup, there is no need to continue use of the bottle.

- Eliminating the bottle is not initially easy. Begin by eliminating the mid-day bottle first, then the evening and morning bottles. The bedtime bottle should be the last to go.

- Do not give the baby a bottle when she wakes up at night.

- For further details, see *Weaning* for information on cup use and how to wean from a bottle to a cup.

Parent Concerns & Tips

What about feeding when the baby is on heart medicine?

- The medications given to control heart function (Digoxin, Furosemide, etc.) do not interfere with feeding.

- It is best to give medications before a feeding, using a syringe or dropper placed directly in your baby's mouth.

- Do not mix any medications in the formula bottle as your baby may not finish it.

- If your baby becomes ill, feeds poorly, or vomits, etc., your baby's medicine should then be adjusted, as per your doctor's instructions.

Tip: Nasal Obstruction and Feeding

Babies, especially in their first year, are nose breathers.

In their first few months (or when they have a cold), they may have nasal obstruction.

If they have a nasal obstruction they will have difficulties feeding when the mouth is "blocked" with a bottle (or breast).

Use saline (0.9%) nose drops to relieve this obstruction (a temporary relief), especially before a feeding, so the baby may feed more easily.

Can I breast and bottle-feed my baby?

- Yes, you can bottle-feed and give expressed milk by the bottle (when you are at work or out, etc.). Use the method described in *Combining Breast & Bottle* to ensure the best feeding method. Be aware of the risks of nipple confusion, etc., if you breastfeed and start bottle-feeding.

Can I use the bottle to feed cereal?

- Feeding cereal in a bottle is not recommend due to choking risks, over-consuming foods leading to obesity, etc. You would need to enlarge the nipple hole in the bottle (see *Cereals* and *Starting Solids*).

Is it okay to thicken formula given in the bottle?

- Your doctor, in the case of babies with gastroesophageal reflux or slow weight gain, may recommend thickening formula in the bottle.
- Formula thickening may interfere with the transition to solid foods. It is probably better to feed small amounts frequently and carefully follow your child's weight gain.
- If it is done, it is important not to thicken the formula excessively, as this may provide increased calories and decreased nutrient intake from other foods.

Recently, my baby cries every time she takes the bottle. What can I do?

- The first question to be asked is if there were any feeding changes recently. For example, has the bottle or nipple been changed? Has the formula been changed? Feeding equipment or methods that have been changed recently may be the cause of your baby's crying after feedings.
- You should check to ensure that the formula is not coming out of the bottle too fast or too slow—a normal flow is one drop per second, at first.
- If the nipple seems to be the problem, then change the nipple to one with an appropriate flow.
- It is also important to assess whether the crying occurs only occasionally during feedings or with each feeding.
- Gastroesophageal reflux may also be a cause for crying since food comes back through the esophagus causing pain and discomfort in your baby.
- Also, formula intolerance may cause your baby to be fussy (with no other symptoms). If your baby is on cow's milk or another formula, discuss with your doctor regarding the use of other formulas (e.g., soy, etc.).

Tip: *Ensuring Comfort*

If you hear a lot of noise coming from your baby while she is feeding, it probably means that she is taking in excess air. When this is the case, hold your baby at a 45 degree angle to decrease air swallowed.

Some babies like to be held in a nursing position while drinking from the bottle. Others find the position disconcerting. Use what your baby prefers or likes.

If your baby is a lazy eater, drip a few drops into her mouth to stimulate her to start nursing.

Do not give a bottle while your baby is in her crib, due to various complications and risks, including the risk of dental cavities, increased risk of asthma (especially if there is a family history), and wheezing development—the baby feeding while lying down causes reflux of the food.

Is there an age limit on bottle-feeding at night?

- To establish a good sleeping pattern, some experts recommend that your baby should not be fed at night after six months of age if she is gaining weight well and growing normally.

- Some babies (especially breastfed infants) may still want to feed at night. If both you and your baby are happy feeding at night, then you may continue to do so, especially if your baby is not gaining weight well, or other problems exist.

- If your baby wakes up and cries at night for a feeding, this may be a manifestation of a sleeping behavior problem. Discuss this concern with your doctor to ensure that nothing else (e.g., ear infection, etc.) is causing your baby to wake up at night. Your doctor can also give advice on how to deal with sleeping related behavior difficulties.

I try to burp my baby in the middle of a bottle-feeding session, but she fusses and wants the bottle. What do I do?

- Not all babies need to burp in the middle of a feeding session.

- Babies are burped when they are young infants. As the baby gets older, she becomes more efficient and may not need to burp at all.

- You should know your baby's behavior and her needs to burp. Some babies are excited when feeding and may get upset when you stop a feeding in the middle.

When will my baby hold her bottle on her own and when should bottle use be discontinued?

- Babies usually begin to hold the bottle on their own around 4 months of age and begin to "feed themselves."

- Begin the use of a cup as early as possible when your baby is holding the bottle on her own and is feeding herself. This teaches the baby to prefer the cup and avoids the problems associated with bottle-feeding after 18 months.

- Formula can be offered after 1 year of age instead of switching to cow's milk, but try to offer it in a cup rather than a bottle. If you do offer it in a bottle, then make sure you do not give any other drinks (e.g., juice) in the bottle to decrease your baby's dependence.

- If your baby seems to use the cup easily, then let her use it more than the bottle.

- The more your baby feeds on her own, the more you will miss the bonding experience that goes along with feeding (and there are always choking risks involved in self feeding).

My baby is a slow feeder and has sucking and swallowing difficulties. What should I do?

- Your baby may require more than an hour to take few ounces of milk and seems not to know how to suck or use her tongue. Saliva may accumulate in your baby's mouth and constant drooling may occur. The baby may be choking or gagging on the formula or breast milk.

- A child with congenital cardiac problems can feed slowly, tire quickly, sweat, etc.

- Difficulties in sucking and swallowing may be the first indication of a neuromuscular problem or other conditions associated with the baby being floppy.

- Many other causes may lead to a slow or poor feeder. In these cases, you must see your doctor immediately, especially if you notice any other abnormalities.

My baby gags when she bottle feeds. What does this mean?

- If your baby seems to be gagging or gulping too fast, then it may mean that the nipple hole is too large (change nipple size if this is the case).

- Sometimes, the baby gags if she has a large amount of food in her mouth, or dislikes the food taste or texture, etc.

- Some babies are born with a strong rooting reflex and have troubles during feedings such as gagging. The gagging reflex continues throughout life to protect against airway blockage.

- Consult your doctor if there are any other abnormalities you notice.

Tip: Bonding

Encourage your partner to bottle feed your baby for the bonding experience.

Tip: Traveling

When you are traveling by plane, giving your baby a bottle when taking off is a great way to stop her ears from popping. Also, remember to pack more bottles than you think you will need, since you never know if the plane will be delayed. The flight attendants will refrigerate any extra bottles, if asked.

Feeding By Schedule or On Demand: Amount & Frequency

General

The amount of formula or breast milk taken varies with each individual and unique baby; her size, activity level, whether she is breast or bottle-fed, infant growth stage, etc. As your baby grows, you will understand and recognize your baby's eating habits (i.e. cries for hunger, etc.). There are often parental questions about whether to feed a baby by schedule or on demand. However, no book can tell a parent how much and how often their unique baby needs to be fed. Typically, breastfed newborns feed about 8-12 times per day and this amount reduces to 6-8 feedings around 2-3 months of age. Bottle-fed babies do not normally feed as often as breastfed infants.

If you feed your baby every time she seems hungry, you are *feeding on demand*. This is a feeding schedule set by the baby, according to her hunger. *Feeding by schedule* is when feeding sessions are planned. The baby is fed at fixed times.

Whether you feed your baby on demand or by schedule, you should always feed her whenever she is hungry. No matter which method works better for you and your baby, the basic point is that you must feed your baby whenever she is hungry, and give her enough breast milk or formula so that she gains weight appropriately.

Clues Your Baby Is Ready to Feed

- Babies may show feeding cues for a while before starting to cry.
- You need to watch your baby for clues that she is ready to feed such as:
  - ❖ Agitation (head moves side to side).
  - ❖ Fussiness/anxiety.
  - ❖ Follows the bottle with "envy."
  - ❖ Tongue or lip movements (a sign that she wants to suck; e.g., sticking out her tongue).
  - ❖ Sucks on her hand or makes sucking motions.
  - ❖ Crying (late sign of when the baby is hungry).
  - ❖ Fists are in the mouth or clenching.

❖ Opens mouth when skin around lips is touched.

❖ Squirming and/or whimpers.

❖ Nuzzling against mother's breast.

- The sleeping baby may show feeding cues even before she wakes (e.g., tosses and turns, suck her hand, fussy, etc.). At some point, your baby will cry for a feeding session.

- Watch your baby for these clues before she begins to cry, since crying may cause your baby to have uncoordinated sucking motions, making it more difficult for you to initiate a feeding session.

Baby's Personality & Nursing Style
- Each baby has a distinct personality and nursing style that will be learned quickly by the mother, regardless of feeding method (on demand and/or by schedule).

- Nursing styles include:

❖ Approaching the breast eagerly.

❖ Feed frequently or less often.

❖ Finish feeding sessions in short periods of time, etc.

- Whatever nursing style your baby has, allow her to dictate her feeding needs. As long as she is gaining weight well and growing normally, the feeding method does not really matter.

- See *Techniques of Bottle-feeding & Related Concerns* for signals on when to stop a feeding session.

Feeding By Schedule or On Demand
Feeding By Schedule
- Feeding on a schedule means your baby is fed every few hours according to her age and weight. You can make a schedule by seeing when your baby feeds every day.

- The amount given at each feeding is determined and affected by the baby's unique needs, weight and hunger, etc.

- Remember that a feeding schedule should not be rigid, but should be somewhat flexible in response to your baby's cues and needs.

- Some infants are naturally more regular in their biological hunger than others. Many irregular babies thrive on a more flexible schedule.

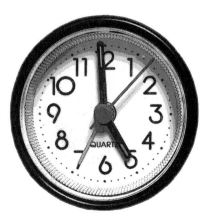

- In the first two weeks of a baby's life, the baby should be woken up to feed about every two to three hours, until feeding is well established. Some babies are more vigorous and will wake up earlier to feed. Others get tired quickly (after the work of feeding) and sleep longer. In this case, you need to wake up your baby and feed her small amounts frequently (if you are breastfeeding, it will stimulate more milk production). If your baby sleeps longer than four hours in the first month and begins to miss feeding times, you may need to wake her up and offer her the bottle or the breast, unless she is healthy and gaining weight well.

- As time progresses, your baby will begin to develop a more regular feeding timetable and may establish her own schedule (naturally becoming feeding on demand).

- There are many reasons why babies cry, so do not assume she always cries because of hunger. You will eventually be able to differentiate a hunger cry from other cries. If your baby's cry changes dramatically, or there are sudden changes in her behavior which concern you, consult your doctor.

- Some babies initially feed better at night—this is normal and it will reverse over time.

- If by the fourth month, your infant is still hungry despite frequent feedings, have a discussion with your doctor regarding your baby's weight gain and the early introduction of solid foods.

- If the baby demands frequent formula feeding and has good weight gain, try distracting her with playtime or give her some water in-between scheduled feedings. She might eat more at the next feeding and be satisfied for a longer period of time.

- Feeding by schedule allows for predictability and security for parents (especially new parents). However, it is not always possible to follow a schedule.

Feeding on Demand
- Feeding on demand means that every time your baby seems hungry, she is fed.

- This is the best and healthiest way to feed a baby, especially with breastfeeding (although probably not in the first month, as you will need to wake up your baby and initiate feedings, as previously discussed).

- A feeding schedule should always be flexible enough to respond to obvious hunger cries.

- There is no definite answer as to whether a baby who is no longer a newborn should be fed on demand or by schedule.

- If you are breastfeeding your baby on a rigid feeding schedule, it may interfere with successful breastfeeding and may put your baby at risk for slow weight gain.

- Remember that breast milk is produced on a supply and demand basis (the more you nurse, the more your body will make).

- In the first weeks of life, frequent unrestricted feedings are crucial to healthy milk supply and the successful establishment of breastfeeding.

- The American Academy of Pediatrics state that babies (especially breastfed infants) need to be fed on demand rather than by schedule. Interference with the baby's feeding cues may lead to slow or poor weight gain, failure to thrive, low milk supply, etc.

- Again, each baby is unique and what works for one may not work for another. Many parents find a middle way that is comfortable for them.

- By three months, many babies have established a pretty regular daily routine of waking up, staying awake, playing, napping, and feeding. Some may just wake up, eat, and sleep. This can vary from day to day for some babies.

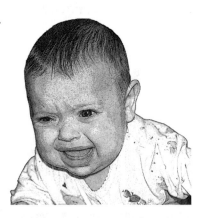

- Feeding on demand allows for the baby to eat according to her appetite, ensuring her nutritional needs are properly met. However, some babies (e.g., premature) may not have the strength to demand feedings.

Tip: Prematurity and Feeding by Schedule or Demand

Some small or premature babies do better on feeding by schedule, since they are found to have less colic, regurgitation, etc.

Feeding Amount & Frequency

Amount & Frequency

- One of the most confusing things when feeding your baby formula is trying to work out how much to feed. There is no single answer for this as it depends on the baby's age, weight, rate of growth, spitting up, and other factors.
- Here a few helpful hints to help you decide how much your baby needs:
  - ❖ Multiply your baby's weight in lb/kg by 2.5-2.7 oz/28-32 ml of formula. If the baby is not eating any solids, the general rule for formula amounts is 2.5-2.7 oz/28-32 ml per lb/kg of body weight. For example, if the baby weighs 6 lb/2.7 kg, she should consume about 15-16 oz/480-500 ml of formula in a 24-hour period.

  - ❖ Consider your baby's age, as the amount of formula your baby needs depends on more than body weight. For example, when starting a full term newborn on formula, try giving about 2-3 oz/60-90 ml at each feeding for the first week. You will soon be able to sense if your baby needs more or less formula.

  - ❖ Do not let solids replace formula too soon. Breast milk or formula should continue to make up most of your baby's nutrition until they are six months old. Complementary foods should start around six months of age.

  - ❖ Let your baby be the guide. Appetites vary, and most babies change their appetites from day to day and month to month.

- The following table gives an *approximate* amount of formula to offer your baby. This is in no way direct and specific for all babies. However, this table will provide you with a general idea of feeding amounts. Consult your doctor about what amount is appropriate for your particular baby.

Age	Feeding / Day	Quantity per Feed
Birth to 1 Week	6-10 feedings	60-90 ml (2-3 oz)
1 Week to 1 Month	6-8 feedings	90-120 ml (3-4 oz)
1 Month to 2 Months	6-8 feedings	120-150 ml (4-5 oz)
2 Months to 3 Months	5-6 feedings	120-180 ml (4-6 oz)
3 Months to 6 Months	4-5 feedings	180-210 ml (6-7 oz)
6 Months to 9 Months	3-4 feedings	180-230 ml (6-7.5 oz)
9 Months to 12 Months	3-4 feedings	210-240 ml (7-8 oz)

Is My Baby Feeding Enough?

At times, you may wonder whether or not your child is receiving enough nutrients to develop properly, especially since babies' appetites frequently change. Here are some factors to help you have an idea of whether your baby is feeding enough (assuming she is a healthy, full-term baby):

- Look at the age and amount to be taken and shown in the previous chart and assess the frequency of your child's feedings.

- In general, a few dirty diapers might be (but are not necessarily) an indication of proper feeding; pale or water-colored urine suggests adequate hydration while darker (apple juice) colored urine suggests that the baby is not getting enough milk. It is easier to judge the wetness of a disposable diaper by comparing its weight to a dry diaper, than by the way the surface of the diaper feels to the touch.

- Orange crystals found in a wet diaper are not signs of adequate fluid intake or dehydration. These are from over-concentrated urine, which is a normal finding, especially in the first few days, but may occur also within the first month. It is not an uncommon occurrence among breastfed infants, during the period that the quantity of colostrum that the baby drinks is low. However, some consider it a sign of slight dehydration if it occurs after 4-5 days, once your milk begins to increase, as the baby should be able to consume sufficient volumes of milk to produce clean urine.

- Other possible signs of underfeeding include:
  - ❖ The skin remains wrinkled in the first month of life.
  - ❖ The baby's face does not seem to fill out.
  - ❖ The baby is unsatisfied, even after a complete feeding.
  - ❖ The baby is hungry quicker than expected.

If you are concerned as to whether your baby is feeding enough, visit your doctor for a growth/weight assessment.

Periods of Growth Spurt

- Growth spurts commonly occur around three weeks, six weeks, and three months of age.

- A baby who had not previously eaten much at night may start waking up and feeding more often to support this increased rate of growth.

- Try not to give formula if you are breastfeeding, as this may keep your breast milk supply from increasing to meet your baby's needs. The resulting lack of breast milk is a common reason why some mothers stop breastfeeding. If you are unsure about the adequacy of your milk supply, consult your doctor.

- Sometimes, the baby will begin to demand more daytime feedings when she begins to sleep through the night. This is usually temporary. If it persists more than a week, it is a good idea to check your baby's weight gain and discuss it with your doctor.

Illness & Feeding

- Many illnesses are associated with a loss of appetite, especially if they are related to the digestive system.

- Extra calories are consumed by your child's fever, or lost with vomiting or diarrhea. This may temporarily affect your child's growth.

- For most brief or minor illnesses, no special diet is necessary, especially if the digestive system is not affected.

- If your baby refuses feedings, do not push or force her. When she begins to recover from the illness, her appetite will return (some children with stomach flu take a while returning to their previous appetite and do best if offered frequent small amounts to drink till they have improved).

- Discuss with your doctor to see if a specific illness requires a change in diet.

- If you (mother) are ill and breastfeeding, it's usually best to continue nursing, as the antibodies in your milk transfer to the baby, boosting her immune system and making the illness milder if she becomes infected.

Tip: Reversal Day & Night Feedings

From the beginning, some babies will sleep a lot during the day and feed more at night. Others feed more during the day.

It is normal for a newborn to feed at night. Within a few weeks, most babies will gradually adjust to more feedings during the day. By the age of 3-4 months, the baby may not need night feeding (yet breastfeeding may still require 1-2 night feedings).

continued

You may be able to improve your baby's sleep by offering more during the day and less at night, until the baby can sleep through the night without any feedings (obviously not for newborns). Try the following:

Naptime during the day can be limited; wake her up to play, feed, change a diaper, massage, talk to, etc.

Distinguish between day and night to produce less stimulation: no noise, keep voices low, no playing, turn off the lights, no television, and no diaper change at night, unless it is necessary.

Nurse more frequently during the day and/or increase the amount of formula offered during the day.

Stretch out the times between feedings at night and gradually decrease the volume of night feedings.

Parent Concerns & Tips

Is it normal for breastfed babies to feed more frequently than bottle fed babies?

- It is not uncommon for many nursing babies to feed more frequently than bottle-fed babies but this is normal and usually does not mean that your baby is not getting enough to eat. If your baby is growing well, you can rest assured that they do not need any supplements.

How often should I make my baby's bottles?

- Some parents make a bottle before every feeding, while others choose to make up several bottles at a time and refrigerate them for up to 24 hours before they are used.

My baby seems to be hungrier than usual lately. Is this normal?

- As stated earlier, a baby's appetite can vary from day to day. As your baby grows older and gains weight, she will probably begin taking more at each feeding and will be able to go longer times during feeding sessions (see *Growth Spurts*).

If I choose to feed on demand, then does that mean that I have to feed my baby every time she cries?

- Babies cry for various reasons and, with time, you will learn what each cry means. Sometimes, your baby simply wants to be held and comforted, while at other times she may be uncomfortable because she was overfed. Eventually, you will learn your child's hunger cues and evaluate the situation before deciding to feed her (e.g., if you just fed her and she cries, she may need to burp, etc.)—see *Crying & Fussing in Relation to Feeding & Nutrition.*

Tip: Formula Feeding & The 32-Ounce/1 Litre Rule

Most experts agree that your baby (older than six months of age) should not be fed more than 32-40 oz/1000-1250 ml of formula.

If your baby wants more than this limit, offer her a bottle of water instead.

If your child is younger than six months of age, it is better to give a bottle than solid food.

Section 3:
Breast & Bottle-feeding: Combination & Weaning

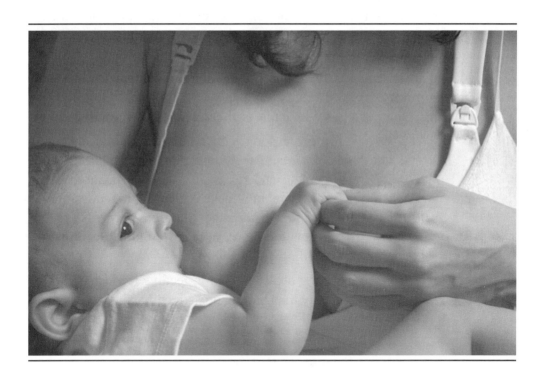

Combining Breast & Bottle-feeding

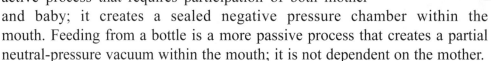

General

Bottle-feeding and breastfeeding are two completely different feeding methods, regardless of any attempts to make bottle-feeding more closely resemble breastfeeding. Suckling from the breast is an active process that requires participation of both mother and baby; it creates a sealed negative pressure chamber within the mouth. Feeding from a bottle is a more passive process that creates a partial neutral-pressure vacuum within the mouth; it is not dependent on the mother.

You do not always have to choose between breastfeeding and bottle-feeding. It is possible to combine both methods, but it is preferable to begin with breastfeeding, as it is easier to switch from breastfeeding to a bottle than the reverse. Mixed feeding allows you to continue breastfeeding while replacing a few feedings with expressed breast milk or formula.

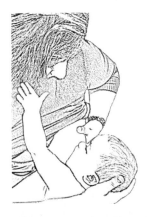

There are some concerns when bottle-feeding a breastfed infant, including nipple preference, breast engorgement and its associated complications (e.g., mastitis), sore or cracked nipples, a reduced milk supply, and a shortened duration of breastfeeding that lessens the nutritional and immune benefits that breastfeeding gives your baby.

Mixing breast and bottle-feeding is much better for your baby than halting breastfeeding altogether (some breast milk is always better than none).

Reasons to Combine Breast & Bottle

Combined breast and bottle-feeding may be needed when the following situations arise:

- The baby is losing weight, perhaps because he is not breastfeeding properly, is not receiving enough milk, was born with malformation (e.g., cleft lip palate), is gaining insufficient weight (e.g., poor prolonged breastfeeding), or does not open his mouth wide enough to achieve a deep latching technique (e.g., dysfunctional suckling).

- The baby has low blood sugar, failure to thrive, dehydration, and/or refuses the breast.

- The mother experiences true low milk supply (see *Low Milk Supply*).

- The mother has to return to a demanding full-time job, has to be separated from her baby for a length of time, needs a short break from breastfeeding, or lacks the desire to breastfeed any longer.

- Drugs that the mother is taking affect breastfeeding.

- The mother or baby has a serious illness. Some mothers are too ill to breastfeed immediately after birth, have extremely sore nipples, or had breast surgery in the past (depending on the seriousness of the problem).

- Not enough breast milk to satisfy twin or multiple babies.

Tip: Pumping Milk

Pumping or expressing breast milk may result in decreased milk production, difficulty re-introducing the breast, etc., and it requires extra time.

When to Start

If you need to introduce the bottle, it is recommended to introduce the bottle to a breastfed infant no earlier than 5-6 weeks of age, if possible. However, each baby is unique and the timing of bottle acceptance varies with each case.

When to Introduce the Bottle to a Breastfeeding Infant

Earlier than 5-6 weeks	Not recommended, since milk production may not be well established yet and breast milk supply or production may be affected.
	Baby may prefer the bottle over the breast, because feeding is easier (milk flow is easier from the bottle than breast).
	Greater risk of nipple preference/confusion.
	Less difficulties for bottle acceptance (especially when starting from day one).
Later than 5-6 weeks	Delay the start of a bottle until after 5-6 weeks of age if you want to breastfeed for a long period of time.
	Less risk of nipple preference.
	Breastfeeding has already been established at this stage.
	May have more difficult transition to bottle acceptance (baby may have developed preference for the breast).

- If you are returning to work and your baby is older than 3-4 months of age, you can smooth the transition and accustom your baby to the bottle by gradually introducing the bottle a few weeks before you begin work (maintain breast milk supply by pumping milk and/or initially using a minimum amount of bottles per day).

- To prevent nipple confusion, it is helpful to use a supplemental nursing system like a feeding cup, medicine dropper, or a spoon to feed your baby instead of a bottle.

Tip: Introducing the Bottle

There is no right time that you must introduce the bottle when combining it with breastfeeding, since you do not know how your baby will respond. For some babies, it is better to start before the age of five weeks, while for others, starting later may ease bottle acceptance. Babies being babies, there is no guarantee of a successful combination at any age.

How to Enhance Bottle Acceptance for Successful Combination Feeding

- Delay using formula until breastfeeding has been well established (usually about three to five weeks).

- There is no single, perfect method to begin supplementing the breast with the bottle.

- The best you can do is to make the process as gradual and natural as possible.

- Begin with giving the bottle instead of breastfeeding at one regular feeding every day, and slowly increase bottle use after a few days.

- Select a nipple with a long shank, wide base, and small holes (ask your doctor or midwife about the varieties available in your region if you have any confusion).

- Select a nipple that most closely resembles the breast nipple.

- Many babies prefer the latex nipple, as it is easier to suck on.

- There are various flow speeds; slow flow nipples most closely reflect the flow speed of breast milk, so they are a better choice for combination feeding. Flow speeds vary between slow, medium, or fast flows—you know that the hole is too big when formula is pouring out in a stream.

- To use the nipple and the bottle correctly, do the following:
  - ❖ Position the nipple fully in the infant's mouth (about 1 in/2.7 cm).
  - ❖ Hold the bottle as horizontally as possible while still keeping the milk in the nipple, so that the baby will have to suck to get the milk out (gravity will not increase the flow).
  - ❖ Offer skin-to-skin contact.
- When combining breast and bottle-feeding, you should use those nipples which most closely resemble the breasts' nipples. Ultimately, whichever nipple you do use will be the choice of you and your baby.
- Resistance to feeding from bottles is rarely a problem in babies younger than a month old.
- Some refuse the formula in the bottle, because breast milk is sweeter, while others refuse what they are not accustomed to.

Here are a few tips on how to get your baby to bottle feed:
- If you are bottle-feeding a newborn, use a *slow flow nipple*. If the flow is too fast, your baby may get frustrated and inpatient, as he has to work harder to swallow the milk.
- Try offering the bottle when your baby is not starving. If your baby is hungry and in a "bad" mood because of it, he may not be so willing to try something new.
- Have someone else offer the bottle. Your baby associates your smell and touch with nursing, and may insist on the real breast if you try to give him a bottle.
- Many babies associate the cradle hold position with nursing, especially newborns. Although some babies will accept the bottle in the cradle hold position, most do better at bottle-feeding if you prop them up on your knees or in an infant seat.
- Offer small amounts from the bottle at first.
- Some babies do not like cold nipples in their mouth, so run the nipple under warm water before you offer it.
- Do not force the bottle into your baby's mouth. Tickle the baby's lips gently until he opens his mouth and takes the nipple.
- Try to bottle feed your baby when he is sleeping. Hold him in a nursing position and feed him a bottle, even if it is only for a little while.

- Avoid giving a bottle where you breastfeed, since the baby associates the location with the feeding method.

(See *Overcoming Bottle Rejection in Breastfed Babies* for further suggestions.)

Relactation

Relactation is the process of returning to partial or exclusive breastfeeding.

- It can successfully occur days, weeks, or months after lactation has ended.

- Dedication, a good milk supply, and a "good baby" will permit you to switch the baby back to breastfeeding alone.

- Generally, the shorter the duration of bottle-feeding, the better the chances of relactation. Milk supply can be re-established with regular stimulation (metoclopramide has been used to assist mothers; however, it is neither necessary nor appropriate in all cases).

- The younger the baby, the greater the likelihood that he will be willing to suckle at the breast (especially if the baby has been previously breastfed).

- It is important that the mother realizes that reality may not follow or meet her expectations of relactation. Mothers should not be disappointed or feel guilty if they are unable to relactate.

- A successful transition from partial to exclusive breastfeeding can be aided by:

    ❖ Pumping your breasts after a breastfeeding session to boost milk production.

    ❖ Gradually halting bottle-feeding. As milk production increases, use less formula.

    ❖ The use of lactation aids, as these may be helpful in the transition period.

    ❖ Halting breastfeeding if your baby is crying. In this situation, offer the bottle and try again at the next feeding.

    ❖ Remember, if you do not succeed with full relactation, any amount of breast milk that you can give your baby is good for him.

- For relactation, consult a lactation specialist.

Parent Concerns

Which formula should I use when I decide to combine the breast and bottle?

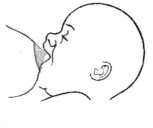

- There is no specific, recommended formula when introducing the bottle in combination with breastfeeding.

- Use the same type of formula that you would have chosen if you had planned to only bottle feed.

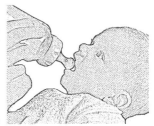

- Talk to your doctor about the best choice of formula for your baby.

Is there such a thing as nipple confusion?

- Young infants fed with a bottle may begin to prefer the bottle, because of the faster milk flow that takes less effort than breastfeeding. Some babies who have begun on the bottle may refuse breastfeeding, a situation called nipple confusion or nipple preference.

- Nipple confusion can occur due to combining breast and bottle-feeding, breast and pacifiers, the age of your baby at weaning, whether or not breastfeeding is established, etc.

- If a baby needs help because of slow weight gain, nipple confusion can be prevented by using alternate feeding methods to avoid artificial nipples. *It is important to remember that the bottle is not the only tool available to supplement feeding.* You may use cups, spoons, feeding syringes, nursing supplements, or bottles. These supplements may involve lapping by the young baby and sipping by the older baby.

- It is important to remember that each baby is unique and will respond differently to combining the breast and the bottle (not every baby is confused, but it is difficult to know in advance how your baby will respond).

Can I mix breast milk and formula in the same bottle?

- Some health professionals do not recommend mixing breast milk with formula in the same bottle.

- It is better to give each one separately (starting with breast milk) so that breast milk does not go to waste if your baby does not finish the mixed bottle.

Tip: Disadvantages of Supplementation

A mother's breast milk production usually decreases with less nursing. Pumping the breasts is a great way to increase breast milk supply.

The baby will receive less of the protective nutrients that breast milk provides.

Weaning

General

*W*eaning from the breast is when you begin to give your baby foods other than breast milk. Most parents define weaning as stopping breastfeeding altogether, which is not necessarily the case. It is a gradual, natural stage in the baby's development. Normally, the need to breastfeed declines as the baby increases his solid food intake, thus leading to the weaning process. Babies wean at different ages; you and your baby will find the right time for this process.

Weaning your baby from the breast is a very personal choice and a time of mixed emotions. Both mother and baby may feel excited by this new freedom and yet, at the same time, feel sadness as they move on to a new stage in the baby's life. Remember that the baby is achieving the milestone of eating solids and feeding from new utensils.

The Right Time to Wean
General

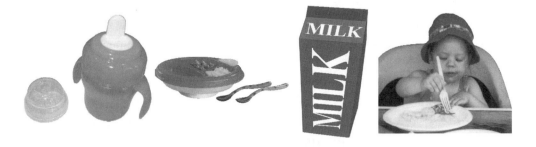

The decision to begin the weaning process depends on what is right for you and your baby. No one else should decide.

- Many mothers assume that the weaning process should begin when the child is one year old, as he does not need to breastfeed any longer. However, breastfeeding is encouraged beyond one year of age, for as long as mutually desired and as long as all nutritional needs are being met.

- Weaning is an individual process and depends on various factors such as work obligations, family support, cultural background, the baby's health status, solid food feedings, etc.

- The simplest, most natural time to wean is when your child initiates the process.

- Resist comparing your weaning situation to other babies and keep in mind that you have provided the best start for your baby by breastfeeding, no matter how early or late you decide to stop (some breastfeeding is always better than none).

Tip: Nipple and Breast or Bottle-Feeding

A bottle with a slow flowing nipple may help diminish the difference between the breast and the bottle.

Weaning During the First Year

- If the weaning process begins before your baby is one year of age, you may need to supplement and/or replace the breast milk with infant formula.

- Common reasons for weaning babies before the age of one year include returning to work, difficulty expressing breast milk or keeping up with the baby's milk needs, if the mother must be away from home for long periods of time, a new pregnancy, job constraints, an increasing lack of desire to breastfeed, concerns about the baby's growth, baby's teeth beginning to erupt, wanting the spouse/caregiver to administer feedings, etc.

Weaning Between 1 & 2 Years of Age

- Both the American Academy of Pediatrics and Canadian Pediatric Society recommend exclusive breastfeeding for at least the first 6 months of life before introducing solid foods (see *Starting Solids*). After 6 months of age, human milk alone will no longer supply all of your baby's nutritional requirements. The iron stores present from the time of birth in the infant are slowly diminishing. Thus, it is appropriate to begin iron-containing solid foods at this time. Delaying the introduction of solid foods beyond the age of 6 months can put your baby at risk for iron and other nutrient deficiencies.

- At one to two years of age, some babies can be more receptive to weaning, as their increased mobility and freedom often distracts them from the breast. Mothers can use this to their advantage and wean with little fuss.

- Waiting until your baby is 18-24 months of age to complete the weaning process helps protect toddlers during a period of frequent infections and illnesses (the breast milk contains an increased concentration of antibodies at this stage of development). This is a great way to relax and reconnect with your toddler.

Tip: Weaning to a Cup

Older breastfed infants can wean directly to a cup.

Weaning Beyond 2 Years of Age

- When your child is older than two years of age, you can discuss the weaning process with him, as he is able to verbalize his feelings.

Types of Weaning and How to Wean from the Breast

Gradual Weaning

- Slow or gradual weaning is the best since it happens naturally and is the least disruptive to both mother and baby.

- The slow weaning process allows time for your baby to adjust to the bottle or cup and have various people involved in his feeding process.

- The gradual weaning process can be described as the *substitution process:*

  ❖ Substitution is usually a process that is recommended when the baby is not very hungry, as this helps ease the weaning process.

  ❖ Begin by substituting one feeding per day with a replacement feeding, starting with the least "favorite" one (e.g., midday meal) of both mother and baby. Usually, the second last one to give up is the one first thing in the morning (typically the best volume of milk production). The last one to give up is the bedtime feeding, because of the comforting factor for both baby and mother.

  ❖ Wait a few days in-between each new feeding before substituting for another breastfeeding session. If your baby refuses the bottle (or cup, spoon, syringe, etc.), try again at the next feeding or the next day. You may introduce it gradually over several days.

❖ Continue to gradually replace breastfeeding until your baby is nursing only once a day (allow the feedings to decrease gradually to help keep you from getting engorgement). Your breasts may feel uncomfortable when beginning to wean, so express just a little for comfort, if necessary.

❖ Begin to skip days between breastfeeding sessions until nursing is eventually stopped. Follow your child's developmental lead and do what is best for both of you.

- Appropriate replacement feedings depend on how old your baby is when he starts to wean. After 1 year, your baby usually should not take much more than 16 oz/500 ml of cow's milk or formula per day. Otherwise, he may not want to eat solid foods and may also develop iron deficiency anemia.

Talk to your doctor about the appropriate formula for your baby, especially if your baby is not yet a year old. Also, look at the replacement feedings suggested below as to what to do after weaning:

- If your baby is feeling frustrated or unhappy with the weaning process, provide him with distraction, extra attention or cuddling (especially at feeding time). Be patient, as some babies make the transition smoothly while others take a little longer.

Replacement Feeding Suggestions

Age	Feeding
Less than the age of one	Continue to give iron-fortified formula.
12 - 18 Months	Use full fat milk (homogenized) as this is needed for proper development. Do not give 2% or low-fat milk.
	If your baby prefers formula, then keep using it instead of milk.

Tip: Helping Your Baby Wean

Change your daily routine. If you have a certain time or favorite chair that your baby associates with breastfeeding, change the usual routine so that he will not be frequently reminded to nurse.

Have the father and/or caregiver take care of your baby at bedtime or nighttime (in case your baby associates nighttime waking with breastfeeding).

Offer your baby substitutions and distractions. When your baby asks to nurse, offer a glass of water, a book, or a favorite activity to get his mind off of nursing.

Continued

Weaning does not have to be an "all-or-nothing" process. Many mothers choose to wean only in the day or night.

If your child continues to nurse for longer than you had planned, do not interpret this as a sign that he is immature, lacks self-confidence, or is overly dependent on you. Instead, you can be reassured that your baby values breastfeeding sessions and finds security and comfort from cuddling during sessions.

Abrupt or Emergency Weaning

Abrupt or emergency weaning means that you stop breastfeeding immediately. It is not recommended, as it may be upsetting to your baby and is usually uncomfortable for you. Avoid abrupt weaning, if it is at all possible. However, abrupt weaning can be necessary for various medical reasons such as when you have to take certain drugs (e.g., chemotherapy, etc.), which are not compatible with breastfeeding.

When weaning abruptly, your breasts will respond by becoming engorged, so express just enough milk so that your breasts do not feel so full, to avoid developing a breast infection or breast abscess. Also, hormone levels drop abruptly, and depression may develop as a result. Support for both mother and baby during this period of time is important for feelings of security and comfort.

Tip: Illness and Weaning

The onset of sudden illness in your child is not a reason to begin the weaning process, as you can pump and store breast milk until your baby is able to accept it again.

Similarly it is not advisable to wean abruptly in cases of mastitis, as you may develop a breast abscess. The milk is still good for your baby, even though you are uncomfortable.

Sudden weaning is difficult for you and your baby, so if you wean suddenly for whatever reason, take the following precautions:

- If your milk is considered safe for your baby, but you cannot breastfeed, pump a little milk to avoid engorgement. This milk can be given to your baby.

- If you are requiring tests where you are taking a medication not compatible with breastfeeding, you can "pump and dump" your milk, until it is considered safe to resume breastfeeding.

- If you must take a medication, long term, that will require you to stop breastfeeding, take analgesics and express enough milk as required for comfort (you can use cold gel packs, cold cabbage leaves, etc., to help relieve engorgement).

- Wear a comfortable, supportive bra and consult your doctor if your breasts become hard and tender (watch for signs of plugged ducts which may lead to mastitis and abscess).

- A mother sometimes needs several days between dropping a feeding or pumping milk before she drops the next feeding or pumping. It depends on the volume of milk she is currently producing.

- If you become ill, take your prescribed treatments and follow up with your doctor.

- Abrupt weaning can be particularly hard on a baby, unless he initiates the sudden stop.

- When weaning between six to nine months, use a cup or bottle (whichever your baby will take).

- If your baby is too young to take a cup, you may need to try several different types of nipples. If your baby has been using a pacifier, choose a nipple similar to the shape of the pacifier.

- If your baby doesn't seem to like the taste of formula, and your milk is considered safe, your breast milk can be mixed with the formula to help him adjust.

- In cases where a mother is hospitalized for surgery, it can often be arranged to have the baby brought to the hospital by a family member for breastfeeding (when the milk is safe). The family member cares for the baby. If the baby cannot be brought to the hospital, a mother can pump her milk and send it home for her baby. Check with the hospital regarding its policy.

- If the baby initially refuses any other foods offered by the mother, it is often helpful if another caregiver feeds the baby.

- Give a lot of attention and cuddling for comfort.

Tip: Decreasing Breast Milk Production

Binding your breasts is not recommended since it may lead to blocked ducts and more discomfort. Talk to your doctor as he may not recommmend Bromocriptine (Parlodel) which is a prolactin suppressant due to reported adverse drug reactions (seizures, strokes, and death).

Natural Self-Weaning

- Self-weaning is when babies decide to stop breastfeeding at some point of time (see *Nursing Strike*). Natural weaning most often occurs around two years of age, but some babies wean earlier.

- This baby-led type of weaning is due to a lack of interest on the baby's part, as they mature and become more interested in their environment and physical activities.

- Many mothers want to wean the baby by one year of age, often because they are uncomfortable with having their older baby tugging at their top to nurse when they are with other people, or because of the negative reaction from family and friends who disapprove. Teething is another reason women give for wanting to wean.

Partial Weaning

- Partial weaning is a natural stage in your baby's introduction to solid foods.

- It is for the mother who wants to continue breastfeeding, yet is unable to provide all feedings by breast (e.g., returning to work, etc.).

- You can choose to express milk to be given to your baby when you are unavailable to breastfeed, or you can have the caregiver give formula while you are away. Your body will adjust to less production during working hours if you start pumping smaller volumes of milk. When you return home, you can breastfeed your child.

- If your baby does not like the taste of formula, you can mix it with breast milk, starting with mostly breast milk and, as he gets use to it, increasing the amount of formula until he is drinking all formula.

Tip: Weaning and Maternal Changes

Some women report that after weaning their babies, they experience improvements in their moods, sexuality, and feel less fatigue.

Weaning from the Breast to a Cup

- When your baby is less than nine months of age, he may wean from the breast to a bottle and then to a cup. However you may introduce the cup as early as six months of age.

- Some mothers prefer breastfeeding until the baby can drink from a cup, avoiding bottles altogether. Other mothers choose to breastfeed for a longer period of time, until the baby himself decides to stop breastfeeding.

- Initially, you may offer breast milk in the cup and then formula. After your baby is one year of age, you may offer whole cow's milk.

- Follow the gradual weaning process to allow your baby time to adjust to the gradual decrease of breast milk. You can begin offering small amounts of formula and gradually increase it until, one at a time, you slowly eliminate breastfeeding sessions. As your baby increases his intake of solid foods the need to breastfeed declines.

- When you have reached the stage where your baby takes 16-20 oz/480-600 ml of milk in a cup and three solid food meals, then the weaning process is considered to be successful.

> ### Tip: Weaning and Bottle Supplementation
>
> Babies who have had frequent bottle supplementation from an early age tend to wean themselves earlier than other babies. This is why it is recommended to avoid bottles for the first 6 weeks, so as to encourage breastfeeding for at least six months, at which time the baby's immune system is more developed. A baby who has never been given a bottle until three to six months of age may not take one easily.

Weaning from a Bottle to a Cup

- When weaning from a bottle to a cup, it is important to remember that the longer one waits in introducing the cup, the harder it is for your baby to give up the bottle.

- Prolonged use of the bottle may pose an increased risk of tooth decay, obesity, etc.

- In order to make the transition from bottle to cup, replace a bottle with a cup once a day. Then wait a few days before replacing more bottles.

- The first bottle to abandon is the midday bottle, then the morning bottle; the hardest to give up is the bedtime bottle.

- Slowly begin to offer water in the bottle and milk, formula, or juice from the cup. If your baby is under the age of one, place less formula in the bottle and offer a cup with milk or juice (see *Cup Use*).

Tip: Bottle Refusal & Alternatives

If your baby refuses the bottle, try the following tricks:
- Have someone else offer the bottle without the mother in the room.
- Try a different type of bottle nipple.
- Try starting a feeding session with the breast and switching to a bottle half-way through the feeding.
- Movement sometimes calms a baby and distracts them enough to be able to take the bottle. Gently bounce your baby by walking around the room or sitting in a rocking chair.
- Watch the milk flow, as a fast milk flow from the bottle may overwhelm your baby. Some babies enjoy a fast flow of milk (see *How to Overcome Bottle Rejection*).
- There are alternatives to the bottle when weaning from breastfeeding such as a cup or spoon. Whole milk and/or solid foods can be given, depending on the baby's age.

When Weaning Is a Problem

- Your baby refuses to eat any solids after the age of six months.
- Your baby has anemia that has been confirmed by a blood test, because he does not take enough iron-containing supplement food.
- Your baby develops cavities from excessive nursing time.
- Your baby is obese from overeating.
- Your baby wakes you too frequently to feed during the night. Your baby is unable to stay with a babysitter, because he will only breastfeed.
- To prevent weaning from becoming a problem, try these tricks:
  - ❖ Try to get your older baby on a schedule of three main meals per day, plus two or three nutritional snacks. When your child wants additional feedings, provide him with extra cuddling, holding, and attention to give him the secure, comforting feeling he may long for.
  - ❖ Also, introduce cup feeding using breast milk, if this was not already begun at six months of age. It is a way to avoid having to wean from a bottle later, and it will make it easier to wean from the breast when the time comes to do so (see *Cup Use*).

Parent Concerns

When should I wean my premature or low birth weight infant?

- Weaning pre-term babies to complementary foods often causes confusion in both health professionals and parents alike.

- It is advised that these babies should be weaned according to their post-natal age rather than their "corrected" age. This is because gut maturity relates more to their actual age.

What type of formula should I use when weaning from breastfeeding?

- This should be discussed with your doctor so that she may recommend a formula that is appropriate for your child.

Do I need to keep offering vitamin D now that I have weaned to formula?

- After having completed weaning from breastfeeding to formula, you do not need to offer any additional vitamin D (unless recommended by your doctor because of premature birth, low birth weight, or other concerns).

- Once your baby has begun on complementary foods and formula, additional vitamins (including vitamin D) are supplied within these foods.

Should I wean from the breast because I am pregnant?

- Women are able to continue nursing while they are pregnant—and they are able to conceive while they are still breastfeeding.

- The mother who is deciding whether to continue nursing during her pregnancy has several factors to consider: her medical history, her physical and emotional comfort level, the nursing child's age, and his need to nurse. If the pregnancy is progressing normally, then the decision of whether to continue to breastfeed is more an individual "parenting" decision, rather than a "medical" decision.

- Each case is unique, and breastfeeding while pregnant must be discussed with your own obstetrician or health professional.

- Nursing during pregnancy will not deprive the fetus of essential nutrients, and nor will it create a harmful "drain" on the mother's body. During pregnancy, it is always important to eat nutritiously, gain weight appropriately, and get adequate rest. A well-nourished mother should have no problem providing enough nutrients for both her unborn baby and her nursing child.

Should I start weaning once my baby has teeth?

- When your child has teeth, it does not necessarily mean that it will cause discomfort for you.

- Keep in mind that not all children bite while they are nursing. However, if you are uncomfortable, change positions more frequently.

- If your child does bite, it is usually because they are teething. You can end the feeding and give a substitute feeding.

- Remember that most children stop biting quickly; it does not mean that you have to stop breastfeeding altogether (see *Biting the Breast*).

Tip: Weaning

Meat and iron-fortified weaning foods should be introduced early to increase iron and zinc intake (e.g., dairy products, meat, rice, wheat, etc.).

The change from breast milk or formula to cow's milk should be made after the age of one year.

Introduce one new food at a time, and leave a few days between each new food.

Persevere with a particular food when it is refused upon first offer.

Do not rush feeding sessions with your baby.

Because of the choking hazard, never put solid foods in a bottle.

If your baby is reluctant to use the spoon, you can use a clean finger with a small amount of food on it to feed him.

Be prepared to continue breast or bottle-feeding if your baby refuses any solid foods.

Will my baby develop cavities from excessive nursing time?

- It is not very common for a baby to develop cavities from excessive nursing time.

- Breastfeeding is usually less of a problem than bottle-feeding at night, because the breast is drawn deep into the baby's mouth, which stops the teeth from soaking in pools of milk.

- There are a few references of an increase of dental caries in breastfed babies over 2-3 years of age who spend long uninterrupted periods at the breast, or breastfeed at night after 6 months of age. Some of these references mention that some babies will develop "dental disease" after the introduction of solids that contain sugar, and that dental caries is also thought to be an inherited trait. Prolonged nighttime feedings and exposure to breast milk may then become a risk factor.

> ### Tip: *Weaning Difficulties for older baby/toddler*
>
> Weaning from breastfeeding may cause withdrawal difficulties for your child (will only increase his desire to breastfeed). Redirect or distract him with new foods or different interactions during his usual breastfeeding time. This is a more positive and effective way to help him (especially good for the toddler age). If your child still wants to nurse, offer the breast, as this will reassure him that you are still there for him.

Overcoming Bottle Rejection in Breastfed Babies

General

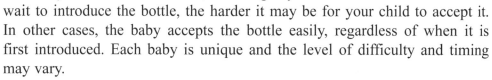

B reastfeeding mothers can breastfeed until it is time to wean. Sometimes, the mother may want or need to combine both the breast and the bottle, or switch entirely to bottle-feeding (expressed breast milk or formula).

Breastfeeding is sometimes associated with bottle rejection. In some cases, the longer you wait to introduce the bottle, the harder it may be for your child to accept it. In other cases, the baby accepts the bottle easily, regardless of when it is first introduced. Each baby is unique and the level of difficulty and timing may vary.

While suggestions to overcome bottle rejection may work for some parents with their babies, it may not work for others. Do not let bottle rejection become a fight. Time and patience are sometimes required when helping your baby overcome bottle rejection, especially with the stubborn baby. For the sake of successful breastfeeding, it is usually better to introduce the bottle once breastfeeding is well established (after four weeks of age). However, if the bottle is started much later than four weeks, your baby may initially reject the rubber or plastic nipples; he knows he likes and what he doesn't like. He'll let you know if he prefers the breast by crying and rejecting the bottle.

Overcoming Bottle Rejection

Here are some tips to improve accepting the bottle, if your baby was previously breastfeeding:

- Consider dropping nursing sessions gradually as a prelude to dropping them altogether.
- Feed when the baby is hungry, or when he is in a good mood (depends on the baby).
- Offer the bottle casually between nursing. Babies may consider it as a snack and not as trying to cheat them out of the breast.

- Get someone else to give the first bottle to your baby when you are not around, at least until the bottle has been established.

- Serve your baby the bottle when he is sleeping, and gradually give the bottle during the day.

- Do not force or make a big issue of it if the baby does not want the bottle right away. Wait and try another day. Be stubborn and continue to try using the bottle.

- If your baby is older, allow him to play with or hold the bottle before he eats.

- Avoid nursing cues such as pulling your baby onto your lap, uncovering the breast in front of him, etc.

- Try using formula or dilute apple or white grape juice instead of water. You may try breast milk in the bottle first—it works for some and not so well for others, but it does remind the baby of the breast milk taste.

- If the bottle is rejected and your baby is old enough, try offering him a sippy cup (see *Cup Use*).

- Be sure to use the right nipple on the bottle. For example, if your baby uses a pacifier, use a similar nipple or change it if the baby "does not like it." Offer a nipple that closely resembles the breast nipple such as the Adiri nipple (see *Nipples*) or try a colorful bottle.

- Try different types of nipples and different sizes of holes. Experiment with various types until you find one that your baby likes.

- Try tilting the nipple into the back of the roof of the baby's mouth, since he will be more likely to accept it this way. You may also tickle the baby's lip with the nipple and allow him to draw the nipple into his mouth. Do not force the nipple into his mouth. If he becomes frustrated, end the session and try again the next day to avoid creating an association of distress with this new feeding method.

- Feed your baby while you are sitting on a bouncing or rocking chair—it may help ease the acceptance of a bottle.

- It sometimes works to distract your baby while you are giving him the bottle.

- If your baby is more than four months of age, try mixing cereal with formula to get your baby used to its taste and texture. Serve the bottle with formula alone afterwards, as he may accept it more easily this way.

- Try serving your baby a sweet formula, since he is used to the sweet breast milk taste, and gradually dilute the formula.

- When feeding your baby with the bottle, try turning him on his side or in a breastfeeding position that he used during the time of breastfeeding, to make the bottle more inviting.

- Warm the bottle, since some babies will not like taking it cold or at room temperature. You may also try warming the nipple along with the bottle (be sure to check the temperature of the milk as well as touching the nipple, before feeding it to your baby by dripping a few drops on your forearm to make sure it is not too hot).

- Make sure whoever is feeding your baby, whether it be you or someone else, is comfortable while feeding. The baby will feel more relaxed and secure.

- Remember, overcoming bottle rejection requires patience, so keep trying and don't get too frustrated. Be aware of your baby's cues and respond accordingly.

Tip: Defeat of Introducing the Bottle

Defeat is when you have tried to use the bottle once every few days for several weeks.

If defeat is your reality, alternate your breast with a cup which can serve to administer other foods.

Remember that the baby can be fed in other ways. Try using a cup (even when your baby is very young), spoon, or eyedropper.

Discuss with your doctor and/or lactation consultant about any possible alternatives to feeding your baby.

When lactation is going well and you have no reason to use a formula bottle, you do not need to use a bottle. Formula may interfere with your breast milk supply and create other problems.

Section 4:
Starting Solid Foods

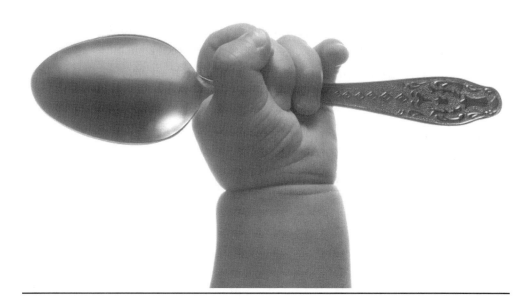

Nutrition at a Glance:
An Age Appropriate Guide to
Feeding Your Baby & Toddler

General

Infants and toddlers grow at a very fast rate, both developmentally and physiologically. It is very important to give your child the right nutrients (and the right amount of them) for normal growth and development.

Breast milk or formula is all your baby needs for the first few months of life. However, as your baby grows, it is important to start a variety of complementary healthy foods at the appropriate time for proper growth and good eating habits for life.

Feeding your baby is the most important thing you can do, but your love, attention, and cuddling are just as important as the feeding itself.

Use *Nutrition at a Glance*'s feeding guide to ensure proper nutrition through every developmental stage from birth to three years of age.

Sequence of Food Introduction

0-4 Months
- Breast milk: Frequent feedings (5-10); baby takes less as she grows.
- Iron-fortified formula: 5-10 per day (16-32 oz/480-960 ml).

4-6 Months
- Breast milk: Frequent feedings (greater than or equal to 5 per day).
- Iron-fortified formula: 4-7 per day (24-40 oz/720-1200 ml).
- Cereal (iron-fortified): Start cereal between 4-6 months (see recommendations); begin with two to three teaspoons of dry rice cereal mixed with breast milk, formula, or water (give once or twice per day and progress to two to four tablespoons twice per day).

6-9 Months
- Breastfeed on demand (greater than or equal to five times per day).
- Iron-fortified formula: About four feedings (24-32 oz/720-960 ml).

- Cereal (iron-fortified): Begin cereals and 2-4 oz/60-120 ml of vegetables or fruits once per day; introduce other grain products (e.g., dry toast, crackers, biscuits, etc.).

- Fruits & vegetables: 1/4-1/2 cup/125-250 g of fruits and vegetables per day; pureed, mashed (e.g., banana, peach, pear, avocado, carrots, squash, sweet potato, etc.), or strained vegetables (yellow, green, orange vegetables), then fruits (or fruits then vegetables); begin with 1 teaspoon and gradually increase to 4-6 tablespoons per day.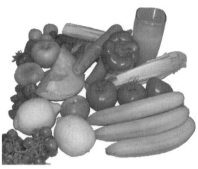

- Protein (egg yolk, pureed meat, poultry, tofu, mashed beans, lean meat, chicken—chewed, chopped, or small tender pieces).

- Dairy (cheese, yogurt, cottage cheese): 1/4-1/3 cup/60-85 g of dairy foods per day.

9-12 Months
- Breast milk (on demand) or formula: 3-4 times per day (16-32 oz/ 480-960 ml).

- Cereal (iron-fortified) and bread (dry toast, unsalted crackers, biscuits, bagels, rice, barley, oats, wheat and mixed cereal, unsweetened hot or cold cereal): 2-4 servings per day (1 serving = 1-2 tablespoons) = 4-8 tablespoons per day (1/4–1/2 cup/60-125 g iron-fortified cereal).

- Fruits and vegetables (banana, peach, pear, avocado, carrots, squash, sweet potato—peeled, soft fruit wedges, and fresh fruits; vegetables can be cooked, mashed, fresh, frozen, or raw if chewed well): 1-2 servings per day (1 serving size = 1-2 tablespoons).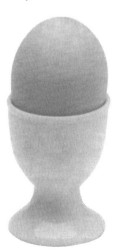

- Protein (lean meat, chicken, or fish, egg yolk, yogurt, cheese, cooked dried beans, mashed beans, tofu; strained, chopped, or small tender pieces): 1-2 oz/30-60 g; you may offer unsweetened juice from a cup (but it is better to give water).

- Dairy (cheese, yogurt with 3.25% milk fat or higher, cottage cheese, grated cheese 1-2 tablespoons per day); combination foods (macaroni and cheese, casseroles).

12-24 Months
- Breast Milk: On demand or 2-3 feedings per day.
- Milk and Alternatives: 2 servings per day; whole milk, yogurt, cheese, cottage cheese; 1 cup/250 ml milk, or 1 1/2 oz/45 g of cheese or 3/4 cup/175 ml of yogurt per serving.
- Grain Products: 2 servings per day; cereal, pasta, rice, bread, muffins, rolls, crackers; 1/2 cup/125 ml of cooked pasta or 1 oz/30 g cold cereal or 3/4 cup /175 ml hot cereals or 1 slice of whole bread per serving.
- Fruits: 3 servings per day; medium fruit, or 90 ml/3 oz of juice (if any) from a cup per serving.
- Vegetables: 3 servings per day (fresh or cooked); ½ cup/125 ml fresh, frozen or canned vegetables per serving.
- Meat and Alternatives: 1 serving per day; fish, chicken, turkey, beef, pork, cooked beans, peas, eggs; lean meat and poultry 2 1/2 oz75 g/1/2 cup/125 ml, or cooked legumes 3/4 cup/175 ml per serving.
- Fats & Oils: Not limited at this age.

3-8 Years
- The following is the recommended daily serving for children aged 3-8 (the smaller portion range is for 3-4 year olds and the larger portion range is appropriate for 5-8 years of age). An example of an equivalent of 1 serving per day is shown for each food group.
- Milk and Alternatives: 2 servings per day; 1.5 oz/45 g cheese, 3/4 cup/175 ml yogurt, and 1 cup/250 ml whole or low fat milk or fortified soy beverage per serving.
- Grain Products: 3-4 servings per day; 1 slice bread 1 oz/35 g, 1/2 bagel 1.5 oz/45 g, 1/2 cup/125 ml cooked pasta or rice, or 1 oz/30 g cold cereal per serving.
- Fruits and Vegetables: 4-5 servings per day; 1/2 cup/125 ml fresh, frozen, or canned vegetables, 1/2 cup/125 ml cooked vegetables (broccoli, peas, mashed potatoes, etc.), 1 cup/250 ml of raw vegetables, 1 medium size fruit , 1/2 cup/125 ml of 100% juice per serving (if any).
- Meat and Alternatives: 2 servings per day; baked or cooked legumes 3/4 cup/175 ml, cooked fish, poultry, or lean meat 2.5 oz/75 g, 1-2 tablespoons of peanut butter, 2 eggs per serving.

- Fats & Oils: Should be limited to 2-3 tablespoons of unsaturated fat each day. This includes oils used in cooking, salad dressing, margarine, and mayonnaise. Use vegetable oils such as canola, olive and soybean. Limit butter and margarine.

*Refer to the websites for appropriate recommendations for healthy eating.

General Tips by Age Group
Birth to 4 Months
- The baby is able to suck, swallow, and protrude her tongue.

- Breastfeeding, iron-fortified formula, or both supply the infant with all the necessary nutrients for the first four months of life.

- Some babies are able to sleep through the night by three months of age. By four months, the eating and sleeping routine are better established and feeding should be "*on demand*" to avoid overfeeding.

- Infants have a rooting reflex, which allows them to search for their food source (e.g., turning towards the nipple for nourishment) and they have a very sensitive gag reflex.

- You may need to burp your baby during or immediately after a feeding, or not at all (see *Burping: Tips & Tricks*).

- Stools at this age vary with breast and formula feeding. Initially, the breastfed infant will have frequent stools with almost every feeding. At two to three months of age, stool frequency decreases. With the formula-fed infant, there are less stools per day (see *Stool Characteristics & Feeding*).

- At this age, your baby may feed two to three times at night, with the rest of the feedings occurring during the day (some babies will feed more at night until they are adjusted to feeding in the day).

Tip: Introducing Solid Food Early

Some parents introduce solid foods earlier than four months of age and, while some babies are able to handle it, it is not recommended. Usually, the child's first reaction will be to spit out the food placed on her tongue, since she still has the natural gag reflex. Your baby's digestive tract and kidneys are still immature and your baby may respond with adverse events (e.g., allergy, etc.).

4-6 Months
- This stage of the infant's life is the *transition period* to starting solid foods (see *Starting Solids*).

- Although the baby can developmentally start solids at this age, it is better to start around six months, since solid foods are not yet nutritionally required and this allows the digestive system to mature (see *Starting Solids* and recommendations for when to start solid foods).

- Your baby's growth rate at this age is slow, but her increased activities increase her need for more energy.

- The tongue thrust and gag reflexes lessen by this age.

- A cup may be offered to your child at about six months of age, although she will likely spill and make a mess of her food.

- If you breastfeed exclusively, then it is recommended to continue breastfeeding until six months of age before starting solids. If you are formula feeding, you may start with iron-fortified cereal between four to six months of age to supplement increasing iron requirements (the iron in breast milk is absorbed better than the iron in formula).

- Introduce a commercially prepared iron-fortified rice cereal as a first solid food since it is easy to digest and least likely to cause an allergic reaction. Later, you may add other grain cereals (oats, barley) to your child's diet, one at a time.

- Use a spoon when feeding your child cereals. Do not feed cereal with a bottle; it is a choking hazard.

- As your baby gets older and develops her eating skills, you can gradually thicken the cereal's consistency by using one tablespoon of mixed cereal and one tablespoon of breast milk or formula (texture should be thick and soup like).

- Infant cereal can be used until your child reaches 18-24 months of age and then you may switch to adult cereal.

- After introducing cereal, you may introduce vegetables or fruits.

- At this age foods should be semi-liquid purees, blended and smooth with no lumps, peeled carefully, cooked/steamed, or boiled and pureed.

Tip: Food Refusal

Your baby may not accept solid foods at the first attempt.

Do not get discouraged; simply offer it again to your child in a few days.

Studies have shown that repeated exposure to foods is needed to enhance food acceptance.

6-8 Months

- Babies are able to manage more textured foods. Food pieces should still be soft and easy to chew.

- You may begin to introduce strained or mashed-textured soft baby foods, beginning with vegetables or fruits.

- Homemade prepared foods or commercially prepared jar foods may be used.

- Your child can be placed in a high chair at the table towards eight months.

- Use fresh or frozen fruits (peaches, pears, prunes, apricots, plums, bananas, apple sauce, and nectarines) or vegetables (squash, sweet potato, avocado, well-cooked carrots, peas, green and yellow beans, broccoli, and cauliflower), or buy strained commercial baby foods.

- You can serve mashed or coarsely pureed cooked fruits or vegetables.

- Introduce each new food, one at a time, when your baby is happy, sociable, and in a good mood.

- Do not use fruits with small seeds such as grapes until at least 24 months of age.

- Watch out for strings in fruits and vegetables such as banana, mango, and broccoli, etc.

- Some babies can handle bread (remove the crust) and baby cookies by seven months of age.

- Foods can be minced or mashed to the texture of cottage cheese. Fruits and vegetables should be peeled carefully and pureed or steamed (with removed ends). Meat must be skinned and have the fat trimmed; it may be poached, cooked, grilled or minced finely (remove all bones).

Tip: Allergies

If there is family history of allergies, speak to your doctor before introducing solids to your child.

8-10 Months

- This age group is also a transition period where the baby moves from pureed to more texture solid foods (mashed or finely minced).

- Introduce your child to chunkier textures; foods should be chopped rather than mashed, and finger foods may be offered.

- Chewing movements are getting better.

- The baby can hold the food and/or her bottle on her own (beginning with finger foods) and drink from a cup.

- Your baby is ready to begin strained chicken, beef, veal, tofu, and meats. Dry toasts also help the baby learn to chew foods and finger foods are appropriate at this age.

- Your baby is still taking breast milk and/or formula and is consuming cereals, vegetables, and fruits.

- You may introduce juice to your child around 8-12 months of age, and help her learn to drink from a cup. Dilute the juice with water and avoid sweet (unnecessary sugar) juices. It is better to use water instead of juices.

Tip: Honey

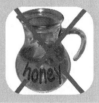

Since honey is associated with botulism (a possibly fatal illness), it should not be given to children under the age of one year.

10-12 Months

- Encourage your baby to eat on her own as self-feeding skills improve and the ability of rotational chewing increases.

- Your baby is now feeding on breast milk and/or formula, cereals, vegetables, fruits, juices, meat and alternatives, more textured foods, milk/dairy products, finger, and table foods.

- At one year of age, you may add fish, whole eggs, and whole cow's milk to your child's diet.

Tip: Separate or Combined Foods

It is good to give your baby separated, individual foods instead of blending them altogether. This helps accustom your baby to different tastes and textures. It is also easier to identify a specific food causing an allergy.

12-24 Months (1-2 Years)

- Your child now sits at the table with the family and enjoys the social aspects of mealtime. With some help, she can use a spoon to bring food to her mouth with fewer spills.

- Your child has progressed from pureed to mash and is now ready for chopped foods.

- Her appetite decreases and her growth rate slows down.

- Her attention span is prolonged while she becomes more independent (learns how to say "No").

- You may serve the following foods to your child:
  - ❖ *Dairy Foods*: soft pasteurized cheese, yogurt, pudding, cottage cheese, etc.
  - ❖ *Grain Products*: Pasta, rice, crackers, pretzels, rice cakes, whole wheat bread, etc.
  - ❖ *Fruits*: apricot, papaya, apples, bananas, peaches, cherries, plums, oranges, grapefruit, etc.
  - ❖ *Vegetables*: yams, potatoes, broccoli, cauliflower, peas, carrots, green beans, etc.
  - ❖ *Protein*: meat, poultry, boneless fish, beans, eggs, tofu, etc.

- You may cut your child's food into tiny pieces, which are then shredded or mixed with other foods.

24-36 months (2-3 Years)

- At this stage of life, your child will be eager to make her own food choices.

- Allow your older child to take part in the food experience by letting her help you prepare foods, and take her grocery shopping with you so she can choose fruits and vegetables, etc.

- Your child's muscle control is much improved, and she can now use a spoon, fork, cup, etc.

- Continue to introduce new foods one at a time, waiting about three days between each new food for allergy identification purposes.

- Offer a variety of foods to your child to ensure a healthy, well-balanced diet. This will also help your child develop good eating habits in the future.

Tip: Dangerous Food

Avoid foods that children can choke on, such as nuts, raw carrots, hard candy, celery, popcorn, chips, etc. Stay close to your child when she is eating and make sure she is sitting down throughout the entire meal to prevent choking. Avoid foods that may cause allergy, such as egg whites, cow's milk and peanut butter—wait until your baby is at least one year of age before introducing these foods.

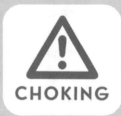

CHOKING

Parent Concerns

How do I know when my baby is hungry or full?

- Your baby will give you clues that she is full by closing her mouth, turning her head away, crying, pushing food away, falling asleep, a slower pace of eating, spitting out, etc.

- Hunger cues include excited arm and leg movements, crying, cooing, looking at the caregiver, opening her mouth, moving towards the food, etc. (see *Feeding by Schedule or On Demand*).

- Over time, you will be able to learn your baby's hunger and satiety clues.

- Stay relaxed and try to feed her again later; do not force feed your child.

I add seasonings when I prepare foods for the family. Is this okay for my young child to eat also?

- While children can begin eating the same foods as the family at the toddler age (two to three years), they do not need any added sugar or salt.

- When preparing the family food, you may leave aside some food for your child with no added seasonings, since children need to learn the natural flavor for foods. However, light seasoning and spices can be added to foods as it may encourage more variety later on (we see this in different cultures). There is no evidence that suggests that only bland foods should be offered and that spicy or more flavored foods should not.

- If you buy commercially prepared foods, it is recommended to use those with no sugar, salt, or seasonings.

How long and how frequently should I feed my baby?

- This varies from one baby to another.

- In general, 2 1/2 oz/75 ml should be consumed by the newborn baby within 15-20 minutes. However, some newborns will initially take 40 minutes to feed—causing their mothers to feel like they are feeding all day.

- Formulas fed babies are able to hold for a longer time between feedings when compared to breastfed babies.
- A general idea of feeding amounts and frequency are given in the chapter *Feeding by Schedule or On Demand*.

My 6-week-old baby has recently become willing to eat a lot. Why is this?
- Your baby is probably experiencing a growth spurt.
- Growth spurts occur at 3 weeks, 6 weeks, and so forth (see *Growth Chart*).
- During these spurts, your baby may require more feedings and increased amounts of food for about a week, or until this period of rapid growth returns to its baseline.
- Growth spurts are another reason why feeding by schedule does not work for babies.

Should I wake up my newborn baby to feed if she sleeps for more than 4 hours?
- A small stomach and liver immaturity requires that your newborn be fed frequently. This means that if she is sleeping more than four hours, you should wake her up.
- Some newborns are "lazy" and, until they get stronger and older, you need to wake them up to feed, especially if they are not gaining weight well.

Which solid foods should be introduced to my child first?
The order of introduction to your baby's diet is as follows:
1) Commercial iron-fortified rice cereal (if homemade, use wholegrain brown rice or millet cereal—you may need iron drops, so talk to your doctor) should be the baby's first food.
2) Fruits (bananas are an excellent first choice food for babies).
3) Vegetables (sweet potatoes are a favorite first food).
4) Avocado.
5) Yogurt.
6) Meat may be introduced around 7 months and is a good source of iron.

How do I know when to add pureed, finger, textured, and table foods to my child's meal?
- There are various developmental indicators, which provide you with cues as to when to introduce each type of food.

Pureed Foods	Finger Foods & Cups	Textured & Table Foods
Tongue thrust reflex has diminished.	Sits on her own.	Chewing movements.
Strong demonstrated ability to swallow.	Grasps for objects, including foods and cups.	Lateral tongue movements (side to side).
Chewing movements instead of sucking movements.	Swallows without choking or gagging.	Pincher grasp (picks up foods between her thumb and finger).
Able to sit up with support.		
Does not gag or choke when given food.		
Opens mouth when hungry and closes it when full.		

Although all babies are different, your baby may be able to manage chewier, more textured foods around seven to eight months of age.

What is a wheat germ?
- This is actually the seed of the wheat kernel and, like all seeds, it is a super-nutritious food.
- Wheat germs are part of the wheat kernel that is removed when whole wheat is refined into white flour or wheat flour.

Can I add water to my child's diet in the first few months?
- While offering **occasional** small amounts of water (about three tablespoon per day) when your baby is less than six months of age will not cause any problems, your baby's water supply comes from breast milk, formula, and other foods once she has started them (around four to six months).
- In the first six months, your baby should receive enough fluids from formula or breast milk, so that she does not require extra water (except in sickness, excess heat, constipation, etc.).
- Once your baby starts solid foods and eats reasonable amounts, her fluids will need to come from sources other than breast milk or formula.

- Between six to twelve months of age, the amount of water offered should probably be limited to 6-12 oz/180-360 ml per day.

- If you have any other concerns about your child's fluid intake, speak to your doctor.

Is there any difference between powder and ready to use formulas?

- The nutritional content in both types of formulas is the same, so you can use either one.

- The difference between these formulas is cost, availability, preparation, method, convenience of use, etc. (See *Types of Formula & Its Preparation*).

Are homemade foods better than jar foods?

- Homemade foods are better than jar foods since you are able to control the ingredients and additives contained in foods.

- It is also less expensive to prepare homemade foods, and you can provide your baby with more variety in content and texture (see *Store Bought Foods & Homemade Foods*).

Is it okay to feed my baby yogurt and dairy products before the age of 1 since milk is started at the age of 1 year?

- The way plain yogurt is prepared may confer some protection, even for most of those babies with cow's milk allergy. It should probably not be started before eight months of age (1-2 tablespoons per day, initially).

- Yogurt and dairy products should **not** be offered to a child with documented milk protein allergy (see *Dairy Products for Infants & Toddlers*).

Are organic products healthier than regular products for my baby?

- Although it is assumed that organic foods are grown without synthetic fertilizers and pesticides, antibiotic treatment, hormones or other additives, they may still contain pesticides and other contaminants from water and soil residue.

- Organic foods are not necessarily more nutritious or flavorful than other foods.

My baby is spitting up a few times every day. Is this normal and will it resolve itself?

- If your baby is growing well, has no persistent projectile vomiting and is just spitting up from time to time (even if food is coming out through her nose), then she probably has physiologic reflux. This means that stomach contents return through the esophagus, because the valve connecting the stomach to the esophagus is still weak. This will improve, as your baby gets older.

- Do not overfeed your baby, as over feeding increases reflux episodes.
- If your baby has reflux and is not gaining weight well, then talk to your doctor about any need for assessment and other management suggestions as related to your child's needs.

What are the risk factors responsible for a child receiving an inadequate diet?

Risk factors for inappropriate nutrient intake are:

- Dietary aspects:
  - ❖ Special dietary requirements (e.g., milk free, gluten free, etc.).
  - ❖ Vegan or vegetarian diet (see *Vegetarianism*).
  - ❖ Inappropriate family diet or dietary restrictions or exclusions.
  - ❖ Prolonged food refusal and lack of dietary variety.
  - ❖ High sugar intake.
  - ❖ Early and inappropriate weaning diet.

- Social aspects:
  - ❖ Low income.
  - ❖ Lack of knowledge.
  - ❖ Irregular family meals.
  - ❖ Poor parent interaction.
  - ❖ Working mother, etc.

- Cultural Aspects and Traditions
- Medical conditions:
  - ❖ Chronic illness.
  - ❖ Mal-absorption.
  - ❖ Nutritional deficiencies.
  - ❖ Feeding difficulties, etc.

- All these factors, singly or in combination, can be reasons for a child's inadequate nutritional intake.

Things to Keep in Mind

- In your baby's first year, the primary source of nutrition is breast milk or formula.

- When offering juice, give it diluted in a cup rather than a bottle, to reduce the risk of tooth decay. Milk and water should be the main source of fluid; there is probably no need for juice at all within the first year of life.

- Microwave safety: When warming food in a microwave, use a microwave safe dish and warm it until it is lukewarm (not boiling).

- If your child has any allergies, always read the labels on food jars to make sure there are no ingredients she is allergic to (e.g., cow's milk protein, wheat, etc.).

- Do not feed your baby directly out of a jar as there is the risk of the dirty spoon creating germ growth in the jar. If your baby wants more food, take the food out of the jar with a clean spoon and put it in a bowl or on a plate.

- Leftover food should not be heated more than once.

- If you are breastfeeding your baby, use vitamin D supplements from when your baby is two weeks to one year of age.

- Offer new foods when your baby is in a good mood and not tired or too hungry. Give your baby time to learn how to swallow these foods and to get used to different tastes and textures (seasoning and spices can be added to foods and may encourage more variety later on). New foods should be offered in the morning and observed the rest of the day for any allergic reaction.

- If your baby refuses a new food, try offering it again in a couple of days. Repeated exposure to a new food enhances the chances of food acceptance (refer to the chapter on a specific food for food refusal suggestions).

- Make meals a happy time for your baby. Never force feed or overfeed her.

- Do not let your baby sleep with a bottle.

- When starting solids, you can offer fruits or vegetables first. There is no evidence that your child will refuse vegetables if fruits are started first. In fact, for some children, the opposite is true.

Starting Solid Foods

General

The introduction of solid food is an important stage in your baby's development. It is an exciting and challenging time for you and your baby. After six months of age, breast milk or formula alone is not enough to meet your baby's needs; additional complementary nutrients are required to support growth, development and to meet your baby's needs.

During the first months of starting solids, the actual quantity of food is of little significance as long as breast or bottle-feeding is continued. Your breast milk or formula should continue to be your baby's primary source of nutrition (at least until the end of the first year of life). Health experts recommend starting solid foods around six months of age since most babies will become developmentally and physiologically ready at this age.

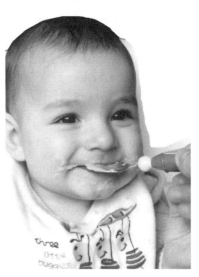

Consider solid foods as an addition, and not substitute to your breast milk or formula, since it is more nutritionally balanced than solid foods at this developmental stage. The baby will be fed and introduced to solid foods slowly as her appetite increases. These new foods allow your baby to experience pleasure in different textures, tastes, and flavors while, at the same time, providing her nutritional requirements. The baby will be fed and introduced to solid foods slowly, as her appetite increases. By the end of your baby's first year, most of her nutrition will come from other sources outside of breast milk or formula. Remember, feeding solids should be a time for social interaction and enjoyment with your baby.

Tip: UK Recommendations for Starting Solid Foods

The Department of Health Recommendations in the UK state that solid foods should begin for most infants around 5-6 months of age.

Clues for Readiness

General Clues

- There is no magic number or time when your child will be ready for solid foods since each child grows and develops at a different rate.

- The decision to begin your baby on solid foods is individual, according to various factors such as the baby's age, weight, hunger status, readiness to start or accept new foods, and other associated medical issues.

- Readiness to start solid foods also depends on the maturity of the baby's digestive tract and the baby's developmental readiness. This type of readiness cannot be assessed or determined by anyone since each baby is different.

- The following points can provide clues to see if your baby is ready to accept new foods (see also *Parent Concerns*):

  ❖ You may use a bit of cereal with formula and place it on the baby's tongue to see the response. If she accepts the taste and does not spit it out, then she is probably ready to begin solid foods.

  ❖ Your baby is able to sit up well when supported and is able to swallow.

  ❖ When your baby is able to hold her head up on her own, you may start to offer other strained baby foods. Chunkier foods should be started when a baby can sit up well on her own (around seven months old).

  ❖ Your baby begins to reach for and show interest in foods on the table. She begins to show excitement when you take away anything from the table that she wants to taste.

  ❖ The baby reaches out and grabs for objects with her thumb and forefinger to move towards her mouth.

  ❖ The tongue-thrust reflex has disappeared, meaning that she no longer pushes solid foods out of her mouth with her tongue. This reflex usually disappears by four to six months of age.

  ❖ The baby has learned to grasp the bottle and the spoon by the age of four to six months.

  ❖ Around five to six months of age, or when your baby is able to express hunger by opening her mouth and sitting forward when food is presented.

Practical Issues

- When discussing cues for readiness to start solids, these will be apparent between four to six months of age. At a later age, most babies will be able to feed on their own. It is not recommended to start your baby on solids earlier than four months.

- When breastfeeding, recommendations include breastfeeding exclusively for the first six months of life and then starting solid foods. However, readiness to start solids can vary (one baby is ready at four months while another is ready at six months), as each baby is unique. Whether it is four months, five months, or six months, each is in the normal range to begin solid feedings. It is a matter of the baby's nutrient needs and her ability to accept it.

- The cues stated above can be more helpful for premature baby or babies that are very small for their gestational age than full term babies, since most four to six month olds born full term are able to start solids. For the premature or small baby, it depends on their biological age and cues of readiness as discussed in this chapter.

When & Why to Start
Reasons Why Solids are Started at 4-6 months of age

- Solids are generally started between the ages of four to six months because there is sufficient muscle control and swallowing ability to handle solid foods.

- The infant's digestive system has developed enough at this stage to be able to break down more complex foods.

- Reasons why health professionals recommend starting solids between four to six months, include the following:

  ❖ The baby's intestine needs to mature enough to handle solids. Between four to seven months of age, the lining of the intestine, which is the body's filtering system, matures and begins to screen for harmful substances, becomes more selective as to what is absorbed, and starts to produce antibodies that prevent entry into the bloodstream of harmful allergens. If food is introduced too early (earlier than four to six months), harmful substances enter the blood and may cause allergies.

  ❖ The baby's swallowing mechanism is not mature until the age of four to six months. The infant develops the ability to move food from the front of the mouth to the back. Before this developmental point, solid foods remain in the mouth and may be spat out; simply wait until your baby is able to swallow.

❖ Between four to six months of age, babies tend to drool. This saliva is rich in digestive enzymes and will help digest the soon-to-come solid foods.

❖ Your baby should be physiologically and developmentally ready to begin solid foods. Physiological changes include the disappearance of the extrusion reflex and the maturity of the renal and gastrointestinal system. Developmental indications of readiness include being able to sit up with support, self-control of hands, and placing objects in the mouth.

❖ The baby is provided with greater protection from nutrient deficiency (e.g., iron-deficiency anemia) as she is recovering enough iron from formula or breast milk. The best immunity from illness a baby can receive is from exclusive breastfeeding, since breast milk contains at least 50 known immune factors.

❖ Delaying the introduction of solids also decreases the risk of food allergies. Studies have concluded that prolonged exclusive breastfeeding or bottle-feeding results in lower incidences of allergies. Waiting to introduce solid foods into your baby's diet helps protect your baby from future obesity since early introduction is associated with increased body fat and weight gain.

Recommendations on When to Start:
Breastfeeding Babies

• The World Health Organization (WHO) changed its recommendations from the infant being exclusively breastfed for four to six months of life to "exclusive breastfeeding for the first six months, with the introduction of complementary foods and continued breastfeeding thereafter," (WHO, 2001).

• The WHO definition of "exclusive breastfeeding" means feeding only breast milk (including expressed milk) and allowing the baby to receive vitamins, minerals, or medicine. Water, breast milk substitutes like formula, other liquids, and solids are not used.

• The American Academy of Pediatrics and Canadian Pediatric Society (2004/05) also recommend exclusive breastfeeding for the first six months of life for healthy term infants, as breast milk is the "best food for optimal growth."

• The American Dietetic Association (2004) states that "for most infants, breast milk and/or formula provides all the required nutrients for about six months after birth and significant but varying amounts thereafter."

- The United Kingdom supports the WHO recommendations, however, reviewed recommendations suggest that infants be managed individually to prevent insufficient growth and other adverse outcomes, and that appropriate intervention be provided. They state that "no complementary foods should be introduced before the end of four months of age." The UK also recommends that the majority of infant weaning should occur at four to six months.
- Infants should be introduced to nutrient rich solid foods, with particular attention to iron, at six months, with continued breastfeeding for up to two years and beyond.

Explanation & Issues for Introduction of Solid Foods
- It is recommended to introduce solid foods at six months of age, especially when there is a family history of allergy.
- For the breastfed infant who is doing well, early solid food introduction may replace a complete, well-digested diet with an incomplete, poorly digested one that can lead to obesity and allergies.
- Some experts say that the six month of age approach may not take a proper account of the special needs of some infants and fails to allow for the different problems present in industrialized versus economically developing countries.
- Some recommend that both breastfed and bottle-fed infants' introduction to solid foods be delayed to the age of six months because of the following reasons:
  - ❖ Better protection from illness.
  - ❖ Baby's digestive system has time to mature.
  - ❖ Less risk of food allergy.
  - ❖ Helps protect the baby from future obesity.

Bottle-fed Babies
- There are no clear recommendations at this point regarding the introduction of solid foods for formula-fed babies, however, starting solids should be considered between four to six months after discussion with your doctor. The four months of age recommendation for starting solids applies more to formula-fed infants than the six months of age recommendation (which applies more to breastfed infants). The reason for this is that

formula is not as complete as breast milk since formula-fed babies are more likely to become anemic than breastfed babies and thus require iron rich foods earlier. It is difficult to absorb more than a certain amount of iron from formula, regardless of how much iron is in it.

- There are no clear recommendations regarding solid food introduction for bottle-fed babies and it is unclear as to why.

Tip: Starting Solids In Premature Babies

This often causes confusion to both parents and health professionals.

Most dieticians recommend weaning to solid foods according to the baby's post-natal age, rather than their post-conceptual age. This is because maturity of the gut relates more to birth date than due date.

The gestational age of a premature baby can be calculated by taking away the number of weeks the baby is born early from their actual age. For example, a 32-week-old baby is unlikely to be ready for solids at four months. Wait another month or two until the corrected age is close to four months (also look at the developmental ability of the baby, as each one is unique).

The decision should be based on physiological and developmental attributes of the infant.

Early Introduction of Solids & the Consequences
Early Introduction (earlier than four months)

- Many times, parents decide on their own that their baby is still hungry and require additional foods. As such, babies may be introduced to solid foods early. Some parents decide to start their child on solid foods before the recommended age of four to six months. Other parents mistakenly believe that early introduction of solids is best for developmental progress.

- The American Academy of Pediatrics (AAP) reports that approximately 1/3 of breastfeeding mothers and about 1/3 of bottle-feeding mothers introduce cereal to their babies at two to three months of age (Kleinman RE. (Ed) 2004, Pediatric Nutrition Handbook).

- Studies show that parents feed cereal to infants less than four months of age because of the following reasons:

  ❖ Baby was not satisfied with breast or formula feeding.

  ❖ Baby sleeps better with cereal.

- ❖ Doctors said to start early.
- ❖ Responding to infant cues.

- Further reasons why parents begin their child too early on solid foods include:
  - ❖ Child has reached four months of age.
  - ❖ The baby has reached a set weight or subjective size.
  - ❖ Baby has begun teething or has increased saliva production.
  - ❖ The breastfeeding mother begins work early.
  - ❖ Parents want to avoid frequent feedings.
  - ❖ Hungry cries, constipation, takes milk too quickly, chews her hands, and changing sleeping patterns are also reasons why parents begin their baby on solids early.
- However, the main reason parents begin early introduction of solids is to "settle" their baby.
- In a poll done by a baby center (website), there were 52,306 responses as to when parents began introducing solids to their babies. The results show that 26% began feeding solids to their infants at less than four months of age, while 57% started at four to six months, 15% at six to eight months and 3% between eight to twelve months of age.
- Whatever the case may be, discuss it with your doctor before starting your baby on solids. Parents need to know the implications of starting their baby on solids too early.

Consequences of Early Introduction
- The consequences of starting your baby too early (earlier than 4 months of age) on solid foods include the following:
  - ❖ A higher risk of allergies, with more severe symptoms and eczema.
  - ❖ Your baby may push any new foods away or will have other responses (spitting up, etc.) as the baby's digestive system is still immature.
  - ❖ Inadequate nutrition and poor growth of your child, because an inappropriate amount of breast milk or formula is given.
  - ❖ Early introduction of starch-containing foods before the age of three months could lead to inadequate hydroxylation of starch in some babies.

❖ Incidences of choking are higher since the baby is not physically ready to begin solids.

❖ Early interruption of the supply and demand milk production in your breast, which may diminish your milk production (if breastfeeding).

❖ Inability of the infant's gut to adequately digest excess carbohydrates and fat efficiently, causing pain, cramping, and diarrhea.

❖ Inability of infant's kidneys to process the greater amount of highly concentrated substance that derives from various solid foods.

Tip: Returning to Work

The breastfeeding mother who returns to work before 6 months and wishes to start her baby on solids can help maintain her breast milk production by still breastfeeding whenever possible, and having the baby's caregiver use solids and pumped breast milk while she is working.

Starting Late

Parents who introduce their children to solid foods after the age of 6 months or within the second half of the child's first year may have the following consequences:

❖ The baby may resist learning new things such as the trick of swallowing or chewing solids (uncommon).

❖ Taste may be more difficult to change at this point.

❖ The baby will prefer more liquids and may refuse solid type foods.

❖ Improper nutrition (especially Iron and Zinc) and slow growth.

The Transition Period

General

• Remember that breastfeeding or formula continues to be your baby's main source of nutrition during the five to six months of age transition period.

• Transition to solid foods is intended to satisfy hunger and provide nutritional complements to your baby's liquid diet. The following are some suggestions to help make the transition easier for you and your baby:

❖ Slowly ease into the routine of feeding your baby solids. Begin by offering solids once or twice a day (1-2 teaspoons) after a feeding. Your baby will be more willing to try something new when she is not very hungry. Offer your baby small amounts (about a teaspoon full) and gradually increase the amount. You may start feeding 1/4 to a full teaspoon of the selected food and slip a tiny bit between the baby's lips to allow the baby to react. A ready baby will take it quickly and not spit it up. If the food continues to slide out, the baby is probably not developmentally 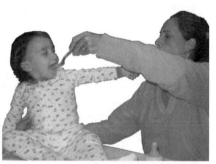 ready to begin solids. If your baby does not accept the spoonful right away, try using your finger as the baby's first spoon; put a dab of food on your finger and place it on the tip of your baby's tongue. If this gets swallowed, place the next dab on your finger in the middle of your baby's tongue.

❖ Give your infant a little breast milk or formula first, then switch to half a spoonful of foods and finally, finish off with more milk. This will help prevent your baby from being frustrated when she is very hungry and it will combine the satisfaction of nursing with the experience of spoon-feeding.

❖ Always use a spoon to feed your baby solids (unless you are thickening the formula for gastroesophageal reflux, as suggested by your doctor). Place the small amount of food on the tip of the spoon and place it in the middle of the baby's tongue. Your baby may react with either a smile or a disapproving grimace.

❖ Watch your baby's reaction when she is experiencing new foods. If the food goes into her mouth willingly, she is ready to accept new foods. If the food comes out and she is grimacing, she is not yet ready to accept solids. Even if the food comes back out of her mouth, she may just need to learn how to close her mouth when food enters. Moreover, it is important to watch her reaction in case of an allergic response.

❖ When introducing new solids to your baby, try offering a new food about every three days (allergic reaction purposes). Make sure to provide your child with various foods from all food groups over the next few months.

❖ Do not add any salt or sweeteners to the baby's food.

- ❖ Do not offer new foods in a bottle that has a large hole in the nipple, since it can cause choking or lead to excessive weight gain (the baby eats larger amounts this way).

- ❖ Minimize the chances of choking by making sure the baby is sitting up either in your lap or in a high chair.

- ❖ Do not force your baby to try a new food. Do not force the food if the baby cries or turns her head away. Let her accept the food at her own pace.

- ❖ Do not start a new food when your baby is tired and cranky. Wait until your baby is happy and alert. If your baby seems hungriest in the morning, consider offering solids at that time. This is especially important for babies with small appetites.

- Remember that rejection of food may simply indicate that the baby's tongue thrust reflex is not yet gone and she cannot move the food from the front to the back of her mouth. Wait a week before trying to feed her again.

- Offering solid foods can take place anytime during the day. When the baby is older, she may want to eat at the table with the rest of the family (it is better for her, too).

The First Meal & Parent Concerns
The First Meal

- Utensils required for the first solid food meal are the following:

  1) Spoon.

  2) Plastic cup.

  3) Bib.

  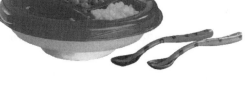

  4) Plastic bowl (e.g., with 3 compartments and suction ring in the bottom to make it difficult for your baby to throw).

  5) Hand or electric food mill or electric blender.

  6) High chair or booster seat.

- The baby's first foods after formula or breast milk should be more of a liquid than a solid. In fact, it should be liquid enough that it pours off the spoon, as thick foods will make your baby gag and choke. Foods should be pureed and diluted with liquid. The texture may be made coarser once the baby is used to eating.

- It is recommended to serve your child iron-fortified rice cereal as a first solid food.

- Rice cereal is easily digested by your baby, provides the iron (30-45% of daily requirements), is least likely to cause an allergic reaction (only rare instances of sensitivity), and is gluten free (a protein that triggers unwanted reactions).

- Mix one teaspoon of rice cereal with one to two tablespoons of liquid. If you prepare the cereal with formula or breast milk, it is more nutritious and will make the food taste more familiar to your baby (making it easier to accept). If you use water, make sure it has been boiled before. Check the temperature before feeding it to your baby.

- Offer your child one to two teaspoons in the beginning and, if she accepts the first feeding, you may offer a little more at the next feeding and gradually increase the amount. In the beginning, you may have to feed with your fingers for first tastes.

- As your baby becomes accustomed to the texture of the cereal, you can gradually make the cereal mixture thicker.

- After feeding your baby rice cereals, it is recommended to try oatmeal and barley cereals next.

- If your baby has a history of constipation or does not like rice cereal, you may start with another type of cereal or cooked/mashed vegetables or fruit (see *Constipation*).

Parent Concerns

Shall I give the same amount of formula or keep increasing it when I start solid foods?
- The baby's peak amount intake at four to six months of age is about 30-38 oz/900-1140 ml per day and it will decrease to 20-28 oz/600-840 ml per day by one year of age. As the amount of solid foods increase, the amount of breast milk or formula taken by your baby will decrease.

What if my baby gags when I start solid foods? Can she choke?
- Gagging is a protective mechanism that tries to keep the food from getting into the respiratory airway to prevent choking.

- When starting solid foods (first rice cereal), some gagging is acceptable until your baby learns to manipulate and swallow food of a different size and texture.

- To make it easier for your baby, you can dilute rice cereal (first solid started) to a thin watery consistency and gradually increase the consistency as the baby is able to tolerate it.

- If your baby experiences frequent gagging (when using appropriate watery textures), then she is either not ready to feed solid foods or the tongue thrust reflex has not yet disappeared. If the gagging persists it may indicate problems, e.g., neurological disorder, swallowing difficulties, etc., so speak to your doctor.

Can I use the bottle for the first solid feeding?

- No, it is not recommended to give your baby her first meal of cereal (solids) through the bottle. You would need to enlarge the hole of the nipple, putting the baby at risk of choking. The baby will also not learn the mechanics or social aspects of eating solid foods. There is also the risk of overfeeding and increased caloric intake.

How should I hold my baby during the first solid feeding?

- When you start introducing solid foods and your baby is already sitting well, you should consider the use of a high chair to sit at the family table. If your baby is ready to eat solid foods but can not yet sit upright if unsupported, then you can place her on your lap in a sitting position; your baby should recline slightly in an upright position, so that she can swallow without choking. You may also try an infant carrier or motionless swing, but they are probably less preferable, as it may not be comfortable for your baby.

When should I offer solid foods—before or after the breast or bottle?

- Some experts would say offer solids first, others say use the breast and bottle first. If you give your baby solid foods first (depending on how much and how often), your baby may take less breast milk. If you breastfeed first, you do not have to worry about giving your baby too many solids (give her as much as she wants). On the other hand, you can start solids first if you are planning on weaning early, or if you are already in the process. It probably does not make a big difference whether you breast or bottle-feed. Once you reach a good amount of solid foods after 4-6 weeks (after having introduced solids), you can start offering solid foods first then see if your child will take the bottle or breast. Otherwise, try breast or bottle-feeding first, then solids.

- Since each baby is different, I would say that whether you give your baby solids before or after breast milk or formula depends on your child's preferences. Some babies need a little milk first to take the edge off their hunger, so they can relax enough to be spoon-fed. Others will take solids first (even in large amounts) yet will take the bottle or breast and start after that. In addition, there is no reason why your baby needs both breast or bottle, and solid foods *every* time she eats, especially when the amount of solid foods taken reaches a "good" amount.

> ### Tip: Food Temperature
>
> Breastfed babies are accustomed to breast milk temperature (about 98 F/36.6 C).
>
> The heating or cooling of foods may not even be necessary for your baby; however, warmed foods sometimes have more flavor as babies will be more comfortable if their foods are at a consistent temperature as well.

Favorite First Solids and Order of Introduction

- Many times, parents ask what to feed their child and at which time of the day. Babies do not know what breakfast, lunch, and dinner is, or any order that food should be given in.

- What you serve and when you serve it depends on your baby's particular feeding behavior and her willingness to take new foods. The order of solid food introduction to your baby's diet is not that important, especially if your baby is starting solids at six months of age. However, if you start earlier than four to six months of age, the order of introduction should start with the less risky solid foods before high risk ones.

- You may introduce solids in this order:
    1) Rice cereal/oatmeal.

    2) Other cereals.

    3) Fruits (one at a time); no citrus fruits until 12 months of age.

    4) Yellow vegetables (e.g., boiled carrots, peas).

    5) Green vegetables (e.g., green beans, broccoli).

- Each baby is different and while some babies develop a taste for sweets, others do not.

- Many babies are born with a sweet tooth. Their tiny tongues are richly supplied with sweet taste buds. Human breast milk is sweet and some breastfed babies may be less likely to accept bland-tasting foods like vegetables than formula-fed babies (of course, each baby is unique).

- Although vegetables are nutritionally superior to fruits, many parents find that babies will more happily eat fruits than vegetables. When introducing vegetables, offer the sweet ones like carrots and sweet potatoes first. Do not worry if your baby likes fruits more—simply offer vegetables at a later time.

- The main goal of starting solids is for the baby to learn how to swallow foods with different textures.

- The following are some first food recommendations:

  ❖ *Cereal:* You may begin offering solid foods with rice cereal. Some suggest that cereal is not necessary for the breastfed baby since both cereal and breast milk are high in carbohydrates. However, it is important to remember that cereal will add about 30-45% of daily iron requirements. It is good for the baby with low weight gain (maybe less so for an obese infant/toddler).

  ❖ *Cooked carrots, sweet potatoes and squash* have good flavor, texture and color.

  ❖ *Applesauce* is an ideal first solid food.

  ❖ *Pears* are easy to digest with its mild flavor.

  ❖ *Bananas* are smooth and sweet (resembles sweetness of breast milk). They can be served uncooked, mashed with a fork, and mixed with formula or breast milk.

  ❖ *Avocado*: Some consider avocado an ideal first solid food since it has a creamy consistency and can be served without cooking.

Tip: Favorite First Foods

Favorite first solid foods include rice cereal, barley cereal, applesauce, bananas, pears, peaches, avocado, sweet potatoes and squash. Yogurt or cheese may be offered when your baby is about eight months old.

Allergies

- According to the American Academy of Allergy, Asthma & Immunology, about two to four percent of children experience allergic reactions to food. The incidence of allergy in early nutritional life is on the rise.

- Some foods are more likely to cause allergic reactions than others. Examples are fish, tomatoes, onions, citrus fruits, spices, nuts, cow's milk, and wheat. These risky foods have various ages at which they may best be introduced to reduce the likelihood of allergy.

- This is why it is recommended to serve new foods in the morning as, if any allergic reaction occurs, you will be able to notice it more easily during the day than at night.

- Particular foods eaten in excess by the breastfeeding mother may also cause allergic reactions in her baby through breast milk.

- Children are more likely to have adverse reactions to food in the first year of life and less after three years of age. The younger the child is when you offer supplemental foods, the greater the allergy risk.

- The following are some signs and symptoms that your baby is experiencing an allergic reaction (see *Feeding & Food Allergy*): runny nose, stuffiness, cold, wheezing, skin rashes, eczema, hives, diarrhea or mucous stools, gas, spitting, vomiting, fussiness and irritability, cranky behavior, poor weight gain (mal-absorption), red itchy eyes and swollen eyelids, bloating and gassiness, etc.

- If there is allergy history in your family, discuss with your doctor regarding when to introduce cow's milk (18 months), egg white (18-24 months), fish and nuts (two to three years).

Tip: Early Nutrition & Allergy Prevention

Eliminate certain foods in the diet during your pregnancy.

Breastfeeding has been beneficial in cases of infants from allergic families.

Maternal avoidance of allergenic foods during breastfeeding is important, especially for those infants at risk.

Also, exclusively breastfeed for six months, or use hydrolysate formula (formula where the protein causing allergy is broken down for better toleration) and introduce solids after six months of age to reduce the incidence of allergy.

Food Refusal, Tastes & Flavors

Food Refusal

- Like everyone, the baby has her own likes and dislikes. Do not worry if your baby is slow in accepting solid foods during the first year of life. Simply continue to offer foods to your baby. It is your responsibility to offer foods at certain times. It is your baby's decision whether or not to take it.

- Allow your baby to run the show, meaning feed your baby when she is hungry or when she wants to eat.

- Babies may reject previously accepted foods, because the food given is "bad," the baby's taste has changed, or they're simply not yet hungry. In these cases, do not force feed or try other foods—leave it for a while.

- Never continue a meal that your baby has lost interest in; this is signaled by fussiness, a mouth clamped shut, food regurgitation, and food thrown around.

- If your baby refuses new foods during the transition period, go back to nursing or bottle-feeding exclusively for about a week or two and then try again. Remember that repeated exposure to food enhances food acceptance.

- When developmentally appropriate, try offering your baby finger foods that they can pick up and feed themselves. Many babies prefer to eat foods right off the table, rather than from a spoon or the mother.

Tastes & Flavors

- Taste buds are located primarily in the mouth.

- Taste buds change their preference with age. While infants and young children prefer sweet foods in most cases, the young infant's sweet tooth diminishes as the child grows.

- Experts report that feeding experiences during the first seven months of a baby's life contributes to their food likes and dislikes. Flavor preferences are therefore established in early infancy and childhood, even before solid foods are introduced.

- Studies show that infants who are exposed to one type of formula (sweet or bland) will reject exposure to a different taste or flavor of another formula. For example, infants who were fed hydrolysate formula preferred foods with a sour taste and aroma, similar to the formula.

Parent Concern

Is it normal that everything I give to my 4 ½-month-old baby comes out?
Yes, this is normal since it is possible that the extrusion reflex is still present and your baby is not yet ready for complementary foods.

Do I have to use all cereal types when first starting solids before giving any other types of food?
If you start offering cereal as a first solid food, there is no specific time for when you should introduce vegetables or fruit. You do not have to use all cereal types before progressing to other types of solid foods. Do not start two food types on the same day. Wait about three days to check for allergic reaction between introducing new foods.

Tip: Taste and Food or Medicine Acceptance

Feeding & Taste

Sweet foods should be placed on the tip of the baby's tongue.

Less sweet foods may be placed on the middle of the baby's tongue.

This increases the likelihood of food acceptance.

Medicine & Taste

To get your child to accept unpleasant medicine, trick the taste buds by letting your child suck on a Popsicle, ice or anything cold which will numb their taste buds before giving them the medicine.

If your baby tends to reject new tastes, place new foods towards the middle of their tongue where there are fewer taste receptors.

After experimenting with various foods at different areas of the tongue, you will be able to find a combination which works for you and your baby.

The Nutritional Staging System

There is a nutritional staging system for baby solid foods to help you choose the right food for your baby. The stages follow your baby's physical development and nutritional needs. It is given by manufacturers as an arbitrary system of grading a food's consistency or lumpiness. The following table outlines the nutritional staging system:

Stages	Developmental Group
Stage 1	This is the first stage in introducing solid foods to your baby's immature digestive system. It includes single vegetable, fruit, liquid grain puree, and cereals.
Stage 2	This includes combinations of flavors such as mixed grain cereals, a variety of fruit and vegetables, and meats with juices. Consistency is close to stage one, but sold in larger jars to meet the appetite of the more advanced infant.
Stage 3	Complex combinations of textures and foods are provided at this stage. Foods have chunkier textures. These may be offered around seven to eight months.
Stage 4	Address toddler nutritional requirements. Include chunkier and textured foods. Assists your child in transitioning to table food.

- The difference in stages is jar size, texture, and the availability of a more diverse combination of foods.
- Remember to check the ingredients listed on each jar for allergy concerns.

Recommendations for Parents

- It is better to make homemade baby foods for your baby, as opposed to store bought foods. It is preferred and recommended to have freshly homemade vegetable meals and fruits.
- Serve natural fruit juices rather than sweetened compounds (see *Fruit Juices*).
- Read the labels on food jars and compare them.
- Buy foods which contain less starch.
- Choose jar foods with no added salt, sugar, or MSG. Avoid these ingredients, along with egg and milk products.
- Do not add salt, sweeteners, butter, or margarine to prepared homemade foods (so that the baby will learn the true flavors of individual foods). Light spicing is possible.
- Avoid canned fruits, since these are usually high in sugar, and canned vegetables containing large amounts of salt.

- Delay the introduction of solids if there is family history of allergies; have a discussion with your doctor.

- Remember, taste may change with age and babies may not like all foods that are given to them.

- When introducing complementary (solid) foods, it is important for parents to know the following:

  ❖ Do not force feed your baby.

  ❖ Avoid over feeding your baby.

  ❖ Incorporate complementary feedings gradually into the infant daily diet.

  ❖ Offer a variety of different foods to your baby.

  ❖ If food is not well received, retry in a few days to a week.

  ❖ Know your baby's cues that signal when she's had enough (e.g., spitting, vomiting, turns head away, seals her lips, etc.).

  ❖ Establish a friendly feeding environment.

- When you buy the utensils required for first feedings, consider the following things:

  ❖ *Spoons*: Plastic-coated spoons are easy on the baby's tender gums and temperature spoons are helpful in telling you when food is too hot for your baby.

  ❖ *Bibs*: Buy big, washable, easy to take on and off, stain-resistant bibs that have either Velcro or snaps on them (large plastic bibs).

  ❖ *Bowls*: Plastic, microwave-safe bowls are the most practical to buy; make it fun for your baby by buying them in different colors and shapes.

Tip: Starting Solids & Type 1 Diabetes Genetics Susceptibility

The relationship between the development of type 1 diabetes and the starting time of solid foods has recently become a research focus. Breastfeeding is strongly recommended for infants at high risk of type 1 diabetes, because of the potential to cause diabetes in infants. The early introduction of most milk feedings has been associated with the development of type 1 diabetes in high-risk infants. Data from epidemiological and animal studies are inconclusive at this point, however it appears prudent to recommend breastfeeding and delay the introduction of non-breast milk feedings until the age of six months for suscepible infants.

Store Bought & Homemade Foods

Store Bought
General

Commercially prepared foods are a convenient way to feed infants. They are an introduction to the texture of adult foods and, at the same time, meet the strict dietary requirements of babies.

Nutritionally, there is no difference between homemade and store bought foods, as the child grows and develops well with both types. Keep your child's diet appropriate for her stage of development and ensure a varied diet.

Availability & Nutrient Content
General

- You will find commercially prepared baby foods in their own sections in grocery and drug stores. You can find prepared foods with organic ingredients in health food stores and, increasingly, in grocery and drug stores. It is more expensive, but if your baby enjoys organic food, it is worth the cost.

- Age appropriate foods will be stated on food labels for when to start your baby on that particular jar of food. Some jars will signify various steps or stages at which you can feed your baby. For example, Step Two usually means you can feed your baby after one month of feeding them Step One. All of this is very confusing and does not have much meaning.

- It is important to check labels and ingredients, because infants do not need ingredients such as sugar, corn syrup, modified food starch, tapioca starch, gelatin or other thickeners (look out for anything containing "ose" on the end of a word/ingredient, as it is a sugar). These additives are used to modify consistency and texture, extend the shelf life of the food, and enhance color and/or flavor. The fewer artificial preservatives, additives, and colorings, the better. Choose products with little or no salt and sugar. The further down on the ingredient list an item is, the less of it there is in the product.

- Keep in mind that an infant's taste buds are still unspoiled and she is completely content with unsweetened cereal, fruits, and other desserts. Sugar (in all its forms) is not only unnecessary, but can undermine the baby's taste for the more delicate flavor of natural sweeteners (e.g., to add sweetener, use natural juice from sweet fruits—better than regular sugar). Sugar gives your baby more calories than needed and accustoms the taste buds to foods that hold less nutritional value. Plain foods will allow your baby to learn various flavors.

> ### Tip: *Effects of Starches and Sugars*
>
> Simple carbohydrates (sugars) have a simple molecular structure whereas complex carbohydrates (starches) have a complex molecular structure made of many simple sugar molecules. Starches get broken down and released into the bloodstream slowly and steadily, while the body digests sugars too quickly and easily. After eating complex carbohydrates (starches), you do not feel hungry for several hours. Try to choose foods that have little or no starch added, as it just fills up the baby without offering many nutrients.
>
> Modified starch is often found in corn, desserts (e.g., tapioca), and junior foods. It acts as a stabilizer in foods to provide desired consistency, texture, and shelf life. Studies show that modified starch has no undesirable effects in the digestion of babies.

For Infants
Cereals

- Cereals are available with some containing about 30% infant formula (check the type of formula to ensure that your baby is not allergic).

- These cereals include barley, rice, oatmeal, cereals mixed with banana and other fruits, rice and pear or orange, and multigrain cereals with mango, pineapple, pear, etc.

Fruits & Vegetables

- The difference in the nutritional value among the various jars of vegetables and fruits available is the concentration of natural fruits and vegetables.

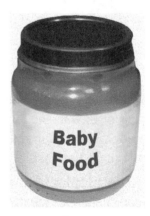

- Fruits and vegetables are cooked and packed soon after being picked, which retains a reliably high proportion of their nutrients.

- Most fruits in jar food contain only the fruit's natural sugars without the addition of more sugar.

- Most green vegetables deliver various vitamins and minerals.

- Compare labels on the jars since something like "chicken and vegetables" will contain more meat than "vegetables and chicken."

- Fruit desserts for the baby contain less nutritional value compared to plain fruits, as fruit desserts contain added sugar or starch.

Meat
- Plain meat provides more protein than mixed dinners like chicken and rice.

Lactose Free Jar Food
The following is a chart of milk and lactose free jar foods for those who are allergic to milk or lactose intolerant.

From the age of 4 Months	From the age of 7 Months
Garden vegetables	Mild Mexican beans
Squash and apples	Vegetarian pasta
Blueberries and apples	Beans in tomato sauce
Apricot cereal	Apple and bananas
Fruit compote	Sweet corn and potatoes
Oatmeal and prunes	Pear and apricots

For Toddlers
- There are a wide variety of jar foods available for the toddler and young child, including fruit or vegetable based foods, and meat and fish based foods.
- Toddlers may enjoy the following foods offered in cans or jars:
  - ❖ *Cereal based foods*: These are pre-cooked cereals with meat, vegetable, or fruit additions. They are usually mixed with high protein foods, and should be given with a non-protein liquid like water. Plain baby cereals are a better buy than cereals with fruit added.
  - ❖ *Pasta*: This is fun, as pastas come in different shapes that may amuse your child.
  - ❖ *Biscuits*: These can be offered dried, or soaked in water or milk.
  - ❖ *Milk-based desserts*: Yogurt or other milk products are the main ingredients in these special desserts, as they have controlled sugar content.
  - ❖ *Drinks*: These may contain special mixes of cow's milk or soy milk.
- Toddlers and young children may also enjoy organic jar foods. Organic foods are made from ingredients that are 100% organically grown and processed, such as fruits, vegetables, whole grains, etc. It should be grown in a certified organic garden.

- Examples of organic jar food include apple, apple and blueberry, sweet potato, carrots, squash, vegetables and pasta, bananas, cereals (rice, oatmeal, rice and banana), etc.

Safety Tips for Buying Baby Jar Foods:
- After buying jar foods, do not feed your baby directly from the jar (place a small amount in a bowl and feed from it) for various health reasons, such as risk of infection. You may also tend to overfeed your baby in order to finish the jar when feeding directly out of it.
- Do not buy or use sticky or stained jars of baby food. Only buy jars with safety buttons (on lid) that are pushed in.
- Once you open a jar, make sure you store it for no more than two to three days, and cover it well. Make sure that the safety seal on the jar was not broken when you bought it. When it opens, you should hear a "popping" sound. If the jar does not make this sound, consider throwing it away, as germs may be in the food.

Advantages & Disadvantages
Advantages
- Jar foods are safe, easy to store and very *convenient* for travel (no need for food preparation).
- Since food comes in ready to use jars, these are already reusable for refrigerated *storage* for leftovers.
- The strained varieties are the perfect consistency for beginner and single ingredient starter foods, which makes it easy to *screen for allergies*.
- Store bought jar foods offer many valuable elements for the growing baby.
- Jar food's *nutrient content* is very similar to homemade foods.
- Appropriate *textures* of foods are recommended according to age or developmental stage.
- Jar foods are available in various flavors and a *variety* of fruits, vegetables, and other foods.
- There is *less pesticide contamination* in baby foods than non-organic produce offered in the markets for adults.
- The ingredients in jar foods are stated. Every ingredient included must be listed on the label, according to regulations.
- There are measures taken to ensure the *hygiene* of jar foods. Manufacturers must follow strict quality control standards and monitor the cleanliness of cooking, storage, and preparation.

Disadvantages

- There are additional ingredients in jar foods, which babies do not require, such as salt, sugar, and modified starch. Additives dilute the nutrient content of foods.

- Commercially prepared foods often have less of a distinct taste to them and feel smoother, so your baby may get used to it and learn to prefer it to "real" food.

- The variety of store bought foods is limited in comparison with homemade foods.

Homemade Foods
General

Virtually any fruit, vegetable, or meat found in the grocery store may be used to prepare your own baby food. Most homemade foods contain more nutrients. There are no added fillers and artificial ingredients. Additives such as salt, sugar, or modified starch dilute the nutrient content of foods. Homemade baby foods can help you provide low-cost, nutritious foods for your baby. If you are nervous about making your own baby food, begin with some of the many soft or pureed grocery foods.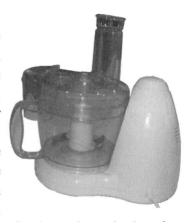

Do not be afraid to experiment with different foods and methods of preparation. Homemade baby foods should be made according to your baby's age, developmental stage, and allergies (if any).

Equipment & Food Safety

Equipment to Prepare Homemade Foods

The following equipment is useful for making baby food—most of it is already in your kitchen:

Equipment	Use
Fork or Potato Masher	You may use a fork to mash soft food (e.g., white or sweet potatoes, squash, carrots, egg yolks, ripe bananas, etc.). A potato masher works well to puree cooked foods.
Strainer	This should have a small mesh where you can push foods through with the back of a spoon. It can be used for juices, soft fruits and vegetables.

Equipment	Use
Food Mill (slightly coarser texture in foods)	Cut food into small pieces and place the cooked food (soft meat, fruits, and vegetables) through the food mill.
Knife	Foods can be chopped or scraped with a knife and then mixed with liquid.
Food Grinder	This may be used to grind up meats.
Blenders	Food items can be blended smoothly for the baby. You may blend until you reach the desired consistency. It is an easy and fast way of preparing baby foods. Most foods may be pureed with a blender. Be sure to remove tough peels and seeds from vegetables and fruits before blending, or they will be ground into the food.
Plastic Ice Cube Trays	These are excellent for freezing extra prepared food. Once the food is frozen, you may place it in containers or freezer bags for further storage.
Steamer	A steamer is great for preparing vegetables, because they will retain more nutrients than if they are boiled. Ensure a tight lid to keep the steam in.
Microwave	Cooking vegetables in the microwave is a form of steaming from the inside out. It is an excellent way to cook while preserving nutrients. Make sure to use microwave-safe and sterilized containers and covers.

In addition to these items, a slow cooker or pressure cooker may prove to be very useful when preparing homemade baby foods.

Food Safety

- Special care should be taken when preparing baby foods, because babies are so vulnerable to germs and illness.

- Always remember to wash your hands and equipment thoroughly before preparing baby food.

- Sterilize the equipment you will use in one of two methods:

  ❖ Boil equipment for 10 minutes in a pot of water to sterilize.

  ❖ If your dishwasher has a cycle which heats the water to 140 F/60 C or higher, you can use it to sterilize your equipment.

- Do not let the baby food sit at room temperature for longer than two hours. Harmful bacteria may grow within the food, so remember to refrigerate or freeze baby food soon after preparing it.

- Make sure to wash the cutting board, especially when cutting between raw and cooked food. These should not come into contact with each other as raw food contains bacteria.

- Also, be sure to cook all meats thoroughly so there is no pink coloration.

- For further details, please see *Safe Feeding & Food Safety*.

Preparing Baby Food

General Preparation

- Prepare fresh fruits and vegetables by scrubbing, peeling, and removing any pits or seeds. Remove all the bones, skin, and fat from meat and chicken.

- Do not use leftovers to make baby food.

- Cook the food in a small amount of water until tender. Use the cooking water if the recipe asks for a liquid (it is sterile and it may contain nutrients that leached from the food into the water as it cooked). Food may be steamed or baked (see following section).

- Do not add any salt, sugar, honey, or any other form of sweetener. Babies do not "know" this sweet flavor and as such, do not need it. Initially, do not use any seasonings. However, as the baby grows, you may add light seasoning. Stay away from strong spices, such as pepper or garlic, which your baby may find unpleasant to eat. Do not assume that making baby food means it has to be bland. Your baby will enjoy the taste of pure foods.

- You may puree or mash the cooked food. Either serve it immediately or refrigerate/freeze it.

Cooking Methods
Baking

- Baking is ideal for starchy, hard foods such as white or sweet potato, squash, apple, and meat.

- You can bake in 350 F/177 C for about 45-60 minutes.

- The heat associated with baking destroys vitamins, but minerals will remain intact.

Boiling

- Boiling is easy, however it loses about 50% of nutrients during this cooking process.

- Make sure to cover the pot to help preserve nutrients.

- Use the cooking water when you need liquid, as there are many nutrients preserved in the water itself.

- Most vegetables require approximately 10 minutes to boil.

- Check the tenderness of foods by piercing them with a fork.

- You may boil chicken or beef to kill bacteria which are unhealthy for the baby.

Steaming

- This is a great way of cooking vegetables and foods, since this cooking method retains more nutrients than boiling does.

Tip: Cooking Baby Food

Steaming is the most preferred method for cooking fruits and vegetables, with boiling being the second preferred cooking method.

Baking is preferred for meats, since more nutrients are retained. Meat purees are best made with plain water. Thus, baking and steaming are the best cooking methods for optimal nutrient preservation.

Microwave

- Microwaving food provides an easy and fast method of cooking vegetables and fruits.

- Nutrient loss is minimal with microwave cooking.

- Never heat or cook foods with a plastic cover in the microwave. Do not let a plastic wrap come in contact with the food, as this may cause toxic chemicals from the plastic to leach onto the food.

- It is best to use a glass dish with a glass lid.

How to Puree

- Puree means to place food through a grinder or a form of equipment which will make the food a liquid-like, smooth texture.

- Some foods, like ripe bananas may be mashed or pureed with only a fork and will not need to be pre-cooked.

- Try the following steps when pureeing foods:

  1) Start by cooking the food items (e.g., vegetables and fruits) until tender, using one of the cooking methods (e.g., steaming, baking, boiling, or microwaving).

  2) Allow items to slightly cool so that you may handle the food without burning yourself.

  3) Cut the food item(s) that you want to puree into small pieces (no larger than 1 inch/2.7 cm squares).

  4) Always save some of the liquid you cooked with, in case you need to thin your mixture—or you can add breast milk or formula if additional liquid is needed.

  5) Process these small portions in a blender or food processor until the texture is smooth (adding liquid when needed).

  6) If necessary, add liquid to obtain desired consistency for your baby's developmental stage.

Tip: The Right Texture

For a very young baby who has just started on solid foods, you must use quite a bit of water to get a very smooth texture. As your baby gets older, she can chew or actually "gum" chunkier foods, to which you will, of course, add less water and puree for less time.

Guide to the Right Texture
Thinning Homemade Foods:

- For the first set of meals, breast milk and formula are good thinners.

- Breast milk may be kept in the refrigerator for about three days and in the freezer for one month.

- Formula may be kept in the refrigerator for about 24 hours but does not freeze.

- Chicken, beef stock, and liquid from steaming fruits and vegetables may be kept in the refrigerator and frozen when mixed with purees.
- Thinners: water leftover from steaming, breast milk, formula, cow's milk, yogurt, broth or apple juice.

Thickening Homemade Foods:
- Thicken the puree when preparing homemade baby food to allow the baby to develop to the next stage of development, namely eating pieces of soft food.
- Mashed potatoes, sweet potatoes, and arrowroot starch are all good thickeners.
- Thickeners: wheat germ, whole grain cereal, cottage cheese, cooked egg yolks, mashed white or sweet potato, and arrowroot starch.

Tip: Thinning or Thickening Food

In order to thin or thicken homemade foods, add the appropriate thinner or thickener (depending on what you need) to the baby's meal for desired consistency and texture, according to your baby's developmental stage.

General Texture Guide
The following table outlines the type of food and texture your baby should be starting according to her age:

Age	Food	Texture
0-4 Months	Breast milk or formula	Liquid
4-6 Months	Add baby cereal	Strained, thick and soup-like
6-8 Months	Add cooked vegetables or soft fruits	Strained or mashed
8-10 Months	Add meats and alternatives	Mashed or finely minced
10-12 Months	Most foods of a wide variety may be eaten at this age	Finely chopped into small pieces for self-feeding

Storing & Freezing

Storing
The following table is a guideline for freezer storage time of homemade baby foods.

Foods	Storage Time
Vegetables	6-8 Months
Fruits	6-8 Months
Cooked Meat or Poultry	1-2 Months
Meat and Vegetable Dinners	1-2 Months
Purees containing Milk	4-6 Weeks
Cooked Legumes or Tofu	2-3 Months

Never freeze foods in glass. It may crack, burst, or leave behind tiny, microscopic fragments.

The Ice Cube Freezing Method
- Place about 2 tablespoons of pureed or mashed food into each cube of a plastic ice cube tray.
- Cover the tray with a plastic wrap and place it in the freezer until they are frozen (usually takes about 24 hours to freeze).
- Take out the food ice cubes when they are frozen and place them in freezer bags.
- Label and date your freezer bags to tell the difference between your foods and storage times.
- If the food is freshly prepared, you may store it in the refrigerator for up to three days.

Warming & Thawing Baby Foods
- Frozen food can be thawed in the refrigerator or the microwave oven on the defrost setting.
- Food that has been thawed should never be refrozen.
- There are two methods of warming foods:
  1) *Stove method*: Place food directly into a saucepan and warm over low heat, stirring often. Make sure to test the temperature of the food before feeding it to your baby.
  2) *Microwave method*: This method usually heats the food unevenly and causes hot spots, even when the food feels cool to you. It is important to stir the food well to prevent burning you baby's mouth. Remember, cover the dish with a microwave-safe cover and not a plastic wrap. Turn

the dish a few times during the heating process to ensure no uneven spots. Allow the food to sit for a few minutes before feeding your baby and test the temperature. It is not recommended to heat pureed meats in the microwave.

- Other methods of warming food include reheating the baby food in a double boiler, egg poacher, or a dish in hot water. Stir food well to distribute heat evenly and test the temperature before serving.

Serving Baby Foods

- Serve the food at a temperature which is no warmer than body temperature. Remember to check the temperature of the food before serving it to your baby.

- Only dip the spoon in the food to the amount your baby will eat at that feeding. It is not good to place the spoon back in the food after your baby has "touched" some of it. This is because your baby's saliva may cause bacteria to grow in the food.

- Refrigerate the leftovers in tightly sealed containers and be sure to use them within a couple of days. You may freeze the leftovers in the ice cube trays until they are frozen solid and then place them into freezer bags.

Advantages & Disadvantages

Advantages

- Homemade food is freshly prepared and less expensive than store bought foods.

- The variety of prepared food is unlimited as you can use many types of food for preparation. Also, the baby enjoys a wide variety of foods and it allows for an easy transition between mashed to pureed foods.

- The amount of additional ingredients or seasonings is controlled (e.g., salt, sugar, starch, etc.).

- You are able to mix prepared food with breast milk or formula, while store bought foods are usually only mixed with water.

- Prepared food can be made ahead of time and frozen for future use.

Disadvantages

- It is time consuming to prepare homemade baby food.

- Parents sometimes use extra salt to suit their own taste, often forgetting that an infant's palate has not been similarly conditioned to the need of salt flavor (ease up on the salt shaker).

Homemade Baby Food: Do's & Don'ts

Do...
- Use the ice cube tray method to freeze pureed food.
- Discard unfinished meals.
- Steam or microwave vegetables and fruits to retain as much vitamins and minerals as possible as opposed to boiling.
- Use fruits and vegetables as close as possible to the time of purchase.
- Remove shells from fruits and vegetables, if you think they can damage your baby. If fruits and vegetables have a thin shell, it is better to leave it on when cooking, as it will keep in nutrients and add nutritional fiber.
- Use corn, canola, or sunflower oil. Do not use butter or saturated fat oil (e.g., palm oil or coconut oil).

Don't...
- Feed nuts, raisins, popcorn, raw vegetables, unpeeled fruits or peanut butter to a child under the age of two years.
- Give honey to a child under the age of one, as there is a risk of botulism (a toxin).
- Serve spinach, beets, or collards to babies under the age of one year, as they are high in nitrates.
- Add salt, sugar, or strong spices to homemade baby foods.
- Use canned vegetables, as they are usually loaded with sodium and additives.
- Place diluted food in a bottle that has a large hole in the nipple, for nighttime feeding, since there are various risks associated with this (bad for teeth, bad habits, etc.).
- Give highly acidic fruits such as oranges, tangerines or pineapples to a baby under the age of one year.
- Force-feed your baby; begin feeding with one to two spoonfuls and let your baby guide you.
- Use fruit or vegetables that are damaged or spoiled.

Microwave Safety
- Do not use jar baby foods or other small jars to heat food in the microwave because the jar may break from the build-up of steam.
- Transfer the baby food to be heated to a microwave-safe bowl.
- Before serving, remember to test the temperature of the food to ensure that it is warm and not too hot.
- Tell your babysitter about the safety precautions and correct use of the microwave for heating and defrosting baby food.

Food with Nitrates
- The following vegetables contain nitrates: spinach, broccoli, rhubarb, cabbage, radish, cauliflower, beets, turnips, and squash.
- When these vegetables are boiled, nitrates leach into the cooking water, which may cause the baby to become ill (difficulty breathing and blue skin).
- In infancy, limit quantity intake (e.g., one to two tablespoons per feeding).
- In young infants, do not add the cooking water from the nitrate vegetables when you prepare baby foods.
- Instead, when preparing baby foods, use breast milk, formula, or boiled water that has been cooled to mix the puree.

Parent Concerns
What does kosher baby food mean?
- Kosher simply means that the food is prepared in accordance with special Jewish dietary laws (e.g., not mixing meat and dairy products).
- These foods meet specific nutritional and hygienic regulations.

What about organic food?
- Organic foods have been grown in a safe and healthy environment using natural fertilizers, free of synthetic pesticides or additives.
- There is no research that conclusively proves that organic food is more nutritious than other foods. However, organic foods provide the following:
  - ❖ Better protection from pesticides that are widely used on a variety of crops; more than 80% of conventionally grown fruits and vegetables tested contained at least one pesticide residue (Pesticide Data Program, 1994-1999).

- ❖ Studies show that some chemical fertilizers, fungicides, and insecticides used by non-organic farmers have been linked to cancer, nerve damage, and birth defects.

- ❖ Since organic foods contain fewer pesticides, you may want to use organic produce when preparing homemade foods for your baby.

- Organic foods contain various nutrients and can be used as a healthy alternative to regularly grown foods.

- Also, there are commercially available organic jar foods, which you can buy. The label should read "certified organically grown" (e.g., organic oatmeal and banana cereal, sweet potatoes, brown rice cereal, garden vegetables, beans, pasta, etc.).

Do I have to warm store bought jar foods?

- No, it is not necessary to warm store bought jar foods. Give at room temperature or, if you want, you may heat the food by placing the amount desired in a cup that is then placed in a pan of hot water. Always stir to distribute the heat evenly and test the temperature before feeding your baby.

What are some practical points I can look for when I buy commercial baby foods?

- When buying store bought baby foods, look at the following:

  - ❖ Date of expiry.

  - ❖ Recommended child's age on the label.

  - ❖ Nutrient contents (in case your child is allergic to a particular ingredient).

  - ❖ Combination of food groups (it is better to buy each separately).

  - ❖ Kosher jar foods (if you keep kosher foods in the house).

  - ❖ Lid is tightly sealed (not broken or previously opened).

  - ❖ Any additives (it is better to buy jar foods without any additives).

  - ❖ Water content (the more water, the more diluted the food).

  - ❖ In the case of cereal, look for whether or not it includes baby formula (since your baby may be allergic to that particular formula).

I am having trouble transitioning from commercial to homemade baby foods. Is there anything I can do?

❖ You can try to mix the first few meals with half commercial food and half homemade food.

❖ As your baby adjusts to this mixture, you can decrease the amount of commercial baby food by a 1/4, so that you slowly begin to offer more homemade foods.

❖ When first introducing homemade foods to your baby, offer her favorite foods (e.g., sweet potatoes and bananas, etc.).

Spices, Flavors & Tastes

General

Spices are strongly flavored parts of a plant that are used in small amounts either as a preservative or flavoring in cooking. Flavor may be defined as a distinctive combination of smell and taste. Tastes distinguish between different flavors in the mouth. There are four basic tastes in the mouth: sweet, salt, sour and bitter. Genetically, most people (including children) prefer sweet and salty tastes and do not like the bitter or sour tastes in foods. However, taste preferences change from day to day, particularly in children.

Children's food likes and dislikes are determined by taste, smell, sight, touch, and the texture of various foods. All of these play a role in whether or not your child will accept a particular food. Studies have shown that feeding experiences during the first year of life contribute to future food likes and dislikes.

Taste Buds

- Taste buds are a group of cells located primarily in the mouth, cheeks, and all over the surface of the tongue. They allow a person to recognize different tastes.

- Taste buds for sweet flavors are located on the tip of the tongue. Salt or sour taste buds are located on the sides of the tongue and bitter tastes are located on the back of the tongue, while the middle of the tongue is neutral.

- Young children's taste buds are more sensitive than adults. This is why children are picky eaters.

- To enhance food acceptance, place sweet foods on the tip of the tongue and less sweet foods on the middle of your child's tongue. If your baby tends to reject new tastes, place new foods on the middle of her tongue, where there are fewer taste receptors.

- Taste buds take a long time to mature and develop, so children's food needs to be simple in texture, flavor, preparation, and presentation.

- If you add seasoning or sweetener to your baby's food (remember, these ingredients are often added to commercially prepared baby foods—check the label), these additional tastes may be *all* that the baby tastes.

- Also, studies have shown that food tastes are stronger when one is hungry since taste receptors are more sensitive.

> ### Tip: Tricking the Taste Buds into Receiving Medication
>
> It is sometimes difficult to get your child to accept an unpleasant-tasting medication. The trick here is to numb your child's taste buds by first giving her a popsicle, ice cream, or anything cold. This way, your child will be more likely to accept the medication.

Tastes at all Ages

Tastes in the Womb

- Taste preferences and future eating habits develop as early as in the mother's womb.

- A baby develops her very first taste buds 9 weeks after conception, but she doesn't perceive the flavor of her mother's diet until later in the pregnancy.

- Unborn babies are able to swallow. Swallowing increases when foods from the mother's diet are sweet rather than bitter or sour. Studies have shown that the fetus swallows up to 4 cups/1 liter per day of amniotic fluid during the last trimester of the pregnancy.

Newborn

- By the time babies are born, they have a very strong sense of taste and already show various taste preferences.

- Newborns generally prefer a sweet taste. For example, a premature baby at 33 weeks has been shown to suck harder on a sweetened nipple than on a plain rubber nipple.

- Taste preferences are further developed through breastfeeding when the newborn consumes breast milk (which is flavored by the mother's diet).

- A formula-fed newborn will experience very little flavor variety, unlike a breastfeeding baby.

Four to Seven months of age

- At this time in the baby's life, solid foods are beginning to be gradually introduced into her diet.

- It is important to introduce new foods one at a time for allergy tracking and to help you understand which tastes and flavors your baby enjoys the most (see *Starting Solids*).

- When you introduce vegetables, start with those that are sweet (e.g., sweet potatoes and carrots) as many babies will prefer the sweet taste.
- Repeated exposure to foods which are not sweet will allow your baby to gradually accept these foods. Once food is accepted, a new taste preference has been developed.

Eight to Twelve months of age
- By this stage in a baby's development, food tastes and preferences are typically established.
- Continue to offer your baby a variety of tastes and textures (see *Textured Foods*). Remember that every baby responds to tastes and textures differently.
- Do not add any additives or sweeteners such as salt, sugar, honey, etc.
- Most babies at this stage will enjoy bland cereals and sweet fruits and vegetables.

Toddler Years
- Normally at this stage in a child's life, most food refusals represent independence and control over food eaten. The child knows what she likes or dislikes and is now able to express these preferences.
- Try offering your child various new tastes and flavors in foods and make the "boring" or "gross-looking" foods seem more appealing (e.g., change presentation of foods, add familiar tastes to these foods, etc.).

Super Tasters
- Super tasters have the most taste buds and are highly sensitive to fatty, spicy, and sweet foods. It is found to be a genetically inherited trait.
- These children basically experience taste much stronger than everyone else. For example, super tasters feel more "burn" sensations from such things as ginger or the carbon dioxide found in sodas. Bitter tastes are bitterer, sweet tastes are sweeter, sour tastes feel sharper, and salty tastes are saltier for the super taster (e.g., grapefruits or broccoli are strong tasting foods that may be refused by the super taster).
- Super tasters tend to stay away from strong flavored foods, fats, and sugars.

- If your child is a super taster, help mask the bitter taste in foods by adding a little oil or margarine to their foods.

- Studies have shown that introducing your child to a wide range of flavors, textures, and tastes early on in life will help her develop good food habits and taste preferences in the future.

- About two thirds of super tasters are females.

- Sensitivity to foods usually declines as your child grows older.

- Consult your doctor or dietitian about providing your super taster child with a healthy, well-balanced diet while being sensitive to her taste buds.

Spicy Foods & Breastfeeding

- One positive aspect of eating a variety of foods while you are breastfeeding your baby is that you are giving her a first introduction to the taste of solid foods.

- The flavor of breast milk constantly changes due to the mother's diet, unlike that of artificial milk (formula) that tastes the same at every feeding.

- Eat a variety of food (well-balanced diet) and allow your baby to enjoy all the tastes and flavors supplied to her through your breast milk.

- Your baby may enjoy the stronger flavors in your breast milk after you eat such foods as garlic or onions. However, highly spiced and seasoned foods may upset your baby's stomach so try to decrease/avoid salty, sugary, or spicy foods. You will know your baby is not enjoying the feeding when she is fussy, irritable, and crying. In some cases, your baby may develop an allergic reaction manifested by a rash, irritability, etc.

- Some health professionals recommend waiting until your baby is at least eight months of age before introducing any types of additives to her diet.

Flavors & Tastes: Suggestions

General Suggestions to Improve Flavors &Tastes

- Many foods taste good when they are served at room temperature (or cold), rather than hot.

- Place sweet foods on the tip of your child's tongue and less sweet foods on the middle of her tongue to increase the chances of food acceptance.

- Avoid excess salting, hot and sour foods, and sugar (it promotes a sweet tooth). If you must sweeten foods with additives, use natural alternatives to white sugar such as maple syrup, honey (only after the age of one year), apple concentrate, etc.

- When oil is required to prepare foods, use canola oil, corn, or sunflower oil as it contains non-saturated fatty acids (soy or olive oil may also be used) compared to more saturated (less healthier) fatty acids. Do not use butter or saturated fat oils (e.g., palm or coconut oil).

- Do not force-feed your child, especially when food appears to taste bad to them. Just keep exposing her to the food—this is proven to gradually enhance food acceptance.

- To help clean your child's taste buds, rinse her mouth with juice, tea, ginger ale, club soda, or salted water before eating.

- Expose your baby to various tastes, flavors, and colored food to broaden her eating habits and future taste preferences.

- Many experts do not recommend the use of spices for the following reasons:
  - ❖ It may be all that the baby tastes (allow your child to become accustomed to natural tastes and flavors before she learns other tastes).
  - ❖ The taste for spices should be acquired (it is not a taste that the baby is born with).
  - ❖ Babies do not expect all foods to taste sweet or salty, etc.
  - ❖ Fosters future unhealthy eating habits.

- These experts suggest that seasoning and spicing in your child's diet should be around the age of four years, once your child has established a healthy and varied diet on her own. This way, you are simply broadening her taste experiences. Toddlers can begin adapting their taste buds to ethnic foods and spices. This is a good age for introducing more diverse flavors and preparing your child for unfamiliar tastes.

- However, other experts suggest that you can use light spicing, meaning very subtle additives such as oregano, basil, cumin, sweet paprika, a little salt, spices or sourness, etc., since these seasonings added to food may even encourage the enjoyment of a greater variety of food later, as seen in various cultures (see also the last question in this chapter's *Parent Concerns*).

Tip: Homemade Foods, Additives, Good and Bad Fats

When preparing homemade baby foods, you have full control of what your baby is eating and you are able to provide healthy and nutritious meals without any additives or sweeteners. Some additives which you may add to make foods more interesting include the following: mint, basil, rosemary, garlic powder, vanilla, pepper, dill, lemon zest, ginger, cinnamon, nutmeg, oregano, anise, oil, butter, or margarine.

Saturated fat (considered "bad" fat) is mostly found in animal products such as meat, poultry, butter, eggs, etc., and in palm oil, coconut oil, etc. Saturated fat clogs arteries, increases chances of heart disease, and interferes with body production of good fat (essential fatty acids that the body cannot produce on its own). Unsaturated ("good") fat is usually supplied by plants and includes oils from vegetables such as corn oil, soya, walnut, sunflower, etc. Hydrogenation of unsaturated fat can transform it into saturated fat.

Meat & Poultry

- These may taste better if they are served cold or at room temperature.
- Marinate the meat or poultry in fruit juice, dressing, or other sauces for more taste.

Fruit

- Fresh fruits are often well tolerated.
- Any type of fruit smoothie, sorbet, or yogurt generally tastes good to the baby's mouth.
- Offer fruity popsicles in your child's favorite flavors.
- Lemon drops or mint may be sucked on after eating fruits to get rid of any lingering taste.

Vegetables

- Use fresh tomatoes when preparing tomato sauce, rather than canned sauce.
- Peel carrots before eating or cooking them to eliminate the bitter taste (or use baby carrots that are already peeled and cut).

Tip: Taste in Children with Cancer

Chemotherapy, radiation therapy, or cancer itself, may cause foods to not taste the same. See general suggestions within this chapter of how to improve tastes and flavors in these cases.

MSG

- Monosodium glutamate (MSG) is an amino acid present in all proteins.

- It is a widely used additive in creating smooth and flavored foods.

- MSG is found in foods such as mushrooms, tomatoes, beef, chicken, corn, fish, and Parmesan cheese.

- Only a small amount of MSG is required to achieve great flavor in original tasting foods. It cannot improve foods that taste bad or bad cooking; it simply makes good food taste better.

- MSG is added to foods before or during cooking.

- Studies show that babies are able to metabolize MSG like adults and that breast milk contains a higher level of MSG than cow's milk. However, MSG is not usually recommended as it could cause adverse effects such as headaches, worsening of asthma, dizziness, tingling sensations, chest pain, etc.

- Thus, look at food labels and watch for MSG in spices, sauces, soups, syrups, and dips; also, look at vitamins, cough syrups, etc., which may contain aspartame and, when eating in a restaurant, ask if soups or sauces contain MSG.

Tip: Starch Fillers

Starches are carbohydrates that are easily digested and contain very little fat.

Food starches help moderate flavor and control texture.

Starches may be present in baby foods in flour form such as rice, tapioca, corn, and wheat and are a great source of calories for growing babies.

The Food and Drug Administration deems starch fillers as safe and suitable for baby food use.

Parent Concerns

Do dental problems have anything to do with tastes and flavors?

- Discuss with your dentist any dental problems that cause bad tastes (e.g., cavities, etc.).

- Do not drink citrus juices (e.g., orange juice, grapefruit juice, etc.) immediately after brushing your teeth with fluoride toothpaste. The chemical mixture of fluoride with citric acid leaves a bad taste in your mouth.

Tip: Food Additives & Child's Behavior

There has been no conclusive evidence linking food additives with your child's behavior. Discuss with your doctor if you have any concerns.

Does food given in early childhood years affect or make a difference in my child's dietary future choices?

- Yes, foods given at early stages in life do make a difference in your child's future choices.

- Your child will learn what the norm for foods is. For example, if she eats foods from your kitchen, then she will learn what normal food tastes like. However, if your child's diet is composed of processed foods, then she will believe that artificial tastes are the norm.

- Despite the fact that your child is born with a sweet tooth (breast milk and most fresh foods are sweet), you can shape your child's taste preferences in the first three years of life. Use this window of opportunity wisely.

- A recent study shows that infants build up a "visual prototype" of foods they have already tried and liked. Babies who are introduced to a wide variety of textures, colors and tastes will be more likely to have broad taste preferences later in life. However, those babies who stick to "safe foods" during infancy will have a difficult time trying new things.

Is there a difference in tastes and flavors between homemade and commercial baby foods?

- The tastes and looks of homemade and commercial baby foods are completely different.

- These variations in tastes, flavors, and colors are due to a variety of external factors; the method of cooking, pureeing or processing, refrigeration, etc. It allows the baby to taste a variety of foods in different textures, shapes, and colors.

Homemade Baby Foods	Commercial Baby Foods
Taste and color variation are common. Stronger in taste (e.g., meats). Fruits and veggies have better taste and "real" color. Different texture. Can control what your baby is eating and know all ingredients (e.g., no additives, etc.).	Processed to a thin and runny texture unlike that of homemade foods. No "real" color.

Is it okay if I eat spices while I am breastfeeding?

- Spicy foods may cause gas in the mother but not in the baby.

- You may eat what you like. However, if you think that the food bothers your baby in some way (e.g., fussy, , irritably cries, wakes abruptly, uncomfortable, wheezing, nasal congestion, mucous or blood in the stool, etc.), make sure it is this particular food (see if your child reacts at least 3 times) before blaming it. Some of the symptoms may represent an allergy to foods such as dairy products, wheat, citrus, etc.

- Remember that in some countries such as Mexico, India, and Thailand, eating hot and spicy foods are the cultural norm and yet not many babies have difficulties.

- The flavor of breast milk constantly changes, unlike that of formula.

- In fact, eating a variety of foods while you are breastfeeding provides your baby with a first introduction to the tastes of solid foods.

Feeding Your Baby with a Spoon

General

Using a spoon is important, because it develops motor expertise and coordination. Eating from a spoon requires a different set of skills than sucking from a breast or bottle. Initially, your baby needs to learn how to use the muscles of her tongue, throat, and lips. However, as your baby grows in independence and starts wanting to feed herself, spoon feeding will promote hand-eye coordination and will help lay the foundation for good eating habits.

Reasons to Switch to a Spoon

- Formula or breastfeeding supplies all the nutrients necessary for the first four to six months; after this time, you need to supply your baby with other nutrients in different foods that will initially require spoon-feeding.

- Beginning your child on solid foods means starting the use of a spoon that will allow your baby to taste or feed. For example, cereals and jar foods ease feedings that contain a more thickened "fluid" food.

- Feeding your child solid foods through a bottle leads to excessive weight gain and increases your child's food intake at each feeding. The baby may choke if she is fed thick foods through a bottle.

> ### Tip: Spoon Use and Motor Skills
>
> The use of a spoon will provide meaning (relative and good use or control of a spoon by your child) for your child at 15-19 months of age, when their motor skills have improved significantly. Good control of the spoon is usually achieved by three years of age.

When to Start & Age/Skill Development

When to Start

- Your baby is ready to begin spoon-feeding when you notice that she is beginning to show interest in food that is on the table (e.g., shows excitement and wants to taste or tries to reach for table food).

- The use of a spoon may begin between four to six months of age and when there is one or more of the following non-specific signs:

❖ Frequent feeding required (baby is often hungry).

❖ Feeds more than 1 liter/4 cups of formula or expressed breast milk per day.

❖ Solids must be introduced and the baby shows interest in solid foods (see *Solids*).

❖ Able to grasp the spoon in her hand.

Signs of Increasing Skill Development

The following are signs of increased skill development in your baby:

• Your baby opens her mouth when she sees a spoon approaching (or reaches for the spoon and puts food in her hands) and is excited to take the spoonful of food. She also looks intently at the food and the spoon.

• Your baby can remove food from the spoon using her upper and lower lips.

• The extrusion reflex has disappeared and your baby's tongue does not protrude after the spoon is removed from her mouth. Food is passed to the back of her mouth until it is swallowed.

• Your baby enjoys and is relaxed during feedings.

• The ability of hand use in babies increases around eight to nine months. Give your baby a spoon and let her play with it at mealtime (practicing).

Age Advancement & Use of a Spoon

The following is an age-by-age guide to your baby's spoon-feeding developments; however, there may be variations according to each unique baby's developmental readiness.

Age	Developments
4-6 Months	Your baby still has the extrusion reflex so she can not take food from a spoon. This usually begins to disappear around this age.
6/8-10 Months	The ability of hand use in babies increases around 8-9 months. Give your baby a spoon and let her play with it at mealtime (for practice).
11-12 Months	Better at placing the spoon in her mouth. You may place the food on the spoon and allow her to place it in her mouth to develop hand-eye coordination.

Age	Developments
12-15 Months	Your child has a desire to feed herself. She may continue to turn the spoon upside down (takes months to master).
15-18 Months	Uses the spoon to feed herself and no longer requires much help as motor skills improve. May continue to spill foods.
18-24 Months	Your child is becoming more skillful at using the spoon. It may be time to allow your child to use a safe, plastic fork so that she may also learn to pick up food with a fork.
24-36 Months	Your baby's spoon skills (and possibly her fork skills) have developed well by this age and will continue to improve. By two years of age, your baby is using the spoon with some spillage and by three years of age, she has better control of the spoon with food.

Which Type of Spoon to Use

General

- The type of spoon used depends on whether you use it to feed your baby or whether your baby uses it on her own to feed herself.

- When you feel that your baby is ready to begin spoon-feeding, choose a small spoon with a long handle (like a coffee spoon) for you to feed your baby.

- The spoon should be small and shallow enough to easily fit into your baby's mouth. It should be easy to grasp and should not have any sharp edges (a curved handle to prevent poking of the eye).

- Use a plastic coated baby spoon, since metal spoons may irritate your child's sensitive gums.

- A spoon that is temperature safe is very useful, since it allows you to know when food is too hot to serve.

- When your baby tries to feed herself, give her a curved handle spoon to decrease the risk of eye trauma.

Types of Spoons

- There are various types of spoons available which include the following:

  ❖ Plastic or silver.

  ❖ Disposable or non-disposable.

  ❖ Short or long handles and with different curves (the longer the handle, the easier to use for the caregiver and the easier it is to reach the bottom of a jar; different handle curves are said to prevent spillage, however short handles may be easier for babies to hold).

  ❖ Color changing spoons that are heat sensitive.

  ❖ Soft tip or touch spoons.

  ❖ Various bowl size spoons.

- Do not use a spoon with a pointed handle.

- Spoons with various shapes or toys that are built on the handle may distract your baby and she will not be able to learn how to eat with a spoon.

- Watch the size of the spoon given to your baby as a smaller spoon may pose a choking risk.

- When removing food from a large container, take out a small amount that you know your baby will finish. Use a clean spoon (one that has not come into contact with saliva or anything else) to prevent introducing germs and causing infection. Also, if you are ill, do not share the spoon with your baby.

Tip: Finger as First Spoon?

The child's first spoon may be your finger, as it is soft and the baby is familiar with its feel. Your finger will also be able to tell you if the food is too hot to serve.

Administration of Food by Spoon

The following are suggestions and tips on when, what, and how to begin administering food to your baby with a spoon:

When

- The first time you try spoon-feeding, do it in the morning so that you can check for any allergic reactions that may occur (caused by a new food).

- Try introducing the spoon when your baby is mildly hungry and not upset.

- Your baby will begin to accept food from a spoon more regularly once she is able to hold food in her mouth without pushing it out with her tongue.

SECTION 4: STARTING SOLID FOODS

What

- Start with more watery food (e.g., formula consistency; soup-like, then offer mashed, etc.) prior to beginning spoon-feeding.

How

- Have your baby sit on your knees with her body straight, when she is expecting the food.
- Place a small amount (1/2-1 tea spoon) of food on the tip of the spoon and put it on your baby's lips, so that she may suck the food off.
- Do not push the spoon into the baby's mouth as this may cause gagging.
- At first taste, the baby may push the food out of her mouth. Simply scoop it up and again place it in-between her lips and mouth. This is normal since your baby is just getting used to both the new taste and taking food from a spoon.
- If the baby is fussy with the spoon, you may also begin by dipping the tip of a clean finger into the food and placing it into your baby's mouth for her to suck on.
- If the baby still protests and shows dislike for the spoon, wait until the next day or after a few days to try again.
- Introduce one food at a time and offer it by way of the spoon for three to four days before introducing another new food. Once your baby has tried a variety of foods, you may spoon-feed her solids throughout the day (breakfast, lunch, and dinner).
- Once your baby is accustomed to the spoon and the food, you may gradually increase the amount offered from 1/2-1 tea spoon to a few tablespoons. Increase the consistency and texture according to your child's age and developmental ability.
- When starting solids and spoon use, mix rice cereal with water, breast milk, or formula to a very watery constituency to make the food more easily accepted. Put a little bit on the tip of the spoon and slip it into your baby's mouth.
- As time progresses, you may thicken the cereal according to your baby's ability to swallow.
- Gradually use various cereals to expose her to different tastes and textures.
- Cereals may be given at any time in the day at your baby's preference.

- At the start of spoon-feeding, you will need to fill her spoon for her to decrease the mess. As the baby develops in age, you can help her take food off the plate and then later let her do the job herself.

- Be sure to place yourself at eye level with your child and not too close to her face. The child should be allowed to come to the spoon, rather than the spoon being brought to the child.

Spoon Refusal: Easing the Transition

- Do not push food into an unreceptive mouth and a baby that turns away. Try again later or use different food after several tries. Your baby may not be ready quite yet, so don't force it on her.

- The best thing to do is begin spoon-feeding with a familiar food. This means that you should start with a small amount of formula or breast milk and then switch to half a spoonful of foods. Finish off with more milk (either expressed breast or formula milk).

- Another method to try is to put a 1/4 teaspoon of selected food on the spoon and slip it onto the baby's lips and see how she reacts. If she is ready for spoon-feeding, she will take it quickly and not spit it up. If the food is being refused, or taken and spit out, then your baby is probably not yet ready for spoon feeding.

- If the baby refuses spoon-feeding, continue formula or breastfeeding exclusively for a week and then retry the spoon.

- Do not be discouraged if your baby is not taking the spoon feedings. It may take as many as 15 tries to get a child to accept new food and to accept taking it from a spoon.

- Allow the baby to take alternate bites from her own spoon as well as from the spoon you hold (use two spoons to help her practice) at around 9-10 months of age.

- After the age of one year, offer finger foods to your child in one hand while she uses the spoon in the other hand to alternate feedings. Alternating between finger feeding and spoon-feeding may help stimulate spoon use.

- Eat with a spoon in front of your baby so that she can see how it is done.

Case Description

Case Description

Jacob is a 10-month-old boy who refuses the use of a spoon. His mother has tried several times to offer him the spoon, but he has refused every time. Everything he is fed is through a bottle (formula, cereal, vegetable, meat, juice, fruits, etc.).

He was born a healthy full-term baby with no complications. He had no oral and muscular motor problems and his weight is normal for his age.

Comments:

- The risk of feeding your child everything through a bottle poses various risks including choking, excessive weight gain, etc.

- Follow the suggestions offered in this chapter if your child refuses a spoon and repeat these methods until you are successful otherwise, you may face more difficulties.

Tip: Keep Trying the Spoon, Don't Give Up

Start the use of a spoon early and keep trying its use despite refusal as studies show that babies may need up to 10-15 tries before acceptance occurs.

- Remember that tasting becomes a way of exploring for your baby, especially as she gets older. Watch out for what goes inside your baby's mouth.

- See chapters on *Starting Solids, Spices, Tastes & Flavors*, etc. for other concerns.

Tip: Spoon Measurements

3 small spoons = 1 tbsp or 15 ml
1 small spoon = about 5 ml
12 drops = about 1 teaspoon

Cereals for your Baby & Toddler

General

Cereals are usually one of the first solid foods introduced into your baby's diet, typically between the ages of four to six months. Cereals add taste, texture, variety, and nutrition to your baby's diet. They are enriched with calcium, phosphorus, iron, and vitamins and supply an immediate source of sugar in the blood.

Cereal is not a required step in the development of a baby's menu, as long as she is growing and gaining weight normally. However, it is a good and effective way to increase iron supplementation. Cereals are also a good source of carbohydrates, calories, and energy.

Types of Cereals

General
- Cereals are available in the following two forms:
    - ❖ *Premixed* baby cereal in a jar is convenient and ready to use.
    - ❖ *Dry* varieties of cereal will need added water, formula, or breast milk. These can vary in consistency to suit the baby and are richer in iron than premixed cereals.

Nutritious Cereals
- A nutritious cereal is like a multivitamin and mineral supplement.
- A nutritious cereal will either say "whole wheat," "whole bran," or "whole grain" on the label. "Wheat," "multigrain," and similar listings do NOT contain the same nutritional value. It must contain the word "whole" before the grain type to ensure maximum nutritional value.
- The quality of the grain is more important than looking at the percentage of vitamins listed on the cereal box.
- Infant cereal is more enriched with iron than adult cereals.
- Cereals with high fiber grain content such as barley, oats, and rye may be helpful for the constipated older infant and toddler.
- Cereals made with the ingredients of formula are a great source of providing your child with about 19 vitamins and minerals. These are easy to prepare—simply add water.

Types of Infant & Toddler Cereals Available

Single Grain Cereals	These cereals include rice, barley or oatmeal.
Mixed Cereals	These include mixture of cereals only or mixtures of cereal, vegetables, and fruits.
Starch Cereals	Barely contain any protein (less risk of allergy). Examples include cornstarch (corn flour).
Crushed Grains	Contains 10% protein. Examples are wheat flour, rice, semolina, and baby's grains.
Grain & Cereals	Cereals and grains include rice, wheat, barley, and rye. Nutritional value is mainly concentrated on iron and group B vitamins. Rice grains are hypoallergenic and easy to digest. Wheat grains are the hardest to digest; the allergy risk due to gluten in these cereals is associated with Celiac disease in the bowels (some studies show that early exposure to wheat cereals increases the risk to develop Celiac disease).

- Multigrain and cereals with fruits add a variety of flavors to your baby's diet. Rice, barley, or oatmeal cereal is particularly good when you add pureed fruits. Try this after your older baby has already started eating fruits.

- Avoid rice cereals that are low in fiber as this can cause constipation. You may need to give high-fibre (brown) rice cereals to help soften your baby's stool, especially with the older infant and child.

- The timeline for the introduction of cereals to the menu are rice, barley, oats, and then the mixed cereals.

Homemade & Commercially Prepared Cereals

The following chart outlines various traits of homemade and store bought cereals:

Homemade Cereals	Store Bought Cereals
If you prepare cereal from grains on your own, consider that these are not iron-fortified, so you would have to consult your doctor about iron supplements for your growing baby.	These are iron-fortified cereals. Convenient, easy to prepare. Good texture. Store open boxes of cereal in a cool, dry place for up to one month (nutrient content begins to decrease later).

Homemade Cereals	Store Bought Cereals
Whole grains in homemade rice and millet cereals may cause digestive problems in your child (e.g., gas) since the baby who is younger than six months of age is unable to digest them.	Well digested by a baby younger than 6 months of age since these cereals are processed and refined (not whole grains).

- Cereals made for older children or adults are not nutritionally formulated for babies. Their texture may be unsuitable and cause choking or gagging in your baby.

Tip: Storing Grains

Store grains and cereals in a cupboard or opaque container since the vitamin content deteriorates when exposed to light.

Suggestions for Homemade Cereals

- Any cereal can be sweetened with pureed fruits that your baby is already used to.
- Plain yogurt may be added to hot cereals since it provides a creamy texture to grain cereals.
- You may add beans to grain cereals before cooking them as it provides a high-protein base for your baby.
- Brown or organically grown brown rice may be used to make natural cereals.
- Brown rice, along with millet cereal, may be served as the baby's first food if given to a baby older than six months of age. At this age, your baby should have the right kind of digestive enzymes to handle the complex carbohydrates in these cereals.

Tip: Use of Millet

Millet is a small, rounded yellow whole grain with a sweet flavor.

It is a tasty alternative to rice cereal.

Millet is naturally high in protein and various essential amino acids.

Suggestions for Store Bought Cereals

- Buy cereals that contain high-fiber grains (barley, millet, oats, rye, whole wheat, etc.), but which have no added sugar, salt, preservatives, or artificial flavors.

- If you buy plain cereals without any added formula, it will give you the choice of whether or not you would like to add breast milk or formula. It will also alleviate allergy concerns, since formula-fed babies may not tolerate the particular type of formula used in a given cereal.

- You can use whole grain organic cereals with no formula added as a first choice cereal or plain refined cereals, which do not contain any hydrogenated fat (saturated fat is considered to be "bad").

- Choose iron-fortified (or those enriched in calcium and B-vitamins) cereals to ensure healthy blood, strong bones, and tooth development in your baby.

- Cereals that advertise "high fiber" content usually contain extra wheat, so make sure your child takes extra fluids when eating these cereals (also, make sure your child is old enough to prevent the problems associated with early exposure to wheat).

- Provide a wide variety of tastes and textures and cereals that are easy to digest.

When & Which to Start

- Cereals are recommended to start like solids (as a first complementary food) at four to six months of age, depending on your baby's weight gain, signs of readiness to begin solid foods, and allergic history.

- If you are thinking about trying to introduce anything other than breast milk or formula before four to six months, talk to your doctor first.

- The American Academy of Pediatrics recommends starting out with rice cereal before introducing cereal with mixed or complex grains such as barley and oatmeal. Rice cereals are the first to be recommended due to the following reasons:

  ❖ Easily digestible by most infants.

  ❖ Less likely to trigger an allergy reaction than other cereals.

  ❖ Easily thinned to a texture not much thicker than milk (when mixed with water, breast milk, or formula).

  ❖ Has no gluten (protein that is associated with Celiac disease).

- A mixed cereal should be added to your baby's diet only after each kind of cereal has been separately introduced and allergies have been ruled out.

- Avoid cereals that contain added fruits and vegetables until your infant is eating multigrain cereals well.

- Use one particular cereal for three to five days before introducing a new type of cereal and watch for allergy reactions or symptoms (e.g., rash, vomiting, diarrhea, breathing problems, etc.).

- The last cereal to be introduced (usually around nine months of age) should be wheat cereal, because it is difficult for your baby to digest and poses an allergy risk (contains glutens associated with Celiac disease and early exposure may increase risk).

- The following table provides a guideline of which grains to give your child according to age. Check with your doctor if you child is younger than six months and you want to start feeding her cereals.

Step 1: 4-6 Months	Step 2: Up to 9 Months	Step 3: 9-12 Months
Single grain infant cereals (rice, barley, oatmeal); start with rice or barley and mix with breast milk or formula.	Mixed grains infant cereal (only after single grain has been accepted).	Continue iron-fortified cereals.
Commercial: Use iron-fortified cereals.	Introduce other grain products (teeth begin to appear); plain dry toast or unsalted crackers (finger foods).	Introduce other plain fortified cereals in combination with breads, pasta, or teething biscuits.
2-4 tablespoons twice per day.	2-4 tablespoons twice per day.	8-10 tablespoons per day.

- Do not use more cereal than is recommended and do not substitute it for important nutrients since you may risk giving too many calories and causing excess weight gain in your child.

- If you breast or bottle-feed and your baby is growing well, start cereals at six months of age (see recommendations in *Starting Solids*) and discuss this with your doctor.

- If your child has constipation, speak to your doctor about starting her on other cereals first (e.g., barley cereal before rice).

Cereal Preparation, Administration & Serving

General Preparation

- Put cereal into a bowl or on a plate.
- You can mix or add it with water, formula, breast milk or various liquids that the baby is used to (e.g., soup, juice, etc.) or vegetables, fruits puree, or yogurt.
- If you do not want to give many calories to your baby, you can mix the cereal with water and diluted juice.
- Initially, make the cereal a runny mixture and later progress to an applesauce like texture.
- Increase the thickness and the amount of cereal depending on your baby's developmental readiness.
- After the age of 1 year, you can mix the cereal with whole cow's milk or diluted cow's milk.

Tip: Wheat Warning

Watch out for mixed grain and/or high fiber cereals that contain wheat.

Administration & Serving

- Start feedings cereals by allowing your baby to lick it from your fingers.
- Ensure that the cereal is not too hot.
- Always use a spoon when feeding cereal.
- At first, give your baby cereals once or twice a day and make sure to offer it after breast milk or formula feeding is finished, so that your baby doesn't fill up on cereal instead of the more nutritious breast milk or formula.
- Initially, start with one teaspoon once or twice per day and gradually increase the amount. The amount of cereal eaten in a meal depends on the baby's appetite.
- If the baby begins to gag, stir in more liquid and try to feed her again.
- Some babies are fed cereal in the morning and their appetite sometimes decreases for the rest of the day. In such cases, use cereals prior to sleep.

- Use a single ingredient, iron-fortified cereal at first, so that you can identify the cause if there is an allergic reaction.

- Once you are certain that the baby is able to tolerate a particular cereal type, you may start introducing other single ingredient cereals (such as barley and oatmeal). Use each type one to three weeks and then switch to other types.

- If there is no allergic reaction, switch to mixed cereal types.

Refusal

- Once you start cereal feeding, try it for a few consecutive days. If the baby is not interested, wait a few days and retry; if the baby still refuses the cereal after several attempts, retry in a few weeks.

- Try other types of cereals, as your baby may not like a particular one. You may try barley or oatmeal if your baby does not like the rice cereal (it is the blandest cereal).

- Once fruits have been introduced into the menu, you may consider mixing the cereal with one of the fruits your baby enjoys.

- If your baby seems to dislike the taste of rice cereal, also try changing the temperature at which you serve it, or change the consistency (adding more or less liquid). To change the flavor, try to prepare the cereal with water, breast milk, or formula.

- Not every baby needs cereal, especially the obese or overweight infant or toddler. However, you may place a minimal amount of cereal for taste and texture learning in other foods. Consider iron sources from other solids such as meat, etc. (see appropriate chapters).

Tip: Iron Supplement & Cereal Refusal

If your baby is refusing iron-fortified cereal when complementary solids are started, discuss with your doctor regarding iron supplements and sources.

If your baby is not eating much cereal initially, do not be too concerned since breast milk or formula provides the major source of nutrition.

Parental Concerns

Why is rice cereal the one that is recommended to start first?

- Rice cereal is an ideal choice for the baby's first solid foods, as it is rich in carbohydrates and contains no gluten (which is associated with Celiac disease).

- It is a good source of protein, nutritional fiber, vitamin B groups (especially niacin and thiamin), iron, and other minerals.

- Rice cereal is among the foods that are relatively safe in not causing allergic reactions (others are potatoes, pears, lettuce, etc.).

- Sometimes, rice cereal is added to infant formula to increase energy (caloric) density or to decrease regurgitation and reflux; however it may result in early satiety (feeling of fullness) which then may defeat the purpose of increasing caloric (energy) intake.

Does cereal have an effect on my child's sleeping habits?

- Normal sleep patterns vary widely; so do not compare your baby to others.

- Some babies sleep through the night (eight consecutive hours) at two to three months of age and others start later.

- There is no convincing evidence that adding cereal to the bedtime bottle helps infants sleep through the night and it is still unclear as to whether we can modify normal sleep patterns at an early age.

- If you notice that your baby is "sleeping well" through the night after feeding cereal before bedtime, then keep it like this as long as your baby is gaining weight well. If there are weight gain issues, then feed your child extra at night to help your baby gain weight.

My baby suffers from constipation after having eaten the rice cereal. What can I do?

- Some babies develop constipation after eating rice cereal.

- Use other types of cereal (e.g., barley or oatmeal) until rice may be tolerated.

- You may want to wait a few days after stopping the use of rice. When you re-start, keep the cereal diluted with extra water and gradually decrease the dilution (according to your baby's stools).

Is there any way I can "fortify" cereals I prepare at home like the way cereals in the store are fortified?
- No, you cannot fortify cereals in the same way as commercially prepared cereals.
- You may add formula, breast milk, wheat germ, etc., to provide an extra "boost" of iron or other nutrients to the cereal.
- Do not forget that once you have added fruits and vegetables to your child's diet, the vitamin C contained in these foods assist in the absorption of iron.
- Speak to your doctor about any medical needs or concerns you may have regarding your child's iron or nutrient intake.

Can I freeze homemade baby cereals?
- Yes, you can freeze homemade cereals using the ice cube tray method that you use for other pureed foods (see *Store Bought & Homemade Foods*).

How do I choose which cereals to give my child?
Ask yourself the following two questions when deciding on cereals to see if they are appropriate for your child and if you answer yes, then they probably are:
  1) Are the cereal pieces or flakes small enough that my baby can manage it on her own with her tiny fingers?
  2) Does the cereal provide various important vitamins and minerals (whole grains, iron, etc.) for my growing baby?

Tip: Cheerios

This is a great choice for finger foods.

Very small pieces make it easy for your baby to grab and place in her mouth.

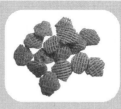

How much cereal is needed for my seven month old baby to get the iron requirements?
- Four tablespoons per day of any type of cereal mixed in with formula will provide about half of your child's daily iron requirements. The remainder of iron requirements should be met through iron-fortified formula, breast milk, and other foods.

Do I still need to feed my baby cereal at 10 months of age or older?

- Because it is iron-fortified and it is an important nutrient for your baby, you may give it to your baby at least once a day at this age.

- Older babies may continue to eat cereal or receive iron-fortified foods from other sources such as meat, poultry, wheat germs, etc.

- If your baby is growing well and eating iron-fortified foods, do not be concerned (talk to your doctor if you are worried).

Is there anything I can add to dry rice cereal?

- Cereal may be prepared with water (especially for excessive weight gaining babies), though it is better to add breast milk or formula, since this will increase nutrient and iron content (especially for babies who experience slow weight gain or growth).

What is the difference between serving my baby brown or white rice?

- Brown rice is usually fuller in nutrient value than white rice since it is not stripped of its outer bran (bran is the broken coat of the seed of cereal grain that has been separated from the flour or meal by sifting or boiling).

- It is rich in vitamins, minerals, and contains three times the fiber of white rice.

- Serve brown or a mixture of brown and white rice to your baby once she is at least nine months old (her digestive system can handle the added fiber).

Should every baby start on cereals at four months of age—does it matter whether or not she is breast or bottle-feeding?

- The American Academy of Pediatrics and Canadian Pediatric Society recommend starting iron-fortified cereals after six months of age for breastfed babies.

- According to some nutritionists, well growing breastfed babies can skip cereals, which are high in carbohydrates, as there is already a high amount of carbohydrates in breast milk. Instead, they should be given other foods, which are high in protein since babies require a lot of protein and cereal has a low protein to caloric ratio.

- Continue nursing or offering formula to your baby to ensure adequate nourishment for growth. Make the effort to supply iron and protein rich foods.

Tip: Starch

Starch is a combination of units of sugar.

It is an important source of energy, especially found in cereals, potatoes (white or sweet), legumes, etc.

Modified starch is typically based on corn or tapioca and is often added to commercially prepared baby foods.

Modified starch acts as a stabilizer in providing consistency, texture, and shelf life to baby food.

It is digested well by babies and is not at all harmful.

What can I do with leftover baby cereal—should I throw it out?
- You may use leftover baby cereal in other recipes such as cookies, biscuits, and pancakes and it can be used as a thickening agent for thin purees or for smoothing out purees (meat).

When do you recommend serving cereal—day or night?
- I noticed that some parents who offer cereal in the morning find it leads to a decreased appetite and their baby will feed less during the day.

- In such cases, I recommend serving cereal at night prior to sleep, allowing the rest of the day for formula, breast milk, or other solid foods.

If I give cereal with added fruits or vegetables to my baby, does she still need whole fruits or vegetables?
- Yes. Cereals with added fruits or vegetables are still considered a *cereal* serving. These do not in any way replace fruits or vegetables in your baby's diet.

Can I feed cereal by the bottle?
- Do not feed cereal by the bottle for the following reasons:
  - ❖ To prevent the risk of choking/lung aspiration from sucking at thick cereal.
  - ❖ To develop feeding skills.
  - ❖ To teach texture and food-moving experience.
  - ❖ For the baby to be able to differentiate between eating and drinking.

How do I get my toddler to eat cereals and can she eat adult cereals?

- Do not feed your baby iron-fortified adult cereals as these are not formulated for a toddler's digestive tract or needs.

- Serve your toddler a cereal that she chooses so that she is more likely to eat it (e.g., take her grocery shopping with you and allow her to pick the cereal).

- Cereal has traditionally been a favorite family breakfast and provides good sources of vitamin B, folic acid, zinc, iron, protein, and fiber.

- Play various breakfast games with your toddler to help her develop muscle skills and hand-to-eye coordination (e.g., finger food train).

Sample Menu (4-6 Months)

These are for early starters (babies less than six months of age) and should be discussed with your doctor.

Breakfast	Lunch	Dinner & Before Bed
Breast milk or formula Infant cereal (1-2 tbsp)	Breast milk or formula Single pureed vegetables (1-2 tbsp)	Breast milk or formula Infant cereal (1-2 tbsp) Single pureed fruit (1-2 tbsp) Breast milk or formula

(You may serve breast milk or formula in-between meals, if necessary).

Helpful Recipes

Homemade Organic or Non-Organic Cereal

Use a blender or food processor to blend uncooked organic or non-organic brown rice until it is finely ground (almost like flour).

Boil about 2 cups/500 ml of water in a saucepan.

Add 2 oz/60 g of the rice flour.

Leave it on minimum heat and stir every 2-10 minutes.

Serve immediately after it has cooled to a safe temperature or store in the refrigerator for two to three days.

This general recipe can be used with other grain cereals such as barley and oatmeal.

For older babies, you can make the cereal thicker by using only 1 cup/250 ml of water, breast milk, formula, and fruits may be added if desired. Be sure to stir consistently to prevent any burning or lumps in the cereal.

Oatmeal & Banana Cereal
Ingredients:
1/4 cup/65 g oatmeal
1/2 cup/ 125 ml water or milk
1/3 ripe banana
1/4 cup/65 ml milk or formula

Directions:
Boil oatmeal and 1/2 cup/ 125 ml of water or milk together for about five minutes.

Stir every few minutes and remove the heat by allowing it to cool for five minutes.

Mash together the banana and remaining milk or formula.

Add to the cooked cereal and stir until smooth.

Serve immediately or store in the refrigerator.

Vegetables

General

Introductory Notes

B reast milk or formula supplies most of the nutrients an infant requires until the age of six to seven months. Vegetables are usually given early in the process of introducing your baby to solid foods so that she will learn to enjoy new tastes, flavors, and textures. Vegetables contain almost no fat, yet they are a good source of energy because of the complex sugars they contain. They do not contain enough protein and calories for the young infant. They are not regarded as being a full meal unless they are included with another food group in order to provide complete and proper nutrients (e.g., meat with vegetables).

The Vegetable Group

The vegetable group includes all vegetables and their juices and consists of both yellow and green vegetables.

Yellow Vegetables	Includes carrots, squash, pumpkin and red pepper. Supplies vitamin A, C, carbohydrates, fiber, and chrome.
Green Vegetables	Includes spinach, beets, lettuce, cabbage, broccoli, celery, cucumbers, green peppers, turnips, peas, asparagus, kale, Brussels sprouts, and Swiss chard.
	Supplies calcium, iron, vitamin B group, fiber, copper and folic acid, as well as vitamin C.
	The greener the vegetable, the more vitamins, minerals and pigments it contains (e.g., broccoli is very rich in vitamin C).

- Beans, lentils, and soy can be included in the protein rich food group.
- Potatoes and yams can be included with foods that are rich in carbohydrates.

When to Start

- You may introduce vegetables a few weeks after your baby has become accustomed to cereals. Most parents start vegetables at five to seven months.
- There is no scientific evidence as to which is better to start first, vegetables or fruits; some infants will prefer the sweetness of fruits and be reluctant to

take vegetables. On the other hand, some babies may start vegetables first and then refuse fruits later. Remember, babies (like adults) have their likes and dislikes.

- It is important to teach children to eat various vegetables from a very young age so that they will develop healthy eating tastes and habits.

Ages of Various Vegetable Introductions

General

- You may start with yellow vegetables such as squash, sweet potatoes, and carrots. They are more palatable and more nutritious than green vegetables.

- Follow up with green vegetables such as green beans and peas, but only after the age of 6 months as they may cause intestinal cramping if the baby's system is not mature.

- The easiest vegetables to digest are carrots, spinach, and white or sweet potatoes.

- Other vegetables you may use are peas, green or yellow beans, cauliflower, and broccoli.

When & What to Start

6-8 months of age	8-12 months of age	Older than 1 Year
Offer pureed and cooked vegetables (yellow, green, orange).	Offer mashed or diced cooked vegetables.	At this stage, you can offer sliced and cooked vegetables as finger foods.
Progress to soft strained or mashed cooked vegetables. Start with one teaspoon and gradually increase to 4-6 tablespoons per day.	You should be feeding 6-10 tablespoons per day at this stage.	Offer some raw vegetables.
Carrots, sweet potatoes, squash, peas, zucchini.	Brussels sprouts, broccoli, eggplant, cauliflower, green or red pepper.	Spinach, tomatoes, cabbage, corn, beets, cucumber, celery, turnips, others*.

*There is a risk of choking when feeding celery, so never give raw celery with strings and make sure there are no celery pieces in pureed or cooked prepared vegetables.

Rhubarb leaves should not be used, because they are poisonous and can be fatal.

Types of Vegetables & Related Properties

Vegetables	Properties
Carrots	Contain beta-carotene (a form of vitamin A), vitamin C, carbohydrates, and nutritional fibers.
	Contains antioxidants that get rid of harmful by-products of the metabolism; studies indicate long-term and positive health effects; other good sources include oranges, kiwi fruit, tomatoes, broccoli, etc.
	Beta-carotene is made more available when carrots are cooked (cooked carrots contain 90% water content), grated, or served as carrot juice; raw carrots have been found to lower cholesterol levels.
	When buying carrots, choose those that are clean and bright orange (indicates a large amount of beta-carotene); they should be firm (not shriveled) and have no decay spots.
	Small or baby carrots are sweeter and tenderer than regular carrots.
	Avoid buying carrots with green spots as these will taste bitter.
Tomatoes	Rich source of potassium, vitamin A, C and E, folic acid, Corotenoids and Flavonoids (antioxidants).
	Most potent antioxidant is lycopen which gives tomatoes its vibrant color (can also be found in guava, watermelon and pure grape fruit).
	Low in calories (20 calories per 3.5 oz/100 g).
	Contains no cholesterol and virtually no fat.
	Water content is about 93-95% and fiber content is 1.2%.
	When buying tomatoes, select those that are firm, plump, smooth and well-formed with good color.
	May be eaten raw or cooked.
	Tomato puree is tomato concentrated juice and tomato pulp.
	The soft inner part of raw tomatoes or cut-up, small pieces makes a great nutritious finger food for toddlers.
Peas/Lentils	Peas and lentils are vegetables that are rich in iron.
	A jar of peas contains about 87% water.
	Important source of protein (especially for vegetarian babies).
	Contains nutritional fibers, calcium, iron, zinc, vitamin B6, and folic acid.

Vegetables	Properties
Peas/Lentils	Whole peas mashed lightly with a fork make a nutritious finger food for older babies.
Corn	Rich in fiber (more in white corn than yellow corn) and carbohydrates. Yellow corn contains more beta-carotene (vitamin A) than white corn. Supplies low amount of calories. Contains no fat and has group B vitamins; also contains cornstarch, corn oil and livestock feed. At room temperature, half of corn's sugar gets converted to starch in one day and heat or cold will stop the conversion. When corn is prepared in salt or boiled in water, most of its nutritional quality disappears. Whole corn kernels are a choking hazard. Very dark-yellow corn means it is old.
Potatoes	White potatoes are rich in carbohydrates. Contain starch, vitamin C, B3, B6 and nutritional fiber. Important source of vegetable protein (especially for vegetarian baby). Among the first vegetables to be used in the baby's menu. Provides a feeling of fullness/satiety. When buying potatoes, select those that are medium-sized, firm, un-shriveled, somewhat smooth and well-shaped; do not buy those with green discoloration. Keep potatoes in a dark area (no light) to prevent green patches from appearing as these patches contain a chemical called solanine (similar to nicotine).
Sweet Potatoes & Yams	There are two varieties of sweet potatoes: 1. Moist fleshed (bright orange flesh that is sweet and moist when cooked). 2. Dry fleshed have an ivory colored flesh which is dry and mealy (like white potato) when cooked. Yams are another type of sweet potato and one of the most complete foods; source of vitamins (especially vitamin A through its precursor of beta-carotene) and minerals (potassium, magnesium, etc.). Yams are moist and have an orange flesh. Dry fleshed sweet potatoes are less sweet than yams (when cooked).

Vegetables	Properties
Sweet Potatoes & Yams	Yams have virtually no vitamin A, but sweet potatoes are loaded with vitamin A.
	Both sweet potatoes and yams are low in carbohydrates, good sources of protein, fiber, beta-carotene, vitamin C, folate and calcium.
	They are more nutritious than white potatoes.
	Pureed sweet potato is an excellent first food for your baby.
Broccoli & Green Peppers	Contains vitamins A and C, calcium, and many other nutrients. Better to serve green peppers pureed or diced raw, because cooking destroys vitamin C.
	When buying broccoli, select those that have medium-sized bunches with small, tightly closed green buds that crowd together tightly (if broccoli has a strong odor, do not buy it).
	When buying green peppers, select those that are firm with a bright color and have thick and smooth skin; only buy those that still have their stems on.

Preparation of Vegetables

General

- Be sure to wash vegetables well with running water (warm water for good pesticide removal) and soap. Peel the vegetable, remove any seeds and rinse again.

- When preparing vegetables and introducing new textures, check the puree carefully for any vegetable bits to make certain that there are no chunks or pieces larger than a small pea. The puree should be very smooth in the first stages.

- Although introducing new textures is important, babies can choke quite easily as large hard chunks are dangerous.

- As your baby's eating abilities advance, you will want her to try new foods with a slightly thicker texture (see *Store Bought & Homemade Foods*).

Methods of Preparation

- Vegetables can be prepared through cooking methods such as boiling, steaming, stir-fry, grilling, pressure cooking, microwaving, baking, or not cooked (raw).

- The best way to keep most of the vegetable nutrients is by steaming.

- Do not use baking soda in the cooking water, as it destroys water-soluble vitamins.

- Do not add salt initially, as this will increase the load on the baby's kidneys.

- Vegetables are most nutritious when they are cooked properly and eaten immediately. If they cannot be eaten immediately, freeze them.

- Make sure foods are thoroughly cooked and mashed.

- Do not overcook vegetables since this will result in nutrient loss. Test the vegetables to ensure that they are fully cooked by piercing them with a fork (you can always add cooking time if vegetables are under-cooked but you cannot do anything if they are overcooked).

- Dilute the pureed vegetable with the cooking water (except in the case of nitrogen rich vegetables). This will keep the minerals and the natural compounds that were washed out during the cooking (heat destroys vitamin C).

- Use as little water as possible during cooking.

- Cooking time for vegetables varies due to size, freshness, age, water content, etc.

- Do not discard the water used for cooking vegetables as it has valuable nutrients which may be used for pureeing other foods like soups and stews.

Boiling
- Boiled vegetables can be minced in a blender, with a fork, or with a plastic grater.

- Initially, your baby will require a runny puree, so mix some leftover cooking water into the puree.

- Add a tablespoon at a time to achieve the desired consistency. All the purees can be made in bulk and frozen.

- Boiling vegetables releases some valuable nutrients into the water.

Steaming
- Steaming vegetables preserves a lot more of the nutrients and taste of fresh vegetables than boiling does.

- Steaming usually takes a few minutes longer than boiling.

- Make sure the water is boiling before placing the vegetables in the steamer and do not pile them up (keep them in a single, even layer).

Microwave Cooking (Steaming)
- Microwave cooking preserves nutrients contained in vegetables.
- Use little or no cooking water when placing vegetables in the microwave.
- Cook in a microwave safe container (microwaveable glass is probably best).

Baking
- Use only a little water to prevent the loss of water-soluble vitamins. Use the remaining water to puree with.
- When baking vegetables, they should be sliced up or baked as a whole (e.g., sweet potato).

How to Puree Vegetables
- Add water to the mixture being processed to achieve consistency depending on your baby's age and ability to eat various textures.
- For most vegetables, use the water in which they were cooked, whether it's from steaming, microwaving, baking, or boiling.
- Pour the water from the cooking pot into a container to pour into the blender.
- Place chunks of cooked vegetables into the bowl of the food processor or blender and add the cooking water.

Tip: Vegetables, Variety and Nutrition

Vegetables that are less processed (raw) are generally better in terms of nutrient value than frozen vegetables.

Remember to serve a whole variety of vegetables, fresh or frozen.

Note that the darker the leaves of salad vegetables, the more nutritious it is.

Do not discard the water that was used for cooking the vegetables as it contains valuable nutrients. Use it for pureeing baby foods.

Vegetable Administration
Feeding
- You can feed vegetables with a spoon or a cup. You can begin serving vegetables that are well cooked, steamed, mashed, or commercially prepared.

- Start with one vegetable at a time and wait a few days before introducing a new one to check for allergic reaction.

- You can start with pureed vegetables and later add ground meat and/ or chicken.

- Start with a few tablespoons of pureed vegetables served once or twice a day.

- On the first day, start with one teaspoon of vegetables and slowly increase to about 1/2-3/4 cup/125-190 g per day by one year of age.

- Only offer your baby the amount that you think she will eat.

- Serve vegetables in a small bowl or on a plate.

- Always serve pureed vegetables with a spoon.

- Begin with placing a small portion on the tip of your baby's spoon.

- Feed one portion at a time and gradually increase the amount as your baby's abilities advance with age.

- Do not force feed your baby—allow her to make her own limits.

- Vegetables can be administered as jar food, homemade foods or soup. You may alternate between jar and homemade foods.

Jar Foods:
  - ❖ Ready to use and convenient.
  - ❖ Not as nutritious as homemade frozen foods (they contain too much added salt).
  - ❖ Do not need to warm jar food (can give at room temperature).
  - ❖ Jar foods include peas, green beans, and yellow beans, mixed vegetables, garden vegetables, squash and sweet potatoes, etc.

Soups:
  - ❖ Make a soup of mixed vegetables.
  - ❖ Soup can be kept for two days and stored in the refrigerator.
  - ❖ Storage for longer periods of time requires freezing in containers.
  - ❖ Use various vegetables that allow the child to know each vegetable and enrich her variety.

- Since vegetables do not have the right nutritional balance to be a full meal, here are a few combinations you can do with vegetables (only use when other age appropriate foods have been introduced): broccoli + carrot + cheese; vegetables + chicken; vegetables + beef; vegetables + ham; and vegetables + bacon.

*Tip: **Finger Foods***

Vegetables make for great finger foods for your baby (see *Finger Foods for Infants & Toddlers*).

Helpful Hints
- Serve raw vegetables as often as possible, or only cook them lightly. Any cooking destroys nutrition, but steaming is best.
- Use vegetable margarine and olive oil instead of butter for spreading and cooking.
- Grill or broil rather than fry.
- Use fresh, natural vegetables or frozen foods over canned foods and, if you do use canned foods, choose ones with no salt or additives.

Best Protein Content	Includes tofu, lentils, beans (black, kidney, and lima), artichokes, and sweet potatoes.
Best Vitamin C Content	Includes sweet green peppers, chili peppers, broccoli, artichoke, sweet potatoes, tomatoes, and Brussels sprouts.
Best Iron Content	Includes tofu, artichokes, lentils, and beans.
Vegetables & Calcium	The combination of cheese and top calcium vegetables (broccoli, tofu, artichoke, rhubarb, beet greens) may deliver a meal that is rich in calcium, which is important in a child's growth development.

Vegetable Refusal
- Do not force your baby to eat vegetables and do not become discouraged if she initially refuses them.
- A very small portion should be offered to your baby so that she is not overwhelmed.
- Try using vegetables that are popular with most children such as carrots, corn, peas, beans and sweet potatoes.
- Try offering your child raw, frozen, or grated vegetables instead of cooked ones. Sometimes, the change in texture, color, and taste can do the trick.
- Serve raw vegetables as finger foods rather than cooked vegetables (see *Finger Foods for Infants & Toddlers*).
- Mix vegetables with breast milk or formula if your baby does not like the taste of vegetables.

- Mix foods up by placing green beans in mashed potatoes or broccoli in the rice with a cheese sauce.

- Disguise vegetables in soups, purees, and sauces.

- You may also place a variety of different colored vegetables on one plate to make it look more fun and appealing.

- You may avoid offering your child green vegetables for a while and, instead, offer red, yellow, orange, and the many other vegetables which are naturally sweet (sweet potato, corn, etc.).

- Use different preparation methods at different temperatures when introducing vegetables to your child again. For example, experiment with sauces or small amounts of dressing to enhance the flavor (see the following recipes).

- Serve dipping sauce with vegetables, since kids enjoy dipping foods in sauces such as melted butter with a little lemon juice.

- Get creative (e.g., corn on the cob) and make eating vegetables fun. For example, make veggie art with your child or allow her to help you prepare vegetables. If your baby is a bit older, take her grocery shopping with you. Children enjoy eating foods that they have prepared.

- Children also enjoy foods that stick to their spoon such as mashed potatoes and rice with cheese sauce.

- Soups are also a good way to get your child to eat vegetables.

- Be a model for your child and show her that you eat vegetables, too.

- Be patient—if your child refuses vegetables, offer her them again in a different way (change color, size, texture, etc.) after a few days.

Vegetables & Risks Associated with Some Vegetables

Carotenemia (Yellow Baby)

- Carotenemia is yellow or orange pigmentation of the skin.

- This is a common condition associated with ingestion of some carotene containing foods, which cause yellow-orange pigmentation of the skin. Pigmentation associated with carotenemia is mainly due to excessive ingestion of carrots or other yellow vegetables such as squash, sweet potatoes, and pumpkin.

- This skin discoloration is harmless.

- It is most obvious in infants at the tip of their nose, palms, soles, nasolabial folds, and forehead.

- Once the offending food that causes this pigmentation is stopped, the skin coloration will disappear in two to six weeks.

- One should differentiate between carotenemia and jaundice.

- Jaundice is a condition in which the bilirubin (a by-product of the liver metabolism) in the blood elevates due to a variety of medical conditions.

- The absence of yellow pigment in the eye sclera (in the eyeball) distinguishes carotenemia from baby jaundice or liver diseases, etc.

Methemoglobinemia (Blue Baby)

- In some places of the world, some vegetables contain an increased amount of nitrate, which is a chemical that can cause "blue baby syndrome," an unusual type of anemia (low hemoglobin count), and methemoglobinemia.

- Potential causes of acquired infantile methemoglobinemia are the consumption of silver beets and the incorrect storage of homemade purees of mixed vegetables (e.g., beets, carrot, pumpkin, green beans, etc.).

- Detection of nitrite in the urine in a blue (cyanotic) infant, suggests the diagnosis of methemoglobinemia.

- Purees of mixed vegetables in cold (refrigerator) storage are not advisable. This type of food should be prepared for immediate use or kept frozen when consumption is delayed more than 24 hours.

- Although the risk is small if these vegetables are given when the baby is more than 6 months of age (though it can occur at an earlier age), some recommend using these vegetables after one year of age.

- Avoid colored greens, mixed vegetables and root vegetables such as beets, turnips, carrots, spinach, and green beans, until the age of one year.

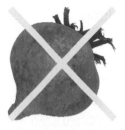 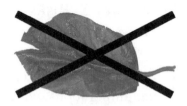

Tip: Baby Food Risks

Manufacturers of baby foods are aware of these risk issues and usually monitor their products for safe levels of nitrates.

Vegetable Allergies
- Symptoms of allergy include rash, vomiting, diarrhea, stomach pain or breathing problems, etc.
- In some cases an allergy reaction is mild, while in others it may be severe.
- A child may react after having contact with a specific vegetable, especially when it is offered raw instead of cooked (see *Feeding & Food Allergys*).
- If you notice that your child has an allergic reaction to a particular vegetable, stop feeding it and speak to your doctor. If your child seems to have a severe reaction, take her to the nearest hospital.

Case Description

Jonathan is a five year old boy with a previous history of allergic rhinitis (sneezing, rubbing the eyes, nose, watery eyes, and no discharge from the nose). His mother complained that when he eats carrots or apples, he develops a rash a couple of minutes after eating and sometimes has loose stool or some abdominal discomfort. Jonathan's mother could not clarify whether or not he has any itchiness of the mouth or throat. There were no other symptoms. She had noticed that when he ate carrots that were cooked, there was no problem. Upon medical examination, everything was normal except for signs of allergic rhinitis in the nose (swollen and pale nasal mucosa). Jonathan was sent to an allergy doctor who did a skin test where the results came out positive for the common environmental allergens mold, grass and ragweed.

Given the complaints, this patient has a history compatible with what is called Fresh Fruit Syndrome or Oral Allergy Syndrome. In these types of allergies, common foods that may cause reaction include *fresh* peaches, apricots, bananas, apples, cherries, kiwis, and vegetables such as carrots, celery and tomatoes. In this condition, the child has frequent history or evidence of associated allergic rhinitis (which Jonathan has). If the fruit is heated or frozen, or the vegetables are cooked, symptoms do not occur.

Vegetables & Fiber
- Fiber is a compound found in vegetables (and not in animal food products such as meat, eggs, or cheese) that your baby does not digest well. Most fibers are sugars that the digestive system is unable to break down.
- Fiber is responsible for the hard texture of skin on fruits and vegetables.
- It is divided into two types:

❖ *Soluble fiber* (e.g., pectin, psyllium) dissolves in water and increases its bulk in the diet. Food sources of soluble fiber are whole grains (cereal, breads, pasta, cakes, muffins), vegetables and fruits with peels, and nuts and seeds. Soluble fiber attracts water and becomes like a gel, which then attracts fat particles, cholesterol, and sugar. As such, it prevents absorption of carbohydrates, sugars, and cholesterol.

❖ *Non-soluble fiber* (e.g., cellulose)*:* Found in cereals and fruit and vegetable skins, legumes (lentils), peas, barley, oat bran, apples, pears, plums, oranges, and citrus fruits; these fibers do not dissolve in water and add bulk to the diet, increasing bowel motility and helping to prevent constipation.

- Despite the fact that fibers are not absorbed into the body, they can have various effects:

  ❖ Liberation of a hormone in the bowel that affects the brain and gives a feeling of fullness. For example, if salad vegetables, bean soup, and rice are eaten, you will be full for 4-5 hours, which may lead to a decrease in calorie consumption.

  ❖ Fibers decrease the risk of colon cancer, cholesterol, diabetes, heart and blood pressure problems, especially in adults.

  ❖ Fibers can cause "gas" which leads to discomfort.

Tip: French Fries

French fries are often served to children between the ages of 9 and 11 months and older. However, children should not be offered French fries below the age of 18 months, as the texture is not yet appropriate for their age group (see *Textured & Table Baby Foods*).

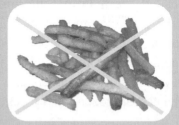

Studies show that approximately 25% of children have one serving of fries at least once per day.

French fries are high in fat and calories and should not be considered a vegetable to be given often to young children.

For a healthier version of French fries, do not deep fry them in oil—lightly brush them with vegetable oil and bake them until lightly browned instead.

Sample Menu

- Always offer breast milk or formula to your baby first, since it is the main source of the baby's nutrition.

- Proteins and meats should be discussed with your pediatrician first before serving them to your child, since some doctors recommend starting these earlier or later (see *Meat & Alternatives*).

- Note that not all babies between six to eight months of age will be eating all of the suggested foods during a given meal time (they can eat more or less than the menu suggests).

- The following sample menu is provided for a child who is between six to eight months of age:

Breakfast & Morning Snack
Breast milk or formula.

Cereal (rice, oatmeal, barley, or mixed).
Fruits or vegetables (avocado, banana, apple sauce, pears, or peaches).

Lunch & Mid-Afternoon Snack
Breast milk or formula.
Cereal (rice, barley, mixed chicken and rice, tofu, and wheat grain).
Fruits or vegetables (squash or pears, pears or banana, sweet potatoes or apple sauce, avocado or green beans, pumpkin or sweet potatoes).

Dinner & Before Bedtime
Breast milk or formula.
Fruits or vegetables (vegetable mix, squash, sweet potato, pear sauce, peaches, banana).
Infant cereal/grain.

Tip: Fresh, Frozen or Canned Vegetables

The nutritional differences between fresh, frozen, or canned vegetables are minimal. Serve whatever is most comfortable for you and enjoyed by your baby. In the first two years of life, some vegetables (broccoli, carrots, zucchini, and squash) must be cooked to be safe enough for your child to eat.

Store Bought & Homemade Vegetable Recipes

Store Bought

The following are some examples of store bought vegetables; use as suggested according to your baby's age.

Vegetables Only	Vegetable Combination
Squash, carrots, peas, green beans, sweet potato, beets, creamed corn, and mixed vegetables	Only use these when other appropriate foods are introduced. Examples include broccoli, carrots and cheese, vegetables with chicken, beef, ham, or bacon.

Homemade Foods

Basic Guidelines for Homemade Vegetable Recipes

Boiling

    1) Peel and slice fresh vegetables for fast cooking (or use frozen ones).

    2) Cook in 1/2-1 inch of water for about 20 minutes, or until tender.

    3) Puree or blend with some of the cooking water.

Steaming

    1) Peel and slice fresh vegetables or use frozen ones.

    2) Steam over boiling water until tender.

    3) Puree or blend with some of the cooking water to get the required consistency.

Microwave

    1) Peel clean and slice fresh vegetables or use frozen ones.

    2) In a microwave safe dish (with water), cook vegetables until tender.

    3) Potatoes need to be pierced several times to allow intense steam to escape (for example, single potatoes generally cook for 3-5 minutes).

    4) Puree or blend with cooking water or add water if necessary.

Sample Recipes for Babies 4-6 months of age

These recipes are for those babies who started solid foods at less than six months of age (see *Starting Solids* for recommendations).

Vegetable Recipe (General)	Sweet Potato Recipe	Carrots Recipe
1. Fresh or frozen vegetables and water is needed. 2. Wash, peel, and slice vegetables. 3. Place vegetables into a steamer or boiling water until tender. 4. Drain and puree with leftover cooking water, breast milk, or formula.	1. Take 1 sweet potato. 2. Steam/boil until tender. 3. Drain and mash using a fork. 4. Add breast milk or formula if your baby likes.	1. Take 1 carrot and 1parsnip; peel and dice. 2. Steam until tender. 3. Puree in a blender and add cooled water, breast milk, or formula.

- Remember, fresh or frozen vegetables are the best to use since canned vegetables may be high in salt.

- Do not use the cooking water to puree or mash if you use vegetables that are high in nitrates.

Sample Recipes for Babies Older than 6-7 Months

Pureed Baby Vegetables	Sweet Potatoes & Yam
3/4 cup/175 ml cooked vegetables chopped into small pieces. 3 tablespoons of water or cooking liquid. In a small bowl, microwave vegetables on high for a minute or until tender. Stir in water and place in a blender for 1-2 minutes until puree is smooth. Serve immediately or freeze in ice cube trays.	Take 1 large sweet potato or yam and preheat oven to 350 F/177 C. Bake the sweet potato or yam on foil lined pan for an hour, turning it after 30 minutes. Pierce it a few times with a fork to ensure tenderness. Cook for another 15 minutes and set aside until it has cooled enough for you to handle it. Peel off outer layer and strain cooked potato in a food mill. Add 5 tablespoons of water, formula,or breast milk to puree it.

- Examples of veggie combinations include squash + apple + sweet potato; green beans + apple or pears; green beans + potatoes with some apple sauce; mixed apple + carrot + rice; mixed sweet potato + yogurt, etc.

Sample Recipes for Babies Older than 1 Year of Age

Vegetable Puree	Vegetable Soup
You may use any vegetable you like.	Need:
Peel and chop vegetables into small pieces or cubes.	8 cups/2000 ml of water 1 small onion
Steam or boil them in a small amount of water until tender.	1 celery stick 2 washed and peeled carrots
Add cottage cheese or plain yogurt to make it a soup.	1 small peeled and washed zucchini 1 washed and peeled potato
Blend vegetables in the food processor to the desired consistency	1 slice of peeled squash 2 small tablespoons of canola oil
Serve immediately or store in freezer in ice cube trays for later use.	Preparation: 　Cut all vegetables into small bits or chunks. 　Place in a pot of boiling water and cook until tender. 　Blend vegetables in the food processor to puree. 　Serve immediately or store in freezer in ice cube trays for later use.

Tomato—Fruit or Vegetable?

- Botanically speaking, tomatoes are a fruit.
- There are many tomatoes available and common ones include the classic tomato, cherry, plum, beef and vine.
- Tomatoes may be eaten raw or cooked.
- Tomatoes are a rich source of potassium, vitamin A, C and E, folic acid, and contain antioxidants (e.g., flavonoids, carotenoids).
- Lycopen is found in tomatoes and provides them with the vibrant color. It is also one of the most potent antioxidants among dietary carotenoids (lycopen is now being studied in reducing cancer risk and heart disease).
- Tomatoes are low in calories at about 20 calories per 3.5 oz/100 g.
- They contain no cholesterol and virtually no fat.
- The water content of tomatoes is about 93-95% and fiber content is 1.2%.
- The largest food fight in the world started out as a single tomato fight in the Spanish town of Bunal, in 1944. It is continued annually by the locals in the town's main square (La Tomatina event).

Fruits

General

Fruits are good sources of energy, water, vitamins (A, B & C groups), minerals (potassium, chrome, etc.) and fibers. They are rich in sugars including fructose, glucose, sucrose, and sorbitol. These natural fruit sugars are more easily digested than the sugars that are added to some fruit juices. Fruits are not a great source of iron; small amounts are present in dried fruits. However, they are excellent complements to cooked cereals, vegetables and yogurt.

The following is a table outlining general fruits and their nutrients:

Avocado	Contains unsaturated fatty acids, omega 3 & 6, and vitamins B1 & B6, protein, niacin, thiamin, riboflavin, zinc, and folic acid. Low in fiber. High caloric content (important for vegetarian children).
Bananas	Contains vitamin B6, nutritional fibers, and potassium. Good source of water. Mature bananas are easy to digest and soft. May cause constipation. Increases serotonin production (hormone for relaxation and satisfaction). Contains tryptophan (helps brain's production of serotonin).
Oranges	Rich in vitamin C. Good source of folate, fiber, and calcium.
Pears	High in sorbitol and fiber content (mostly vitamin C and some fiber contained in the skin). Good for constipation.
Prunes	Contain vitamins A and E, minerals (calcium and iron), and high in fibers. Large amounts of sorbitol (sugar that loosens the stool).
Apples	Very good in fiber content (soluble fiber) and pectin (lowers cholesterol level). Contains cancer fighting flavonoids. Use fresh apples for best results in nutrients.
Apricots	Contain protein, calcium, iron, vitamin A and K, folic acid, and zinc. High beta carotene, potassium and fiber content (especially in dried apricots).

Cantaloupe	High in vitamin C, beta carotene, and potassium content.
Dried Figs	High in calories and carbohydrates. Contain nutrients including calcium, fiber, potassium, and protein.
Grapefruits	Low in calorie, high in fiber content and vitamin C. May cause problems when taking medication particularly in adults.
Kiwi	Good source of vitamin C, especially when eaten out of the peel.
Mango	High in fiber, vitamin C, calories, and beta carotene.
Cranberries	Offered as a fresh fruit, dried fruit, juice, or sauce. Contain no cholesterol and almost no fat. Low in sodium. Contain antioxidants and phytonutrients that protect against diseases and infections (e.g., ulcers, gum disease, urinary tract infections, cancer, aging, heart disease, etc.).
Dried Fruits	The term "dried" means that the water has been removed from the fruit. As such, bacteria, mold, and yeast cannot grow as they require certain amounts of moisture. Dried fruits contain natural sugar, which may promote tooth decay. You should limit your child from eating large and frequent quantities of dried fruits. There is a significant amount of vitamin lost during the drying process, especially vitamins A and C. However, they are still a healthy snack for toddlers, if used occasionally. You may re-hydrate dried fruit to prevent your child from choking by cooking until tender and then cutting it into small pieces.
Citrus Fruits	Citrus fruits include oranges, grapefruits, lemons, clementines, mandarins, tangerines, pommelo, etc. These fruits are full of vitamin C (an essential nutrient that repairs tissue damage, heals wounds, and prevents scurvy), potassium, folate, and sodium and are cholesterol-free. They help fight against diseases such as heart disease and birth defects (when the mother consumes citrus fruits), due to their high level of antioxidants. Citrus fruits should not be introduced to your child until at least one year of age, because they commonly cause food allergies and reactions (e.g., rash, etc.). As such, begin with a small amount over the course of several days and monitor for allergic reactions (hives, wheezing, difficulty breathing, etc.).

- Fruits rich in vitamin C, fiber, calcium, and folic acids include oranges, cantaloupe, apricots (dried), strawberries, papaya, kiwi, grapefruit, mango, and avocado.

When to Start

The baby is ready to begin strained fruits between the ages of six to seven months. You can introduce fruits about two weeks after introducing vegetables (if vegetables are introduced first) and offer one fruit at a time, three days apart. The following table outlines examples of fruits you may introduce to your child at the appropriate ages:

Early: 7 Months-1 Year	Late: 1 Year & Older
Bananas, nectarines, pears, apple, avocado, prunes, plums, peaches, apricots, cantaloupe, pineapple (at 9 months), honeydew melon, and papaya.	Oranges, tangerines (citrus fruits), kiwi, grapefruits, grapes, berries, cherries, strawberries, mango, and watermelon.

Which to Start & How Much

Which to Start

- When starting fruits, use peeled, cooked, or canned fruits that have been strained or blended. It is best to feed your baby cooked purees of fruits (apples, pears, etc.).

- A very soft or mature banana is usually one of the first fruits introduced to your baby because it is soft and easy to digest. Bananas are also the only fruit which can be served raw to a child six to eight months of age.

- Each fruit should be given *alone* and three days apart from the next, so that your baby will gradually learn its taste and in case of an allergic reaction you will have enough time to see if it develops.

- Initially, it is best to allow the baby to enjoy the taste of fruits without any additives (biscuits, cheese, etc.).

- You may mix fruits only after each fruit has been eaten on its own or separately, so that you know that your child is not allergic to the fruit(s).

Tip: Canned Fruits and Syrup

When serving canned fruits, use ones which are packed in water or the fruit's own juices, since those packed in syrup are very high in sugar content. Canned fruits should be stored in plastic or glass containers after they have been opened.

How Much to Offer
- Start with one teaspoon on the first day and gradually increase the amount to six to eight tablespoons per day by the age of one year.
- In general, it is recommended to start with mashed fruit two to three tablespoons, once a day, either between meals or with formula or breast milk.
- Always feed pureed fruits from a spoon.
- The following are recommended fruit portions per age group:

6-9 Months	Offer 6-7 tablespoons of pureed, cooked, canned or fresh, ripe fruits per day.
9-12 Months	Offer 7-10 tablespoons of soft, fresh fruits (peeled, seeded, and diced) or canned fruits (packed in water or juice), per day.

Store Bought & Homemade Fruit Preparation

Store Bought Fruits
- There are many store-bought or jar foods which offer fruits. Many of these are ready to use, requiring almost no preparation on your part.
- If you choose to feed your baby canned fruits, buy those in their natural juices. Canned fruits that are packed in their own juice are already cooked in the canning process (puree and serve). If these come in sugary syrup, rinse the fruits before pureeing.
- Some babies enjoy jar foods, because of their sweetness and texture.
- Examples of commercially prepared fruits include the following: apple sauce, prunes, pears, peaches, plums, banana/apricot/plums/prunes with tapioca, pear with pineapple, apple and blueberry, fruit dessert, cherry vanilla pudding, banana apple dessert, organic fruits, etc.

Tip: Nutrition for Older Babies

For older babies, you can peel and dice fruits into small pieces and serve immediately as finger foods. Make sure the fruits are very soft and ripe to prevent choking. Be sure to buy fresh, natural, or frozen fruits over canned fruits.

Homemade Preparation
Cleaning Fruits:

- Soak and scrub all fruits under running water (washing is not half as effective as scrubbing fruits).

- Use a brush to help remove bacteria, pesticides, and chemicals.

- Remove any peelings, cores, or seeds from the fruits.

Cooking Fruits:

- To prevent choking, fresh fruits must be cooked until they are soft and then pureed. Bananas, papayas, and avocado can simply be peeled, mashed, and served. Mash fruits with a fork or crush to soften. Do not use the blender, since it destroys important nutrients, including Vitamin C. Use some of the cooking water to puree the fruit, as it contains valuable nutrients.

- Most fruits (including apples, pears, peaches, plums, and apricots, etc.) can be prepared using one of the following methods:

Boiling	Wash, peel, and cut fruits into small pieces. Remove core, seeds, or pits in fruits. Add 1 cup/250 g of fruit to 1/4-1/2 cup/85-125 ml of boiling water. Allow to boil until tender (10-20 minutes). Do not add any sugar. Blend or puree until smooth. Serve immediately. Refrigerate what was used or freeze the rest.
Steaming	Wash, peel and cut fruits into small pieces. Remove core, seeds, or pits in fruits. Steam fruits for 15-20 minutes. Blend or puree until smooth. Serve immediately. Refrigerate what was used or freeze the rest.
Microwaving	Wash and cut fruits into small pieces. Remove core, seeds, or pits in fruits. Place in small glass or microwave-safe bowl with 2-3 teaspoons of water and cover tightly. Microwave for about 1-2 minutes until fruit is tender. Stir and test to make sure that 'hotspots' will not burn your baby. Allow to cool and peel fruits. Mash or puree until smooth. Serve immediately. Refrigerate what was used or freeze the rest.

Storing Fruits:

Keep fruits in their whole shape (refrigerated, whole or uncut) until you are ready to use them. Cut-up fruits can be refrigerated for only one to two days. Any fruits which have been cooked and/or pureed should be kept in the refrigerator for no longer than one full day and then discarded. Raw fruits can be frozen and pureed fruits can be frozen in ice cube trays for up to two months. Ripe fruits should be kept in the dark since light destroys the vitamin C content. Throw out leftover fruits which have touched the baby's mouth or spoon.

Fruit Refusal

- Many young infant and toddlers refuse to eat fruits. If one type of fruit is refused, respect this choice since there may be another fruit that she likes.

- Studies have shown that continued exposure to a particular food will enhance acceptance of the rejected food. Continue to offer your child the rejected or new fruit every couple of days, in a non-stressful environment.

- Use various preparation methods (described previously), portion sizes, and fun ideas (using many colored fruits on one plate) to get your child to accept a rejected fruit.

- If your child continues to refuse fruits offered, try adding fruits to various recipes of food you make, whenever possible. This is called the "hidden" method since your child does not know that fruits are in the food (e.g., fruit salad, snack mix, chopped fruits in cereal, etc.).

- Another way to get your child to eat fruits is through drinking them by offering 100% fruit juice and fruit smoothies. It is an easy way of ensuring your child receives the recommended fruit servings (4-6 oz/120-180 ml of fruit juice provides one to two servings of fruit).

- When pureeing your cooked fruit, try using breast milk or formula instead of the cooking water. This will provide your child with a familiar taste mixed with the new flavor and provides a nutritional boost, too.

- Leave a bowl of bite-sized fruits on the table so that your child may have the option of snacking on these.

- Let your child pick the fruits when she goes grocery shopping with you.

- You can try to mix pieces of fruit with yogurt or serve the fruit with a dip. Use yogurt with fresh or frozen fruits.

- Mix any chopped fruits with jello or offer fresh, washed, and peeled raw fruits.

- Serve apple sauce instead of whole fruit.

- If your child refuses citrus fruits, offer alternative sources of vitamin C (strawberries, cantaloupe, vitamin C rich juices, broccoli, etc.).

- Do not force-feed your child or turn foods into a "reward and punishment game."

- Do not overwhelm your child with huge portion sizes. Instead, give a small slice and allow your child to ask for more.

Parent Concerns

Why is serving my child a fresh fruit better than fruit juice?

- Fresh fruits offer more nutritional value than fruit juice since many nutrients are lost in the juicing process. Also, children tend to get full from the juice more quickly than from fresh fruit and will be less likely to eat a proper, healthy meal. Remember that fruit snacks or drinks made with "real fruits" do not count as a fruit serving.

How can I keep fruits fresh?

- You may sprinkle lemon juice on fruits to keep their freshness, since lemon acts as an antioxidant to keep fruits from oxidizing (turning colors).

Is the skin of fruits important to eat?

- Much of the fiber in fruits is contained in the skin (especially in apples, peaches, and pears). You can serve the fruit with the skin to get its full fiber value.

Is there such a thing as too much fruit?

- Yes, there is, since eating too much fruit or juice may cause your child's stool to become acidic. She may also experience painful, bright red diaper rashes.

More to Know

All fruits grow above the ground, either on trees, vines or shrubs. Fruits such as avocados, eggplants, tomatoes, pumpkins, rhubarb, and cucumbers are classified by botanists as fruits and not vegetables.

"An apple a day keeps the doctor away." Is this true?
- More and more these days, it seems to be true.
- Apples are a great source of fiber and contain antioxidants and phytonutrients, which protect against infections, cell damage and diseases.
- Soluble fiber contained in apples is known to reduce blood cholesterol levels.
- The British Medical Journal published a study that was conducted in 1996, which showed that of 5000 participants, those who ate the most apples had the lowest incidence of heart disease.
- Studies have also proven that it does not matter how you get your apple source, whether from the fruit itself or from apple juice—either is good.

My infant has sore gums from stomatitis. Can she eat all fruits?
- Stomatitis is an inflammation of the throat and gums, usually caused by a viral infection. You may offer your child various fruits, however do not serve acidic fruits (e.g., grapefruits, etc.) as they can sting and burn.

Can I freeze fruit purees?
- Yes, you can freeze fruit purees in much the same way you freeze veggie purees, however some fruits will not freeze solid (prunes, apricots). Other fruits will turn colors upon freezing such as pears, apples, and bananas. It does not mean that the fruit is rotten, it is the natural oxidation process the fruit goes through when frozen.

What can I use to make puree?
- You may use leftover cooking liquid, breast milk, or formula to make a puree.

When I buy bananas and avocados, what should I look for?
- When buying bananas for your child, select those that have smooth skin. Bananas are better served when they are slightly ripe with a small amount of brown spots on the skin.
- When buying avocados for your child, select those that are dark green and have a bumpy texture. Avocados should be firm yet gentle when you press upon it. When you open the avocado, it should be green and a little yellow around the pit.

If I introduce fruits first, will my baby then reject vegetables?

- You have the choice of introducing either fruits or vegetables first. It does not matter which food you introduce first to your child.

- Every baby is different and has specific taste preferences that develop over time.

- Despite the fact that fruits are sweet, your child will learn to accept and enjoy the taste of vegetables as well.

- When introducing new foods, it is always important to introduce them gradually and repeated exposure to new foods will enhance acceptance.

- However, many babies do prefer green vegetables over yellow vegetables, which is a great way to begin introducing vegetables after fruits, and many babies enjoy vegetables over fruits (see *Vegetables*).

Case Description

Alex is an 11- month-old boy, who was healthy until he began eating tomatoes, beets, and strawberries. Each time Alex ate tomatoes (either raw or in soup), he developed an itchy rash on his face and chest. The same thing would happen when Alex ate beets and strawberries. He presented with recurrent hives, rash and itchiness located in the knees, armpits and chest. There were no other symptoms (shortness of breath, wheezing, vomiting, etc.).

Comments:

- Fruits and vegetables sometimes cause a variety of allergic reactions. This is why it is recommended that citrus fruits and some vegetables be introduced at a later age.

- When a child has an allergy to any citrus fruit, delay the introduction of any other citrus fruits. There is a higher risk of developing allergies to more than one citrus fruit.

Tip: Fruit and Food-borne Diseases. Wash Thoroughly

Fruits and vegetables tend to cause food-borne diseases more often than poultry and eggs. Potential contaminants found in these products include salmonella, E. coli, and the hepatitis A virus (The Medical Post, Jan 17, 2006). (See *Safe Feeding & Food Safety*).

Sample Menu (6-8 Months)

Breakfast & Mid-morning:
Breast milk or iron-fortified formula
2 tablespoons of strained fruits

Lunch & Mid-afternoon:
Breast milk or iron-fortified formula
2 tablespoons of pureed meat (see comments below)

Dinner & Before Bed:
Breast milk or iron-fortified formula
2 tablespoons of strained vegetables
2 tablespoons of infant cereal
Breast milk or iron-fortified formula (before bedtime)

- The order of when to give vegetables, fruits, cereal, or meat during the day is of no importance.
- Some recommend starting meat and alternatives before the age of eight months.
- You can mix cereal with breast milk or formula.

Helpful Homemade Recipes & Combination Ideas

Fruits & Yogurt (for ten months or older)
Ingredients:
1/4 cup/85 ml plain yogurt
1/4 cup/85 g cooked, unsweetened fruit
Directions:
Combine both yogurt and cooked fruit.
Mash all the lumps until smooth, if necessary.
Serve immediately.

Banana Puree & Rice (babies starting on solids)
Ingredients:
1 ripe banana
1-2 teaspoons of baby rice
2 tablespoons of breast milk or formula
Directions:
Mash the banana until smooth.

Mix the rice and milk; stir in the banana.

Continue mixing for runny puree or stop mixing for firm puree.

Puree with Pears & Apples
Ingredients:
1 ripe pear, peeled and sliced

1 apple, peeled and sliced

Directions:
Cook both pears and apple in a small saucepan with one tablespoon of water, over a low heat.

Remember to stir occasionally until tender.

Puree in blender and serve.

Fruit Combination Ideas (about 6 months of age or older)
1) Apple + cereal: Blend apples or apple sauce together with rice or oatmeal cereal.

2) Apple + pear sauce: Blend apples and pears together.

3) Banana + avocado: Blend bananas and avocado together and add to the baby's cereal.

4) Pumpkin + cereal: Blend pumpkin puree with rice or oatmeal cereal.

5) Pumpkin + bananas: Blend pumpkin puree with bananas.

Fruit Combination Ideas (eight months & older)
1) Apple pie: Blend cereal, apple sauce, and yogurt together and mix well.

2) Pumpkin pie: Blend pumpkin puree with cereal and yogurt and mix well.

Fruit Juices

General

Juice is not necessary for infants and should definitely not be used to replace breast milk or formula. Fruit juice (along with fruits and vegetables) should not be considered a meal, but rather, part of a meal or snack. More than 90% of all infants consume fruit juice by the time they reach the age of 1 year.

Fruit juice can be a healthy source of vitamin C and an extra source of water for infants. It contains a small amount of protein, minerals, and calcium. There is no fat, cholesterol, or fiber (unless there is pulp) contained in juice.

Types of Juices

General

- The type of juice and its content (carbohydrates, sorbitol, fiber, etc.) affect your baby's ability to digest, absorb, and tolerate the juice.
- Types of juices include apple, pear, peach, prunes, apricot, banana, grape, etc., and mixed juices.
- Apple and pear juice contain a great amount of sorbitol, which may cause gas and stomach distress in infants.
- Orange and grapefruit juice contain more natural vitamin C than any other juices.
- There are two types of juices: store bought juices that are convenient and ready-to-use and homemade juices that need to be prepared.

Store Bought Juices

- In order to be considered fruit juice, the Food and Drug Administration (FDA) mandates that the product be 100% fruit juice.
- Products labeled "fruit or juice drink," "juice beverage," or "juice cocktail" are probably mostly sugar and water and only 5-10% juice.
- Check the ingredients label to make sure you are getting only fruit juice. There are companies that manufacture special juices only for infants. These do not contain any added sugars or additives, and they are more expensive than regular juices.
- Look for juices that contain 100% fruit juice labels. The most nutritious type of juice will say 100% fruit juice fortified with vitamin C.

- Choose juice that has a description of "unsweetened" or "no artificial flavors or color added." If sugar or glucose is mentioned in the label, then that juice is not the best choice for your baby. Anything called "drink, punch or ade" has little or no fruit juice.

- Look for juice that offers calcium and vitamin C (not only calories) and pick juices from jars that are made especially for babies.

- Remember to immediately refrigerate any open bottles that contain unused portions. Opened bottles of baby juice need to be tightly covered and placed in the refrigerator. Do not leave open jars at room temperature.

- Also, the safest juice available for infants and children is pasteurized juice, because the pasteurization process eliminates bacterial contamination. Unpasteurized juice may contain pathogens (e.g., Escherichia coli and Salmonella organisms) and these may cause serious illness.

- You may use a family size jar of unsweetened juice or use frozen unsweetened juice. Dilute the juice with an equal amount of water prior to serving.

Tip: Juice From Roadside Stands

Do not use apple cider or juice bought from roadside stands, as it may not be safe for your baby (risk of infection).

Homemade Juices

- Appropriate natural juices are grapes, oranges, bananas, apples, peaches, pears, tomatoes, melons, etc.

- Freshly squeezed juice contains more vitamin C than those made from concentrate, canned, or frozen juice.

- Do not give unpasteurized "fresh" juice. To pasteurize juice and kill harmful bacteria, boil it for three to five minutes. Do not leave the pasteurized juice at room temperature. Place it in a sterile container and refrigerate no longer than two days (see *Safe Feeding & Food Safety*).

When & Which to Introduce

Here is a table of the types of juices you may give your baby according to her age.

7 Months-1 Year	1 Year and Older
Grape, apple, pear, peach, banana, cantaloupe, honeydew melon, and apricot juice.	Kiwi, strawberry, berry, mango. Citrus: orange, grapefruit, tangerine, lime, and lemon juice.

- Juice should not be introduced into the infant's diet before the age of six months. Offering juice before introducing solid foods risks replacing healthier breast milk or formula with less nutritious food. It can interfere in the breastfeeding process by filling the baby up so that she nurses less. Excessive amounts of fruit juice (especially given in the first few months) leads to poor nutrition.

- Introduce juice at nine months of age or later (breast milk, formula, and water are better), when your baby is able to drink from a cup. It is better to incorporate juices in the meal with a cup than in a bottle used between meals, due to juice's high sugar content (bottle use increases the risk of cavities).

- Do not give juices throughout the day, but rather at set times (e.g., snack or mealtimes). Avoid giving any juice at bedtime.

- For the toddler, the best time to take juice is at regular snack times that are not too close to mealtime since it may spoil her appetite.

- It is good to offer some juice with iron-fortified cereal, as Vitamin C in the juice will help increase iron absorption.

How to Introduce & How Much

- White grape juice is recommended as the introductory juice in most infant diets as it is the most intestinal-friendly juice; it is easily digested and absorbed, contains no sorbitol, and the sugar content is easiest on the immature intestines. It may even help in the alleviation of IBS (Irritable Bowel Syndrome) and is less likely to cause recurrence of diarrhea.

- Apple juice is also recommended as a choice for beginner juice, because it is well accepted and pleasing to a baby's taste buds. It is fortified with vitamin C, which may help babies absorb more iron.

- Introduce only one fruit juice at a time, about three days apart.

- You may dilute the juice in order for the baby to get used to a lighter "sweet" taste. While diluting juice is a common practice, there is no clear rationale for this. It is recommended mainly if your baby likes juice and consumes a lot of it (I recommend diluting when first introducing juice into your baby's diet, as juice is less and less recommended to be given in the older infant and child, if to be given at all).

- At first, dilute one ounce of juice with 3 oz/90 ml of water for a total of a 4 oz/120 ml serving. Gradually increase the total quantity as your baby grows older.

- Mix juice with water (half juice, half water) to minimize effects on teeth, stool, etc.

- Children from the age of 6-12 months should get no more than 4 oz/120 ml of juice per day. Children from the ages of 12 months-4 years should receive 4-6 oz/120-180 ml. Older children should be limited to 8-12 oz/240-360 ml of juice per day.

- Comment: These amounts may vary year to year with Canadian or American recommendations, so talk to your doctor. However, it is clear at this point that the less juice offered (if at all, or diluted) at any age, the better.

- Do not give excess juice amounts at any age, as it takes the place of food and nutrients the baby/child needs.

Tip: Cranberry Juice and Urinary Tract Infection

Cranberry juice is considered to be effective in the prevention and help in the treatment of urinary tract infections due to its ability to prevent bacterial adhesion in the lining of the urinary tract. You need more than the juice alone to help in treatment for both children and adults.

Problems, Concerns & Benefits

Poorly Balanced Diet & Its Effects

- Fruit juices generally do not contain many vitamins and nutrients (other than vitamin C and some are calcium fortified).

- Excessive amounts of juice creates a poorly balanced diet, since drinking too much juice will fill your child and decrease their appetite for more nutritious foods. It may also contribute to damaging the enamel of the teeth, leading to tooth decay. Further, loose bowel movements, constant diarrhea, and obesity may occur as a result of drinking too much juice.

- Excessive consumption of juice may also irritate the skin, causing diaper rashes worsened by diarrhea. Excess apple juice causes loose bowel movements and constant diarrhea.
- Remember that milk is a major source of calcium in the infant and toddler's diet and as such, it is important to offer milk during meals and snack time rather than juice.

Tip: Juice Vs Whole Fruit

Juice is not necessary for infants, as it offers no nutritional benefits over whole fruits (juice contains no proteins, calcium, fat, or iron). It is important for parents to realize that juices are not nutritious and should be limited, particularly if it is the one food item your child likes.

Irritation of the Intestine
- Juices that contain Sorbitol and those with a high fructose to glucose ratio (excess fructose ferments in the large intestine) may cause irritation of the intestine (diarrhea and abdominal pain).
- During these intestinal illnesses, you may administer juice that contains no Sorbitol, such as citrus, strawberry, raspberry, blackberry, and white grape juices.

Benefits
The following can be considered some benefits of juice:
- Children who do not like to eat any fruits usually enjoy fruit juices (6 oz/180 ml of fruit juice = 1 serving of fruit).
- Children who do not like to drink plain water can drink fruit juice with diluted fluoridated water. It is a good way to give your child fluoride.
- Using 100% fruit juice (with added calcium) may be beneficial in children who do not drink milk or have a milk allergy, do not eat foods that are high in calcium, etc.
- Fruit juices help in the treatment of constipation and iron absorption (especially important if your child is anemic).

Parent Concerns
How can I limit the amount of juice my child drinks?
- Juice is highly addictive for young children. In order to limit the amount of juice your child drinks, try the following:

❖ Offer juice less often.

❖ Dilute the juice with water and gradually add more water everyday.

❖ Serve whole fruits or small snacks instead of juice.

❖ Serve milk or water instead of juice.

What if my baby refuses juice?

- If your baby refuses juice, it is not such a "big deal" as fruit juices are not considered a necessity in the infant diet. You may go directly to fruits and vegetables.

Do I have to dilute juice when I give it to my baby?

- If given before one year of age, it is recommended to dilute the juice. In fact, some suggest diluting juice at any age.

- If your toddler drinks an excessive amount of juice, you may begin to dilute the juice to decrease the ingestion of empty calories, improve her appetite and the intake of more nutritious foods.

- If your toddler drinks a very small amount of juice, you do not need to dilute it.

What do I do if my baby has diarrhea, gas, and stomach pain from fruit juices?

- Some juices such as pears, apples and prunes contain significant amounts of the sugar fructose and sorbitol, which is non-absorbable and leads to diarrhea, gas, and stomach pain. This is due to fermentation from the existing bacteria in the large bowel.

- In these cases, decrease juice intake or eliminate it from your child's diet.

- Usually, diarrhea is associated with excessive juice intake (grape juice is better tolerated than apple or prune juice).

Can a rash occur in the anal area from juice?

- Large amounts of fruit juices sometimes irritate the anal skin area and cause anal rashes due to acidic stools. Decrease the use of fruits or dilute juices and/or eliminate it entirely from your baby's diet to stop the rashes. Consult your doctor.

Tip: *Mouth Rash From Juice*

A rash sometimes develops around the mouth in some infants after having been fed freshly squeezed citrus juice. This is most likely contact allergic dermatitis and is uncommon. See your doctor.

Is commercial baby juice okay to use?

- There are commercial baby juices available specifically for infants and toddlers that are okay for use.

- They are more expensive than regular frozen or bottled juices.

- Avoid unpasteurized juices and do not use regular bottled or canned vegetable juice since they are high in sodium (use low sodium vegetable juice).

Why can I give my constipated baby apple juice and not apple sauce?

- There is a difference in contents between apple juice and apple sauce.

- Apple sauce contains a higher level of pectin (soluble fiber that firms and bulks stool) and leads to constipation.

- Apple juice contains more sugars and liquids and has a mild laxative effect that has been proven to provide some relief from constipation (it also helps children absorb more iron).

Extra Helpful Tip: *Juice & Constipation*

If you think your baby is constipated and she is younger than 6 months, you can give her 2-4 oz/60-120 ml of water or diluted fruit juices (grape, pear, apple or prune) 1-2 times per day, in consultation with your doctor. If your baby is older than 6 months of age, giving peas, beans, peaches, pears, cereals, and strained prunes will provide high fiber content.

Textured & Table Baby Foods

General

Texture refers to how smooth, thick, thin, or lumpy a particular food is. By 8-9 months of age, many infants are able to progress from simple pureed or strained foods to textured and table foods. At 8-12 months, most babies will use their fingers, try to use utensils (spoon, cup) to feed, and most will want to eat table foods.

Textured and table foods introduces your child to a wide variety of stimulating foods. As your baby enters the toddler years, you will find them both challenging and rewarding. The introduction of textured foods into your baby's diet is a significant developmental stage as it impacts your baby's eating habits and preferences and allows her to master the skills of swallowing and chewing. It is a time of ongoing discovery and occasional frustration.

It is important to offer age appropriate food textures. Feeding problems and nutritional issues may be due to the fact that some parents present foods that are inappropriate for the development feeding skills of the young child for fear of choking, convenience of faster feeding, lack of knowledge, etc. Foods that are not well tolerated by a toddler (e.g., those that present a challenge in chewing) are often perceived as food resistance. As such, many parents will pressure a child to eat them. Toddlers can and will learn to eat a variety of foods that are texturally appropriate for their age with time, patience, and a consistent approach.

When to Start & Readiness for Textured Foods

- Each child is unique and different, so there is no specific time to introduce textured foods. It is dependant on your child's developmental stage and readiness.

- Eight to twelve months of age is the average time period when babies are introduced to textured foods. During or after this time, she will be learning how to chew. Most parents will know from previous experience or intuition when their baby is ready to begin textured foods.

- Generally, if your baby is able to eat small slices of food without gagging or choking, is mashing with her jaw, moving food around in her mouth, and clearly enjoys this type of food, then she is ready for textured foods.

- The presence or absence of teeth is not a necessary factor or sign of readiness to start textured foods as many infants mash the food between their gums, palate, and tongue.

- If you are unsure about your baby's readiness for textured foods, wait a couple of weeks until you feel she is ready.

- It is important for you to continue feeding your child iron-fortified cereal, breast milk, or formula during the first year, and continue to offer finger foods (e.g., ripe banana, cooked vegetables or fruits, soft bread, etc.) while progressing with textured and table foods.

- Chewing entails large pieces of food that are broken down into smaller pieces for the food to be swallowed easily. Learning to chew may prove to be a difficult task for a child who has been eating pureed foods for a long period of time. However, textured foods must be introduced into your child's diet to allow for oral muscles and speech development. Offer your child foods that are easy to chew such as grilled cheese sandwiches, sliced pieces of cheese or chicken, cottage cheese, apple sauce, bananas, hot cereals, pancakes, cooked green beans or carrots, chopped cucumbers, etc.

How to Choose Textured Foods

- The choice of which textured foods to choose depends on food softness, size and variety.

  Softness: Foods should be soft enough to be easily mashed and dissolved in the baby's mouth without the use of teeth; these foods include fruits (bits of bananas, grated fruit), vegetables (mashed potatoes), pieces of cheese or grated cheese, meat, fresh bread, etc.

  Size: Pieces should not be larger than 1/4 inch/0.75 cm (nothing bigger than a pea) to decrease the risk of choking; e.g., pasta can be cut into smaller size pieces prior to serving.

  Variety: Choose a variety of textured foods to help your baby develop familiarity with a range of tastes and textures.

  Textures: The consistency ranges from pureed and blended table foods (commercial baby foods), mashed and lumpy foods, ground, chopped to regular textured table foods such as:

  ❖ Pureed and blended table foods (foods that form a paste or thick liquid) such as apple sauce, blended meats, vegetables and fruits. The baby is ready to eat these foods when she is clearly able to suck and swallow, uses a spoon to feed, and does not gag when swallowing thick purees.

❖ Mashed and lumpy foods (foods that keep some of their texture and consistency) are slightly blended or mashed with a fork, including mashed potatoes, bananas, fruits and vegetables. The baby is ready to eat these foods when she is swallowing without gagging, closing her lips when moving food around or swallowing, and has an up-and-down chewing movement.

❖ Ground and chopped foods (not blended to keep some of the food's original texture and consistency or chopped into bite-size pieces or finger foods) are easy for your baby to chew; these include scrambled eggs, cottage cheese, pieces of crackers, ground meat, chopped fruits that are raw or cooked, etc. Your baby is ready to eat these foods when she is able to chew in a rotary pattern (usually around 18 months). Before this time, your child is able to chew soft foods with their front teeth.

❖ Regular foods (cut up or left in its original form) include vegetables, fruits, and, basically, all types of foods. Your baby is ready to eat these foods when she is able to close her lips, keep the food in her mouth, and she is biting through the food.

The following are examples of starter food choices. You may chew or mash it first to assist your baby in eating these foods.

Vegetables	Cook vegetables until soft. Use wax or green beans, carrots, zucchinis, potatoes, etc.
Fruits	Prepare the fruit by slicing and cutting it into small pieces less than 1/4 inch/0.75 cm in diameter. You may use ripe bananas, peaches, pears, seedless grapes, apricots, plums, melon pieces, avocados, etc. (after about 1 year of age).
Soft Cheese	You may serve cheddar cheese that is grated, sliced, or cut into small pieces.
Pasta & Grains	Soft pasta is usually a baby's favorite. You may serve macaroni, fusili, spaghetti, linguine, and penne; serve it plain with butter or sauce.

Making the Transition

Here are some suggestions to help you make the transition from pureed or strained foods to more textured foods in your baby's diet:

- Do not stop all pureed foods at once, as the introduction of more textured foods should be gradual (e.g., you can mix some textured foods into your baby's smoothly pureed baby food). Continue offering some pureed foods at the same time; introduce one textured food at a time.

- When beginning to introduce a new textured food, offer a few spoonfuls of a familiar texture first and then offer the new texture (feed your baby with a spoon and never feed solid foods or new textured foods through the bottle). Introduce mashed or lumpy foods in the beginning and slowly progress to ground textured foods. You can begin with tiny, soft, unnoticeable lumps in foods and in time, your child will be able to control these lumps in her mouth and swallow them.

- Encourage your child to try new foods by offering her textured foods in various colors, shapes and sizes. Introduce foods your baby enjoys or are her favorites since these provide her with some form of familiarity and she will be more likely to accept new foods that have a flavor she is used to.

- To prevent choking, remove all the bones, skin, pits, and seeds from fruit, fish, poultry, or meat and avoid nuts or seeds.

- Grind, mash, cut, or moisten foods for young infants and toddlers.

- Cut rounded foods into short, thin strips instead of round pieces to make it easier for your child to handle and swallow. Cook foods until they are soft enough to chew and swallow.

- As solid foods continue to be increased into the child's diet, breastfeeding or formula decreases to two to four times per day at 6-8 oz/175-250 ml each.

- Always feed your baby in a seated position, so that she is comfortable and you are comfortable feeding her.

- Never rush the feeding session, especially when introducing new textured foods.

- Provide a happy and relaxed atmosphere when feeding your child new foods.

- Be patient and encourage your child while she is learning all of these new textured foods.

Tip: Messy Eating

At about seven months of age and older, your baby may be able to hold her own bottle, cup, and/or spoon.

You have to realize that any of these feeding methods are messy, however they help develop coordination and motor skills. As such, encourage your child to feed herself and do not get upset if the baby is a messy eater (most babies are!).

To prevent a mess, offer simple finger foods that do not pose much of a messy risk such as Cheerios, etc. You may use bibs and paper spreads on her chair or on the floor to prevent a mess from happening.

Be sure to praise and encourage your child for being able to eat on her own.

Difficulties Associated with Textured Foods

Textures Causing Difficulties

- *Thin* liquids or textured foods are sometimes difficult for children to swallow. In this case, you should thicken the food a little bit to make it easier for your child to swallow. You may use the following food items to thicken foods: infant cereals, pureed fruits or vegetables, powdered milk, yogurt, pudding, apple sauce, commercial thickeners, etc.

- *Thickened* liquids or textures move slower in its transition from the mouth to the throat, allowing the child to take her time swallowing.

- If your child experiences difficulty swallowing *dry* or *lumpy* foods and foods that do not dissolve, you may serve pureed foods, fruits or vegetables or you can mix these textured foods with moist, mashed vegetables or fruits.

- To make a *smooth* texture for your child, blend foods well in a blender or food processor with formula, breast milk, or water for moistness and smoothness, especially when first introducing these foods to your child.

- You may use the following food items to thin food texture: water, liquid milk or formula, pureed fruits or vegetables, ketchup, mayonnaise, juices, etc.

Gagging or Choking

- *Gagging* can be defined as experiencing a regurgitate spasm in the throat to a particular food or a reflexive response to an introduced food (e.g., new textured foods). It is a protective mechanism against aspiration for chunkier food textures rather than for pureed foods or liquids (coughing also helps prevents aspiration from foods entering the lungs).

- *Choking* is defined as an airway blockage of the lungs caused by foreign objects or foods.

- Both gagging and choking are signs that your child is having difficulty swallowing the food offered. Common causes of gagging and/or choking include the following:

  - ❖ Serving your child the wrong texture at an inappropriate age or developmental stage.

  - ❖ Feeding technique may be too aggressive for your child (e.g., placing the spoon too far back in her mouth).

  - ❖ Behavioral response or a way of getting attention.

  - ❖ The angle your child sits at during a feeding session may influence how she swallows (see *Making the Transition* in this chapter for helpful suggestions).

Dysphagia

- *Dysphagia* refers to feeding or swallowing difficulties that occur in infants.

- Symptoms of dysphagia may include difficulty breastfeeding (latching onto the breast), problems with suck-swallow routine or age-appropriate feeding skills, avoiding certain textures, and coughing, choking, or gagging associated with feedings.

- Risk factors for dysphagia are premature birth, neurological problems, delayed introduction of textured foods, and syndromes that affect mouth, esophageal, and pharyngeal structures.

- If your child experiences any of these symptoms, speak to your doctor for further evaluation and treatment.

Parent Concerns

I am worried about my baby choking. When is it safe for me to go from no lumps in foods to some lumps?

- This transition period of moving into more textured foods always makes parents feel anxious and nervous.

- Babies are different and many are able to start managing textured foods around seven to eight months of age.

- Eight to ten months of age is a good time to introduce lumpier textures (e.g., adding mashed or grated foods to smooth purees).

- Ensure that the food pieces are soft, easy to chew, and of small sizes.
- Encourage your infant/toddler to develop hand–to-mouth coordination and mouth and jaw development by offering finger foods (e.g., cooked carrot sticks, pieces of soft fruits, vegetable sticks such as zucchini, potato, etc.).

Do store bought baby foods provide the same texture as homemade foods?
- No, store bought baby foods provide little variety in texture.
- Smooth pureed baby foods (starter or beginning labeled jar foods) are suitable for up to eight months of age.
- Foods that are labeled for juniors are suitable for babies older than eight months of age since they have soft lumps (not much texture).
- The textures in store bought baby foods do not provide your baby with much practice in learning how to chew and/or swallow.

My baby prefers the smooth textures of store bought baby foods. What should I do?
- You can try to prepare homemade foods that have a smooth texture, however you will not be able to get the smoothness of jar foods due to the manufacturing process.
- Some babies get used to the smooth jar food and refuse more textured foods.
- Slowly increase the texture in homemade prepared foods to help your baby gradually accept the more textured foods.

May I continue to give my baby pureed foods while at the same time offering her lumpier foods?
- It is okay to continue offering pureed foods as long as she is not refusing or resisting the changes to more appropriate foods for her age, like textured foods.

How do I know when my baby is ready for table foods?
- Consider table foods as food for adults that may be safely offered to your child when she is an older infant or toddler.
- Remember that your baby does not need to have teeth to accept table foods.
- If your baby seems interested in table foods, offer her these foods in a safe and appropriate manner (e.g., small pieces, use of a spoon or cup, etc.).

Which children are likely to have difficulties with chewing or swallowing when offered textured foods?

- Children with special needs (e.g., premature babies, those with neurological problems, cerebral palsy, Down's syndrome, etc.) may have difficulties chewing or swallowing more textured foods.

- If your baby seems to have difficulties chewing or swallowing, discuss it with your doctor.

Homemade & Commercial Textured Foods

Preparing Homemade Textured Foods

When preparing homemade baby foods, select the setting on your blender or grinder, watch as it processes, and stop the machine when you see a lumpy or chunky texture (that your baby is ready for) or allow it to continue blending for a smoother texture.

Fruit Breakfast
Ingredients:
2 tbsp of rice baby cereal
2 tbsp of peach puree
2 tbsp of pear puree
1 tbsp of mashed cooked rice (mashed with a fork)
2-3 tbsp of breast milk or formula

Directions:
Mix all of these ingredients together and warm slightly if you desire.
Serve for a great textured cereal.

Apples & Carrots
Ingredients:
2 tbsp of apple puree
2 tbsp of carrot puree
1 tbsp of chopped pasta or spaghetti

Directions:
Mix all of these ingredients together and warm slightly if you desire.
Serve for a great textured meal.

> **Tip: Do Not Serve These Foods in the First Year of Life**
>
> Citrus foods (oranges, grapefruit, tomatoes), honey, fish, and foods that pose a choking risk such as hot dogs, peanuts, grapes, raisins, popcorn, etc.

Commercially Prepared Textured Foods

- Many companies who make baby foods label their jars according to each developmental stage in a baby's life.

- Read the label carefully before choosing a jarred food for your baby.

- Each stage (e.g., Stage 2 or 3) signifies the food's texture; however, this is sometimes misleading.

- Babies must be gradually introduced to the later stages in jar foods by being given various foods one at a time. Typically, babies begin with purees and slowly begin feeding with other textures before finally arriving at soft table foods.

- Smooth pureed foods that have Stage 1 or Starter foods on their labels are recommended for babies up to the age of eight months.

- Foods that are labeled Stage 2 or Junior foods contain soft lumps and are recommended for babies a little older than eight months of age.

- When you are unsure of what type of jarred food your baby is ready for, consult your doctor for further advice and recommendations.

Sample Menu (8-12 Months)

8-10 Months

Breakfast (7-8 am)	Cereal + formula or breast milk
Snack (10:30 am)	Fruit
Lunch (12-1 pm)	Meat products with soup
Snack (4 pm)	Cheese or cottage cheese or mixed fruits with mixed vegetables
Dinner (6:30 pm)	Vegetables (e.g., mashed potatoes, squash, etc.)
Snack (before bed)	Cereal and formula or breastfeeding
In-between meals	You may use formula or breastfeeding

10-12 Months

Breakfast (7-8 am)	Cereal and formula or breast milk
Snack (10:30 am)	Fruit
Lunch (12-1 pm)	Rice, diced chicken, cooked pear
Snack (4 pm)	Cheddar cheese or crackers
Dinner (6:30 pm)	Vegetables, pudding, breast or formula feeding
Before bed	Cereal and pear, cooked carrots and pieces of fruits or spaghetti, meats and mashed potato
In-between meals	You may use formula or breastfeeding

Meat & Alternatives: Legumes & Fish

Proteins

Every function in living cells depends on proteins. Protein is the major component of building muscles, tendons, skin, hair, enzymes, eyes, and a variety of other organs and processes. The building blocks of protein are *amino acids*. *Complete protein* contains essential amino acids (there are 23 amino acids in total, of which 9 are essential and 13 are non-essential). *Incomplete protein* is protein that is missing one or more of the essential amino acids, (plant source proteins). The *essential acids* are those which are needed in order to live, but that are not manufactured by the human body. They must be consumed in food. Offering a healthy variety of foods will ensure that your baby/toddler receives all the necessary amino acids.

Infants need a lot of protein for growth. In the early months of a baby's life, an adequate supply of protein comes from either breast milk or formula. Meat, legumes, and fish provide proteins. Animal proteins are better tailored than plant proteins (incomplete protein) to meet the needs of the growing infant. The daily Recommended Dietary Allowances (RDA) for protein, in grams is the following: 0-6 months =13 g; 6-12 months =14-18 g; 1-3 years =16 g; and 4-6 years=22-24 g. The following table will provide a general outline of how many grams of protein are contained in certain food servings:

Food Serving	Grams of Protein
1oz/30 g serving of cheese, lean meat, fish or poultry	6-8 g of protein
1 cup/250 ml of cow's milk or soy milk	6-8 g of protein
2 tablespoons of peanut butter, an extra-large egg or 1/2 cup/125 g tofu	8 g of protein
1/2 cup/125 g beans (pintos, kidneys or garbanzo)	7 g of protein
1 cup/250 g cooked pasta	5 g of protein
1/2 pita	3 g of protein

Meats

General

- Meat provides additional flavor and variety to a baby's menu, is a good source of iron, vitamin B12, and zinc, and the best *complete* source of protein available. All of these play an important role in the baby's intellectual development and more. It is important to introduce meats at an early age (usually about 6-8 months) due to the baby's need for protein and iron (in addition to breast milk and formula in the first year of life).

- Healthy meat alternatives that provide protein include tofu, beans and other legumes, nuts, seeds, eggs, and dairy products. Fish (only given after the age of 1 year due to allergy risk) or poultry are also excellent alternatives.

- The following outlines the ages by which you can introduce fish, meat, and poultry:

  6–9 months of age: Poultry (chicken, turkey, etc.), beef, and lamb
  1 year: Lean fish (flounder, sole, cod, catfish, haddock, etc.), pork, liver, and fatty fish (sardines, halibut, tuna, bluefish, salmon, etc.)

- Almost all meats are rich in iron; these include turkey, beef, pork, veal, lamb, steak, ribs, and chicken.

- Processed meats are not recommended, along with bacon (high in saturated fat and low in protein), ham, sausage, salami, bologna, precooked luncheon meats or other meats that contain nitrates, salt, or other additives.

- Many children develop anemia from iron deficiency and vitamin B12 deficiency (particularly vegetarians with a prolonged abstinence from meat) when not enough meat and alternatives are consumed. This may also result in decreased zinc levels, which can affect your child's short-term memory, learning, and concentration. These effects may last for years (shown in studies of children from 9-15 years of age).

> ### Tip: Getting Enough Iron
>
> Iron-fortified cereal and meat are the best iron sources for your infant. Although some recommend eggs as a good source of iron, the iron in eggs is not well absorbed.

Availability, Preparation & Administration
Availability

- Jar meats are a good source of protein and vitamins (2 1/2 oz/75 g of commercially prepared meat can provide about 50% of an infant's recommended daily protein allowance).

- It is better if there are no nitrates or MSG (monosodium glutamate) contained in commercially prepared baby and adult meats, as are often found in chicken, lamb, and beef (all with broth).

- When buying meat, choose fresh and natural meat. Ground meat should be bright red and clean, not darkish red or brownish red. Also, choose meat with the lowest amount of fat.

Preparation

- Before cooking the meat, you need to remove excess fat and cut the raw meat into small pieces to ensure that it is thoroughly cooked (no pink parts). Remove any and all bones from fish (boneless included), poultry, and meat.

- Meat may be placed into a food processor, which will cut the meat into more small bits rather than just shredded pieces.

- For the meal to be thick and cause satiety, you should start cooking the meat (until soft) and the legumes, and then add the vegetables. You may puree all of these in a blender later on.

- You can use a meat thermometer to test that the meat has been thoroughly cooked. Internal temperatures of ground meat should reach at least 160-180 F/71-82 C in the center and ground poultry should reach at least 180 F/82 C in the center.

- The processed meat or ground food can be mixed with broth and/or water to the desired consistency.

Administration

- Start offering meat with one tablespoon daily and gradually increase the amount to about six to eight tablespoons per day by the time the baby is twelve months of age.

- You may begin with chicken, using a tender piece of the thigh, leg or breast meat. Other choices include soft beef prepared in shepherd's pie or stew. Also, meat or legumes are usually given together with vegetable soup.

Tip: Handling Meat Safely

Wash everything thoroughly in very hot water using antibacterial soap (hands, utensils, etc.).

Keep a separate cutting board for meat than the one you use for all other foods.

When shopping for meat, shop for it last so that it remains cold longer and place it in the refrigerator as soon as possible. Keep meat, poultry, and fish away from all other groceries and bag the meat separately. Tie the bag to contain any leaking liquids.

Do not leave raw or cooked meat at room temperature for more than a few minutes.

Do not keep uncooked frozen meat in the freezer for longer than three months.

Do not keep cooked meat in the refrigerator for more than 24 hours.

Never refreeze meat, poultry, fish or any other food once it has been thawed.

Meat Refusal

- Some infants refuse to eat meat, because of its texture and taste. It is generally not a favorite food among infants and children and acceptance may take longer than for other foods.

- The following are some suggestions for dealing with meat refusal:

  ❖ Try offering meat that is pureed, slightly warmed, or mixed with a favorite vegetable.

  ❖ Offer meat in less recognizable forms (e.g., sausage, corned beef, meat sauce, etc.).

  ❖ Try different types of homemade prepared chicken and fish (e.g., minced, mashed, etc.).

  ❖ Do not overwhelm your child with large portions. Serve small amounts with favorite foods (e.g., meat with vegetables or mashed potatoes, etc.).

  ❖ Continue to offer your child various types, textures, colors, shapes, etc., of meats and alternatives.

- Do not worry if your older infant refuses meat initially. They can receive protein from other foods that satisfy protein needs (both complete and incomplete), such as rice, cottage cheese, avocado, milk, grain cereals, fresh fish or poultry, and well-cooked mashed legumes (lentils, chick peas and soy beans), eggs, tofu, peanut butter, etc. Various combinations of protein alternatives may help your child get proteins that will include essential amino acids that your infant/child cannot produce on her own.

- Combine these foods to make complete proteins:
  - ❖ Grain cereals and legumes: Rice with lentil or tofu.
  - ❖ Seeds: Hummus and tahini, peanut butter and lentils or bread, or hummus, tahini and bread altogether.
  - ❖ Milk products and seeds: Cheese or yogurt with peanut butter and sesame, milk and oatmeal, cheese with macaroni or bread.
  - ❖ Milk and seeds, milk and grains.

> ### Tip: Meat Allergy
>
> Allergy to meat is rare. Children with meat allergy may react to just one type of meat such as beef, chicken, lamb, etc. The most common symptom of meat allergy is a skin reaction.

Legumes

General

- A *legume* can be defined as anything that grows in a pod. It is derived from the leguminous plant, which is a family of plants that bear seeds in pods.
- Legumes are an important source of proteins from vegetable origins, but their nutritional value is not complete (they do not supply all the necessary amino acids). They contain vitamin B (thiamin, niacin, riboflavin) and iron.
- Legumes are usually added to the baby's menu at about 8-9 months of age.
- Legume groups include beans (soy, white, lima, brown, pinto, garbanzo, etc.) and lentils (red, yellow, green).
- Lentils, like other legumes, provide carbohydrates, protein, vegetable fat, vitamins and minerals. They are digested slowly and provide a feeling of satiety or fullness (due to the soluble fibers).
- Beans are a source of vitamin B6, niacin, riboflavin, potassium calcium, iron, and folic acid. They are high in fiber and contain no cholesterol.

> ### Tip: Hummus
>
> Hummus is a mix of oil, garlic and mashed chickpeas, sometimes called garbanzo beans and is among the legume family. It contains vitamin B3 and iron and is rich in nutritious fiber. Hummus is a great source of vegetable protein, which is especially important for the vegetarian baby. It may be nutritionally blended, dried or spread with chick peas, olive or canola oil, pureed sesame seeds and tahini lemon juice. It may be spread on a pita or whole grain cracker.

SECTION 4: STARTING SOLID FOODS

Legume Preparation
General Preparation

- Clean legumes by rinsing them under cold running tap water using the sink hose.

- It is best to keep legumes in water for a few hours so that they will not ferment and become sour before boiling them for two to three hours (this, however, is not very practical).

- After frequent changing of the soaking water or prolonged cooking, legumes are easier to digest, and produce less gas and less abdominal pain. Cook legumes slowly until they are soft.

- You can grind uncooked, dried legumes into a powder (which will make for quicker cooking).

Cooking Beans

- There are many types of beans, such as kidney, lentils, lima, soy, etc.

- Beans can be eaten raw, sprouted, or cooked.

- Soaking beans is not completely necessary; however it does have some advantage.

- Soak the beans for approximately 2 to 5 hours, which will leach out some of the gas. You need to throw the soaking water out and replace it with new water before cooking. Also, before cooking the beans, remove any cracked or discolored beans from the bunch.

- Place the beans over low heat for cooking (beans take a long time to cook) and always cook beans by simmering, not boiling (can cause shells of beans to separate).

- Cook beans with no cover for a firmer texture or with a covered pot for a softer texture for your baby.

- You can test the beans to see if they are finished cooking by tasting them or squeezing a bean between your thumb and forefinger (if the inside is hard, the bean is not finished cooking).

- Once the beans are thoroughly cooked, soft, and tender, you may offer them to your child as a finger food or as part of a meal (e.g., with vegetables, etc.).

- Cooked beans can be kept in the refrigerator for three to five days.

Soy Beans

- The single most important bean in the world is the soy bean.

- It has the highest protein content and is known to have the most complete amino acid balance (closest to the actual human need) in a vegetable, so that it can be considered a complete protein in and of itself.

- Soy beans are also excellent sources of iron, calcium, potassium, essential oil (linoleic acid), and vitamin E and they lower cholesterol.

- Soy beans do not make ideal foods for babies, because they are hard to digest and they are high in fiber. However, when given in moderate amounts, they provide important vitamins, protein, and minerals. These beans also help the baby develop a taste for food that may be very beneficial for them in their diet when they get older.

- These beans are usually integrated into other foods such as tofu, soy sauce, and soy milk, shown in the following table:

Type of Food	Description
Tofu	Known as soy bean curd. Soft, cheese-like substance full of proteins, that can be used in place of meats. Great source of iron and calcium and is 95% digestible (good for the sensitive stomach). Can easily be used at home by slicing it into small cubes, blending it with bananas or other fruits and serving it with a spoon, mashing tofu with cottage cheese, avocado or hummus; tofu does not have to be cooked, because it is made from cooked soy beans. Great as a finger food for babies. Considered one of the more appropriate and recognized baby foods.
Soy Sauce	Fermented sauce made from soy beans, roasted grain, water, and sea salt. Brownish liquid usually used to season food while cooking or at the table.
Soy Flour	Made from whole soybeans that have been roasted and ground. Contains iron, protein, vitamin B, and calcium and is free of gluten. Useful in home cooking and some are defatted to keep the flour fresh (loses all its fat content). Gives baked goods a protein boost and keeps them from going stale.
Soybean Oil	Worlds most widely used edible oil, containing omega 3 fatty acid and no cholesterol. Found in nearly 80% of edible oil consumption in foods like mayonnaise, meat products, frozen foods, etc.
Soy Sprouts	Excellent source of proteins and vitamins. Can be used like other green vegetables in prepared foods.

Soy Allergy

- Many children are allergic to more than one legume with soy allergy being the most common allergy in infants (less than 1% of the population is allergic to soy).

- Allergy symptoms may include eczema, swelling, nose congestion, asthma, anaphylaxis, canker sore, digestive problems, diarrhea, red eye, breathing problems, lowered blood pressure, itchy hives, hay fever, etc., and are diagnosed with a skin allergy test.

- Foods containing soy products that should be kept away from your soy allergic child include soy sauce, some infant formulas, baked goods, vegetable broth, etc.

- Other names for soy products to avoid include miso, natto, okara, textured soy flour or protein, tofu (soybean curds), vegetable protein, yuba, tempeh, mono-diglyceride, edamame, etc. Also, soy is frequently used as a component of another ingredient such as hydrolyzed plant protein, lecithin, monosodium glutamate (MSG), soybean oil, margarine, etc.

- Alternate sources for nutrients found in soy products include alternate protein sources (e.g., meat, fish, poultry, cheese, eggs, etc.), omega-3 fatty acids (salmon, tuna, walnuts, canola oil, cow's milk, whole grain bread, etc.), folate (e.g., green leafy vegetables, beans, lentils, etc.), iron (e.g., meat, poultry, beans, green leafy vegetables, etc.), calcium (cow's milk, cheese, yogurt, etc.), vitamin D (salmon, egg yolk, etc.), zinc (e.g., meat, whole grains, vegetables, etc.), fiber (whole grains, fruits, vegetables, etc.) and B vitamins (bread, cereals, pasta, rice, etc.).

- Most children outgrow soy allergy by the age of two years, while a rare few keep this allergy into adulthood.

Tip: Beans, Family History of Allergy and G6PD Deficiency (Favism)

G6PD deficiency is the lack of glucose-6-phosphate dehydrogenase, an enzyme present in red blood cells. It is most common and frequent amongst African Americans, but also occurs in Greeks, Italians, Chinese, and Sephardic Jews. Also, boys are usually affected while the female carrier is rarely affected.

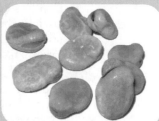

Children with G6PD must be careful to avoid fava beans as the quality of the bean may affect your child's response.

Continued

Raw beans are more likely to cause the reaction than cooked, frozen, or canned beans.

The maturity of the beans is important as young beans are more likely to cause a reaction.

Moreover, children with G6PD should avoid drugs (aspririn, quinine, etc.), antibiotics and chemicals (e.g., methylene blue, naphthalene, etc), etc. Upon exposure to these chemical agents, a severe clinical condition may develop, which causes destruction of the red blood cell (acute hemolysis). This leads to anemia and other clinical consequences of jaundice, lethargy, abdominal pain, vomiting, and prostration to shock. Between these episodes, children seem normal with no symptoms.

Fish

General

- Fish is high in protein content, a good source of energy, and contains vitamins B12, B6, B3, niacin, and iron.

- 60% of the brain is fat and 1/3 of it is omega-3 fatty acids. Fish such as salmon, tuna, and mackerel supply this fatty acid, which has an effect on the emotional and intellectual development of a child.

- The various types of fish include salmon, tuna, mackerel, swordfish, tilefish, pollock, cod, sea bass, founder, sole, halibut, haddock, ocean perch, trout, herrings, sardines, anchovy, oysters and lobsters, shark, rock fish, pike, squid, snapper, yellow tail, etc.

- Fish is usually introduced after the age of one year (due to allergy risk and mercury). Some experts suggest waiting later than that, while others believe it is safe to begin adding fish into the diet as early as 9-10 months of age.

Preparation/Administration

- It is recommended to have fish 2-3 times a week, feeding 2-3 fish balls at first. Meat should alternate with fish about 4 times per week.

- When you first introduce fish to your child, select one of the "white flesh" types, such as flounder, haddock, cod, and sole. These are considered the safest to introduce with the lowest allergy risk and are easily digestible.

- It is very important to remove the bones prior to giving it to your child, as bones may cause choking (canned fish is safer than fresh fish).

- You may poach, bake, or steam the fish and then puree it as you would any other meat and you may serve tuna in its own water or in a light broth.

- When preparing fish, choose low-fat cooking methods such as broiling and steaming to avoid unnecessary fat and calories.

- Fish should be cooked thoroughly until it is white, flaky, and separates easily from the bones. Puree the cooked fish immediately and keep at room temperature for no more than a few minutes (freeze immediately after).

Fish Risk

- Offer fish with low mercury levels such as canned light tuna, salmon, catfish, etc.

- The FDA (March 2004) advised pregnant women, nursing mothers, and children to limit fish to two meals per week. Avoid swordfish, shark, king mackerel, swordfish, and tilefish altogether and limit fresh or frozen tuna to one meal per week (www.cfan.fda.gov/~dms/admehg3.html). A Health Canada Advisory (May 2002) offered slightly different guidelines; women of childbearing age, pregnant women, and children should eat no more than 1 meal per month of shark, swordfish, and fresh or frozen tuna. The advisory does not apply to canned tuna, which must meet Health Canada's commercial regulation guidelines of 0.5 ppm of mercury.

- Do not offer canned fish for adults to your baby as it contains too much salt.

- Raw fish may contain parasites.

- Some fish may have high nitrites content and may be contaminated with bacteria (listeria), such as smoked fish (salmon), trout, or white fish. BE CAREFUL.

Fish Allergy

- Amongst other foods (milk, eggs, soy, nuts, etc.), fish also has a high tendency to cause allergic reactions. This is the main reason why it is important to introduce fish after the age of one year.

- Shellfish, crabs, shrimps, lobsters and "bony" fish are high-risk allergenic foods; therefore delay their introduction until your child is three years of age or older.

- If your child suffers from fish or shellfish allergy, it is better to avoid all fish and its products (including caviar, Caesar salad, Worcestershire sauce, imitation seafood (e.g., sushi), oysters, scallops, clams, etc.). However, some children are able to tolerate certain types of fish while being allergic to other types.

- Be careful with fried foods in restaurants, as the deep fryer may be used to fry fish, prawns, and other shellfish, contaminating your child's chicken or French fries.

- Altogether, it is better to avoid all seafood restaurants and seafood in general if your child has an allergy.

Case Description

Ethan is a ten year old boy who began eating canned fish when he was one year old with no problems. At 18 months, Ethan tried baked, fresh fish and developed a generalized rash on his face and hands along with swelling and itchiness that disappeared after two hours. When he was four, his parents took him to a Chinese restaurant where he was served chicken soup with corn. This soup was probably made with utensils that touched fish or seafood. As a result of the restaurant food, Ethan developed a severe rash, facial swelling (his eyes closed from the swelling), itchiness, fussiness, and cried a lot. He was taken to the hospital and treated with anti-allergic medications.

In the hospital, he had no breathing problems, wheezing, stridor (barky cough), etc. The rash was resolved within 45 minutes of treatment.

When he was six years old, Ethan developed itchy eyes and nose and was diagnosed with environmental allergies. He was then taken to the hospital for skin allergy testing for fish and seafood and an Epipen was given to his parents in case of an allergic reaction.

At the age of eight, Ethan was found positive in allergy testing for cod, halibut, herring, salmon, sardines, sole, tuna, bass, and trout. He also tested positive for allergies to mixed grass, various trees, and mold.

Recommendations for Ethan included avoiding all fish and carrying an Epipen in case of a life-threatening reaction to one of his many allergens.

Parent Concerns

Is meat sterilized by radiation dangerous for my baby?
- Radiation is a method used to decrease the risk of acquiring infection due to bacteria (e.g., E. coli, listeria, etc.). This is done by treating the uncooked meat and meat by-products. It is not dangerous and does not affect the taste of meat.

If meat looks normal, does this mean it is okay for my baby?
- No, meat can look and smell normal yet it may be contaminated with bacteria.

When can I introduce liver to my baby?
- Liver may be introduced at10-12 months of age (it may first be introduced with a vegetable puree). It is a good source of vitamin A, B, protein, and iron. Do not offer liver more than once a week due to its large amounts of iron.

What are some examples of commercial baby foods I can buy?
- There are various commercial baby foods available and some examples include:
  - ❖ Meats: beef, ham, veal, turkey, chicken, etc.
  - ❖ Meat and Vegetables: chicken or beef or turkey or ham with vegetables.
  - ❖ Legumes: peas, green beans, etc.
  - ❖ Other: chicken noodle, macaroni tomato beef, turkey rice, beef egg noodle, etc.

Do the mercury levels in fish affect pregnant women or newborn development?
- The University of Rochester's Medical Center studied 779 mother-infant pairs from an Indian Ocean Island nation where individuals consumed 11 fish and meat portions in an average week. The study did not find that the infants showed any effects from mercury, despite the high levels of fish in their diets (Medical Post, March 2006).

Sample Menus

Meal	8-10 Months	10-12 Months
Breakfast	Breast milk or formula Infant cereal (3-4 tbsp) mixed with breast milk 2 tbsp mashed fruit	Breast milk or formula Infant cereal (5 tbsp) 1/2 slice whole wheat toast
Mid Morning	Breast milk or formula	Breast milk or formula
Lunch	Strained or blended meat	Junior meat (4-6 tbsp)

Meal	8-10 Months	10-12 Months
	(2 tbsp)	Junior fruits (3-4 tbsp) and/or juice
	Strained or blended veggies (2 tbsp)	Junior vegetables (6-8 tbsp) Breast milk or formula
	Breast milk or formula	
Mid Afternoon	Breast milk or formula	Breast milk or formula
Dinner	Strained or blended meat or fish (2 tbsp)	Pureed veggie and meat combo (8-10 tbsp)
	Mashed potatoes or veggies (2 tbsp)	1/2 slice whole wheat toast Junior fruit (3-4 tbsp)
	Strained or blended fruits (2 tbsp)	Breast milk or formula
Bed time & Snacks	Breast milk or formula	Breast milk or formula + cereal

- When selecting meats for your baby, choose the following: chicken breasts, thighs or legs, beef (fresh lean ground beef, top sirloin), boneless pork tenderloins or center cut pork chops, turkey breasts, thighs or legs, etc.

Recipes

Fun with Fish

Ingredients:
8 oz/220 g fish fillets
4 oz/120 ml whole milk

Directions:
Pour milk into a large frying pan that is placed on the stovetop.
Gently heat milk (do not boil) and add fish fillets.
Allow the milk with fish to simmer for 5-10 minutes over low heat.
Take out the fish and allow it to cool.
Use the milk to blend or puree the fish.
Serve immediately or refrigerate.

Great Meat Balls

Ingredients:
8 oz/220 g lean ground beef
1/2 cup/125 g mashed potatoes

Directions:
Mix the beef and potatoes well.
Make small balls out of the mixture.
Place the meatballs on a baking sheet to bake at 350 F/177 C for about 15-20 minutes.
Once they are baked and cooled slightly, serve immediately or freeze.

Chicken & Rice Mix

Ingredients:
1/4 lb/110 g ground chicken
1/2 cup/125 g chopped sweet potatoes
1/2 tea spoon parsley
1 cup/250 g rice
3 cups/750 ml water
1/2 cup/125 g chopped zucchini

Directions:
Place chicken and water in a pot on the stove and allow to boil for about two minutes.
Add all the remaining ingredients to the pot.
Allow simmering for 30 minutes or until tender and soft (make sure to cover with a lid).
Serve immediately or freeze.

You may follow the same recipe for legumes and/or meat alternatives with dried legumes instead of chicken (canned beans and legumes are already cooked, so do not re-boil; these can be mixed with water and left in the pot for about 20 minutes until soft).

Tip: Tasty Combination Ideas

Tofu, blueberries, and bananas.

Tofu, avocado, and peaches or pears.

Beef or turkey or chicken with apple sauce and/or carrots or sweet potatoes.

Meat or chicken with mashed vegetables and/or fruits.

Dairy Products for Infants & Toddlers

General

Dairy products are generally defined as foods derived from milk (cow, goat, and sheep) and are also referred to as milk products. Dairy products are required as a part of a healthy, well-balanced diet and for strengthening the fast-growing bones of young infants and children. Surveys consistently show that milk products (and the subsequent calcium intake) are under-consumed (about 2 instead of the recommended 3-4 servings in 9-18-year old children). Dairy products are nutrient-rich foods that provide calcium, especially, but also other important minerals and vitamins.

Types of Dairy Products

Milk

- Milk provides essential nutrients including calcium, vitamin D, A, B12, riboflavin (promotes skin and eye health), phosphorous (strengthens bones) and other minerals.

- Infants and young children need fat for their growing bodies, so offer your baby whole milk (3.25% milk fat) after the age of one year and until at least two to four years of age, as recommended by your doctor (see *Cow's Milk* for recommendations).

- Here are some of the milk varieties that offer different calorie and fat content:

Types of Milk	Fat Content (%)
Whole Milk/Homo	3.25
Reduced Fat Milk/2 %	2
Low Fat Milk, Skim or Non-Fat Milk	1 or less
Chocolate Milk	Various fat contents
Evaporated Milk	6.5
Evaporated Fat Free Milk	0.5 or less
Sweetened Condensed Milk	8 or less

Yogurt

- Yogurt is a fermented (curdled) milk product that contains live bacteria. These bacteria are friendly as they produce vitamin B in the intestine and fight harmful bacteria. Yogurt also normalizes bacteria in the colon (large intestine).

- Like milk, yogurt provides protein, calcium, vitamins, and other minerals essential in the growing child. Some experts suggest that yogurt aids in digestion, prevents diarrhea, and fights against infections and various diseases.

- There are groups of "believers" and medical experts who believe that yogurt has the following characteristics:

  ❖ Yogurt can boost your immune system.

  ❖ Prevents diarrhea in children on antibiotics.

  ❖ Prevents certain types of cancers.

  ❖ Prevents vaginal yeast infections in mothers and women.

- Some studies suggest that yogurts containing active bacterial culture are effective in decreasing the incidence and duration of diarrhea (*Dig. Dis Science* 2003 48:2077-82).

- The culturing process of bacteria in yogurt produces enzymes that digest the milk protein, which makes yogurt less allergenic. This is a reason why some milk allergic children are able to tolerate yogurt. Similarly, yogurt contains the lactase enzyme that lactose intolerant children need, meaning that some lactose intolerant children may also be able to eat yogurt without symptoms.

- Yogurts come in various fat and flavor contents, including low fat (0.5-2% milk fat), non fat (less than 0.5% milk fat), added fruit flavors, and yogurt beverages.

- Yogurt is a textured food that many young children enjoy. The best type of yogurt to offer your child is plain yogurt, since it contains more calcium and has no added sugar compared to flavored or added ingredient types of yogurts. However, some babies do not enjoy the acidity of plain yogurt, so try another type of yogurt that may include fruits.

- Whole milk organic yogurts are also available and can be given to your child.

- You may offer yogurt to your child as a dip, topping, shake, or smoothie; it is one of the more versatile foods.

- Children with milk allergy should not eat yogurt made from cow's milk. However, they may be able to eat yogurt that is made from non-cow's milk (soy)—read the labels carefully and ensure that your child is not also allergic to soy.

Tip: Buying Commercial Yogurt

When buying yogurts, words that contain "live or active culture" signify a healthy type of yogurt.

Yogurts that are pasteurized (including words such as "pasteurized", "stabilized" or "heat treated") may kill beneficial bacteria and should be avoided.

Avoid yogurt with sugar, flavors, gelatin, and artificial sweeteners, as these interfere with beneficial bacterial activity.

Buy plain yogurt with no additives, including no fruits.

Do not buy old or expired yogurt (check the expiry date).

Buy whole milk yogurt initially and after one year of age, you may buy low fat yogurt (since the baby needs the fat, initially).

You may add your own flavoring to yogurts, using plain yogurt as your base and adding fresh fruits, natural jam, canned fruits, honey (for babies older than one year), and pureed, cooked sweet potato.

Cheese

- Cheese can be made from various milks including 2% fat, 1% fat, skimmed, non-fat milk, etc.; various processes produce the array of cheeses available today (more than 400) including cottage, cheddar, Edam, havarti, Monterey Jack, provolone, mozzarella, feta, Swiss, gouda, etc.

- Cheese provides calories, protein, vitamins A, B2 & B12, calcium, phosphorous, and zinc and ranks as one of children's most preferred snacks.

- You may add cheese to your child's diet after the age of eight months. Buy only natural and non-processed cheese for your child (e.g., parmesan, cheddar, feta, Swiss, mozzarella, ricotta, cream cheese, etc.).

- Check the expiry date on the package. Look for expiration clues such as molds on the cheese (that are white, blue, pink, green flecked or have furry patches). Its color should be uniform from the center to the edge (white cheese becomes yellow as it gets old).

Tip: Ideas for Adding Cheese to the Child's Diet

Melt cheese over other foods such as vegetables.

Add parmesan cheese to pasta.

Slice cheddar or Swiss cheese and offer as finger foods or serve with crackers.

Add cheese to meat or vegetable purees.

Ice Cream

- Ice cream and frozen yogurt are nutritious dairy products that contain protein, riboflavin, calcium, and other essential minerals and vitamins.
- Calorie and fat content vary depending on the type of milk used (2%, 1%, skim, non fat, etc.) and added ingredients (cream, egg yolk solids, sweeteners, natural, or artificial flavors, etc.).
- Ice cream comes in wide varieties such as reduced fat, low fat, light, and fat free ice cream.
- Children may be offered ice cream between the ages of twelve to eighteen months.

Tip: Other Types of Dairy Products

Milk-based desserts, cream, butter, quark, knir/kefir, pudding, whey, etc.

When to Start

- Milk products can be gradually introduced in the child's diet at eight to nine months of age.
- Do not give cow's milk until your child is one year old. However, yogurts, cheeses, and other dairy products can be offered in small quantities starting around eight to nine months of age.
- You may begin by offering one to two tablespoons of a particular milk product per day, making the process gradual.

- Good first choices for milk products are plain yogurt, cottage cheese, grated hard cheese, etc.

Calcium & Dairy Products
Why Calcium Is Needed & How Much
- Calcium is necessary for various reasons including:
  - ❖ Strong bones and teeth.
  - ❖ Body cell function.
  - ❖ Nerves and muscles function.
  - ❖ Contributes to normal blood clotting.

Daily Calcium Requirements for Infants, Toddlers, & Children

Birth-6 Months	210 mg/day
6 Months-1 Year	270 mg/day
1-3 Years	500 mg/day
4-8 Years	800 mg/day
9-18 Years	1300 mg/day

- The calcium requirement for infants totaling 400-600 mg/day equals two to three servings of beverages and foods rich in calcium (e.g., one serving is equivalent to 1 cup/250 ml of milk, fortified juice or yogurt, one inch cubes of cheese, etc.).
- Breastfeeding your baby at least four times per day will provide your baby with the calcium she requires.
- Calcium fortified soy milk is a good substitute for regular milk.

Dairy & Non-Dairy Sources of Calcium
Dairy Sources
- The following are approximations of servings and calcium amounts:
  - ❖ *Yogurt*: Fruit flavored; 3/4 cup/180 ml) = 300 mg of calcium. Plain; 3/4 cup/180 ml = 300 mg of calcium.
  - ❖ *Cheese*: Firm cheese (cheddar, Swiss); 1 inch/2.5 cm cube = 300 mg of calcium. Processed cheese slices (regular or low fat); 2 slices = 250 mg of calcium.

- ❖ *Cottage Cheese*: 1 cup/250 g = 150 mg of calcium.

- ❖ *Milk* (skim, 1%, 2%, whole, buttermilk, chocolate): 1 cup/250 ml = 300 mg of calcium.

- ❖ *Pudding with milk*: 1 cup/250 ml = 300 mg of calcium.

- ❖ *Ice Cream*: 1/2 cup/125 ml = 75 mg of calcium.

- ❖ *Yop*: 1 1/2 bottle/120 ml = 300 mg of calcium.

- ❖ *Minigo*: 2 containers/60 ml = 300 mg of calcium.

Non-Dairy Sources

The following table outlines non-dairy sources of calcium amounts:

Calcium fortified cereal and grains	Cereal: 1 cup/250 g = 100-200 mg Bread: 2 slices = 50 mg
Vegetables	Broccoli: 1 cup/250 g = 100 mg Collards, Rhubarbs: 1/2 cup/125 g = 170 mg Blackstrap Molasses: 1 cup/250 g = 170 mg Kale, Spinach, and Turnips: 1 cup/250 g = 200-250 mg
Fruits & juices	Calcium fortified juice: 1 cup/250 ml = 300 mg Orange juice: 1 cup/250 ml = 50 mg (fortified 1 cup/250 ml = 300 mg of calcium) Soy beverages: 1 cup/250 ml = 300 mg
Legumes	Soybean nuts: 1/4 cup/65 g = 110 mg Beans: 1 cup/250 g baked = 150 mg Tofu: 3 oz/90 g = 190 mg
Fish & seafood	Sardines: 3 oz/90 g = 370 mg Salmon: 3 oz/90 g (canned) = 180 mg Tofu: 3/4 cup/165 g = 300 mg
Nuts & seeds (sunflower, almonds, hazelnuts, cashews, walnuts, tahini, etc.)	Sesame seeds: 1 oz/30 g = 280 mg Almond butter: 2 tbsp = 80 mg Almonds: 1 cup/250 g = 300 mg

Signs of Low Calcium
- The following are signs and symptoms of low calcium levels (hypocalcemia) in children:
    - ❖ Seizures, loss of consciousness.
    - ❖ Bizarre behavior and irritability.
    - ❖ Headaches, vomiting, and mental problems.
    - ❖ Abdominal cramps, diarrhea.
    - ❖ Dental problems and defective nails.
    - ❖ Skin rashes and yeast infections.
    - ❖ Photophobia (difficult looking at light).
    - ❖ Chronic conjunctival infection (persistent eye infection), and cataract.
    - ❖ Spontaneous muscle contractions and larynx spasms.

Tip: Increasing Calcium

In the case of low calcium, you may need calcium supplements, appropriate dietary habits and, sometimes, additional vitamin D (vitamin D sources include fish, liver, fortified milk and cereal, etc.). Remember that multivitamins do not always contain calcium.

- The following interfere with calcium absorption:
    - ❖ Foods high in oxalate chemicals (e.g., strawberries, blueberries, sweet potatoes, spinach, berry juices, tea, cola, peanuts, chocolate, almonds, parsley, etc.).
    - ❖ Citric acidic foods (e.g., citrus fruits and juices, etc.).
    - ❖ High fiber diet (see *Vegetarians*).
    - ❖ Foods high in phosphor (e.g., meat, poultry, corn, potatoes, etc.).
    - ❖ Foods high in phytates (e.g., wheat bran and germs, barley, oats, corn chips, rye bread, nuts, sesame seeds, rice, beans, soybeans, bran and wheat cereals, etc.).

Tip: Calcium Absorption

Calcium absorption is 60% from breast milk, 40% from cow's milk formula and soy formula, and 30% from cow's milk.

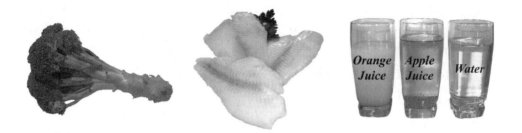

How to Boost Calcium Intake
- The following are suggestions to help you boost your child's calcium intake:
  - ❖ Eating small amounts of calcium-containing foods frequently provides better total calcium absorption (e.g., calcium tablet of 50 mg should be split and taken twice daily instead of all at once).
  - ❖ The lactose contained in milk facilitates better calcium absorption.
  - ❖ Vitamin C and D containing foods improve the absorption of calcium.
  - ❖ Use various preparation methods to add calcium to your meals (e.g., add sesame seeds to salads, etc.).
  - ❖ Eat fruits and vegetables that are low in oxalate and phytates (e.g., broccoli, kale, mustard, etc.).
  - ❖ Eat dairy and non-dairy sources of calcium to provide a healthy, well-balanced diet.

Dairy Issues & Concerns
Dairy Food Refusal
- Young children's appetites constantly change.
- Dairy food refusal is usually a phase which passes with time.
- If your child refuses dairy, try the following helpful tips in dealing with dairy food refusal:
  - ❖ Stay calm and do not force your child to eat.
  - ❖ Offer new dairy foods with foods your child is already accustomed to.
  - ❖ Do not overwhelm your child with large portions. Serve small sizes of dairy products and refill the plate upon request.
  - ❖ Encourage your child to eat on her own or with you at the table.
  - ❖ Vary the shape, size, texture or preparation method when serving dairy foods to your child (e.g., pizza bites or pockets, mozzarella sticks, grilled cheese, cheese strings, parmesan, etc.).

- Allow your older child to participate in dairy food selection and preparation since she will enjoy the experience and be more willing to try it.

Tip: Helpful Ideas for Dairy Food Refusal

Try to make soup, oatmeal, or other hot cereal with milk instead of water.

Pour milk over cold cereal for breakfast or snacks.

Incorporate milk into a fruit smoothie or milkshake

Milk Allergy
- Milk allergy is a response to one or more proteins found in milk or dairy products and can be due to immune or non-immune mechanisms.

- This allergy usually begins in the early infancy stages, however most babies outgrow it within the first few years of life.

- Introducing dairy products into a child's menu before the age of 1 year when there is family history of milk allergy is not recommended. Before the age of 1 year the risk of developing an allergy is high.

- Symptoms of milk allergy include skin reactions, nausea, vomiting, diarrhea, and respiratory system reactions including a runny nose, itchy and watery eyes, wheezing, shortness of breath, etc.

- If your child has a milk allergy, you must be very careful to read labels on foods you buy to avoid giving your child any milk proteins (many are hidden in various foods). Milk proteins to watch out for include butter, casein or anything such as, cheese, curds, lactoferrin, lactose, margarine, natural flavoring, whey, yogurt, etc. (see *Cow's Milk*).

- You can replace milk with water, broth, or juice when preparing homemade foods.

- Some babies are able to handle soy milk; however babies who are allergic to cow's milk may be allergic to soy milk as well.

- Nutritional needs must continue to be met even without milk or dairy products in the diet.

Non-dairy Foods which Are High in Calcium
- Dark greens (collards, parsley, mustard, dandelion, turnips, spinach, broccoli, etc.).

- Beans (chick peas, navy, or pinto beans).

- Nuts and seeds such as sesame or sunflower seeds, almonds, hazelnuts, cashews, etc.
- Calcium fortified cereals, foods or beverages (e.g., juices).
- Seafood (salmon, sardines).
- Artichoke and papaya.
- Vitamin C foods such as orange juice, tomato, etc. help improve the absorption of calcium.

Lactose Intolerance

- Lactose intolerance is when the digestive system is unable to completely break down the sugar called lactose found in milk.
- Common symptoms of lactose intolerance include nausea, cramps, diarrhea, bloating, gas, etc.
- Children who are lactose intolerant must not consume any dairy products and should avoid any milk proteins found in foods (e.g., cheese, candy, whey, casein, hot dogs, curds, pizza, sour cream, yogurt, etc.).

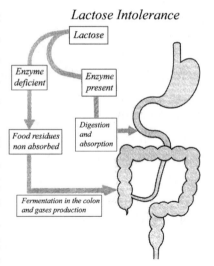

Lactose Intolerance

- Eliminating dairy products to treat lactose intolerance should be considered a last resort. This is because avoiding milk and milk product lower the intake of calcium, vitamin D, and proteins, all of which are important for the growing child. A lactose free diet may actually increase the risk of inadequate bone mineralization (varied amount, timing, type of dairy product can make a difference). Many children are able to eat small amounts of lactose throughout the day or consume it with other foods (tolerated without any symptoms).
- Foods rich in calcium may still be given to your child such as green leafy vegetables, sesame seeds (may be added to shakes, soups) etc., and you may even need to provide calcium supplements (speak to your doctor about your child's calcium intake).

Osteoporosis in Children

- Osteoporosis is a disease characterized by low bone mass and deterioration of bone tissue, which results in fragile bones and fracture risks.

- Osteoporosis sometimes has no early symptoms but, later, the young child experiences dull or sharp pains in her bones or muscles.

- There are two important minerals that children must receive for normal bone formation and these are calcium and phosphate. The body uses these two minerals to produce bones. If the child does not get enough calcium in her diet, bone production and tissue may suffer.

- The following suggestions are ways to help keep your child's bones healthy:

  ❖ Proper nutrition and physical activity (muscles get stronger the more we use them).

  ❖ For toddlers and older children weight bearing activities such as walking, running, dancing, playing tennis, hiking, basketball, gym, and soccer are great for the bones.

  ❖ Serve foods rich in calcium and vitamin D.

- Playing outside with your child is great, since she will receive vitamin D from the sun.

Tip: Nutritional Calcium is Much Better than Calcium Supplements

A study that evaluated 19 studies involving 2859 children aged 3-18 years who received either calcium supplements or placebo, showed that calcium supplementation has very small effects on bone mineralization in children. This suggests that a balanced diet that includes calcium and weight bearing physical activities are healthier for your child than offering calcium supplements. Overall, nutrition is important.

Other Issues

The following issues are associated with dairy products and all assert the same message: serve your child dairy products in moderation!

Dairy Products & Cholesterol	Cholesterol is a type of fat needed for various body functions, however, too much cholesterol is not good.
	It is found in full fat dairy products such as milk, cheese, and butter.
Dairy Products & Iron	Dairy products are deficient in iron, and a diet rich in them may cause iron deficiency in your child.

Dairy Products & Diabetes	Diabetes is a disease where blood glucose levels are above normal. Most of the food consumed is turned into glucose or sugar for our bodies to use as energy. The pancreas (near the stomach) makes a hormone called insulin to help glucose get into the cells of our bodies. One has diabetes when the body cannot produce enough insulin or cannot use its own, causing the sugar to build up in the blood. Symptoms of diabetes include excessive thirst and urination, very dry skin, tiredness, tingling, infections, extreme hunger, and weight loss.
Dairy Products & Colic	Colic is defined as crying for an extended period of time. Some doctors and medical experts believe that milk allergy causes colic, while others disagree and believe that the general cause of colic is unknown. Some parents do claim that removing dairy products from their infant's diet results in the colic getting much better, sometimes disappearing completely.
Dairy Products & Kidney Stones	Kidney stones are hard, stone-like masses that can form in one or both kidneys and are usually painless, although they sometimes cause pressure, pain, and infection. The most common type of kidney stone is calcium stones made of calcium and oxalate, which are chemicals found in certain foods. A diet rich in calcium and oxalate may increase the risk of calcium stones forming in the kidney.

Parent Concerns

If my child is lactose intolerant, can she eat dairy products?

- Most people with lactose intolerance are able to tolerate a small amount of dairy products, including milk.
- If your child is lactose intolerant, you may try to include dairy products in the following way:
  - ❖ Offer small portions (e.g., 1/2 cup/125 ml of milk or use lactose reduced milk).
  - ❖ It is easier to digest milk when it is mixed with other foods.
  - ❖ You may try adding over the counter enzyme drop tablets to milk to break down the lactose (or buy milk with lactaid if you take milk).

❖ Offer low fat or hard, aged cheese that has the lowest lactose content, or yogurt.

When can I introduce cheese into my child's diet?

- Cheese may be introduced to your child at eight months or older.

- If your baby cannot grasp the cheese yet, offer cheese that is mashed, easy to grasp, or melted over foods (e.g., vegetables, meat, etc.).

- You may also try offering cut up biscuits mixed with cottage cheese or offer small pieces of cheese as finger foods.

When can I introduce yogurt into my child's diet?

- Plain yogurt may be introduced at eight months of age.

When should I begin introducing dairy products when there is a family history of milk allergy?

- When there is family history of milk allergy or lactose intolerance, dairy products should not be introduced until after the age of one year.

- Use food sources other than dairy products (see appropriate sections throughout this chapter) to provide the daily calcium requirements for your child.

What are allergy symptoms to dairy products and are they the same as cow's milk allergy symptoms?

- Yes, allergy symptoms to dairy products are similar to those of a cow's milk allergy.

- Symptoms may include vomiting, diarrhea, rash, abdominal discomfort, bloody stool, etc. (see *Feeding & Food Allergy*).

My baby refuses cow's milk. Is it okay or enough to provide only other dairy products?

- Babies do not need cow's milk; however they do need enough calcium.

- As long as the daily required amount of calcium is supplied through other dairy and/or non-dairy products (see appropriate sections), it is okay for your child not to take cow's milk.

- Remember, it does not matter whether or not your child is breastfeeding or bottle-feeding as long as she receives adequate amounts of calcium.
- If you have any concerns about your child's calcium levels, consult your doctor.

If I use dairy products with whole milk, will my baby get fat?
- No. Whole (or homo) milk should be used with dairy products until at least the age of two years.
- Do not give your child 1%, 2%, or low fat milk before two years of age.
- If you are concerned about overweight issues with your child (under two years of age), speak to your doctor.
- After two years of age, if your child is overweight, you may offer 1%, 2%, low fat or skim milk.

Why is it recommended to introduce dairy products at 8 months of age and cow's milk at 1 year?
- Cow's milk is introduced at the age of 1 year, because it is associated with various problems such as bleeding in the digestive system, iron deficiency anemia and its consequences, etc. (see *Cow's Milk*).
- Even after the age of one year, the American Academy of Pediatrics suggests offering only a small amount of cow's milk to provide calcium requirements (16-20 oz/500-620 ml for children aged one to three years).
- Dairy products, especially yogurt, are easier to digest and are less allergenic than cow's milk. These products are better tolerated and can be introduced at the age of eight months to supply additional calcium.

Are white spots on my child's nails a sign of low calcium intake?
- White spots on your child's nails do not indicate calcium deficiency.
- Small white spots on the nails are the most common form of Leukonychia, which is a whitening of parts or of the entire nail.
- Picking and biting of the nails are a prominent cause in young children and nail biters.
- In most cases, when white spots appear on a single or a couple of fingers or toes, the most common cause is injury to the base (matrix) of the nail. When

this is the case, white spots may disappear after around eight months (the time necessary for nails to re-grow completely).

- White spots showing up on all or nearly all nails for long periods of time (months or years) can be due to several reasons, such as zinc deficiency, etc. Whitening of the entire nail may be a genetic condition or a side effect of some medication (e.g., antibiotics sulphonamides type).

- Whitening or discoloration of the nail in bands or "stria" may be caused by physical injury to the nail matrix (e.g., excessive nail "tapping" or slamming a car door, etc.). It may also be caused by liver disease, chemotherapy treatment, etc.

Tips: Dairy Product Fun

There are many options available to you when preparing homemade dairy food meals or snacks. Simply play with all of the various dairy products available to you and mix and match with vegetables and fruits. Blend all of the ingredients together or simply mash them together until desired texture and consistency.

Sample Menu (1 Year Old)

Breakfast & Morning Snack

Whole milk or formula

Cheese (1 oz/25-30 g; e.g., cheddar cheese)

Half an egg

Quarter fruit (e.g., banana, apple, orange)

Small bite size crackers

Lunch

Pasta (25-30 ml or 2 tablespoons)

Pasta sauce (tomato; 5 ml)

Whole milk or formula

1-2 cookies (oatmeal or tea cookies)

1/3 cup/85 ml of cereal or iron-rich oatmeal (1/3 cup)

Dinner

1 slice of bread

Vegetables (1-2 oz/30-60 ml of e.g., broccoli; 1-2 meatballs or spinach, vegetable soup, cooked carrots, etc.)

1/4 fruit

Whole milk or formula

- Spread whole milk or formula throughout the day's meals and snacks to amount to 16 oz/500 ml per day.

Finger Foods for Babies & Toddlers

General

Finger foods are any bite-size foods that your baby can pick up and eat on her own.

From the age of eight to ten months, the baby develops skills to hold food in her hand, chew, and swallow. Your baby will gradually learn texture, color, and aroma of various finger foods. Finger foods will encourage your baby to begin independence (self-feeding) and develop fine motor skills.

At first, most babies will hold the piece given to them (e.g., piece of bread) in their fist and may mash it that way. They will slowly learn to coordinate each individual finger for picking up the food and transporting it into their mouth. A baby develops fascination with small objects and wants to do it "on her own." The pincer grasp, which is holding of an object between the thumb and the forefinger, develops in a baby between the ages of nine to twelve months. As babies develop their ability to put things into their mouth, parents need to be more cautious and aware about food and other items which may cause choking.

Tip: Messy Eater

Keep your sense of humor whenever she spills or makes a mess with the food.

It is important to allow the baby to play with food to teach her texture, smell, and taste.

Prepare all that is needed for your baby's meal before placing her in the high chair (the high chair is always better than at a table).

To reduce the mess, place food directly onto the high chair tray. Keep bowls out of the baby's reach.

Always give small amounts of food at a time.

Keep a wiper on hand for quick cleaning of your baby's hands.

When to Introduce & Signs of Readiness

When to Introduce

- Your baby is probably ready for finger foods when she either grabs the spoon you are feeding her with or takes the food directly off your plate. This usually happens between seven to nine months of age.

- At first, your baby may just take the food with her hands and bring it to her mouth but, eventually, she will use the pincer grasp to pick up food.

- You should probably wait until your child is able to sit up well without any support. She should also have the coordination to hold and bring food to her mouth with a thumb-finger grasp (at about nine to twelve months of age).

- Ensure that everything you give her is soft, easy to swallow, and can break down into smaller pieces. Supervise your child when she eats, in case of choking.

> ### Tip: Waiting for Teeth to Introduce Finger Foods
>
> You do not need to wait until your baby grows teeth to begin finger foods.
>
> Regardless of whether or not your baby has teeth, she is not going to be able to begin actually chewing foods until she reaches a much older age (chewing for the baby is just mashing food between her gums).
>
> Also, if your baby is not gagging or choking, then the texture of finger foods you are offering is fine.

Signs of Readiness
8-10 months of age:

❖ Picks up objects with thumb and forefinger.

❖ Able to transfer objects from one hand to the other.

❖ Places everything she touches in her mouth.

❖ Jaw moves in a chewing motion, etc.

10-12 months of age (in addition to above):

❖ Swallows food easily.

❖ Has more teeth.

❖ Trying to use a spoon, etc.

How to Introduce

General Aspects of How to Introduce Finger Foods

- Foods that qualify under the category of finger foods are foods that have a swallowable consistency, or ones which will dissolve in the mouth without the need for chewing (or are soft enough to be "chewed" by the gums). Start with foods that have been well received in pureed form in earlier feedings.

- Cut finger foods to small pieces. The size should be no bigger than 1/4 inch -0.75 cm to prevent choking (e.g., small pieces of cookies, crackers, natural cheese, etc.).

- When first introducing finger foods, choose soft fruits (pears, peaches, bananas, etc.) or steamed vegetables.

- You may place a few pieces of finger foods onto your baby's high chair and continue offering them as your baby is eating them.

- Start by offering your baby's favorite food (e.g., sweet potatoes) to help enhance first acceptance. Add new foods gradually and, if your baby rejects the food, then try again at a later time.

- At the beginning, only give your baby 2-3 bits of finger food at a time to prevent her from stuffing her mouth and risking choking.

- Teething babies may enjoy eating frozen banana, dry bread crusts, melba toast crackers, etc.

- Try to offer a selection of flavor, shapes, colors, consistencies, and textures (e.g., cooked, ripe, raw peeled, grated, cubed, diced, baked, dry, steamed, etc.).

Tip: Smooth Introduction of Finger Foods

The following are a few suggestions of how to smoothly introduce finger foods:

- Do not offer too many pieces at a time (limit to 2-3 pieces).

- Introduce finger foods one at a time (slowly introduce new ones).

- Transition to finger foods over a seven to nine month period.

- Continue feeding soft, pureed baby foods.

- Always supervise your child when she is eating (especially on her own).

- Feed your baby in a high chair (or make sure she is in a seated position).

- Offer spoon-feeding before finger foods since she may refuse to use a spoon as she gets used to eating with her fingers.

Types of Finger Foods & How to Serve
Fruits

- You may offer peeled raw fruit (e.g., pear, peach, banana, etc.) or chunks of ripe fruits.

- Make sure you remove any seeds and pits inside fruits.

- Harder fruits (e.g., apples) may be grated or served in small bite size pieces.
- Toddlers may be served small pieces of dried fruits in moderation, as these are a good source of iron.
- Watch your child carefully, as there is a risk of choking.

Vegetables
- Vegetables have to be well cooked to very tender (e.g., green beans, potatoes, carrots, yam; broccoli should be cut in half or crushed).
- You may choose to steam vegetables such as broccoli, cauliflower, peas, etc., or offer soft cooked or grated carrots.
- Raw vegetables that may be served include ripe avocado, cherry tomatoes, etc., which are cut into small pieces.

Dairy Products
- Cheese can be grated or cut into small cubes and offered.
- You may also choose to offer bites or strips of melted cheese on bread.

Meats & Protein
- You may cook and give small pieces of chicken, beef or fish after 1 year of age (e.g., fish sticks, etc.).
- Meat or meatballs must be soft and cooked in a sauce.

Bread & Cereal
- You can offer pieces of toast, whole grain crackers, rice cakes, cooked pasta, whole grain cereals (e.g., Cheerios, etc.).

Finger Food Refusal
- At first, if you see that your baby is not interested in finger foods, wait a week or two before retrying.
- Offer these foods when the baby is very hungry so she is less likely to get distracted. Some babies may get frustrated quickly if they are hungry. In this case, offer finger foods as a snack or after she has eaten other foods.
- You may need to experiment with different foods to find what works for you and your baby.
- For some babies, it is fun when they put a certain food into their mouths and make noises with it (e.g., Cheerios cereal).

- Try changing the way you are offering these foods (offer a variety of shapes, colors, and textures). You can offer finger foods before giving breast milk, formula, or other baby foods.

What to Avoid: Red Flags

Do **not** offer an infant or young child (until three to four years of age) the following as they may cause choking:

- Spoonful of peanut butter.

- Nuts or popcorn, dried fruits (e.g., raisins).

- Uncooked peas or celery.

- Candies, chewing gum, and marshmallows.

- Hot dogs or meat sticks, chunks of meat or poultry.

- Other hard, round food or raw, fresh vegetables (large pieces of raw carrots, fruits such as unripe fruits, cherries, apples, pears and grapes).

- Avoid foods that are hard or slippery and those that do not break easily into small pieces. These are all choking hazards.

- Homemade bread dissolves in the infant's mouth, however some commercial bread becomes pasty and it is possible that your infant may choke on this bread.

- Teething biscuits, bagels, pretzels, and breadsticks may cause choking. Use them only for infants with good biting, chewing, and swallowing skills. Also, only use them for children who are at least one year old, and when they are sitting up and supervised by an adult.

Sample Menu (8-10 Months)

Breakfast (7-8 am)	Breast milk and/or formula + cereal
Snack (10:30 am)	Fruit pieces
Lunch (12-1 pm)	Soup with well cooked meat
Snack (4 pm)	Cottage cheese and/or cheese bits Mixed fruits or vegetables (offered as sticks, cubes, etc.)
Dinner (6:30 pm)	Vegetables
Before Bed	Breast milk and/or formula + cereal
In-between meals and/or snacks, you may offer breast milk and/or formula.	

Tip: *Examples of Finger Foods (use according to your child's developmental age and ability)*

Whole-wheat bagel; whole grain bread or toast; lightly toasted bread, cut up and spread with vegetable puree for extra vitamins.

Rice cakes or other crackers that become mushy in the mouth.

Well cooked pasta of various shapes and sizes.

Cheese—Swiss, Cheddar, Havarti, Edam are all good choices cut in slices, string cheese or grated cheese.

Chunks of ripe banana, ripe pear, peach, apricots, and cantaloupe.

Cooked to very tender: carrots, white or sweet potato, yam, broccoli, cauliflower, peas (see preparation/administration for cooked foods) which must be cut in half, crushed, or peeled.

Pieces of scrambled eggs (later than one year of age).

Small pieces (pea-size pieces) of chicken; mini chicken.

Soft meatballs (pea-size pieces) cooked in a sauce or soup; mini meatballs.

Cereals like Cheerios.

Slices of canned fruits (peach, pear, and pineapple).

Peeled plums, peaches, avocado, and mango wedges.

Flaked fish sticks.

Cut up grapes, cherries (pits and seeds must be removed); cut up raisins, apricots, and shaved, dried prunes.

Small cubes of tofu.

Cup Use

General

Cups provide a way to offer liquids (such as water, juice, breast milk, formula, etc.) to a baby or older infant and child. It is sometimes used as an alternative to bottle-feeding for a breastfed baby who requires supplementation or is unable or unwilling to breastfeed or drink from a bottle. It may also be used as an alternative feeding method for a baby whose mother is unavailable, ill, or resting sore nipples.

Cup feeding is an alternative for pre-term or special needs babies who cannot get enough milk from the breast. A baby who is having difficulties latching onto the breast can use the cup while she improves her breastfeeding skills. Cup feeding is less likely than bottle-feeding to interfere with establishing a better breastfeeding routine (the use of a bottle should be avoided, as it may cause nipple confusion). It provides an alternative to babies who have cleft palate (an opening in the roof of the mouth in which two sides of the palate did not fuse as the unborn baby was developing).

There are several advantages to using a cup instead of a bottle:

Advantages of Using the Cup	Disadvantages of Using the Cup
Baby controls the feeding.	No sucking opportunity.
Does not require much energy on the baby's part to learn to cup feed.	Amount in the cup may be lost (spilling when used at an early age, so expect a mess).
More of an oral experience as cup feeding stimulates tongue and jaw movement.	
Promotes good eye contact and improves baby's hand-to-mouth coordination.	
Provides another method to administer fluids (water, juice, breast milk, formula, etc.).	
Prevents bottle dental caries with cup use rather than continuous use of a bottle.	

- You can use fluids inside the cup such as water, juice, breast milk, formula, cow's milk (over one year of age), yogurt, etc.

- If your baby cannot yet consume juice or cow's milk, you can offer the sippy cup in-between feedings with small amounts of expressed breast milk or formula each day.

Types of Cups

- There are various types of cups (sippy, small adult cups, adult, etc.) that you can try since each baby may like a different type of cup (just like bottles and nipples).

- The type of cup used is not overly important, although the younger the baby is the more you will need to help her hold the cup.

- Each baby has her own preference for the cup. Some babies do well with the usual sippy cup (a training cup with a screw or snap on the lid and a spout that allows your child to drink without spilling), while others refuse the spout and prefer a cup with an "indented" lid (almost no lid at all). Some prefer the infant straw-type cups and yet others prefer the juice box type containers.

- Some of the following are general guidelines when offering a cup to your child who is first learning:

  ❖ Use a cup that has a sipper with a spout since your baby will not be able to drink successfully from a regular, adult cup until she is well into her toddler years.

  ❖ The cup needs to be spill proof (sipper cups are good for this purpose) as well as drop proof (plastic), so that it does not crack or break if it is dropped.

  ❖ The bottom of the cup should be heavy so that it will not tip easily and should have one or two handles for your baby to hold with (easier to hold the cup).

  ❖ Some baby cups have different spouts attached to them to allow for varying liquid flows.

  ❖ "First Years" disposable sippy cups are great when introducing a cup to your child as they can be thrown in the dishwasher after each use. However, these cups wear over time, leak, and sometimes crack.

❖ Cups with soft tips seem to be successful when transitioning from the nipple of the breast. Some babies enjoy cups with softer and longer mouthpieces when transitioning from the bottle to the cup.

❖ Many babies and toddlers take to cups with soft spouts easily.

Tip: Cup Selections

A cup with a spouted lid offers good transition from suction to sipping. The "spill-less" cup does not spill when it tips over.

When to Start Cup Use

- Your baby may be ready to begin drinking from a cup between the ages of 5-9 months. Some enjoy a sippy cup as early as five to six months of age, while others are not interested until one year of age. However, most babies are probably ready for cup use between the ages of seven to nine months.

- Some babies may resist using a cup if it is started later than the age of 1 year. Starting early use of a cup is better than starting later, since an older baby may understand that we want her to forget about the bottle and/or formula. It is also better to start early, as it can take months to learn to drink significant amounts from a cup.

- Note that the baby may start the use of a cup as early as two months of age, however gagging will occur less frequently when the baby is able to sit without support.

- A six month old baby, who is sitting up without any support and is using both hands for play, is developmentally ready to begin learning to drink from a cup.

- When the baby becomes "bored" with the bottle and plays with it (usually around seven to nine months), she is ready for the cup.

- Around four to six months of age, babies seem interested in cups while watching other family members drink from it. However, they do not yet have the motor skills to handle it well.

- Premature babies can be fed with a cup of breast milk or formula beginning from birth.

Tip: Starting to Use the Cup

Your baby will be able to form her lips around the edge of a cup and drink (as long as you hold the cup in the beginning) between six to nine months of age.

How to Ease the Transition

- Begin the transition gradually by adding a sippy cup during bottle-feeding.
- In the beginning (at about six months), let your baby take small sips from a cup while you hold it.
- Initially, fill the cup with water (it's less messy) and later (when better control of the cup is achieved), use formula, expressed breast milk, or diluted juices.
- When your baby becomes better coordinated, put a little more fluid into the cup.
- Do not try to hold the cup for her; instead urge her to use it even if she is only able to take a sip.
- You may use a small amount of fluid in the cup and pour drops slowly into her mouth. Remove the cup and allow her to swallow. Stop when she becomes upset or turns her head.
- Initially, use the cup in midday, then in the morning. The bedtime feeding bottle is the last one to abandon (see *Weaning*).
- Remember that the baby may just want to play with the cup for the first several weeks.
- Also, note that babies love to imitate, so drink from a cup in front of them.
- Do not use the cup initially when your baby is hungry, tired, upset, stressed, etc.
- Do not show the bottle when trying to wean to a cup.
- Offer colorful cups to your baby when first introducing the cup.
- Encourage your baby to use the cup when you think she is ready.
- If your baby refuses the cup, try a straw first, since some babies get the hang of drinking from a straw easier than a cup (drink from a straw first to show her how it is done).
- Change the liquids you offer in the cup, since some babies only like to drink water or juice from a cup and prefer milk or formula in a bottle (babies associate these with breast or bottle-feeding).
- If the baby refuses, postpone the use of a cup for a few weeks and retry at a later time.

Tip: Moving From A Sippy Cup to Regular Cup

Although it can vary from child to child, most can use regular cups by two to three years of age, when they can hold a cup without spilling liquid.

How to Offer the Cup: Gradually Mastering It

- Start with a small amount (1 tablespoon of water) of breast milk or formula in the cup, and then gradually increase the amount.

- Hold the baby in your lap and show her how to drink. Begin by holding the baby in an upright position.

- Protect your baby's clothes with a towel or soft cloth in case of spills.

- Bring the cup to your baby's lips and place the edge on the outer corners of her upper lip (gently resting on her lower lips with tongue inside the cup).

- Do not pour the milk into your baby's mouth as this may cause her to spit it up or gag. Simply tilt the container a bit and let her reach for it with her tongue. If she wants more, give her time to swallow and offer more.

- Allow your baby to set the pace for feeding from a cup. Stop after several minutes so that your baby will not be tired.

- Until about nine months of age, your baby will use the same sucking method used for the bottle on the cup.

- At ten to fifteen months, your baby will hold the cup in both hands. Gradually, she will become more skilled at taking several continuous swallows without support.

- At fifteen to eighteen months, your baby may have already learned to how to really drink from a cup. Once she becomes fairly skilled in cup use, try giving her an uncovered plastic cup and fill it with a small amount of water. Expect a lot of fluid to dribble from the sides of her mouth until a tight seal between her lips and the cup is learned.

- By eighteen to twenty-four months, your baby will be able to hold the cup with both hands but there will still be some spills. Do not make her feel bad should she spill some fluids. Tuck a small towel between her neck and bib to prevent drips.

Tip: What Not to Do

Do not allow your baby to take the sippy cup to bed.

Always clean your baby's cup thoroughly (prevents the buildup of bacteria and mold).

Do not offer cow's milk in a sippy cup until your baby is one year of age.

Do not always refill your baby's cup with milk or juice. If she had her amount for the day, offer her water when she is thirsty or would like to drink from the cup.

Cow's Milk

General

Cow's milk has a higher amount of proteins and minerals than formula or breast milk (which may lead to stress on the baby's kidneys). It is low in vitamin C and iron, which are integral in the infant diet. Cow's milk should not be used to replace breast milk or formula during the first year of life, but it may be introduced as an ingredient of solid foods in the rest of the baby's diet (e.g., yogurt, cheese, if no evidence of allergies has been previously noted).

It is not recommended to start cow's milk until *after* one year of age. Babies who are less than one year old and consume cow's milk are at a higher risk of iron-deficiency anemia (which may lead to learning and psychomotor developmental delays) and allergic reactions. If cow's milk is consumed, especially in the early months of life, tiny amounts of bleeding may occur in the digestive tract. Over a long period of time, this causes iron loss, which may lead to anemia. As such, parents are advised not to rush using cow's milk, even during the second year of life.

Weaning to Cow's Milk After 12 Months

Types of Milk to Use & Fat Concerns

- Some experts claim that low fat diets need to be encouraged for children above two years of age, to maximize the likelihood of future dietary habits and reduce the risk of obesity and heart disease. Others are concerned that this approach, particularly in toddlers, may provide insufficient energy for normal growth and development. Overall, reduced fat and skim milk should not be used for children under two years of age, because milk is a key fat and energy source for this age group. Reduced fat variety can be encouraged for preschool children, aged three to four years. However, each child's case needs to be assessed within the context of growth, eating patterns, and family history.

- The following are daily fat requirements for children: 30-40% energy from fat for one to three year olds; 25-35% energy from fat for four to eight year olds; and 20-25% energy from fat for the age of nine and up.

- Weaning is the process of replacing breast milk or formula in your baby's diet with other foods.

- When you wean from the bottle or the breast to cow's milk at the age of one year, use whole cow's milk rather than skim milk, non-fats, or low fats. Your child needs whole cow's milk due to its higher fat content, which is important in maintaining good weight, proper growth, and brain development.

- Vitamins A and D are also better absorbed from whole cow's milk.

- Also, never feed unpasteurized milk to your baby as bacteria in this milk may seriously affect your baby.

Intake Amount

- Limit your baby's milk intake to 16 oz/ 500 ml per day.

- It is better to serve it in a cup at set times, such as at mealtimes.

- Use a gradual approach when transitioning from breast milk or formula to cow's milk. Begin by mixing a small amount of cow's milk into your baby's cup of formula or breast milk. Gradually decrease the amount of formula or breast milk and increase the amount of cow's milk.

- Excessive amounts of milk will lead to increased calories and a decreased appetite for other foods, since too much milk can be too filling.

Cow's Milk Refusal

Try the following tips if your baby refuses cow's milk:
- Offer milk in a small, colorful cup and provide a straw with that cup.

- Try offering soy milk.

- Replace milk with yogurt, milk soups, or cheese.

- Add milk powder to mashed potatoes, hot cereal, minced meat, pureed legumes, and blended fruit.

- If powdered milk and liquid are not accepted, add vitamin D supplements and/or other sources of calcium such as cottage cheese, tofu, cooked broccoli, rhubarb, and cream of wheat (see *Dairy Products for Infants & Toddlers*).

- Mix yogurt with ketchup, herbs, sun-dried tomatoes, and chopped garlic and serve it as a dip for raw vegetables (kids will enjoy anything as a dip).

- Make grilled cheese sandwiches in pitas, cut them into wedges and serve them with soup or salad for dinner.

- Make fruit smoothies in the blender and serve while your child is watching television.

- Food substitutions for cow's milk include: canned fish (salmon, herring) for calcium and vitamin D; broccoli, etc., for good sources of calcium (see *Dairy Products for Infants & Toddlers*). Alternatives also include rice milk, which now come in different flavors and are often calcium and vitamin-fortified, calcium-fortified orange juices and hypoallergenic formula. You can also try fresh organic soy milk and soy cheeses, and yogurts and cream cheeses.

Cow's Milk Allergy

General

- Some babies develop cow's milk allergy before the age of one when they are given formula or cereal with a cow's milk base formula. Most will manifest a true allergy upon their first exposure.

- Cow's milk is made up of protein, carbohydrates or sugar, fat, vitamins, minerals and water. It is the milk protein that causes cow's milk allergy.

- The estimated prevalence of cow's milk allergy varies from 2.2 to 5.9%.

- Allergenic proteins in cow's milk include casein and whey proteins. Allergic reactions occur when our bodies react to these proteins as if they were a foreign substance.

- Recommended starter infant formula's is based on cow's milk and is the most frequently administered protein in the infant diet. As such, it is not surprising that cow's milk allergy is the most prevalent allergy in formula-fed and breastfed (if mother consumes enough dairy products) infants.

- Most milk sensitive children outgrow their allergy before the age of three and the remission rate is above 80% between the ages of three to six years.

Symptoms of Allergy

- Cow's milk allergy may result in a wide variety of symptoms. This fact frequently complicates its recognition, which leads to a misdiagnosis or confusion with other diseases.

- Symptoms of cow's milk allergy can be due to an IgE mediated reactions or non-IgE mediated reactions. IgE is the immunoglobulin of the type E that may be produced by a sensitive infant/child as a response to milk exposure. As such, it may produce certain symptoms.
- This is different than lactose intolerance (which is due to an enzyme deficiency preventing proper digestion and is not an immune response).

IgE Mediated Symptoms (milk protein allergy):
- Usually occurs within minutes or two to four hours after milk ingestion.
- Can include skin reactions such as hives, swelling, vomiting, abdominal pain, diarrhea, and occasional respiratory symptoms (e.g., wheezing).
- Hives and redness may spread to the face and the rest of the body.
- May include anaphylaxis, which occurs immediately after cow's milk ingestion, in which breathing may be impossible due to swelling of the face, mouth, and tongue, and wheezing and hypotension. Seek immediate medical help, as this can be fatal.
- Worsening of eczema may sometimes be the sole presenting sign of cow's milk IgE mediated allergy.

Non-IgE Mediated Symptoms (milk protein intolerance):
- This reaction is less understood.
- Symptoms are often delayed and can develop hours or days after ingestion. Some of these children have higher incidence of chronic skin rashes and respiratory symptoms.
- Common symptoms are those of the digestive system, which include vomiting, chronic diarrhea, protein losing enteropathy (protein loss in the bowel) that can lead to swelling in the legs or other areas (edema) of the body, sudden pallor, and colitis.

Cow's Milk Allergy: Label Watch
- It is very important to know for certain if your baby has a cow's milk allergy because if she does, you must ensure that all milk and milk products are removed from her diet.
- The following labels and names are **not** a complete list of what to avoid or look for, however, they are some suggestions to help you:

❖ The milk protein may be a hidden ingredient in various foods and these include: butter, cream, all cheeses, yogurt, ice cream, puddings, breads, pancakes, waffles, mashed potatoes, croutons, many baking mixes, cereals, granolas, some lunch meats, many frostings, etc. Avoid foods that contain curds, custard, half & half, hydrolysates of casein, whey lactoglobulin, etc.

❖ Names to watch out for when reading labels which contain milk proteins are margarine, sweet or sour cream, malted milk, lactose, non-fat or organic milk solids, curds, whey in all forms, lactalbumin, whipping cream, nougat, puddings, milk shakes, hot dogs (sour), some canned tuna, etc.

❖ Any foods, which contain the word "casein" in their label, should not be given to the milk sensitive baby. Variations of this word include caseinate, ammonium caseinate, calcium caseinate, hydrolyzed caseinate, sodium caseinate solids, zinc caseinate, etc. Basically, anything with "casein" in it should be taken out of the infant diet.

❖ Ingredients which may indicate the presence of milk protein include: chocolate, Simplesse, caramel colors, brown sugar, high protein flour, luncheon meats, sausages, milk kosher food ("D, K, U, COR, MK" on the label all indicate the present of milk protein), etc.

Diagnosis & Treatment
• The diagnosis of IgE mediated cow's milk allergy is usually made with a positive prick skin test or by measuring the blood concentration of specific IgE antibodies. The diagnosis of cow's milk induced enteropathy (non-IgE) is made by combining patient history together with clinical response to elimination and re-challenge, as there are no laboratory tests to confirm the diagnosis (see *Feeding & Food Allergy*). The following are some measures to treat allergy:

❖ Avoid and be aware of various labeling with hidden sources of milk proteins or lactose.

❖ Calcium supplements must be considered in an infant's dietary intake, if a milk allergy prevents sufficient calcium intake in the diet.

❖ Toddlers with milk allergy may react to toys and bedding which are contaminated with milk.

❖ In most cases, children are able to tolerate traces of milk protein in baked goods. Strict avoidance of traces of milk protein is usually unnecessary for cow's milk induced enteropathy (non-immunologic response) as the threshold of triggered reaction usually involves a higher amount of milk protein (but some will react to small amounts).

❖ Children who experience an anaphylactic reaction must strictly avoid milk protein. Further, an Epipen must be available at all times in case of an otherwise fatal exposure to milk.

❖ In infants with documented cow's milk formula allergy, your doctor will suggest a replacement formula, which may be hypoallergenic extensively hydrolyzed (rather than partially hydrolyzed) formula or formula of extensively hydrolyzed protein or amino acid mixtures (CPS, AAP and European recommendations).

❖ If the mother is breastfeeding, partial or complete elimination of dairy products may be required depending on the baby's symptoms, so discuss this with your doctor (see *Infant Formula: Which to Use & How to Choose*).

Issues with Cow's Milk
Cow's Milk Allergy & Lactose Intolerance

• Milk, infant formula, breast milk, and dairy products all contain a type of sugar called lactose. Those who are lactose intolerant are unable to properly digest this type of sugar in their bodies.

• Avoiding both cow's milk and lactose in a child's diet is very challenging.

• Parents of children with cow's milk allergy do not have to avoid lactose-containing foods as long as they have no dietary intolerance to lactose.

• Lactose intolerance is a deficiency of a digestive enzyme (lactase), which results in milk sugar lactose remaining undigested and then being fermented by the gut to produce lactic acid. This causes gas, bloating, flatulence, abdominal pain, diarrhea, and nausea. These symptoms usually occur several hours after ingestion of lactose.

• It is treated by substituting lactose-reduced milk or by ingesting lactose enzyme (Lactaid) with milk products.

• Depending on the degree of lactose intolerance, some lactose intolerant children may tolerate yogurt, goat milk, and natural, aged cheeses (cheddar, Swiss). Avoid fresh, unripe cheese (mozzarella, cream and cottage cheese, ricotta).

SECTION 4: STARTING SOLID FOODS

Cow's Milk Allergy & Colic

- Infant colic is a common condition among infants and usually resolves by the age of three to four months. The cause is not known.

- Colic is usually recognized by bouts of inconsolable crying, often for hours at a time, for no specific reason.

- In trials of cow's milk based formula, avoidance may be necessary.

- Your doctor may suggest using other formulas (e.g., hypoallergenic, extensively hydrolyzed formula, etc.) for a short period of time to rule out cow's milk as a possible cause of colic.

- Re-introduction of cow's milk at a later time is often possible.

Cow's Milk Allergy & Eczema

- Eczema is a condition affecting the skin. There are different types of eczema, depending on the root causes of the problem. However, they all have one thing in common: they result in dry, itchy, red, and cracked skin, which may become sore and bleed because of scratching.

- Up to 80% of individuals with eczema end up with other allergic diseases, either allergic rhinitis or asthma.

- At the present time, there is no evidence that eczema is caused by an allergy. In a small number of patients, certain foods (such as milk protein, eggs, chocolate, etc.) seem to aggravate eczema and avoiding the food seems to improve the condition.

- If eczema is severe, a trial of cow's milk avoidance may be necessary to see if it helps improve the symptoms

- To determine a definite relationship between eczema and cow's milk, re-introduce milk on several occasions and document the reactions. This is important to do, as eczema episodes come and go at various times and is not necessarily related to foods since there may be other things that may predispose for it (heat, scratching, etc.).

Tip: Treating Eczema

Bathe baby daily and keep soaking time limited to10minutes.

Bathe your child with warm, not hot, water. Use small amounts of mild soap.

Add about 1/2-1 cups/125-250 ml of gentle bath oil to the water during the middle of the bath.

Continued

Avoid excessive scrubbing. Keep all fingernails short and clean.

Wash off residue of irritating foods and clean baby's face after eating tomatoes, oranges, and strawberries.

Be sure to use a moisturizer immediately after the bath. Make sure the moisturizer does not contain alcohol, as this may dry the skin.

Place a humidifier in the home to moisten the air if your home is dry.

Dress your child in mostly cotton clothing, as this is least irritating to the skin.

Medications as prescribed by your doctor (e.g., antihistamines, anti-inflammatory, antibiotic, etc.).

Remember that there may be times when the eczema emerges for no apparent reason.

A Word About...

Goat Milk

- Like cow's milk, goat's milk is not recommended until at least the age of one year. It should not be used as a substitute for breast milk or formula.

- Goat's milk is high in sodium, chloride, and potassium, which may cause gastrointestinal bleeding, anemia, and poor growth in babies.

- Goat milk is deficient in folic acid and iron, which may lead to anemia (iron deficiency and megaloblastic type).

- Further, 95% of infants with cow's milk allergy are usually allergic to goat's milk as well.

- According to the Food and Nutrition Board Institute, goat's milk fails to meet the recommended daily intake for vitamins and minerals such as vitamin C, niacin, folic acid, vitamin B12, and copper.

Organic Milk

- Organic milk is a healthy type of milk, because babies have immature systems and need the very purest and safest of foods.

- Organic milk is nearly completely free from synthetic pesticides and chemical fertilizers.

- Certified organic milk means that no hormones or antibodies were fed to the cow and the milk was protected from pollutants during processing.

- Make sure that the milk is pasteurized, as unpasteurized milk is dangerous to your baby.

Soy Milk

- Soy milk contains phytoestrogens (an estrogen-like hormone) found in plants such as whole grains, potatoes, dried beans and apples.

- Soy milk is a good alternative for children over one year old who won't drink milk or who are raised as vegetarians. Also, it is good for those that are allergic to cow's milk but are able to tolerate soy milk.

- Make sure to buy a vitamin-fortified, whole-fat variety (enriched soy milk) to ensure that your child is getting the nutrients she needs.

- Ensure that your child's diet contains other sources of calcium-fortified foods, since soy milk contains phytates which may decrease the absorption of calcium and other minerals.

Tip: Soy formula & Milk Allergic Child

There is a one in four chance that the child who is allergic to cow's milk is sensitive to soy milk as well.

You may use hypoallergenic formulas as an alternative to soy or cow's milk.

Even better, and particularly for the child with severe milk allergy and soy intolerance, use extensive protein hydrolysate formulas such as Nutramigen or Neocate.

Case Description

Lauren is an 8-month-old girl who was breastfed until the age of five months. She has a history of eczema. She then began on cow's milk based formula, which resulted in swollen eyes and face, hives, and breathing difficulties the first time she was fed. Lauren was taken to a local hospital and treated for allergies. It was then recommended to start Lauren on a soy type formula. Around the age of nine months, she was introduced to egg yolks, upon which she developed breathing difficulties, swelling and hives after just a few minutes. Later, during an examination, Lauren looked well and no findings arose, other than eczema. She was sent to an allergy skin test that came positive for milk, eggs, and peanuts. Lauren was diagnosed with a milk allergy as well as allergies to nuts, peanuts, and eggs. An Epipen was prescribed to Lauren, in case of inadvertent exposure and a severe life threatening allergic reaction.

Conclusion:

- Lauren has multiple allergies.

- The original formula given was based on cow's milk to which Lauren developed allergies. Also, due to Lauren's severe allergic reactions to eggs, her parents were advised to take a test for the MMR vaccine.

- MMR vaccines contain traces of egg and therefore, she was tested prior to administration of the vaccine (recommendations regarding testing for MMR vaccines have since changed).

- Also, physical contact alone with cow's milk is enough to produce an allergic reaction since Lauren's older brother once accidentally poured milk on her face and she quickly reacted with swelling, hives, vomiting, and a rash.

- At the age of 3 1/2 years, Lauren was given a repeat skin test that confirmed her allergy to peanuts and nuts, but not to eggs and milk.

- At the age of six years, Lauren was able to tolerate eggs, but she maintained her allergy to tree nuts (almond, hazelnut, walnut, cashews, brazil nuts, etc.) and peanuts.

Cow's Milk & Constipation

- The frequency, consistency, and appearance of bowel movements will depend on the food your baby is eating.

- Constipation is a condition where stools become firmer and harder.

- Pediatric constipation, which is not usually thought of, is sometimes due to cow's milk.

- In most cases, both physicians and parents will think of diarrhea and vomiting as associated with cow's milk allergy.

- There is no difference between whole milk, low fat, or skim milk in respect to their ability in causing constipation.

Discuss with your doctor whether a trial to place your child on a cow's milk free diet is worthwhile and observe to see if easier bowel movements result.

Milk & Bone Health

- Suboptimal dietary calcium intake during childhood may predispose children to increased fracture risk due to inadequate bone mass.

- Long-term avoidance of milk has been associated with small stature and poor bone health. In fact, children who constantly avoid milk have almost a three times greater risk of fracture than those who drink milk.

Increased physical activity combined with a calcium-rich diet will help reduce the risk of fracture and build strong bones (Klakyarf, H.J., *Nutrition Today* 41:171-177, 2006).

Milk & Obesity

Your doctor may advise you to reduce the fat content in milk by switching from whole fat milk (3.25% MF) to reduced-fat milk (1-2% MF), after your child's second birthday.

Cooking Milk Free

- Substitute another liquid for milk.
- When a recipe calls for milk, try soy milk as a substitute.
- Use unflavored, unsweetened, vitamin enriched, full fat soy milk for best results and for maximum nutrition.
- To substitute for creams, use an unflavored soy milk creamer.
- If your baby has a soy allergy, try water, chicken stock, beef stock, or fruit juices.

For the lactose intolerant, you may use lactaid milk or lactaid dietary supplements.

Parent Concerns

My toddler refuses to drink milk. How can I replace her calcium needs?
- Milk provides calcium, protein and calories, however children are able to receive these nutrients from other sources, including dairy products such as yogurt, cheddar cheese, cottage cheese, calcium-fortified juice, cereals, leafy green vegetables (green pepper, broccoli), etc. (see *Dairy Products for Infants & Toddlers* for more details).

What do I do if my child is taking excessive amounts of milk per day?
- Excessive amounts of milk will interfere with your child's appetite for other foods and increase the risk of iron deficiency anemia.
- It is not recommended that your child use more than 16 oz/500 ml of milk per day.

- Try to decrease the amount of milk your child takes by gradually diluting the milk with water or serving it in a cup. Gradually offer more water instead, with occasional fruit juices.

- Do not offer milk in the bottle frequently and do not allow your child to walk around or sleep with a bottle full of milk.

Is soy milk better than cow's milk?

- Cow's milk is usually better than soy milk, unless it is enriched because soy milk has 30% less proteins than cow's milk and is short on vitamins A, B12, folate, zinc, and calcium. Soy milk also has less fat than cow's milk. However, enriched soy milk may be better as it is fortified with calcium and vitamin B12. It produces less allergenic risk than cow's milk.

- Soy milk is usually used in children who refuse cow's milk, those who are allergic to cow's milk but can tolerate soy, or those who are vegetarians.

- Soy milk contains phytoestrogens which raises concerns about hormonal imbalance effects (see *Infant Formula: Which to Use & How to Choose*).

My child does not like milk. Is it appropriate to give toddler formula?

- Yes, it is appropriate to serve toddler formula since it has all the vitamins and minerals necessary and does not have the negative effects of cow's milk (risk of anemia, decreased appetite, etc.). However, do not exceed 16 oz/500 ml per day, as your child may be too full on formula to eat a healthy well-balanced diet.

My child prefers drinking chocolate milk to regular milk. Is this okay?

- Chocolate milk is okay for your child to drink, however, it should be used in moderation, as it is sweet and high in calories. You do not want your child to develop a heavy taste preference for sweetened foods, beverages, or flavors.

Are there are any reasons when cow's milk should be used before the age of one year?

- There are no reasons why cow's milk should be used before the age of one year, as the associated health risks are too high.

- Some parents consider giving their child cow's milk before the age of one because it is cheaper than formula or because the child prefers the taste of cow's milk to formula or the child does not like formula anymore (before the age of one year).

- Serving your child cow's milk will not save you much money, since your child will take other solid foods to her diet and fewer feedings are required as she gets older and closer to one year of age.

- If your child refuses formula except for cow's milk, speak to your doctor before you risk serving cow's milk too early in your baby's life.

- Some experts recommend that cow's milk not be introduced until 18 months of age because of the various risks involved (the later cow's milk is introduced, the better; see *Iron Deficiency*).

Are there any nutritional differences between organic and regular milk?

- There are no nutritional differences between organic and regular whole milk. Organic milk simply suggests that the cow was not fed on grass/grains that contained any fertilizers, pesticides or herbicides. Typically, the cow is not given large-scale, preventative anti-biotics or growth hormones.

If and when will my baby outgrow her milk allergy?

- Most babies outgrow milk allergies between 2-8 years of age (typically around age 4). During the period of time when your baby has milk allergies, ensure that she is consuming enough calcium and a well-balanced diet.

I am breastfeeding my baby and have a family history of milk allergy. Will this affect my baby?

- If you have family history of milk allergy, it is better to minimize consumption of cow's milk if you are breastfeeding your baby.

- Eliminate cow's milk or foods containing cow's milk in your own diet if your baby develops symptoms such as recurrent diarrhea, spitting up, blood and mucus in the stool, gas and other symptoms of allergy such as hives, swelling, etc. Elimination of milk from the diet depends on the severity of symptoms in your baby, so discuss this with your doctor first.

- Ensure that your calcium intake is appropriate in your diet if you have to stop taking milk or milk products for your baby's sake.

I do not see blood in my baby's stool. Does this mean that my baby does not have a milk allergy?

- No, this does not mean that your baby does not have a milk allergy as you may not be able to see the blood in the stool.

- If the blood is "hidden" in your baby's stool, it is known as occult and is sometimes only found through lab tests.

- Skin allergy tests may be done to confirm a diagnosis of cow's milk allergy, but not for enteropathy (see *Feeding & Food Allergy*) along with other symptoms of a possible milk allergy or enteropathy.

Are cold symptoms a manifestation of cow's milk allergy?

- Cow's milk allergy may appear as "hay fever" at any age, which includes symptoms such as stuffiness/nose obstruction, cough, and a runny nose that seems to persist for a long period of time. When cow's milk is eliminated from the diet, all of these symptoms may disappear or resolve themselves. However, it is important to remember that a prolonged runny nose may be a manifestation of other medical causes (e.g., common colds, etc.) and it is not easy to suspect allergy on the basis of this one symptom alone. Do not stop giving milk during your child's cold (or as asthma flares up), as there are no repeated studies that confirm that milk worsens the cold or asthma attacks. However, it is possible that some people who drink milk may have increased mucus production and any fatty foods may produce a sensation of thicker secretion in the back of the throat.

Tip: Reflux & Milk Allergy

With reflux, you must wait a longer period of time than colic (e.g., 2-3 weeks) to see improvements of any symptoms caused by a milk allergy (if this is the cause). Spitting up alone is unlikely to be a result of a milk allergy.

Which milks are not recommended for my child?

- Do not use 2 or 1% skim milk before the age of 2 (babies need full fat contents until they are older).

- Do not give unpasteurized cow or goat's milk since there is a risk of harmful bacteria.

- Soy milk may not contain enough calcium, protein, and fats, so do not serve to a child less than two years of age, unless it is enriched soy milk.

- Canned or condensed milk should not be given in the first year of life.

My child enjoys formula instead of cow's milk. Can I still feed her formula after the age of one year?

- Yes, you may continue to feed your child formula even up to the age of two years or more, if your child does not like cow's milk. It is probably better to continue with formula since it supplies many nutrients important for the toddler during their picky eater timeframe. Also, formula supplies iron and there are less risks of iron deficiency and its consequences.

Eggs

General

Eggs are an important source of proteins (a large egg provides 6 g of proteins) and are mostly used for tissue growth (have an increased biological value). Eggs contain amino acids necessary for brain development, along with vitamins B12, folic acid, and zinc. Omega 3 & 6 are fatty acids that are important for good eye and brain development. Some chickens are fed these added nutrients and then produce eggs which contain these fatty acids (they will be labeled on the carton). Choline, which is also present in eggs, is important for nerve transmission and memory. Moreover, eggs have a high satiety effect, meaning that your child will feel full after consuming eggs.

Eggs may be considered a "natural" multivitamin (although they are high in cholesterol). An egg contains about 75 calories, 4.5 g of total fat, and 13 vitamins and minerals, although they are not a good source of iron. Due to their high protein content, eggs are included in the meat, fish, poultry, nuts, and bean group of the food pyramid.

It is suggested to consume 3 eggs per week, after the age of one year, as part of a healthy diet. It is recommended to start out with egg yolk, rather than egg white, at about the age of nine months. Egg yolk contains a higher proportion of the egg's vitamins and is less allergenic than the egg whites. If there is history of egg allergies in your family, it is safer to introduce eggs between eighteen to twenty-four months of age.

Author's Comment:

Although it is suggested introducing egg yolks at nine months of age and egg whites at one year of age, I believe there is no significant difference between these two ages. The baby at risk of developing an allergy to egg yolk or egg whites can develop it at nine months or at one year of age (even if she is a bit older and stronger).

It is impossible to completely separate the yolk from the egg white without some traces of egg whites, which may still lead to allergic reactions. To put it simply, one should start a whole egg around ten to twelve months of age. Moreover, I recommend providing the missing proteins from eggs through meat, which can be introduced from six to nine months of age (and also provides additional iron). In fact, meat allergies are rare compared to egg allergies.

Availability, Safety & Preparation

Availability

The following table outlines the types of eggs available in the market today.

Types of Eggs	Information
Standard Eggs	Most commonly used. Available in white and brown shells. Color of the egg is determined by the breed of the chicken. No nutritional difference between white or brown shelled eggs.
Organic Eggs	Ingredients in the chicken's diet are grown without any pesticides, fungicides, herbicides, or commercial fertilizers. More expensive than regular eggs. There is no nutritional difference between organic and inorganic eggs.
Quality & Appearance	Grade AA are eggs that have thick, firm whites. Grade A eggs are like the AA, however whites are only somewhat firm. The appearance of an egg in terms of its color varies due to many factors, so when buying or cooking eggs, ensure that they are safe by understanding what each color means: cloudy white (very fresh), clear egg whites (aging), pink eggs (spoiled and should not be used or eaten) and blood spots (ruptured blood vessels in the yolk of an egg and not necessarily unsafe to eat). Yolk color varies in yellow shades depending on the hen's diet. For example, if the hen was fed yellow-orange plants, the yolk will be a dark yellow.

Egg Safety

- Before buying eggs at the store, make sure to check the eggs for dirt, cracks, etc. Buy clean eggs with un-cracked shells from a refrigerated display case.

- Store the eggs in the refrigerator in their original carton to protect them from odors and damage. Eggs should always be kept in the coldest section of the refrigerator (near the back or middle to lower inside shelf of the refrigerator; never on the refrigerator door) at 40 F/4 C or slightly below.

- Be sure to refrigerate eggs away from any meat or product that may drip juices onto the eggs.

- Hard-boiled eggs, leftover cooked eggs, or egg mixtures should be refrigerated immediately after cooking and may be stored in the refrigerator for up to one week in a tightly covered container.

- Eggs should only stay at room temperature for no longer than two hours. After this time, they must be discarded.

- Never cook eggs in their shells in the microwave, as they will explode.

- Do not serve raw, uncooked, or out-of-date eggs to your child and it is important to remove all of the eggshells, especially any small pieces that may be inhaled into the baby's respiratory system.

Egg Preparation

- Eggs may be offered in any one of the following forms: hard-boiled, soft-boiled, sunny side-up, scrambled, and omelet.

- Handle eggs safely by washing your hands, utensils, and all equipment before and after contact with eggs (always wash your hands after handling raw eggs).

- When feeding eggs to your child for the first time, begin with a small amount of egg yolk, as it is thought to be less allergenic than egg whites.

- It is usually recommended to start with a hard-boiled egg, because it is more hygienic and easier for the baby to digest.

- Begin with a mashed, hard-boiled egg yolk and do the best you can to separate the white part of the egg from the yellow (the egg yolk and white area separate best when the egg is cooled). One method of separating the yellow and white part of the hard-boiled egg is to take out the white area with your hands and cut off the outside yellow layer. Serve the middle of the yellow part of the egg (ensures that no white part is consumed along with the yellow area of the egg).

- It is not advised to fry the eggs, particularly the egg yolk, as it is rich in cholesterol and fat and may injure blood vessels in the body. However, if you decide to fry the eggs, then use a low burner with a protective core. Also, use canola oil or a bit of butter or soft margarine (possibly even with water).

- You may mix in one teaspoon of wheat germ or milk when scrambling eggs to increase their nutritional content.

- Eggs should be cooked thoroughly until the yolk is firm and scrambled eggs should not be runny.

- After your child accepts this without any signs of allergy, you may proceed to offer a combination of egg yolk and egg whites at about 1 year of age.

- If you give scrambled or full eggs at first, you will be mixing the yolk and egg white.

- It is recommended that your baby is fed an egg every one to two days (limit cholesterol intake to 300 mg per day), especially if she does not eat any type of meat. Remember that eggs are also an ingredient in other foods (e.g., cakes, etc.).

Egg Cooking Safety & Salmonella

- When cooking eggs for young children, make sure the eggs are cooked thoroughly. Eggs which are lightly cooked or served raw may contain salmonella (bacteria) or other forms of bacteria that may make your child sick.

- Salmonella is destroyed by heat, so when eggs are handled, refrigerated, and cooked properly there should be less risk of bacterial contamination.

- If eggs are used in other food recipes, be sure to dilute the eggs with liquid ingredients (e.g., milk) and cook the egg mixture to 160 F/71 C. High cooking temperatures destroy bacteria that may be present.

- Some recipes ask for whipped, raw egg whites, which may contain salmonella. These are okay to use as long as they will be baked or cooked at a high temperature to kill the bacteria present.

- Raw egg whites may be replaced with pasteurized egg white products. However, all egg products must be pasteurized, meaning that they are quickly heated at a required temperature for a certain period of time. This destroys possible bacteria present in eggs, such as salmonella.

> **Fun Recipe: Cheese Omelet (Older than 1 Year of Age)**
>
> Ingredients: 3 eggs, 3 tbsp of water, 2 tbsp of grated cheese (Swiss, Cheddar, Havarti), and 2 tbsp of butter
>
> Directions:
>
> Beat eggs lightly with added water.
>
> Melt the butter in a pan.
>
> Add the eggs to the pan and lightly stir together.
>
> Add the cheese to the eggs and cook for 1-2 minutes.
>
> Switch sides of the omelet to cook the other side well for another 1-2 minutes.
>
> Once the omelet has been thoroughly cooked, place it onto a dish and serve.

Egg Refusal

- Many children experience phases of food refusal. It is a normal part of growing up and asserting independence, however there are things you can do to help your child accept a new food (egg) such as the following:

  ❖ Eat eggs in front of your child, as she is more likely to try it when she sees others enjoying it.

  ❖ Do not force your child to eat eggs when she does not want to. Simply offer her another food for the time being and re-try in a few days.

  ❖ Keep offering eggs in various forms (e.g., hidden in other foods or added to cooked foods, etc.) on several occasions. It can take about 5-15 tries before a child will become familiar with and accept a new food.

  ❖ Offer small portions of eggs when she is hungriest, as she may be more likely to accept it.

  ❖ Praise and encourage your child when she shows interest in foods.

- There is also the option of replacing eggs with other protein meals such as cheese, yogurt, meat, fish, legumes, etc.

- Also, the following substitutes can be used when preparing homemade foods requiring the ingredients of eggs:

  ❖ 1/2 mashed banana for muffins and cookies.

  ❖ Tomato paste or mashed potatoes to bind ingredients when necessary.

  ❖ 1 oz/30 g of mashed tofu instead of an egg.

  ❖ In baking products, use 1 tablespoon of soy flour or cornstarch, etc.

Egg Allergy

General

- Egg allergy refers to an overreaction of the body's immune system to proteins found in eggs, especially in egg whites. Egg allergies are usually less severe than peanut allergy.

- Symptoms of egg allergy may occur right after the child consumes eggs or a couple of hours later. These symptoms may include the following: rash, hives, itchiness, swelling in the face and/or lips, shortness of breath, wheezing, vomiting and nausea, diarrhea, etc.

- Egg allergy is diagnosed after exposure to eggs (or foods containing eggs) leading to a rash or any of the above symptoms.

- Typically, egg allergy is confirmed through skin allergy tests. A weak egg extract is placed on the child's forearm and if the area reddens or swells, it is considered to be a positive allergic reaction to eggs.

- Most children outgrow allergy to eggs between the ages of two to eight years.

Safety for the Egg Allergic Child

- If your child has an egg allergy, do not give eggs until the allergy disappears (known by a negative allergy test). A nutritionally balanced diet should include other foods such as meat and alternatives (e.g., chicken, fish, etc.).

- Be careful of "hidden" eggs in foods such as: cakes, cookies, mayonnaise, ready-made schnitzel, ice cream containing egg yolk, pasta, Caesar salad, custard, pies, pancakes, waffles, salted foods, soup, soft drinks, baby food, battered foods, buns and breads, French toast, puddings, salad dressings, quiche, burgers, mayonnaise, marshmallows, muffins, pretzels, waffles, doughnuts, anything fried, meringue, cookies, chicken nuggets, some vaccines (e.g., MMR), etc.

- Make sure you read the labels of food or baking products carefully. Some indicators of foods, which contain egg products, include the following: egg whites, powdered egg, albumin, globulin, livetin, lysozyme, anything that begins with "ovo" (ovoglobulin, ovotransferrin, ovovitella, etc.), ovalbumin, simplesse, vitally, silica albuminate, etc.

- For extra safety for the egg allergic child, follow these tips:
  - ❖ Tell the day care or school staff that your child is allergic to eggs and explain the use of the Epipen (when it should be used and how to administer it).
  - ❖ Be sure to let everyone around you (family and friends) know that your child is allergic to eggs.
  - ❖ Teach your child not to share foods with anyone.
  - ❖ When eating outside of the home, be careful and watch what your child eats.
  - ❖ Re-introduce eggs only after allergy tests were done to confirm that the allergy has resolves (usually, children outgrow egg allergy by the age of five years).

- Many children with egg allergies are able to tolerate baked goods without any problems. Egg products that are cooked for long periods of time at high temperatures may be more easily accepted than less cooked egg products.

- Also, children with mild reactions are likely to develop a tolerance earlier than children who have severe reactions.

Tip: Likelihood of Coronary Artery Disease

Researchers find no correlation between coronary artery disease (CAD) and the consumption of eggs by children. Egg intake does not seem to increase the likelihood of your child getting CAD.

Vaccines & Eggs

General

- Some vaccines are made with eggs or egg compounds.

- These vaccines may not be given if your child has egg allergies. Your doctor will decide what vaccines your child can take or should not take.

- Adverse reactions occur more often with vaccines such as yellow fever and influenza, which are grown in embryonated eggs. For example, the MMR (measles-mumps-rubella) vaccine, which is the most widely used in Canada, is grown in chicken embryo cell cultures. Even with extensive purification, it may contain traces of avian proteins resembling proteins present in hen's eggs.

- Recent studies show that anaphylaxis may occur after the administration of the measles vaccine to persons with hypersensitivity to eggs, but also in those with no history of egg allergy. The cause of allergy is suspected to be from gelatin or neomycin, which are included in the measles vaccine.

- Skin testing for egg allergy cannot predict who will react and who will not react to vaccines.

Egg Allergy & Vaccines

- *MMR Vaccine:* For persons with a mild egg allergy and no previous anaphylactic reaction to hen's eggs (urticaria, swelling of the mouth and throat, difficulties breathing, hypotension), the MMR vaccine may be given with professional observation of your child for a half-hour.

- In patients with severe egg allergy (anaphylactic reaction), it is recommended that, if the vaccine is given, it should be in a place where anaphylaxis can be taken care of and where the person may be observed for at least 30 minutes after the immunization (e.g., hospital).

- *Flu vaccine* should not be given unless it is absolutely necessary, regardless of whether or not your child has mild or severe allergy to eggs. It should not be given to children with a known anaphylactic or hypersensitivity reaction to eggs resulting in hives, swelling of the mouth and throat, difficulty breathing, and shock.

- *Flu vaccines* can be done if a skin test is done to the flu vaccine prior to its administration and is negative. A risk benefit analysis should be done in every patient (e.g., patients with chronic diseases such as asthma, cardiac, etc.) in which the vaccine is particularly recommended.

- Ultimately, your doctor will decide when your child should be given a particular vaccine and/or the need to consult an allergy specialist.

Case Description

Leora was a 16-month-old baby who developed a rash around her mouth and became cranky and aggressive when she consumed eggs or egg products. Her mother was unsure as to whether or not Leora had had previous episodes of mild rashes around her mouth, especially since she showed no other symptoms such as swelling in the face or difficulty breathing.

There was no family history of any type of food allergy or symptoms of allergy related to the nose or eye. However, Leora had mild skin eczema.

Leora's examination was normal. She was sent to an allergy doctor for confirmation of egg allergy. Allergy skin testing done by a specialist confirmed the diagnosis of a milk allergy, also a slightly positive test for egg allergy. Leora also had skin tests done for MMR vaccines to see if these could be given to her and was found to be negative. Thus, Leora had the MMR vaccine with no adverse effects.

Leora seemed to have a mild egg allergy. It was suggested to hold off on egg products until a skin allergy test was re-done to see if she has outgrown the allergy. Two years later, she tested negative for the allergy and was able to include eggs in her diet.

Tip: Eczema and Egg Allergy

Patients with eczema have a higher incidence rate of egg or other food allergies.

Parent Concerns

If I am allergic, will my child be?

- If the parent has no allergy, the child has a 15% risk of developing an allergy.
- If the parent has an allergy, the child's risk of developing an allergy increases to 20-40%.
- Lastly, if both parents have allergy, the child has a 40-60% risk of developing an allergy.

If and when are egg allergies outgrown?

- Allergic reactions to eggs are usually outgrown by the age of five (range two to eight years), however, a few children may retain the allergy into adulthood.

My child is allergic to egg whites. Can she still eat egg yolk?

- Egg white cause the allergic reaction, since it contains most of the allergenic proteins in the egg.
- It does not make a difference which part your child is allergic to, since it is difficult to separate the white from the egg yolk. Even the smallest amount of egg yolk may trigger a severe allergic reaction in your child.

If my child is allergic to eggs, what can I replace this ingredient with when baking?

Eggs are an important ingredient in baking and cannot be used when your child is allergic to eggs. For each egg substitute, use one of the following to replace it:

1 teaspoon of baking powder, 1 1/2 tablespoons of oil or water

1 tablespoon of vinegar, water, or baking powder

1 teaspoon of yeast dissolved in 1/4 cup of warm water

1 packet of unflavored gelatin, 2 tablespoons of warm water

1/2 large mashed banana

Can I use raw eggs in recipes without eating them raw?

- Raw eggs always carry the risk of salmonella infection and as such, are not recommended for use. However, when raw eggs are used in a recipe that will be baked or cooked at a high temperature, the heat will destroy any contaminating bacteria.

If my child is allergic to eggs, can she eat chicken?

- Typically, chicken may be tolerated well when your child is allergic to eggs. However, this should be discussed with your doctor or allergy specialist, since some proteins contained in eggs and chickens are similar and may cause an allergic reaction in your child.

What temperature is required to cook eggs?

- Cooking temperature should be high enough that it destroys possible bacteria in the eggs.
- For example, a pasteurized whole plain egg without any added ingredients may be cooked at a temperature of 140 F/60 C for about 3 1/2 minutes.
- For immediate egg consumption or use, cook at a temperature of 145 F/62 C for about 15 seconds.
- When eggs are used in a recipe with other foods (e.g., milk, sugar, etc.), cook the egg mixture at a temperature of 160 F/71 C for a few seconds to destroy all possible bacteria.

My baby has been diagnosed with egg allergy and I am breastfeeding. Should I stay away from eating eggs in my diet?

- Yes, you should stop eating eggs in your diet when your baby has an egg allergy. You may resume eggs in your diet after you have stopped breastfeeding your baby or she has outgrown her allergy.

Tip: Cholesterol & Eggs

Fat, cholesterol, and about 44% of the proteins are found in egg yolk.

The white part of the egg has more than half of the proteins, vitamins, and minerals.

1 large egg contains about 213 mg of cholesterol.

Eggs contain the highest quality of food protein.

When considering cholesterol levels in your child, it is important to know how much cholesterol she is getting from other foods such as milk, cheese, yogurt, meat, etc.

The question of cholesterol in the young child is unclear and while saturated fat has never been placed with a limit, your child's intake should probably not exceed 300 mg/day.

Section 5:
Issues Related to
Feeding & Nutrition

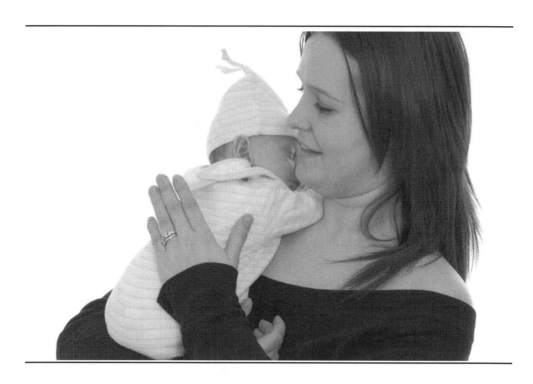

Burping

General

Burping gets rid of the air that babies sometimes swallow during a feeding or when crying. Every baby is different—some babies require burping with every couple of ounces they are fed, while others can go entirely without being burped. In some babies, infrequent burping may lead to spitting up, crankiness, gassiness, restlessness, and irritability. Even though there are babies who could benefit from burping, some babies simply cannot elicit a good burp (even with lots of help on your part).

When to Burp

General

- There is actually no reason to burp every baby. While burping is optional for some babies, it is not necessary for others.

- Young babies naturally fuss and get cranky when they swallow air. As such, babies are burped to take out excess air after a feeding. If the baby swallows air during a feeding, it may cause discomfort and burping can help relieve that discomfort (babies feel better after burping).

- Some babies stop feeding in the middle of a session or slow down the feeding process mainly because they need to burp; a well-burped baby may be able to eat more. However, if the baby does not burp, there is no reason not to resume the feeding.

- If your baby falls asleep and does not burp, there is no need to wake him up. Sometimes, your baby may awaken due to gas. Simply picking him up to burp him may put him back to sleep.

- If you spend about 10 minutes or more trying to burp your baby after each feeding and your baby is still unable to burp, then it is probably unnecessary to burp him.

- Your baby may be more likely to burp after a large feeding.

- When your baby only has a "snack feeding," it is not always necessary to burp him.

- In general, try to burp the baby frequently as he may not show any clear signs of discomfort. The pause and change of position alone will slow the gulping and reduce the amount of air the baby swallows.

- As your baby grows, you will not have to worry about burping him during or after every feeding. Many parents stop burping their babies between 4-6 months of age. After this age, many babies are able to burp easily on their own.

- The only benefit of burping is a decrease in discomfort and regurgitation (if there is any). Mothers should pay attention to their baby's "language" (signs the baby gives) and they will learn when their babies need to be burped.

The Breastfed Baby
- Breastfeeding babies take in less air than bottle-fed babies, because their mouths form an airtight seal around the nipple. Also, breastfed babies can control the flow of milk from the breast. They suck with a slower rhythm that allows them to better coordinate their breathing and swallowing techniques.

- Do not worry if your baby rarely burps, as long as he seems comfortable. Keep the breastfeeding session as calm and leisurely as possible.

- Some babies do swallow air when the breast is very full and the milk flow is fast, so try burping your baby when this happens.

- Burp your baby in the middle of a feeding when switching breasts and after a feeding (if your baby falls asleep at the breast, you do not need to disturb him with the burping routine).

The Bottle-Fed Baby
- If your baby is bottle-fed, try burping him after each 2-3 oz /60-90 ml or as necessary, according to his possible signs of readiness.

- If the baby has gas or is spitting up a lot, burp him more frequently.

- When the baby is formula-fed, burp him in the middle of the feeding since formulafed babies suck more air than breastfed babies, resulting in more gas.

Identifying Signs of Readiness to Burp

- The more conscious you are of your baby's feeding habits, the easier it is to identify when your baby is ready to burp. Here are a few signs that tell you that your baby is ready to be burped:
  - ❖ Squirming and grimacing when you lay your baby down.
  - ❖ Painful facial expressions.

❖ Pushy, fussy noises your baby makes while feeding.

❖ If your baby is content, then the need to burp has past (if he needed to burp at all).

How to Burp Your Baby

• Patience is required to burp your baby; there is no "right" way of burping your baby, as each baby is unique.

• Take your time trying various burping techniques and positions until you find the technique that works for you and your baby.

• Choose a position which is comfortable and convenient for you and your baby.

• You may even vary the positions from time to time for excitement and stimulation purposes for the baby.

• Remember to use a towel or bib on your shoulder or your baby's chin, since he may spit up.

• No matter what position you use, always remember to support your baby's head and keep it and the chest higher up than the rest of his body.

• There are various positions and technique you may use to burp your baby, including:

1) Over the Shoulder Burp

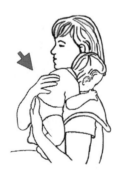

❖ This is the most common method used to burp a baby.

❖ Hold the baby in an upright position with his head on your shoulder.

❖ Make sure that your baby's upper belly is against your collarbone.

❖ Support his head and back with one hand.

❖ Gently pat the baby's back with the other hand.

2) Over the Lap Burp

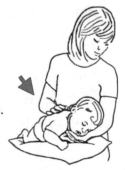

❖ Lay the baby on your lap with his back up.

❖ Support the head so that it is higher than the chest.

❖ Gently pat or rotate your hand on the baby's back.

❖ This may also be done by sitting the baby on your lap.

❖ Support the baby's chest and head with one hand.

❖ Pat the baby's back with the other hand.

3) Burp and Switch

❖ Some babies burp if they change sides.

❖ This may help avoid a large spit up of food.

4) Knee to Chest Burp

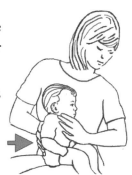

❖ Sometimes babies need help not only getting the air out of their stomachs, but also getting the air out their intestines.

❖ The knee-chest position requires flexing the baby's knee up against his chest.

❖ This helps the baby pass excess gas.

5) Baby on Left Arm

❖ Place the baby face down on your left arm (make sure he has space to breathe).

❖ Place your hand on his stomach and pat him on the back until he burps.

Tip: Crying and Burping

When your baby is crying, he will not be comfortable enough to burp. You may try changing positions or techniques or even just walk around while you are burping him. Some parents find that bouncing the baby a little while walking seems to help.

Helping Your Baby Swallow Less Air

- Position the bottle so that no air gets into the nipple during a feeding.

- When feeding the baby, position yourself in an upright position and your baby in a semi-upright position, so that he swallows less air.

- Try out different bottle and nipple shapes, which may help your baby swallow less air (different types of nipples may reduce or increase air swallowing). For example, babies with cleft palates swallow a lot of air during feedings. In these cases, use the Haberman, Nuk, or other nipples that decrease air swallowing.

Parent Concerns

My baby spits up when he burps. Should this be a cause for concern?

- Regurgitation or "spitting" up is very common during the baby's first few months of life and about 40% of normal, healthy babies spit up, usually right after a feeding (when trying to burp).

- The elastic-like muscle at the entry to the stomach that closes to prevent liquids from being pushed back up is not fully developed until the ages of 6-12 months. As a result, the valve is easily pushed open by food, liquid, or air in the stomach, which results in regurgitation (spit up).

- To avoid regurgitation, do not move your baby too much or too vigorously after feeding.

- Occasional regurgitation does not have any influence on the baby's nutrition.

- However, if the baby is regurgitating a lot and not gaining any weight, discuss with your doctor.

- Frequent regurgitation or projectile vomiting could signal a problem and you must speak to your doctor.

Do I need to burp my baby at night?

- Burping is usually less necessary during nighttime feedings, because babies are more relaxed at this time and swallow less air.

- If your baby needs to burp at night, you can simply try to place him over your hip as you lie on your side. Burp him and then switch sides.

- The knee-chest position (described earlier) may be used at night.

How do I know when my baby needs to burp?

- You will know your baby's burping habits and cues with time.

- Some of your baby's cues may include the following: irritability, fidgety behavior, slowing or stopping the feeding session, discomfort or uneasiness, pulling off the breast or bottle, etc.

- Some babies may be able to burp easily using one of the positions mentioned previously. With time, you will be able to find the position that allows your baby to burp.

- To decrease air swallowing during a feeding, feed your baby before he starts to cry and if you are bottle-feeding, be sure to hold the bottle appropriately (45 degree angle).

- Remember, that babies do not need to burp with every feeding, however it is worth putting in the effort after a large feeding session.

- As the baby gets older and more efficient at feedings, burping will become less of an issue.

How can I put my baby to sleep when he is taking a long time and not burping?

If your baby does not burp for a while after a feeding and you need to put him to bed, place him on his side and place the baby's mattress one notch higher at the head of the crib or discuss with your doctor.

Tip: After Burping

Some well-burped infants will probably be able to eat more at each feeding and sleep for longer periods of time.

If you interrupt your baby's meal to burp him when he does not need it, you will have a crying, frustrated baby on your hands.

Hiccups & Feeding

General

Hiccups are frequent, sudden, and involuntary contractions of the diaphragm muscle (the large muscle that separates the chest from the abdominal cavity) and the muscles between the ribs. This results in sudden intake of air terminated abruptly by closure of the glottis (the upper part of the respiratory airway). It may be considered a primitive reflex. Symptoms of hiccups include a funny, silent, or loud noise that is sometimes accompanied by discomfort.

In babies, hiccups are benign in the sense that they are not indicators of a problem, nor do they cause problems of any kind. They are common in the first few months of a baby's life and lessen in frequency as the infant gets older. They occur particularly during or after a feeding and seem to be more distressing for the parents than for the baby. Some babies seem to have more hiccups than others.

Causes for Hiccups

- Many times, there is no clear or apparent reason for hiccups. However, over-distension of the stomach in infants could be an important triggering factor for hiccups as it seems to cause irritation and stimulation of the nerve in the diaphragm.
- Over-distension may result from air swallowing (this is more common in bottle-fed than breastfed babies), vigorous sucking, over-feeding, or rapid ingestion of fluids.
- Infrequently, hiccups are caused by medical problems such as pneumonia or drug reactions, etc.
- Everyday hiccups are usually a result of inhaling too much air, eating spicy foods, or drinking too quickly.

Tip: Infants & Toddlers with Hiccups

Infants and toddlers with hiccups can do well with a bottle of formula or nursing. The sucking and swallowing motion helps to interrupt the hiccups.

Who Hiccups?

- In the early months of life, it is normal for healthy babies to hiccup frequently. Babies often hiccup even before birth, particularly during the third trimester of pregnancy. It is sometimes noted on prenatal ultrasounds and is completely normal.

- Hiccups are more common in premature babies, probably because of the baby's immature central nervous system.

- Hiccups are also frequent among babies with gastroesophageal reflux (the return of food to the mouth) or "silent" reflux. Persistent hiccups or coughs may be signs of reflux.

- Babies hiccup more frequently than older children, probably due to the relative immaturity of their internal organs. Persistent hiccups or chronic hiccups in older children and adults have various causes and different treatment methods that are not in the scope of this discussion.

- Any child can get hiccups that last for no more than a few minutes.

Hiccups & Feeding

- Do not delay a feeding simply because your baby has the hiccups. A feeding may actually help the hiccups disappear.

- Hiccups do not interfere with the baby's eating habits; however, they may distress your baby if he is in the middle of a feeding.

- If your baby always gets the hiccups after a feeding, then the culprit could be overfeeding and/or excessive air swallowing. When overfeeding is the cause of hiccups, try to feed your baby either smaller portions more frequently, or on demand, rather than on schedule.

Duration of Hiccup Episodes

- Hiccups are usually brief episodes (seconds to minutes) that occur at a frequency of 4-60 per minute and remain somewhat constant in babies and toddlers.

- A hiccup bout involves recurrent hiccups that may last up to 48 hours.

- Persistent hiccups are defined as hiccups, which continue longer than 48 hours but less than 1 month.

- Finally, hiccups are considered intractable when they last more than two months.

- Some lengthy hiccup durations are more of a concern in older children and adults, requiring further assessment by a health professional.

Dealing with Hiccups

- When an infant/child has the hiccups, there really is not much a parent can do but simply wait patiently until they disappear. Consider hiccups as another newborn reflex.
- Babies certainly do grow out of hiccups. They get less frequent as the child grows older.
- Most episodes of hiccups are self-limiting, lasting seconds to minutes.
- There are ways to help your baby deal with hiccups and these can include the following:
  - ❖ Try to get your baby to burp or relax and, if the hiccups stay longer than 5-10 minutes, a few sips of water may help.
  - ❖ Try to feed your baby with a bottle or with the breast when he has the hiccups as this may help get rid of them. However, sometimes you may have to wait to resume a feeding until the hiccups are gone.
  - ❖ If your baby hiccups often, feed him before he is hungry and burp him during the feeding.
  - ❖ It is a well-known fact that frequently burping your child helps reduce the frequency of hiccups (see *Burping*).
  - ❖ Comforting or distracting your baby may sometimes help get rid of hiccups.
  - ❖ The American Academy of Pediatrics recommends that you mix 1/4 teaspoon of sugar in 4 oz/120 ml of water and let your baby have a few sips.
  - ❖ Gripe water may help in reducing and ridding your baby of hiccups (it contains safe, natural ingredients).
  - ❖ For infants, anise seeds are also said to help with hiccups. Use only regular anise seeds (avoid the plants). Pour a cup/250 ml of boiling water over a teaspoon full of anise seeds. Give your baby the anise infused water (1-2 teaspoons) once it has cooled.
  - ❖ Check the nipple on your bottle since the hole of the nipple can sometimes be the wrong size and may cause hiccups. A rapid flow, slow flow, or no dripping at all may cause air swallowing, which, in turn,

causes hiccups. When bottle-feeding, bend the bottle more and more as it empties, so that the nipple will be full of milk at all times (so there is less to no air).

❖ For more serious cases of hiccups in older children and adults, doctors usually treat them with tranquilizers and muscle relaxants or hypnosis. In severe cases, surgery to the phrenic nerves may be suggested.

Tip: Hiccups Purpose

Hiccups' original purpose was to dislodge food caught in the esophagus. We all get them and most of us hate them. Although annoying, regular hiccupping disappears before 1 year of age.

Oral Thrush in the Breast & Bottle-fed Baby

General

Yeast infections are common among nursing mothers and their babies. It most commonly occurs in babies under the age of 12 months. Infants and children can get yeast infections in the mouth (oral thrush) and on the skin (e.g., the diaper area in infants), while mothers can get thrush on the nipples, and/or vagina.

Thrush is caused by the overgrowth of the yeast Candida Albicans, single-celled fungal organisms that live naturally and harmlessly in the mouth, intestine, skin, and vagina. Conditions such as hormonal changes, broken skin, vaginal birth when the mother has vaginal yeast, etc., can lead to various yeast infections, including oral thrush.

Thrush is transferable between mother and child (vagina–breast). Some babies are simply more susceptible than others to the fungus. Bottle-fed babies actually have more thrush than breastfed babies.

Symptoms & Effects on Feeding

Thrush in the Baby's Mouth

- Oral thrush does not actually bother many babies. Fussiness, irritability, and poor feeding occur in infants only if the infection is painful, but this is rare.

- There are usually no symptoms in the baby to attract the mother's attention, except for small, milky-white patches or coating on the inside of the mouth, cheeks, or gums. These patches cannot be wiped away unless they are scraped off (which may cause bleeding). If these small patches are present, it usually spreads to a few different places in the mouth.

- The following table may help parents differentiate between milk and thrush:

	Milk	Thrush
Removal	Wipes away easily. Milk on the tongue comes and goes with feedings.	Does not come and go. Not removed easily. May bleed with removal.
How It Looks & Location	Thin white coating on the tongue.	Usually visible on the inside of cheeks, lips, gums, and tongue. Thick, white coating on the tongue (resembles cottage cheese).

Skin: Diaper Rash & Thrush

- Pustular or red spotty diaper rashes may appear, as an extension of the infection throughout the digestive system (from the mouth).

- These diaper rashes usually do not respond to preventive diaper rash creams.

- Some babies are diagnosed with oral thrush by the presence of a nappy rash alone (caused by the same fungus). Nappy rashes may be due to yeast infections in the mouth (oral thrush) that have travelled through the digestive system into the diaper area.

Thrush on the Mother's Breast

- Oral thrush can be passed on from baby to mother and, in most cases, mother to baby.

- Symptoms of oral thrush on the mother's breast include the following:

  ❖ Burning sensations in the nipple or breast during or after a nursing session (even in the absence of other symptoms or signs of infection).

  ❖ Sharp, shooting pains from the nipples to the chest wall or back.

  ❖ Nipples may appear pink, shiny, oozy, crusty, or flaky.

  ❖ Small, white blisters may occur on the nipple.

- There is a difference between pain from a poor latch and pain from a candidal nipple infection. In most cases, the pain (often described as "stabbing" pain) that is associated with a poor latch remains limited to the nipple and areola area. With candidal nipple infection, pain may radiate to the mother's back or shoulder area and, often, the breast. Also, pain associated with candidal infection often occurs after a period of pain-free nursing while pain from a poor latch develops soon after birth.

- It is sometimes possible that the mother has bacterial mastitis (breast infection) along with a yeast infection. Symptoms of bacterial mastitis include a high fever, red streaks on the breast, hot spots on the breast, and flu-like symptoms (see *Mastitis*).

- You may ask yourself the following questions to help you identify whether you have a yeast infection overgrowth on the breast (consult your doctor if you have any concerns):

  ❖ Do you have a cracked nipple that does not heal?

  ❖ Did you have a yeast skin rash under your breasts during pregnancy?

❖ Do you feel shooting ("stabbing") pains in your breast?

❖ Have you had a painful breastfeeding experience lately?

❖ Have you or your baby recently been on antibiotics (sometimes treatment increases the risk of yeast infections)?

❖ Do you have diabetes?

❖ Does your baby have thrush or yeast diaper rash (which may give some indication that the mother is also infected)?

Effects of Thrush on Feeding

- There can be breastfeeding difficulties if thrush is present in either the mother or both baby and mother, since the yeast can be passed back and forth between the mother's nipples and the baby's mouth.

- When nursing, infected babies may pull off the breast, nurse poorly, and refuse to latch on to the breast.

- When your baby suffers from oral thrush, he may experience pain which may affect his appetite and prevent him from feeding properly.

- If you or your baby has thrush for a long period of time, the baby may have slow weight gain because of feeding difficulties that is due to both of you.

Predisposing Factors of Yeast Infection for Mothers & Babies

General

- Usually, thrush occurs in the mouth of most babies for unknown reasons.

- General factors that may encourage the growth of Candida, include poor nutrition, an illness that has lowered resistance, diabetes, use of immunosuppressive drugs, and vaginal birth to a baby when the mother has yeast, thrush present in the breastfeeding mother, pacifiers, oral use of antibiotics, and other associated infections in the mouth.

Causes for Infants/Children

- Most babies contract oral thrush during their delivery. When babies pass through the vagina (infected with yeast), they swallow yeast on the way and infections may occur at any time (usually 7-10 days after birth).

- It has been suggested that oral thrush in babies and maternal breast Candidiasis are early common complications after birth in mothers who received intrapartmum antibiotics (*Obstetrics Gynecology*, July 2005).

- Babies may contract oral thrush due to the following possible reasons:

  ❖ Prolonged sucking on a bottle or pacifier.

  ❖ Poor hygiene of bottle equipment.

  ❖ Immune system is not fully developed (increases risk for developing infections).

  ❖ Infant/child with severe malnutrition, cancer, steroids, or other suppressive immune system treatment.

  ❖ After a viral infection with throat inflammation and superimposed yeast overgrowth (especially in a condition called stomatitis); decreased resistance during infection may encourage yeast growth.

  ❖ Antibiotics given to the baby (can cause oral and peri-anal diaper rash).

  ❖ Pacifier use.

Tip: Diseases and Oral Thrush

If an older child gets thrush in the mouth or has ulcers that look like they may be thrush, these may be signs of another disease. If this is the case, then consult your doctor. Some children with throat infections (e.g., stomatitis) may develop an ulcer and thrush in the mouth. Others with depressed immune systems (from diseases or medications that decrease the immune system) may develop oral ulcers and thrush.

Predisposing Maternal Risk Factors

- The following are risk factors for yeast infections in both mothers and babies:

  ❖ Vaginal yeast infection in the mother during pregnancy or in delivery.

  ❖ Antibiotics given to the mother during pregnancy, labor, and delivery, or shortly before or during the time that yeast symptoms appeared.

  ❖ Long term and frequent use of steroids given to the mother and/or infant/child.

  ❖ Maternal use of oral contraception, and pregnancy itself.

❖ Allowing damp nursing pads or bras to stay up against nipple tissue for a long period of time or using plastic-lined nursing pads that prevent good air flow to the nipple area.

❖ Breakdown of normal skin, friction and trauma (allows Candida Albicans to invade), or nipple injury due to poor latch.

❖ Diabetes in the mother (large amounts of sugar encourage the growth of Candida).

Treatment

General Treatment

- Healthy children with mild oral thrush may not need any treatment at all.

- If you are breastfeeding, it is important that you and your baby be treated at the same time, even if only one of you presents symptoms of oral thrush. Both breasts should be treated simultaneously with anti-fungal ointment to prevent the infection from spreading back and forth between mother and baby.

- It is recommended that the breastfed infant (or any infant with symptoms), be treated with oral and anti-fungal medications (e.g., Nystatin).

- Discuss with your doctor if your pain persists after a few days of treatment, as you may need to change treatment or add additional medications (ointment or oral medication).

- Oral thrush may recur, but there is no need to be concerned as it is very common and has no major side effects.

- The following are anti-fungal medications that kill Candida germs on the inside of the mouth for mother and/or baby:

Nystatin

- Nystatin comes with droppers to place liquid drops inside the mouth and onto the affected areas.

- This is repeated until the white spots have cleared.

- These drops should be given to the baby after a feeding and not before, as the medication may be washed away with the feeding.

- A cotton swab may be used to apply the medication to other areas of the mouth, using care not to insert a swab that has touched the baby's mouth back into the bottle.

- A clean swab should be used each time you dip into the bottle or a small amount may first be poured into a cup, with any left over medication being discarded after that particular application.

- The medication's directions say to apply Nystatin four times a day, but because yeast grows back fast (in about 90 minutes), it is important to apply Nystatin more often.

- In some cases, resistance to Nystatin occurs.

Gentian Violet

- While gentian violet was once a common form of treatment for oral thrush, it is no longer used as much. There is a concern that it may induce the development of cancer, however these studies have been mainly based on animals that were given large amounts everyday over a long duration.

- There is also a concern about the alcohol gentian violet contains (it is dissolved in 10 % alcohol). However, the amount the baby receives is small and most of it is not swallowed.

- When treatment to Nystatin is resistant, some professionals may still recommend using a 0.25-0.5% solution that is applied to your nipples twice per day for three days.

- If the pain is due to a yeast infection, lessening of the pain occurs within the first few hours after the first application of gentian violet.

- If you use gentian violet for your baby, take a clear ear swab, dip it inside the gentian violet and place it inside of the baby's mouth. It takes a few seconds for it to spread around the baby's mouth. Apply a small amount once per day (for three to seven days) and do not overuse. You may apply Vaseline to your baby's lips before using it to try to avoid purple stains (when a baby is placed on the breast while using gentian violet, it may stain the mother's nipple and areola).

- Any nipples on bottles or pacifiers should also be boiled and treated with gentian violet.

- It is effective, works quickly, but it is messy (stained clothes may require a few washes before it is removed).

- *Comment*: As a pediatrician, I have prescribed gentian violet for children in the past and have not noted any related side effects.

- Consult your doctor prior to use.

Diflucan (Fluconazole)

- This prescribed medication is a strong pill (used to treat severe and stubborn infections) and should only be used under supervision by your health professional.

- It also exists as a pediatric suspension for the infant/child.

- Diflucan should not be used as a first time treatment.

- Diflucan has an 86% rate of successful treatment compared with Nystatin, which has a 46% success rate.

- There have been no complications from exposure to Diflucan while breastfeeding your baby.

Ketoconazole or Itraconazole

- Ketoconazole is another anti-fungal medication that can be taken by mouth.

Ointment Combinations

- These are ointments that include an antibiotic, anti-fungal, and steroid (anti-inflammation) all in one such as those used for mastitis in the mother.

- Some use this combination even when there is no evidence of mastitis in combination or alone with gentian violet. However, these do not treat the baby's mouth.

Comment: I have used Daktarin (miconazole) Oral Gel in babies with oral thrush and found that it works well (quickly). If it is available in your area, consult your doctor about using this medication.

Tip: Acidophilus Capsules

Acidophilus capsules have been used to prevent or treat infection with candida albicans. However, scientific evidence of any effects is unclear, so I suggest using it as a complement to other treatments.

Additional Prevention & Treatment Measures

The following are some comfort measures and hygienic guidelines for you and your baby while you wait for the treatment to work.

- Both mother's and baby's hands should be constantly well washed.

- Regularly sterilize all items that come in contact with the baby's mouth (e.g., teethers, toys, pacifiers, nipples, feeding equipment, etc.) in boiling water for about 20 minutes, as these items may also harbor yeast. It is generally better to replace feeding equipment after 1 week of treatment.

- Breastfeeding should be continued throughout the treatment process (do not stop feeding). Take extra care with nipple hygiene when breastfeeding, so that they do not become infected.

- Throw away damp nursing pads and thoroughly wash all damp bras. Change your bras daily if they become wet, as damp nipples are good breeding grounds for yeast. If you have a yeast problem, it is better to simply avoid breast pads altogether (if possible) and, if they are needed, use disposable breast pads.

- Pump milk for a few days should breastfeeding become too painful (you may use Ibuprofen for the pain). Your doctor may advise you to throw away any breast milk that you expressed and stored while you had thrush, because the yeast can contaminate your breast milk and yeast is not destroyed by freezing.

- Sometimes, an application of vinegar and water solution to the nipple and areola of the breast can help clear candida. Mix 1 tablespoon of vinegar to 1 cup/250 ml of water. You may do this at the end of each feeding and air dry (avoid using soaps and lotions).

- When the baby has a yeast diaper rash, diaper wipes should not be used. Use water and washcloths instead, and place your baby in cloth diapers. These seem better during an infection (your doctor will prescribe ointment to treat the diaper rash).

- When washing infected clothing from either the mother or baby, hang the clothing outside to dry since sunlight is known to kill yeast. Hot water over 122 F/50 C also kills yeast (e.g., dishwasher, sink, laundry, etc.). Additionally, white vinegar can help kill yeast, so add this to bath water or washing machines when cleaning clothes, etc.

- Even though thrush symptoms may seem to have disappeared after a couple of days of treatment, continue treatment (as recommended by your doctor) for about 4-14 days, since yeast may still be present (without symptoms).

Case Description

David is a fifteen-month-old boy who just finished a seven day treatment with antibiotics for an ear infection. Prior to visiting the doctor's office, he developed a diaper rash that lasted three days (with loose stool). David's mother said that she used the usual cream and powder, but it did not help his diaper rash. She also stated that when she washed him, he cried every time she touched the area of the diaper rash.

Upon examination, David had a diaper rash with red areas of blood and pustulc satcllitc (a lcsion arca that signifies evidence of a yeast infection) that was painful when touched. David's other body parts were normal, including his throat, which had no evidence of oral thrush.

The suggested treatments for David include:

(1) Change diapers frequently.

(2) If the room is warm, leave David's diaper area to air dry when possible.

(3) No powder, as it increases yeast growth.

(4) No Vaseline, as it is irritating and may cause more blocked skin glands.

(5) The use of a medical cream, as directed by your doctor.

Comments: Diaper rash with yeast can occur when your baby is taking antibiotics and has loose stools. Many times, parents use powder thinking it will help, but it only worsens the situation. Once inflammation or yeast infection occurs, you need appropriate medical cream for treatment and not the usual Barriere cream. Also, do not use your usual cream for treatment at the same time as any other medical creams that are prescribed by your doctor.

Diaper rash with yeast can sometimes be very painful and requires medication for the pain (locally or orally), so consult your doctor.

Parent Concerns

Is thrush dangerous or a serious cause of feeding problems?
For the baby:

- The baby may not even be bothered by the infection. Sometimes the mouth is sore, but it is rarely very painful.

- Thrush is not at all dangerous and there is no need for concern. However, if it affects feedings patterns in your baby, he is probably in pain.

- Bouts of thrush are usually short-lived (it clears up within a few days to a few weeks).
- Follow your doctor's instructions for treatment, including pain relief, and it will pass like any other infection.

For the mother:
- For the breastfeeding mother it can sometimes be a frustrating situation, as yeast can linger. Some mothers experience so much pain that they stop breastfeeding.
- A worsening problem is a treatment resistant strain of yeast, making it more difficult to get rid of and causing a longer duration of pain. Also, the yeast strain may enter the milk ducts and the standard Nystatin does not work.

When should I see the doctor?
Consult your doctor when the following situations arise or occur:
- ❖ Your baby is fussy, has difficulty swallowing, or has feeding problems.
- ❖ You have symptoms of sore or cracked nipples, and your baby has symptoms of oral thrush as well, whether you notice thrush in your baby's mouth or not.
- ❖ Your baby is irritable and has a diaper rash, with or without any oral thrush seen in the mouth.
- ❖ Thrush lasts longer than 10-14 days, even with treatment.
- Other concerns or questions that you need to raise with your doctor:
  - ❖ Chronic, persistent and/or recurrent oral thrush (it can be a symptom of an immune deficiency).
- Thrush can be a very tenacious infection and may take 2-3 weeks to see results, so do not become quickly discouraged over the course of treatment. Continue treatment for a few days after the patches have disappeared to ensure complete resolution of the infection.

My nipples are not sore or cracked, but I experience pain when I breastfeed. Could it still be thrush?
Sometimes, thrush can exist even when the nipple is not sore or cracked. Speak to your health professional if you experience pain when you breastfeed or have a cracked nipple that is healing slowly.

My baby has thrush. Can he still go back to day care?

- Babies and children with thrush can still go to day care or school. However, careful hand washing and cleaning must be done at all times (not only when the baby has an obvious infection).

- Make sure that your baby is not given any pacifiers or is sharing bottles, etc. (speak to the caregivers).

Can we protect our baby from developing thrush?

No one can protect your baby from developing thrush, since almost everyone has Candida in their bodies. You can follow the hygienic measures and other preventive aspects previously discussed.

Are all diaper rashes associated with thrush?

- No, they are not, since diaper rashes are very common in infants and toddlers.

- In fact, most diaper rashes are not associated with yeast infection.

- Diaper rashes are red, swollen, or bumpy patches around your baby's diaper area that may cause him discomfort.

- Your doctor will be the one to assess whether there is a yeast infection on the diaper rash.

- With prolonged inflamed rash and moisture, yeast has a tendency to grow. Your doctor may prescribe a combination of anti-inflammatory and anti-fungal creams.

- Be sure to change your baby's diapers frequently and clean the area well after each bowel movement. You may also use super absorbent disposable diapers and allow the diaper area to air dry (bare bottom when possible). Do not use any powders (e.g., Talc, etc.).

Why does my baby have recurrent oral thrush?

- Some babies have a tendency to develop recurrent oral thrush or fungal diaper rash.

- There is no clear reason for this, especially when your baby/toddler is growing normally.

- Use the preventive measures suggested in this chapter. If thrush (oral and other skin areas) is recurrent or persistent, consult your doctor.

I have nipple thrush. Can I give my baby expressed breast milk?

- Use of refrigerated or expressed milk during thrush-episode treatment may not be a problem for your baby.

- You could dilute the defrosted "thrush" milk by mixing it with expressed, "non-thrush" milk. You may heat the defrosted milk to kill most or all of the Candida present.

- If it is possible, give your child milk that was expressed and frozen prior to the mom developing thrush.

Nutrition & Diet: Important Factors in Oral Health

General

Oral diseases begin at a very early stage, usually from the time bacteria begins to live in the oral cavity. As new teeth begin to grow and the diet of the infant and/or young child becomes more sophisticated, the bacteria produces acids and toxins that are harmful to the hard and soft tissues in the mouth.

Your child's baby teeth usually start to appear between six to twelve months of age. These are the baby's primary (first) teeth, an important aspect to having healthy adult teeth as they hold a space for permanent teeth (which develop somewhere between the ages of six to twelve years). Poor oral health and an improper diet can result in bacteria in the mouth reacting with sugar to form acid, which then eats through the enamel covering the teeth.

Diet and nutrition play key roles in keeping good oral health and preventing disease.

They have two different meanings; *diet* refers to eating habits and patterns of food intake, while *nutrition* refers to how the body uses nutrients for its growth, function, and maintenance.

Tip: When to Start Cleaning Teeth

It is good to start cleaning teeth as soon as they erupt from the gums. You can wipe the teeth with a soft washcloth or with a moist piece of gauze. You may later use a soft infant toothbrush so that your child becomes accustomed to the sensation.

How Nutrition Affects Oral Health

- Maintaining good nutrition is important in the initial growth and development stages of oral tissue, as it leads to good future oral health and resistance to disease.

- The prenatal period has an effect on your child's future oral health. A baby's teeth begin forming before birth; so ensure that you receive adequate nutrition and proper oral health.

- Malnutrition during the critical initial life stages of a pregnancy (prenatal nutrition) may result in enamel hypoplasia. It is an underdevelopment or incomplete development of the teeth, since formation of the primary teeth occurs at around 3-4 months into pregnancy. It can also lead to higher risks for cavities (caries) and tooth eruption.

- Nutritional deficiencies throughout a child's life may impact on healing and increase the chances of oral infections or diseases. It is a determining factor in the progression and severity of periodontal disease (around the tooth; e.g., bacterial infection of the gums and the surrounding tissue in the child's mouth).

- In the prevention and treatment of periodontal diseases, it is important to continuously supply the body with adequate nutrients such as protein, vitamin C, iron, zinc, and calcium. The following table outlines various vitamins and minerals and their role in oral health:

Vitamins & Minerals	Role in Oral Health
Vitamin A	Required for gum health. Maintains the integrity of mucous membranes in the mouth.
Vitamin C	Required for periodontal, gum health, and collagen production. Assists in healing wounds and the prevention of bleeding gums.
Vitamin D	Important for the development of healthy bones, teeth, and jaw growth.
Vitamin B2 (Riboflavin)	Vitamin B2 deficiency causes changes in mucous membranes of the mouth (angular chelitis and glossitis).
Calcium & Phosphorous	Calcium helps in the formation of teeth and bones. Phosphorous is required for energy production, metabolism and the development of healthy bones.
Zinc	Required for the repair of damaged tissues and metabolic processes. Aids in healing wounds.
Fluoride	Important for strengthening bones and teeth.
Iron	Required for energy and blood production. Iron deficiency causes glossitis (red, painful tongue).

How Diet Affects Oral Health

Dental Caries (ECC)

- Diet plays an integral role in the development of early childhood caries (ECC), an infectious bacterial disease and form of tooth decay in the primary teeth of infants and toddlers (usually between the ages of one to three years). It is mainly due to bacteria known as streptococci mutants that are passed from the parent to the child through frequent intimate contact (usually transferred from the mother's mouth to the baby's mouth during a feeding session, especially when using a spoon). The earlier the child's mouth is colonized with a mother's oral bacteria, the greater the risks.

- It affects about 10 % of preschool aged children in Canada. The child who experiences ECC tends to remain high risk and usually develops caries in his permanent teeth.

- Appearance of ECC may be as follows:

  ❖ In mild cases, the child's teeth will have a chalky, white appearance.

  ❖ In moderate cases, the teeth will look like a stained brown color and may even be partially eroded.

  ❖ In the most serious of cases, teeth will be dark brown or even black, with partial or full loss of the tooth's crown.

- Parents need to control their child's food intake, since most children enjoy foods full of sugar and sweet drinks. These are the greatest causes of tooth decay, especially if they remain in the child's mouth for a long period of time.

- Insufficient fluoride is also a contributing factor in tooth decay. It is necessary for the strengthening of teeth and bones and should be included in the infant's diet soon after birth. It works by coming in direct contact with the tooth enamel (the outside of the tooth).

- In most cases, fluoridated municipal water, fluoridated toothpaste, and dentist applied fluoride may be adequate for decay prevention. Parents must check with their doctor and local health department to find out whether their drinking water contains fluoride and the amount of that fluoride. In cases where well water is used, it should be tested to assess the amount of fluoride (safe levels are 0.3 ppm of fluoride or less).

- Sources of fluoride vary. Even if your local supply of water is not fluoridated, your child can receive adequate amounts of it from other sources including:

❖ Municipal water supply.

❖ Toothpaste.

❖ Foods and formula prepared with water.

❖ Vitamin preparation.

❖ Some soft drinks and fruit juices.

❖ Seafood.

❖ Dentist applied topical fluoride, etc.

- The ingestion of too much fluoride during the formation of the first or permanent teeth can cause a white to brown mottling of the permanent teeth, which may become dark stains. If too much fluoride is absorbed in the blood stream, it attacks the enamel on the inside of the teeth and causes fluorosis. Fluorosis is not a big health problem and it can be avoided. It occurs in babies or young children who excessively swallow fluoridated toothpaste. The developing teeth in babies and young children are more susceptible to fluorosis so do not use fluoride rinse before your child is six years old.

Tip: Pregnancy and Fluoride

Fluoride supplementation for pregnant women has not been proven to reduce the incidence of dental caries in the infant.

Preventing Tooth Decay

The following are some suggestions to help prevent tooth decay in your child:

- Ensure that your baby receives adequate amounts of fluoride in his water supply.

- It is suggested that, at nap or bedtime, you not use a bottle that contains formula or breast milk as they contain sugars (you may use plain water instead). Frequent nighttime bottle-feeding, when saliva flow is at its lowest, significantly increases the risk of ECC (the more saliva, the more protection). The bottle should only be used for feeding purposes and should not be used as a pacifier.

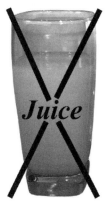

- Do not leave the bottle with the formula or breast milk in the baby's mouth for a long period of time.

- Gradually eliminate the bottle after one year of age. Start offering cup use from the age of six months and on.

- Breastfeeding may lead to tooth decay if your child constantly falls asleep at the breast with milk in his mouth (breastfed babies tend to have less cavities than bottle-fed babies).

- Never dip soothers in anything sweet.

- If your baby is on liquid sweetened medication, rinse and brush his mouth with clear water after the medication is given.

- Choose foods carefully and avoid those that contain large amounts of added sugar. Snacks for toddlers should be low in sugar (avoid sweets such as candies, raisins and dried fruits, etc.) and avoid snacking continuously.

- Processed sugars are not good nutrients as they increase the risk of plaque formation and allow acid producing bacteria to remain longer on the teeth. Avoid excessive intake of simple sugars and refined or cooked combinations that include cookies, potato chips, doughnuts, and some breakfast cereals.

- The number one source of refined sugar is soft drinks (soda pop). They have no nutritional value and are clearly associated with tooth decay. Chemical erosion of the teeth may occur, since soft drinks contain phosphoric, citric, and carbonic acid.

- When offering juice, it is better to dilute the juice with water (even 100% juice) and offer it in a cup, rather than in a bottle. Do not offer any sugary fruit punches or carbonated drinks.

- Give sweet foods during the meal and not alone between meals. Fruits between meals are preferred as they are better than sweets. It is better to use formula or water between meals, and not juices or sweet drinks.

- If your child takes sweets or snacks high in carbohydrates in-between meals, offer pieces of cheese (e.g., Swiss, cheddar), as bacteria thrives in an environment rich in carbohydrates (sugars). Use aged, natural cheeses (contains protein, calcium, phosphorous and fatty acids), which affect the growth of streptococci bacteria and decrease the risk of caries.

- Make sure your child eats a well balanced diet, especially one that is rich in calcium, vitamin C, and vitamin D, all of which are essential for good dental health.

- Hygiene, teeth cleaning, and dental follow-up is important (do an early follow-up for infants at risk).

Tip: Nursing Bottle Effects

Nursing bottle caries primarily affects the upper anterior teeth and the posterior teeth, but other teeth may be affected as well. It tends to spare the lower front teeth, because of the shielding of the lip and the tongue.

How Oral Health Affects Nutrition

General, Oral Surgery, and the Wired Jaw Patient

- Oral pain, problems in the oral cavity, and dental diseases act as major contributors to poor diet and nutritional habits, failure to thrive, weight loss, and malnutrition.

- A child who has undergone oral surgery (oral impairments or braces known as wired jaw application) requires a special diet to support post surgical needs. At this time, nutritional deficiencies are at a high risk until eating habits resume in full.

- Oral surgery may interfere with or even prevent chewing, during a period when the child has increased metabolic requirements. Patients may only be allowed liquids during the first days of their recovery and then slowly graduate to a soft diet.

- Consult your doctor if there are any concerns after oral surgery in regards to your child's nutrition.

The Child with Special Needs

- Special needs children are at a high risk of developing tooth decay since they have various feeding difficulties and use many medications that are sugar-based.

- Often, food stays in these children's mouths for a long period of time, making them more susceptible to tooth decay or bacteria forming in the mouth.

- Parents must provide extra care and attention to special needs children and closely monitor their oral health and eating habits.

> ### Tip: *More Oral Diseases*
>
> There are more diseases associated with oral involvement, which may include the following: Diabetes Mellitus Type 1, hematologic disorders (anemia, acute lymphoblastic leukemia), varicella-zoster, pseudomembranous candidiasis (thrush), aphthous ulcers, herpangina, and hand, foot, and mouth disease.

More to Know About Dental Health

Neonatal Teeth

- Natal teeth are teeth that are present at birth, while neonatal teeth are teeth which emerge through the gingiva during the first 30 days of a baby's life. These teeth usually emerge in the lower front area, though they may occur in other areas as well (teeth in the back region are not common and may be correlated with other syndromes or diseases). Because these are normal primary teeth, a new primary tooth will not replace them once they are lost.

- Normally, teeth present at birth or neonatal teeth can be kept. However, in some cases your doctor may remove these teeth if they are loose and pose the risk of your child swallowing the tooth. In most cases, neonatal teeth are loose or mobile.

- If they are actually teeth and not a remnant of development, it is a good idea to maintain them. Talk to your doctor regarding treatment for your baby, especially if they are moving too much (hyper mobile).

Baby Teething

- When babies are born, they have primary teeth that are not yet visible and have not broken through the gums yet—this process is called teething.

- Most babies begin teething around the age of six months; by the age of three years, a baby's teeth are usually fully developed (10 teeth on the upper area and 10 on the lower area). Many parents report drooling in their babies that start at about three months of age.

- Symptoms of teething may include irritability, fussiness, sleeplessness, loss of appetite, swollen gums, crying, increase in drooling, etc.

- Irritability and discomfort can probably be associated with teeth eruption. However, if your baby has a high fever or diarrhea, consult your doctor, as this is not caused by teething (although most parents will attribute it to teething). Also, sore or swollen gums can be a sign of local inflammation. Sometimes, with teeth eruption, there is bleeding around the teeth and blue discoloration that will resolve once the teeth erupt and blood has been dissolved. Some infants may even refuse to feed or withdraw from the breast or bottle when they start to feed, due to gum tenderness around erupting teeth.

- The following are some suggestions for helping your baby with erupting teeth:
  - ❖ Use soft or pureed foods like pudding, apple sauce, etc.
  - ❖ Avoid frozen bananas or Popsicles.
  - ❖ Use medications for pain or soothing of the gums. Use topical anesthetics as little as possible due to the risk of methemoglobinemia (blue discoloration of the skin and red blood cell destruction).
  - ❖ Try massaging the gums with a clean finger for 1 or 2 minutes. You may use wet washcloths, teething biscuits, or teething rings.
- Consult your doctor for medical advice if you are concerned, especially if your child has a high fever and any other symptoms.

Tip: Teeth and Table Food

Babies do not need teeth for table food.

Teething & Breastfeeding
- When your baby is teething, he usually loves to bite down on anything (including the mother's nipple).
- Do not overreact, as the baby may get scared or discouraged from nursing. Instead, calmly remove your baby from your breast and firmly say, "No biting," then allow him to latch on again.
- If your child continues to bite, end the nursing session and after a few feedings like this, your child will stop biting (see *Biting the Breast*).
- Teething may cause your baby to seem disinterested in feeding, since swollen gums sometimes makes sucking a painful experience. Let the baby chew on a soft, clean warm washcloth for comfort.

Iron, Vitamin & Fluoride Supplements
- Some iron and vitamin supplements, particularly those in liquid form, stain the teeth.

- To prevent staining of the teeth, apply drugs towards the back of your baby's throat. Toothpaste containing baking soda and/or hydrogen peroxide can be useful in removing stains on the teeth caused by supplements (see *Iron & Iron Deficiency*).

- The Canadian Dental Association does not recommend giving fluoride supplements to children below the age of 3 years. Supplements are to be given only by your doctor or dentist in high risk situations such as the following:

  - ❖ Dry mouth, for various reasons.

  - ❖ Increased dental disease incidence in the family.

  - ❖ Use of medications/syrups containing sugar over long periods of time.

  - ❖ Local water does not contain fluoride and you are exclusively breastfeeding. If the water has 0.3-0.6 ppm fluoride and your child is between three months and three years of age, then he does not require supplements. However, if your child is three to six, then he requires supplements. If the water has more than 0.6 ppm, then no supplement is needed at any age (provided that the child drinks 0.5+ oz/15+ ml of water per day).

Dental Visits
- It is important to find a dentist who specializes in treating infants and young children (including those with special needs).

- Parents should take their children to visit the dentist after the first tooth erupts, usually between six to twelve months of age (visit earlier if there are problems or concerns).

- At risk infants or young children may need to visit the dentist every two to three months to ensure proper oral hygiene.

- The earlier the visit, the better the chance of preventing dental problems.

General Tips for Oral Health & Teeth
- Decrease the risk of the acidity that leads to tooth decay by educating your child to brush his teeth, especially after eating sugar or carbohydrates.

- Supervise your child, discourage toothpaste swallowing, and use a pea-sized amount of toothpaste, especially if the child is less than three.

- Teach the child to spit up toothpaste, and to avoid swallowing it.
- Do not share toothbrushes (germs transfer easily). Replace it as the bristles become flattened with use.

Parent Concerns

My child has stomatitis and has difficulty eating. What can I do?

- Stomatitis is an inflammation of the mucous lining of the mouth, which may include the cheeks, gums, lips, tongue, and floor or roof of the mouth. It is a common infection in children, usually occurring between six months to three years of age. Symptoms may include fever, drooling, irritability, tongue or mouth sores, redness, swelling, difficulty swallowing, and gum bleeding. Viral infection is the most common cause of stomatitis, along with malnutrition, vitamin deficiency (especially vitamins B & C), cheek biting, braces, or jagged teeth. With infectious cause of stomatitis, treatment includes analgesics for fever and pain, local anesthetics for the mouth, and anti-inflammatory medication if there are canker sores in the gums or mouth. Various dietary measures such as using soft foods, jello, soup, cottage cheese, pudding, no acidic foods, etc., can help ease the pain.

What happens if my baby loses a tooth too soon?

- If your child loses a tooth prematurely for various reasons (e.g., tooth decay), the permanent tooth may erupt at an angle, causing crowding of the adult teeth. Further, it may also affect your child's speech, his chewing ability, and the use of his tongue.

Can I let my older infant chew on a frozen biscuit, if he seems uncomfortable from teething?

- This is not recommended, since the biscuit can break apart and your child may choke. You may offer your child a chilled (not frozen) teething ring instead of a biscuit. Avoid fluid filled teethers, since they may contain liquids that are poisonous (in case your child swallows them). Older children may eat cold foods such as plain yogurt or unsweetened apple sauce.

The Pacifier & Effects on Feeding and Nutrition

General

Sucking is a natural behavior that allows babies to feed and grow. Some babies enjoy sucking without feeding and will exhibit sucking behavior when they are tired, bored, or in need of comfort. Pacifiers usually satisfy the baby's need to suck and it should only be used in-between feedings (not as a substitute for a feeding).

The use of pacifiers is a controversial issue among medical professionals. A recent Canadian report states that up to 84% of infants use a pacifier at least some of the time, proving that it is widely used in today's culture. Until more conclusive evidence is available, either for or against the use of pacifiers, their use should be the parents' choice.

When to Start & Stop Pacifier Use

- A baby suckles on the breast differently than on a pacifier. In the early days, when you and your baby are getting used to breastfeeding, the use of a pacifier can cause nipple confusion (this is less of a problem if your baby is bottle-feeding, or if you have ample breast milk production). Avoid pacifiers until breastfeeding is well established. Otherwise, this can lead to ineffective suckling, breast refusal, colic, etc.

- An exception for the early use of the pacifier is for premature or sick babies in the hospital, who may use it for comfort.

- If the baby uses a pacifier after six months of age, limit its use to nap time or nighttime, so that it will not interfere with socializing and vocalizing during the day.

- Plan to stop pacifier use around twelve months of age. Begin by limiting the amount of use, and only use it for comfort. Remember, the longer it is used, the harder it is to break the habit.

- Do not punish your child if he does not give up the pacifier.

- Praise your child when he has given up the pacifier.

Pacifiers & Their Effects

Pacifiers & Their Effects on Feeding

- Pacifier use may result in poor latching technique, sore nipples, and a difficult start on breastfeeding. Try to avoid the pacifier until your newborn baby learns to latch onto the breast properly and you have milk supply.

- A study on the effects of the pacifier, when introduced early at two to five days, showed that pacifier use in the first month of life was detrimental to breastfeeding. These findings support the recommendation to *avoid* exposing breastfed infants to pacifiers during the first month of life. However, some babies may tire from nursing in the initial breastfeeding stages and some parents use pacifiers to help calm the baby until he learns to breastfeed appropriately. Try rocking or cuddling your baby first, and if he is still irritable and crying, then offer the pacifier. You may seek advice from your doctor.

- The use of a pacifier while still breastfeeding can lead to decreased intake of breast milk, so do not give a pacifier instead of a feeding. It may mix up how the baby sucks on the breast and/or may stop the baby from feeling hungry. Offer the pacifier in-between or after feedings, when you are sure the baby is not hungry.

- It is better not to use the pacifier when the baby is not gaining weight or is nursing poorly, as it interferes with good feeding habits, so discuss this with your doctor.

- Some studies show that pacifier use is associated with early weaning. Other studies, however, have concluded that pacifier use may be a marker of breastfeeding difficulties or reduced motivation to breastfeed, rather than a true cause of early weaning.

- To decrease your baby's dependence on the pacifier and to win him back to breastfeeding, try the following:

  ❖ *Feed him more frequently*: Sucking on a pacifier will not meet your baby's nutritional needs.

  ❖ *Eliminate distractions during nursing*: If you need to, nurse in a quiet room.

  ❖ *Establish a routine*: Try a daily nap and nursing routine where you go to a quiet room, then lie down and nurse him, much as when he was first born. This peaceful reconnection is likely to get him back to the breast.

  ❖ *Offer your finger*: If he does not want to feed on the breast, let him suck on your finger periodically, instead of on the pacifier.

❖ *Nursing on the move*: Use a baby sling, etc., to nurse your baby while moving around, as this may distract him from his desire for his pacifier.

> **Tip: Premature Stoppage of Breastfeeding**
>
> According to many studies, pacifiers and thumb-sucking are associated with the premature stoppage of breastfeeding.

Parent Control

- The Canadian and American Dental Association recommend pacifiers over thumb sucking, because it is easier for the parent to control the sucking habit. Parents can control the use of a pacifier better, as it is harder to control thumb sucking. When it is time to remove the pacifier, you simply take it out. However, with thumb sucking, you can't really do anything (you certainly cannot cut off his thumbs!). Also, using a pacifier has the advantage of freeing the baby's hands so he can explore the world around him.

- However, some will argue for the practicality of thumb sucking over pacifier use:

  ❖ Pacifiers tend to get lost because they often fall on the floor. The baby cannot lose his thumb—it stays right where it is.

  ❖ As long as you keep your baby's hands clean, you do not have to worry about germs. There are more germs on pacifiers, as they always fall onto unclean surfaces.

  ❖ Also, thumb sucking tastes better to babies than pacifiers do. Thumbs are the same temperature as the breast (if you are breastfeeding).

Dental Problems

- Prolonged use of the pacifier can lead to dental problems.

- Malocclusion, gingival recession, and teeth mal-alignment may occur if the baby is still sucking on a pacifier after the age of two years.

- Some studies found higher occurrences of open bite and posterior cross bite in two to five year old children who used pacifiers. The longer the use, the stronger the association.

Pacifiers & Analgesic (Comforting) Effects

- The pacifier is used as a simple comfort measure in painful procedures for both full term and premature babies (e.g., small procedures like blood tests, vaccinations, after circumcisions, etc.).

- If the baby is gaining weight well, you may allow your child to use the pacifier when needed and in moderation, if it seems to soothe him or relieve anxiety (e.g., crying).

Tip: Colic and Pacifiers

Some babies with colic find it soothing to suck pacifiers in-between feedings.

- However, some researchers say it is better for the baby to learn to comfort himself, rather than be dependent on an artificial aid, which is under the parent's control.

- In many instances, parents "push" the pacifier into the baby's mouth just to "shut him up." Parents must first determine if their baby is hungry or if he needs to be cuddled or rocked, etc. Try other methods of calming your baby down, such as pushing the stroller back and forth, consoling, etc. As a last resort, parents may use the pacifier.

Pacifier Use in Sleep & Sudden Infant Death Syndrome (SIDS)

- A pacifier may interfere with the baby learning to fall asleep on his own. It may also cause an interruption of sleep (e.g., when it falls out, the baby cries for it, waking you up as well).

- If your baby is breastfeeding and likes to fall asleep while sucking, let it be the breast rather than a pacifier (the breast is the best pacifier).

- There is an increasing body of evidence that shows that pacifier use is associated with a reduced risk for SIDS. There are various explanations for this, but the exact reason is still unclear.

Pacifiers & Ear Infections

- Pacifier use has been reported to be one of the risk factors for the development of ear infections.

- This risk is increased with prolonged and frequent use of the pacifier. Therefore, restrict its use in the early months of life, when the need to suck is strong and the risk of middle ear infections is high.

Pacifier Safety

Choosing a Safe Pacifier

- The best pacifier is the safest pacifier. Current pacifiers are made of latex or silicone and various health branches monitor the safety of pacifiers.

- Select one that is appropriate in terms of size for your child's age and one that cannot break (choking hazard). It should also have a firm base (1 1/2 inch/4 cm across) with ventilated holes so that your baby's nasal passages are not obstructed (this also prevents facial rash).

- It is better to have a single piece pacifier than one with multiple parts.

- Choose a smaller pacifier for a newborn and buy the larger size when your baby grows.

- Test the pacifier first to see that it cannot be pulled apart. Every pacifier should have a large, rigid shield to prevent the baby from placing the entire nipple fan inside his mouth.

- The type of pacifier will depend on your baby's preferences, but it must contain all the safety features discussed.

- Have a few of the same pacifiers on hand in case of a break or tear (babies usually prefer the same type of pacifier to be used).

Cleaning Pacifiers

- Always sterilize the pacifier (same methods as nipple and bottle sterilization) before use for about five minutes. Make sure it is cooled down before giving it to your baby.

- Keep it clean by washing it with hot, soapy water after each use.

- Always check for cracks or tears before giving the pacifier to your baby. If you see a crack or tear, throw it out (it is a choking and germ risk).

Safety Tips

- Never tie a pacifier around a baby's neck, as it may cause strangulation and death. Instead, use clips with short ribbons attached to it.

- Never attach a pacifier to a crib, carriage, playpen, or stroller. Never put the pacifier on strings.

- Never make your own pacifier out of bottle nipple caps or other materials. It can cause choking and death.

- Do not give a pacifier right after administering medication. Sometimes, the material in the medication can cause the material in the pacifier to break down.

- Do not let your child chew on a pacifier, as it can break apart leading to choking and death. Less drastically, chewing can cause problems with his teeth.

- Do not let an older child use pacifiers for long periods of time during the day.

- Do not dip pacifiers or nipples in sugar or honey.

Parent Concerns

I would like to give my baby a pacifier, but he does not want it. What should I do?

- Try a variety of nipple shapes and pacifier features (e.g., elongated, round, gel filled, orthodontic, etc.) since your baby may have distinct preferences.

- When the baby is in a good mood, place the pacifier gently into his mouth. Do not offer the pacifier for the first time when he is upset or hungry, as it will only frustrate him.

- Most babies refuse the pacifier initially, so continue trying. Also, remember that he may prefer his thumb for sucking, or nothing at all.

Is there an association between thumb sucking and thumb infection?

- Frequent and prolonged thumb sucking can be associated with inflammation of the thumb and yeast infection, since bacteria in the mouth and persistent moisture may lead to bacterial and fungal infection.

- Consult your doctor about treatment for thumb inflammation and/or infection (e.g., antibiotics, anti-fungal cream, and/or anti-inflammation cream).

My baby gags after sucking his thumb. Is this normal?

- Yes, this is normal, since some babies place their thumbs so far back in their mouths that they may gag (or even vomit).

- Try to offer a pacifier to your baby (if he accepts it) instead of the thumb until his sucking instinct diminishes (around nine months of age).

- Offer new activities to your older baby to distract him from thumb sucking.

- Do not forcibly take his thumb out of his mouth, as this may encourage him to continue sucking his thumb.

Summary

There is no clear consensus on the effects of pacifier use. However, it is recommended for premature babies to decrease stress (especially in the hospital). The decision to offer a pacifier is a personal parental choice. If you decide to use the pacifier, make sure it is used appropriately and safely. For example, if you are breastfeeding, you may want to delay the use of a pacifier in case of nipple confusion, decreased milk production, and early weaning. You should wait until breastfeeding is well established. Also, do not use the pacifier to replace feedings or to "shut up" your baby's cries. See the section on effects of the pacifier on your baby (SIDS reduction is among one of the important effects of the pacifier and its use). Should you decide to offer a pacifier to your baby, discuss with your doctor the pros and cons of early or late pacifier use (see following chart). You may offer the pacifier at any age (see previous points for limitations or reasons for early use). While some babies accept the pacifier easily, others are simply not interested.

Consider the following pros and cons when deciding whether to use a pacifier early or late, and depending on whether your baby is breast or bottle-fed. Discuss with your doctor before use.

Pros of Pacifier Use	Cons of Pacifier Use
Decreased risk of SIDS.	Safety risks.
Control is better than the thumb.	May interfere with breastfeeding & weight gain.
Comfort/analgesic effects.	Dental problems with prolonged use.
Frees the baby's hands to explore.	May interfere with sleep patterns.
May satisfy the baby's need to suck when not feeding.	Possible increased risk of ear infections.

Gastroesophageal Reflux

General

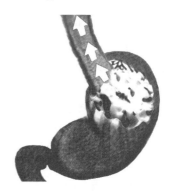

Gastroesophageal refers to the stomach and esophagus (tube that connects the mouth to the stomach) and reflux means to flow back or return. Gastroesophageal reflux occurs when stomach contents reflux, or back up, into the esophagus during or after a meal. A ring of muscle at the bottom of the esophagus opens and closes to allow food to enter the stomach. This ring of muscle is called the lower esophageal sphincter (LES). Reflux can occur when the LES opens, allowing stomach contents and acid to come back up into the esophagus.

Gastroesophageal reflux (GER) is a common problem in infants, usually beginning in the first weeks of life. Almost half of all infants have symptoms of reflux two or more times each day. Most infants with reflux will effortlessly spit up a short time after eating and will have no other problems. When a baby throws up or spits up after nearly every feeding and numerous times between feedings, parents often become concerned and worried that there is something wrong with their baby's stomach. Parents may be concerned that their baby is not keeping enough food down to grow; is allergic to milk, etc. Fortunately, in the vast majority of cases, none of these are true. Almost all babies with GER will ultimately outgrow this problem. However, there are a small number of infants and children who have either various associated symptoms and complications of the different types of reflux, whether it is the simple type or complicated reflux.

Clarification of Definitions

- Often times, parents are unclear as to whether their infant/child is regurgitating or vomiting. Regurgitation and vomiting are not specific to GER and may be symptoms of other underlying diseases.
- If your infant seems well in other ways (e.g., gaining weight and happy), then regurgitation and occasional vomiting is probably not a major concern (discuss it with your doctor, anyway).
- However, it is important to be able to distinguish between regurgitation and

vomiting, because vomiting may be a manifestation of a serious illness that requires immediate medical attention, especially if it is persistent or recurrent.

- *Regurgitation or spitting up* is the passage of gastric content from the stomach and esophagus that is a passive or effortless event. The end point of the gastric material that has refluxed up the esophagus is commonly the pharynx (the cavity behind the nose and the mouth).

- *Vomiting* is when the stomach content is forcefully expelled from the mouth. The following may be, but are not necessarily, associated with vomiting: a new symptom, uncomfortable during vomiting, abdominal pain, acts or looks sick, etc.

- *Projectile vomiting* is when your baby brings up stomach content in a forceful way. The amount of milk or food can seem large on the floor, but is usually the amount of the last feed. Babies with simple GER may occasionally have projectile vomiting. There are other unclear reasons for projectile vomiting (e.g., allergy, severe urinary tract infection, etc), but one, which is not uncommon, is a condition called pyloric stenosis.

- *Pyloric stenosis* is the narrowing of the pylorus (outlet) from the stomach into the small intestine. As the pylorus gets narrower, only a small amount of food enters the intestine, while the rest is vomited. It is more common in boys and symptoms usually appear between three to five weeks of age. If your baby is under two months of age and has pyloric stenosis, he may initially experience recurrent regurgitation progressing to projectile vomiting (around four to six weeks of age). In such cases, speak to your doctor immediately. It is important to realize that many babies with pyloric stenosis may start with regurgitation, which will progress to projectile vomiting.

Types of Reflux

Physiological Reflux

- This type of reflux is defined as regurgitation (passive, effortless, or non-forceful) or the passage of gastric content from the stomach and esophagus. It is not associated with complications or systemic illness of the child (i.e. babies have no other problems, except for making a mess).

- Physiological reflux is common (40-60%) in infants between one to four months of age, but decreases to 1% as symptoms resolve by four year of age. About 1/2 of all babies up to three months of age spit up at least once per day.

- Infants with physiological reflux are commonly referred to as "happy spitters" and they are characterized by frequent spitting up. This usually peaks at two to four months of age and occurs right after a baby eats, but it may also occur one to two hours after a feeding. The liquid that is regurgitated is usually made up of saliva, gastric juices, and milk. If the baby was just fed and regurgitates, the liquid looks very similar to milk. If the milk has been partially digested, it may smell like sour milk and look curdled.

- These infants are usually healthy and continue to grow and develop appropriately.

- For most babies, simple reflux gets better when they start to sit, while others improve when they start to stand. Many babies outgrow spitting up by seven to eight months of age and most have stopped spitting up by twelve months of age.

- The cause is considered to be the immaturity/relaxation of the valve or muscle at the upper end of the stomach, allowing stomach contents to pass through and result in regurgitation or vomiting. In addition, other contributing factors may include the following:
  - ❖ Short and narrow esophagus which allows the passage/regurgitation of stomach content into the esophagus.
  - ❖ Delayed emptying of the stomach in the young infant.
  - ❖ The diet of the baby is more liquid so there is more of a chance for regurgitation.

- Worsening factors for the above may include:
  - ❖ Overfeeding is a major cause for regurgitation. If the baby has eaten more than his stomach can hold and has a weak valve, regurgitation or vomiting can occur.
  - ❖ Air swallowing from over-anxious sucking through holes in the nipple of a bottle, burping, and moving the infant vigorously after a feeding may all lead to regurgitation or even vomiting.

Gastroesophageal Reflux Disease (GERD)
- GERD is also called pathologic GER. It is defined as regurgitation of gastric content (back up, refluxes) into the esophagus with accompanying symptoms and possible complications.

- GERD is a common pediatric problem affecting infants, young children, and adolescents which does not receive the awareness and attention it deserves. In an October 2005 survey, 80% of adults had never heard of GERD and, if they had heard of it, they did not understand or know anything about it.

- GERD occurs in a small number of babies (about 1 in 300 infants) for whom reflux is more frequent and is a chronic and severe disease.

- In pre-term infants, children, and adults transient relaxation of the lower esophageal sphincter (LES) leads to the development of GERD.

- In older children, it is not completely understood, but appears similar to that of the adult.

- GERD can be classified as primary or secondary:
  - ❖ Primary GERD occurs in isolation and is not associated with other diseases.
  - ❖ It is a motility problem of the lower esophageal sphincter dysfunction.
  - ❖ Secondary GERD results from other related causes/risk factors such as premature or critically ill infants, children with various conditions that put infant at risk for GERD such as, Cerebral Palsy or other neurological abnormalities, syndromes (e.g., Down Syndrome), Cystic Fibrosis, food allergy, especially cow's milk protein allergy (however, there is not a clear and full consensus on this association), etc.

- There are many medical reasons responsible for regurgitation and vomiting which are beyond the scope of this discussion (e.g., malabsorption, narrowing of the esophagus, other causes of feeding intolerance, oral pharyngeal dysphagia, etc.).

- In infants with *GERD*, regurgitation is the most noticeable manifestation. In mild GERD, symptoms can range from multiple episodes of drooling and spitting up gastric content to projectile vomiting.

- In severe *GERD*, regurgitation can be recurrent or associated with vomiting and can lead to inconsolable crying, aversive behavior associated with feeding (e.g., irritability, arching, refusal to feed, choking or gagging with feeding, etc.), frequent burping, bad breath, and abdominal pain.

- Complications of GERD include growth failure, respiratory problems (e.g., pneumonia, stridor, cough, etc.), esophagitis, behavioral changes, vomiting of blood, etc.

- The following table outlines worrisome symptoms of reflux disease in infants 0-24 months of age and 2-12 years of age, that may indicate complicated reflux (GERD), so speak to your child's doctor or health care professional if any of the following occur:

0-24 Months	2-12 Years
Vomiting associated with green or yellow fluid or appears like coffee grounds or blood.	Vomiting associated with blood, green, or yellow fluid.
Poor weight gain or failure to thrive.	Poor weight gain or weight loss.
Severe crying and irritability related to feeding.	Frequent sensations of food/liquid coming up into the back of the mouth.
Difficulty eating or persistent food refusal.	Frequent discomfort in the stomach or chest.
Difficulty breathing or breathing stops (turning blue) associated with vomiting or spitting up.	Trouble swallowing or painful swallowing. Wheezing, asthma, chronic cough, or recurrent pneumonia.
Excessive drooling.	
Repeated bouts of pneumonia.	
Chronic cough or wheezing.	

- Additional signs that reflux may be complicated in the infant/young child include chronic nasal or sinus congestion, chronic ear infections, Sandifier's syndrome (where the baby arches the neck and back to relieve reflux pain), irritability and pain (shortly after feeding begins), burning and scarring of the esophagus (esophagitis; inflammation of the esophagus from acid reflux), erosion of dental enamel and bad breath, laryngitis, etc.

- In summary, the following table outlines the basic difference between gastroesophageal (simple) reflux and gastroesophageal reflux disease (GERD). Parents should remember that GER is usually normal for full term normal infants and only becomes complicated when the worrisome symptoms for GERD are noticed. If these signs are present in your child, consult your doctor for further evaluation.

GER (no associated complications)	GERD
Regurgitation with consistent weight gain. No signs or symptoms of esophagitis (inflammation of the esophagus). No respiratory complications.	Regurgitation with poor weight gain or weight loss. Persistent irritability and crying during or after feedings, irritable after feedings.
No neurobehavioral symptoms (e.g., Sandifer's Syndrome—tilting of the neck and back).	Difficulty swallowing, iron deficiency, pyrosis (heartburn) in children.
Content during and after feedings.	Respiratory problems from aspiration.

GER (no associated complications)	GERD
No anemia.	leading to recurrent wheezing, pneumonia, chronic cough, and stridor. May have blood tinged vomiting.

Silent Reflux
- Silent reflux refers to gastroesophageal reflux (simple) or GERD without any outward or typical symptoms. This could mean that a child is not regurgitating, vomiting, or appearing uncomfortable, but is experiencing a reflux episode.
- Silent reflux is when the contents of the stomach only go as far as the esophagus and are re-swallowed, causing pain (due to back flow of stomach acid content) but no regurgitation.
- Some children may swallow the reflux material instead of throwing it up. This can be more damaging as the reflux material burns the esophagus on the way back down.
- Silent reflux is difficult to diagnose because of its "silent" characteristics. However, the following are symptoms which may indicate silent reflux: irritability and pain, poor sleep habits with frequent waking, arching of the neck and back (during or after feedings), frequent hiccups, anemia, apnea (stopped breathing), excessive drooling, problems swallowing, gagging and choking, respiratory problems (bronchitis, wheezing, asthma), poor weight gain or weight loss, erosion of dental enamel, etc.

Diagnosis of Reflux
- The doctor will talk with you about your child's symptoms, examine your child, and recommend tests if needed to determine if reflux is the cause of the symptoms or its complications.
- Usually, no diagnostic tests are necessary when the child is active and gaining weight appropriately. Various medications may be tried initially without running any tests to see if symptoms improve. If the medications do not help, your doctor may decide to do tests and x-rays to check the esophagus, stomach, and small intestine for problems and to rule out other possible causes and complications.
- Tests may include the following:
  - ❖ *Esophageal PH Probe study*: A tube is placed through the baby's throat to measure the acid level at the bottom of the esophagus.

❖ *Upper GI or barium swallow*: The baby will swallow a barium mixture (which makes images on the x-ray easier to see) and an x-ray will be taken. It is not as invasive as the PH probe study. This test will show if there is reflux and its degree, as well as any other abnormalities of the esophagus/stomach (e.g., Hiatal hernia, blockage, etc.).

❖ *Scintigraphy or milk scan*: The baby is given liquid mixed with a radio-labeled powder, which is detected by a scanner. This shows the baby's reflux episodes as well as the normal emptying of the baby's stomach.

❖ *Endoscopy*: An endoscope (a small flexible tube with a very tiny camera) is inserted through the mouth and down the esophagus and stomach, which allows progression through the esophagus for the examination of the sphincters and narrowings or ulcers in the area (due to back flow acid leading to inflammation, narrowing and ulcer of the esophagus). The lining of the esophagus, stomach and parts of the small intestine can be examined and biopsies (small pieces of the lining can be painlessly obtained to look for abnormalities such as inflammation, etc.).

❖ *Manometry*: A manometer measures the pressure inside the esophagus with a thin tube that has tiny openings at various locations. These openings sense pressure as the baby swallows and the esophagus contracts. Results are shown on a computer and this process allows the doctor to see whether the esophageal pressure is normal or abnormal.

Treatment
Management of Simple Reflux
- Treatment depends on the child's symptoms and age and treatment is sometimes started without the need of any tests. When there are no significant health problems (e.g., poor weight gain or weight loss, etc.), infants will benefit most from little to no treatment. However, the following are some suggestions for helping your infant with simple reflux:

    ❖ Allow your baby to rest more frequently during feedings.

    ❖ Feed your baby before he becomes hungry or upset.

    ❖ Feed smaller amounts more frequently. Avoid overfeeding, which makes regurgitation worse.

❖ Burp your baby during a feeding (every 2 oz/60 ml), but try not to interrupt his feeding rhythm.

❖ Do not move your baby vigorously after a feeding (milk will leave the stomach more quickly, making back up less likely).

❖ The nipple hole in the bottle should not be too big or too small.

❖ Eliminate tobacco smoke exposure in the baby's environment as it promotes reflux (lowers the lower esophageal sphincter pressure).

Treatment of Complicated Reflux (GERD)
- In addition to the above measures the following should also be included:

  ❖ *Thickened feedings and formula* are especially recommended for the infant or very young child. Feedings are thickened with 1 tablespoon of dry rice cereal per 1 oz/30 ml of formula. This may be useful in the management of the full term infants with GERD. Commercial formula that is pre-thickened with rice starch is available, so you may discuss this with your doctor.

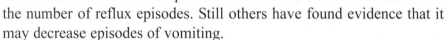

  ❖ However, literature is unclear regarding its efficacy for treatment of GERD. Some suggest evidence of improvements in feeding and sleeping. Others find inconsistent evidence of improvements in the number of reflux episodes. Still others have found evidence that it may decrease episodes of vomiting.

- *Formula*: The North American Society for Pediatric Gastroenterology Hepatology and Nutrition (NASPGN) guidelines emphasize that, in most infants with symptoms of GER, changing from one type of formula to another does not decrease symptoms.

  ❖ However, a small subset of infants with GERD may be allergic to cow's milk protein, which will result in a dramatic decrease in vomiting within 24 hours. In such instances, a two week trial of hypoallergenic formula should be considered (amino acid formula is more effective than extensive hydrolyzate formula—although more expensive, it has a better taste). Infants with cow's milk protein allergy can also be sensitive to soy protein.

❖ Changing from a traditional lactose based formula to a hypoallergenic formula is preferable to changing to a soy formula. Infants who are having difficulty achieving adequate growth may require higher caloric density formula.

Positions and Effects on Regurgitation & SIDS

Discuss with your doctor position recommendations, your baby's reflux severity, and the risk of SIDS, as there are new recommendations from NASPGN.

- *Supine* (lying flat on one's back): This may lower the risk for SIDS and should be the adopted and preferred position, upon discussion with your doctor.

- *Prone* (lying flat on the abdomen or face down): It is currently discouraged for the treatment of GERD in infants less than 12 months, because the risk of SIDS generally outweighs the potential benefit of prone sleeping (contrary to earlier medical opinion). The prone sleeping position for GERD is only considered in unusual cases, where the risk of death from severe GERD and complications outweigh the potential increased risk for SIDS (only adapt this position after discussion with your doctor).

- *Side lying*: This position may also decrease the reflux, however it is also associated with increased risk of SIDS.

- *Upright seated*: This position causes increased pressure in the abdomen and is associated with increased GER episodes. As such, this position should be avoided. Do not place your infant (as historically advised) in an infant seat after a feeding.

Tip: Avoid Increased Pressure to the Abdomen

Avoid swings, slings, strollers, chairs, and any other device that increases pressure in the abdomen.

- Have your child eat small meals more often and avoid large meals before exercise. Avoid eating two to three hours before bedtime.

- Help your child lose weight if he is overweight, as it increases the risk of reflux.

- Avoid certain foods and liquids for the older baby and child, which are known to cause reflux. Here are examples of foods you may want to avoid (talk to your doctor first):

❖ *Vegetables*: Tomatoes or tomato juice, corn, cucumbers, and turnips.

❖ *Fruits*: Apples, bananas, and citrus fruits.

❖ *Beverages*: Milk and carbonated beverages.

❖ *Starches*: Beans, oats, and tofu (avoid these in large quantities).

❖ *Miscellaneous Foods*: Vinegars, chocolate, honey, black pepper, foods with high fiber or fat content, and spicy foods.

- If your baby is not growing well or develops persistent signs and symptoms of abnormality (e.g., lung problems from aspiration, wheezing, arching, irritability, etc.), your doctor may suggest the following:

  ❖ Medication to decrease stomach acidity (neutralize it or increase bowel, esophageal, and gastric motility).

  ❖ Follow up with a specialist (e.g., gastroenterologist).

  ❖ Surgery may be required to tighten the lower esophageal sphincter or feeding tubes, etc., in severe cases (where medical treatment fails to control GERD).

Reflux & Other Conditions

Reflux & Asthma

- Reflux has been shown in many studies to worsen and sometimes, even cause symptoms of asthma. Studies estimate that anywhere from 30-90% of all asthmatics could also have some degree of reflux.

- Asthmatic children sometimes present with silent reflux.

- There is no conclusive evidence as to whether reflux triggers asthma or if the asthma triggers reflux. However, effective treatment of reflux can improve symptoms of asthma.

- Here are some possible indicators that your child may have both asthma and reflux:

  ❖ Asthma symptoms worsen after feedings.

  ❖ Persistent cough that gets worse when lying down.

  ❖ Excessive spitting up.

  ❖ In these cases, controlling the reflux can usually control asthma.

Reflux & Milk Allergy

- Cow's milk allergy or sensitivity can occur in infants who are younger than one year. Allergy may be mistaken for existing reflux.

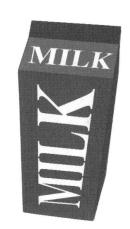

- If regurgitation or vomiting is caused by milk allergy, symptoms usually disappear when cow's milk protein is eliminated from the baby or nursing mother's diet (if she consumes dairy).

- Discuss with your doctor switching to hypoallergenic formula, as this may eliminate reflux that is associated with milk or soy protein intolerance.

Reflux & Colic

- When a healthy child cries uncontrollably for an extended period of time (e.g., more than three hours per day), it is a condition called colic.

- It is estimated that up to 25% of infants have colic. It usually begins between the third and sixth week after birth and tends to disappear on its own by the third month (sometimes later).

- Some experts believe that reflux is the most common cause for colicky babies, even though no conclusive evidence of this theory has been found.

- Silent reflux is often mistakenly diagnosed as colic, because the baby does not spit up.

- Here are a few symptoms to help you differentiate between colic and reflux:

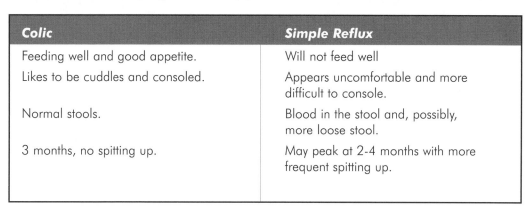

Colic	Simple Reflux
Feeding well and good appetite.	Will not feed well
Likes to be cuddles and consoled.	Appears uncomfortable and more difficult to console.
Normal stools.	Blood in the stool and, possibly, more loose stool.
3 months, no spitting up.	May peak at 2-4 months with more frequent spitting up.

Parent Concerns & Tips

How does GERD differ in young children from older children and adolescents?

- Reflux in children is age-specific with characteristic signs and symptoms based on maturational age and size, as well as the severity of the disease.

- Young children usually do not report heartburn to their doctor. Rather, the parents of the child observe the symptoms of reflux such as irritability during or after feedings, arching, inconsolable crying, etc.

- The older child or adolescent will present with more typical symptoms of reflux including heartburn, chest pain, early morning nausea or abdominal discomfort, etc.

My baby is breastfed. What can I do to minimize regurgitation/reflux?

- Reflux is much less common in breastfed babies than in bottle-fed babies.

- Even when breastfed babies have reflux, they have shorter, fewer, and less severe reflux episodes than bottle-fed babies. The reason for this is that breast milk leaves the stomach much quicker than formula, leaving less time for back-up into the esophagus.

- Breast milk is best for the baby with reflux, as it is less allergenic than formula and is digested twice as fast.

- Try the following suggestions if you are a breastfeeding mother:

  ❖ Eliminate foods from your diet that make reflux worse (e.g., fatty foods, caffeine, spicy foods, citrus foods, etc.).

  ❖ Feedings should not be "short" but, rather, for as long as the baby wants to hold onto the breast.

  ❖ The baby is encouraged to suck at the breast as long as possible with each feeding, even after the breast is relatively empty, since sucking produces waves of muscle contraction in the esophagus that move food towards the stomach.

  ❖ Try lots of skin-to-skin contact with a fussy feeder or even breastfeeding while moving (rocking or walking) your baby.

  ❖ A good latch onto the breast can minimize air swallowing and help a spitting up or colicky baby.

  ❖ Do not interrupt active suckling to switch breasts.

❖ Make sure your baby is comfortable and relaxed (the more relaxed, the less reflux).

- Be assured that breastfeeding can and should continue.

Will changing my baby's formula help with the reflux?

- About one third of infants experience formula changes to help with reflux.

- Mothers feel that their infant's reflux may disappear with a change in formula. However, this is not the case in many situations.

- With simple reflux, parental comforting is all that is needed if the baby is gaining weight well and is healthy.

- Remember that using iron-fortified or non-iron-fortified formula makes no difference to colic, regurgitation, vomiting, fussiness, and stool frequency.

- It is also important to note that true allergy to cow's milk or soy based formula occurs in less than 2% of infants and is unlikely to present with only regurgitation and/or vomiting. Formula intolerance triggers more vomiting than regurgitation.

- If allergy is suspected, a trial of switching formulas to extensively hydrolyzed, hypoallergenic formula, or soy formula, may be considered (after discussion with your doctor). If your baby's symptoms do not disappear, then it may be possible that he has soy allergy (if using soy formula), or lactose intolerance (it is rare to have congenital lactose intolerance).

- A premature baby has a higher chance of reflux; however, don't exclude the possibility of allergy or formula intolerance.

Tip: To Change, Or Not To Change, Baby's Diet

The question parents need to ask themselves is this, "Must we change the baby's formula to ensure adequate weight gain?" If the answer is no, and the baby appears to be healthy, educate yourself about other possibilities and consult your doctor.

How can I relieve my stress when my baby has reflux?

- You must understand that infant reflux is a common problem and many parents have a difficult time with their babies.

- Emotional stress sometimes takes place and puts a strain on your family, because of the unbearable guilt you feel when you are unable to stop your baby's regurgitation, vomiting, and pain.

- To relieve your stress, begin by educating yourself. Read all the suggestions made in this chapter. You will be the best advocate for your baby; by understanding infant reflux yourself, you are already helping your little one. You may further discuss this topic with your doctor.

My doctor does not seem concerned when I tell him about my child's reflux. Why is this?

- Simple reflux, as defined in this chapter, is a common daily condition seen in the doctor's office.

- It is upsetting (especially to parents), because reflux may persist for a while, and your doctor may consider it to be normal

- Your doctor knows your baby's physical status and weight gain. If everything is normal, he will explain to you that the situation is transient and will resolve on its own as the baby gets older.

- If your baby has other symptoms of complicated reflux (as mentioned in this chapter), discuss this more seriously with your doctor to assess the need for evaluation and treatment.

Does teething or the pacifier make reflux worse?

- No, teething or the pacifier does not make reflux worse. It simply increases saliva production. Since saliva is alkaline, it may neutralize and help the acid that comes up with reflux of stomach contents.

- Some experts believe that when babies are teething, they tend to drool more and swallow a lot of that extra saliva, causing regurgitation.

My 5-month-old baby spits up a lot these days and he ate much more when he was younger. What could be the reason for this?

- When regurgitation starts at this age or older, consult your doctor to rule out reflux conditions or any other illnesses.

- The cause of regurgitation depends on various factors. Some can be assessed by questioning such as:

  ❖ Did you stop breastfeeding and start on formula? (possible allergy)

  ❖ Does your baby have mucus or blood in the stool? (milk allergy)

  ❖ Any medications taken recently by the mother (if breastfeeding) or by the baby?

❖ Is your baby in a period of growth spurts?

❖ Does he swallow more air when he is feeding (causes increased regurgitation)?

- In any case, you should discuss this concern with your doctor and remember that simple reflux can peak at two to four months of age.

How can I tell the difference between simple reflux and complicated reflux?

- Complicated reflux has all the symptoms of simple reflux. However, these symptoms are worse, and have the following, additional symptoms: irritability worsens after each feeding, poor feeding, spitting up blood, frequent hiccups (more than usual), excessive drooling, cough, wheezing (due to chronic acid reflux), etc.

- These symptoms, along with your doctor's assessment of growth, recurrent infections and problems (e.g., dental erosion, respiratory difficulties, etc.) will help in the diagnosis of complicated reflux.

What does it mean if my baby has food coming out of his nose when he spits up?

- In many babies with simple reflux, stomach contents come out through the nose.

- This is usually not dangerous and does not indicate the severity of your baby's reflux.

- It can sometimes happen after a feeding with burping. It is probably related to the amount of air swallowed and pressure the stomach contents are refluxing back in the direction of the esophagus.

Do toddlers have reflux?

- In most cases, reflux disappears by the age of one year and/or when babies begin sitting up, standing, walking, and have solid foods introduced, along with maturation of the valve (at the connection between the esophagus and stomach).

- However, reflux sometimes persists longer in a happy and growing toddler. In these situations, medications may be prescribed, along with possible investigations of your child's digestive tract to rule out other potential illnesses.

Case Description

Anna, aged 3 1/2 months, had recurrent regurgitation and vomiting on and off since she was six weeks old. She was feeding and gaining weight well on cow's milk based formula. Anna was a full-term baby with no birth complications who weighed 6.4 lb/2910 g at birth. At 3 1/2 months, her weight was 15.8 lb/7200 g.

Anna was diagnosed with William syndrome (associated with heart abnormalities, low calcium levels, low birth weight, small head, minor anomalies in the face, dental problems, low performance score, etc.) after a heart murmur was noted. This was confirmed by chromosome analysis and a consultation with a geneticist.

Anna had an upper GI and small bowel follow-through test that showed no evidence of gastroesophageal reflux.

Conclusion:

The radiological test was done to see if there is evidence of gastroesophageal reflux or if there were any other causes of vomiting due to a digestive tract abnormality (especially because the patient had an associated syndrome where feeding problems can arise). Anna was simply overfed, resulting in her being overweight and having an associated simple gastroesophageal reflux.

Stool Characteristics of Babies & Toddlers in Health & Diseases

General

Stools are solid wastes composed of undigested foods, bacteria, mucus, and dead cells that pass through the rectum as bowel movements. Parents are often preoccupied with their child's stool, wondering what is normal and how frequent or consistent it should be. Babies' bowel habits are individual and over time, you will get to know your baby's routine.

Most babies with apparent stool problems are either perfectly normal or have minor, temporary difficulties that will pass with time. Stool problems rarely represent a more serious problem. Education on the range of infant stool characteristics may alleviate concerns parents have about formula intolerance or underlying (gastrointestinal) bowel diseases.

Age & Normal Stool

Premature Babies

- Premature babies may have one to six stools per day.

- Their stools seem to be more semi-solid watery in consistency than those of full-term babies.

Newborn Babies

- First stools in newborns (first month) comprise of a very dark, black, sticky material called meconium, which was in the baby's intestines during pregnancy. It is excreted in the first 24 hours (a baby who is still passing meconium stools or no stools at all after the 4th or 5th day should be evaluated by a health professional). After it has passed, there is a yellow-green transitional stool.

- Transitional stool is loose and sometimes seedy in texture (particularly among breastfed babies). It may occasionally contain mucus or traces of blood which were swallowed during the delivery.

- After 3-4 days, the stool will change according to what your baby is fed:

- *Breastfeeding*: Mustard color, loose consistency, and watery stool. Sometimes, it is seedy, mushy, or curd-like. At first, your baby may have a bowel movement with every nursing—this is not diarrhea.

- *Formula-fed babies*: The color of the stool is pale yellow (curd like) to yellow brown, or light brown to brown green. If iron is included in the formulas, the stool may be black or dark green. Formula-fed babies' stools will be less frequent and smell more prominently than that of breastfed babies.

Beyond the Newborn Period

- Breastfed babies range from 1-7 stools or more per day in the first 6 weeks.

- After six weeks to three months of age, the breastfed baby can go from several bowel movements per day to about 2-4, or he can even go several days without any bowel movements. At this age, the bottle-fed baby can have one to three stools per day. This variation in stool frequency is considered normal.

- From six to twelve months of age, the introduction of various solid foods will result in changes of color, odor, consistency, and frequency of stools. The stools become drier, darker, and less frequent than before (about three per day).

- Between one to three years, most infants will have only one or two stools per day, while eating usual family meals.

- Between three to five years, stools will be similar to those of an adult, except in size; frequency will be about 1 per day.

> ### Tip: Bowel Frequencies
> A study of bowel frequency in healthy children showed that:
> - The number of bowel movements decreases very quickly after the first month.
> - After the age of three years, the change in daily frequency is significantly less.
> - Infants who combine formula and breastfeeding have a stool frequency closer to that of formula-fed infants.
> - The higher frequency of bowel movements in breastfed infants is not well explained. It is possible that it is due to a more frequent activation of the gastrocolic reflex in breastfed infants, most of who feed on demand. This reflex stimulates the baby to have a bowel movement.

Factors Affecting Stool Consistency

It is evident that fluid balance, diet, and timing all come into play when determining stool consistency. Many parents wonder how it is possible for their babies' stool consistency to change day-to-day when the child is on the same diet. There are many factors which affect stool consistency:

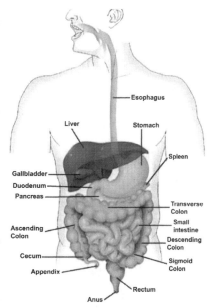

- *Fluid intake*: If the child consumes enough water or other fluids, he eventually exceeds the bowel's ability to re-absorb the water, thereby producing a loose stool (the unabsorbed fluid passes out with the stool).

- *Insensible fluid loss*: This is fluid lost through the skin and breathing. It is affected by body temperature and the rate of breathing. The more fluid lost, compared to the amount taken in, the more it may have a significant impact on stool consistency. For example, a child with a high fever may lose a lot of fluid through the skin and breathing, resulting in a firmer stool.

- *Sugar intake*: Consumed sugar influences stool consistency, so when too much sugar is given, diarrhea may result. Also, sugar in some juices causes more loose stools than other juices.

- *Food intake*: The type of fiber (soluble versus insoluble) and the amount influence stool consistency (see *Vegetables*).

- *Length of time stool remains in the colon*: The longer the stool stays there, the firmer the stool will get due to re-absorption of water in the colon (part of the bowel). Children hold stools back for a variety of reasons (e.g., constipation, psychological, etc).

Normal & Abnormal Stool Patterns

Hard Pellets & Constipated Stool

- A baby becomes constipated only when the stools are hard, pebbly, infrequent, and painful to pass (consistency is more important than frequency).

- Constipation is a common problem in childhood, and a significant number of children develop chronic constipation. Aggressive treatment should begin shortly after constipation begins to lessen the likelihood of chronic constipation.

- Hard pellets can sometimes be due to constipation.

- A complication of constipation is Encopresis, a watery mucus or liquid stool which oozes around the constipated stool. Parents sometimes think that their child has diarrhea, when this is not the case. The problem and treatment for Encopresis is the same as for constipation (see *Constipation*).

- *Bloody diarrhea*: Bloody diarrhea occurs when the baby's bowel (intestine) is infected by a particular microorganism or in inflammatory bowel disease (e.g., ulcerative colitis, etc). This type of stool is different than red, bloody streaks in the stool because these blood streaks, which occur in stool during diarrhea, may occasionally represent an association with a more severe condition.

> ### Tip: The following signs may be an indication when stool becomes diarrhea:
>
> *Watery stools which may contain blood and/or mucus, bad stool odor, abrupt increase in stool frequency, baby is not feeding well, acts sick or feverish, etc.*

Stool Colors
- Whether your baby is breast or bottle-fed, minor changes in stool color occur day-to-day and are of no significance.
- Exposure to air may cause the stool to change to a green or brown color; this is normal.
- Parents often change their baby's formula because they believe their baby is not properly digesting the current formula because of variations in stool color.
- Talk to your doctor before making any formula changes.

The following is a list of various stool colors and their significance:
White Stool
- This color results because there is a decrease in the bilirubin and urobilinogen excretion from the liver to the bowel (due to obstructed canals in the liver).
- White stool results from a condition called congenital extra hepatic biliary atresia.
- If you notice a white stool and your child is jaundiced (yellow skin), consult your doctor immediately.
- A light white color stool may occasionally occur in normal babies and toddlers with colds.

- Pale stool may occur with Hepatitis (inflammation of the liver) and other symptoms may include dark urine, yellow skin, and whitening of the eyes.

Green Stool
- Green stools result from an oxygenation of bilirubin (giving the yellow color of the stool) to biliverdin. It also means that food moved quickly through the large intestines (rapid transit) and did not have enough time to be affected by the bile secreted by the liver.

- Causes of green stool may include the following:
  - ❖ These types of stools are more common in babies who are given formula with 12 mg of iron per liter formula such as Enfamil with iron, Prosobee, Nutramigen, Carnation, etc. It occurs up to 50% of the time.

  - ❖ In breastfed babies, green stools can occur normally. Green stools are not a sign of overfeeding (yellow stools in breastfed babies occur about 90% of the time).

- In the first few days of life, stools will look greenish-brown, this is meconium stool and there is no reason for concern.

- Green stools also occur when the baby has the stomach flu (also called Gastroenteritis). In this case, the color is caused by a very rapid passage through the bowel associated with moderate to severe diarrhea.

- A urinary tract infection with a bacterium called E. Coli may be associated with green stools.

- Green stools can occur with taking drugs such as Indometacin, or vitamin supplements.

- In some breastfeeding mothers who take iron supplements, the baby's stool may become green.

Watery/Runny Stool
- If your child's stool is watery and there are sudden changes of smell, colors, and frequency, consult your doctor.

- Frequent watery stools occur when the baby has bowel infections (Gastroenteritis) and when the baby has a milk allergy.

Black Stool
- Black stools usually occur if the baby is bleeding from the digestive system or is taking iron salts, supplements, or drugs (e.g., charcoal, Indometacin, etc.).

Red Streaks & Bloody Stool
- The bloody streaks come from the lower intestine or rectum.

- This occurs in cases of anal fissure (tiny cuts around the circumference of the anus) or a milk allergy. The mechanism of dietary protein transferred from the mother's ingestion of cow's milk may cause enterocolitis (inflammation of the bowel or bleeding) and can be a sign of cow's milk allergy in your baby.

- Red streaks in the stool sometimes occur in the breastfeeding baby whose mother is on a dairy or soy product diet. If this is the case, talk to your doctor, as you may need to eliminate dairy products and then observe the stools to see if they improve. This may represent food sensitivity/milk allergy in the baby.

- With cessation of the mother's ingestion of milk, the disappearance and re-introduction of milk to the mother's diet may lead to blood in the stool again, meaning that your baby is possibly allergic to milk.

- Sometimes, babies ingest blood through breastfeeding from a mother with a cracked nipple, and that blood passes to the baby's stool.

- Consult your doctor about the various causes of red streaks in the stool; in most cases, however, it is not a major concern.

Tip: Food & Color of Stool

Orange colors	Carrots
Red colors	Beet or Beet Juice
Black streaks/strands	Banana
Small dark "objects"	Blueberries or raisins
Light green pellets	Peas
Yellow pellets	Corn
Seeds	Tomato, cucumber, melon
Sandy stools	Cheerios, oatmeal cereal, pear, etc.

Mucus Stool

- Mucousy stools can result if the baby eats certain fruits like bananas. It may indicate an irritated colon, and may also point to a food allergic reaction.

- Another reason may be that the baby has intestinal infections/inflammation (e.g., stomach flu, colitis, etc.) or a condition called irritable bowel syndrome (IBS).

- Stool may be described as a jelly-like mucus and blood stained in a condition called intussusception, which is bowel obstruction (occurs more often in children under two years of age). Symptoms associated with this condition may include severe stomach pain attacks, crying and vomiting. Consult your doctor immediately.

Stool Odor

- Stool odor rarely has any medical significance.

- Odors come from the breakdown of food in the diet.

- High protein diets produce more noxious gas than carbohydrate diets, due to the type of product breakdown.

- Internal illness or infection may also change the way food is broken down, thereby causing an unusual foul odor.

- Pale, floating, or foul smelling stool occurs in diseases associated with malabsorption such as Celiac disease, Cystic Fibrosis, inflammatory bowel diseases, etc.

Tip: Celiac Disease

Celiac Disease is a digestive disease caused by sensitivity of the small intestine to the protein gluten, which is found in wheat, barley, rye, and, perhaps, oats. The food is not absorbed properly. Symptoms gradually develop after the baby has started on solids, particularly those that contain wheat (e.g., cereals, breads, crackers, etc.). Symptoms include weight loss or weight gain, a very pale, floating stool that has an unpleasant smell, lack of energy, etc. The treatment for Celiac disease is a gluten free diet.

Stool Patterns, Parent Perceptions & Switching Formula

- Perceived intolerance to infant formula is a frequently reported parental reason for switching formulas. It may be related to perceived symptoms of constipation, fussiness, abdominal cramps, and excessive spitting up or vomiting.

- There is a progressive change in stool consistency, frequency, and color from breastfeeding to weaning to formula. Stools become firm as the infant weans from the breast to the formula. The stool is less yellow and more greenish-brown.
- The following are stool patterns with various formulas:
    - ❖ The composition and/or processing of cow's milk-based iron-fortified formulas affect stool characteristics.
    - ❖ Whey predominant formulas (not casein predominant formula) are associated with loosened stool (whey and casein are types of proteins found in cow's milk and are the main proteins in some formulas).
    - ❖ Levels of iron in formula affect stool color: higher iron content produces a higher incidence of green stool compared with a low iron formula.
    - ❖ In general, soy formulas tend to produce firmer stools than other formulas, so these can be good for a bout of diarrhea.
    - ❖ The developmental stages and growth of your child as well as the introduction of solid foods may affect changes in stool color.
- The general point is that infants may have various tolerances to formulas. Some formulas may be presented to the mother as "less constipating."
- When parents are concerned about their baby's stool, changing the formula is not necessarily the answer. Your infant's stool color, for example, is often a reflection of what he eats, and the type of formula may change the color. The color of the stool is not important if your baby is healthy and growing well. If he is not growing well, then stool color only becomes significant in the context of other symptoms.

Case Descriptions

Case Description 1:
Alena is an eight month old girl who had no immediate problems at birth. She was breastfed for the first six months of life. Alena's mother decided to introduce lactose-free formula into her diet, since her stool was soft. At this point, Alena began to experience recurrent coughing episodes with occasional mild wheezing (she has shown improvement in these symptoms since she was treated). There is family history of asthma and, over the last few months, Alena's mother noted a persistent, bulky, frequent, and foul smelling stool.

Alena has a good appetite, is gaining weight well and has no symptoms of vomiting.

Due to her mother's stool description, a sweat chloride test (assessment of sodium sweat amount after stimulation) was done. This showed that Alena had a much higher amount of sodium than normally expected, which led to the consideration of a diagnosis of a disease called Cystic Fibrosis. There is increased fat in the stool in this disease, so stools were collected for assessment over a 24 hour period, which confirmed a high amount of fat in the stool.

With genetic testing, Alena was confirmed to have the Cystic Fibrosis mutation and both her parents were carrying this genetic mutation as well. Cystic Fibrosis is an inheritable disease, whereby the abnormal gene is inherited from both parents (who may be carriers with no symptoms). Although the genetic mutation is present from birth, symptoms may not appear until months or years later.

Recurrent chest infections and secretions of sticky mucous in the lungs cause progressive lung damage. It also causes deficiencies in pancreatic enzyme secretions which help in food digestion and nutrient absorption in the intestine; their absence causes the type of stool described in Alena.

A diet high in calories, protein, and vitamin supplements is recommended. Treatment of lung problems, infections and/or wheezing, etc., will include antibiotics, inhalations, physiotherapy, and treatment for various further complications.

Conclusion: This case is an example of when stool characteristics can be an important factor in diagnosing a serious disease.

Case Description 2:
Michael is a six month old boy who is breastfed and gaining weight well. There was some irritability and frequent green stools noticed. Michael's appetite was good with no other symptoms (e.g., vomiting, wheezing, etc.).

Michael's mother brought him in for a routine checkup, and stated that she recently noticed that his stool was grass-green. Upon examination, everything seemed to be normal and there was no evidence of a throat infection or dehydration. Because of the green and loose stool of increased frequency, a urine test was done and confirmed a urinary tract infection.

Michael's infection was treated with antibiotics and he also had other tests done, such as an ultrasound of the kidneys, etc. This was to confirm that there was nothing wrong with his kidneys that predisposed him to infections. These tests proved to be normal.

Conclusion: Frequent, green, loose stools, with or without vomiting, fever, irritability, etc., may sometimes be evidence of a urinary tract infection, which can be confused with the stomach flu.

Tip: Diseases & Stools

Stool characteristics may vary with diseases, such as the following:
- Diarrhea of infectious causes.
- Intolerance to carbohydrates.
- Cystic Fibrosis (stool tends to be oily and difficult to flush, as it tends to float).
- Malabsorption syndrome (fatty, watery or sticky stool, though it may be normal).
- Celiac disease (large volume of stool, floating in toilet water, etc.).

Parent Concerns

My one-month-old breastfed baby passes stools every time he feeds. Is this normal?
- This is normal since some babies have reflex (gastrocolic reflex) that tends to push the food out through the stool.
- This usually improves after the first six to eight weeks of life.
- However, if your baby develops diarrhea, you may need to consult your doctor.

Can occasional and short (1-2 day) episodes of green stool occur?
- Infants and toddlers with rapid transit of bowel contents may have green stools.
- In most cases, it is normal to have these short episodes, as they may be a short-lived bowel infection.
- If the amount increases or is persistent, consult your doctor.

Why does the transition to solid foods produce changes in my baby's stool?
- Stool color, frequency, odor, and consistency may be affected by many factors.

- As solids foods are introduced, they affect stools in the following ways:
  - ❖ More fiber gives a softer consistency.
  - ❖ Sugars in fruits and vegetables affect bacteria in the large bowels.
  - ❖ Fat contents affect contractions of the intestine.
  - ❖ Addition of constipating foods may increase the firmness of the stool.
  - ❖ Increasing fluid intake softens stools.
  - ❖ Cereals sometimes make for harder stools.
- Bacteria in the bowel will prosper if different sugars are introduced in the baby's diet, and stool odor can change due to gases produced by these bacteria. These, for example, can occur after stomach flu and should improve within two weeks.
- Furthermore, you can observe stool changes with various foods given to your child (see previous *Stool Color & Foods* chart).

Some babies fuss and push just before they have a bowel movement. Is this normal?
- Babies muscles related to bowel movements are not fully mature at birth, so some babies seem to make an effort and fuss before a bowel movement. Sometimes, changing positions may help (a semi-reclining position in your lap or in an infant seat).
- There is no need for any treatments unless your baby has a real struggle and seems very uncomfortable. Consult your doctor regarding your concerns.
- Be assured that your baby will outgrow this problem.

Conclusion
- Changes in the diet can be associated with different bowel movements.
- Changes in color, smell, consistency, and content are usually of no concern if they only last a few days. However, if there are additional symptoms or if the abnormal stool persists, see your doctor.
- Remember, any medications (e.g., iron) that you or your baby are taking can affect stool appearance and consistency.
- Consult your doctor when the following occurs:
  - ❖ Baby has a persistent green stool.

❖ Baby has a persistent foamy stool.

❖ Red stools (especially with abdominal pain or vomiting).

❖ Stools contain mucus.

❖ Blood in the stool, especially if the amount of blood is large.

❖ Difficulty passing stools.

❖ Newborns with white stools and jaundice.

❖ Pale, floating stool, in the toilet and foul smelling stools.

❖ Fatty stools (may be evidence of malabsorption problem).

❖ Bloody stools in diarrhea (may be caused by various organisms, especially bacteria such as E.coli, Salmonella, campylobacter, yersinia, etc., some of which may lead to severe complications).

Constipation

General

Constipation is generally described as the passage of hard stools. Any definition of constipation depends on how often the child normally passes stools and the normal consistency of them.

Constipation is a common problem for children, but it is usually temporary and no cause for parents to be concerned. It is one of the most over-reported symptoms associated with pain, pushing, grunting, bleeding, etc., (16% of toddlers are reported by their parents to be constipated).

In healthy children, the number of bowel movements changes with age and diet (breast or bottle-fed, solid food introduction, etc.). Newborns may average several bowel movements per day. In older, healthy breastfed infants, there may be weeks between bowel movements, but the stools are soft. By around age four years, a child may average one bowel movement per day. Nonetheless, it is not correct to assume that a bowel movement everyday is "normal." There is no "right" number of bowel movements, as each person's body finds its own normal pattern, which depends on many factors. In general, two or less bowel movements per week may be a sign of constipation.

Causes of Constipation

General Mechanisms

- To understand constipation, it helps to know how the colon (the large pipe in the intestine) works. As digested food moves through the colon, the colon absorbs water and nutrients from the food, as it becomes waste or stool. Muscle contractions push the stool towards the rectum and by this time, the stool is semi-solid (because most of the water has been absorbed). Constipation occurs when the colon absorbs too much water or if the colon's muscle contractions are slow, causing the stool to move through the colon too slowly. As a result, stools can become hard and dry.

- Constipation arises when feces remain in the colon for a long period of time, possibly due to a "sluggish" colon (less motility), a low fiber diet (produces less stimulation in the colon), and obstruction in the digestive tract, which may not allow for an easy stool evacuation.

- Large stools stretch the intestine, causing muscle tone to become weak. To complicate matters, the passage of hard and large stools (through a narrow rectum) can tear the anal wall and create anal fissures. This is indicated by a history of pain and defecation with crying (when passing stool) and "holding back" (when on the toilet). Streaks of blood may be seen in the stool or on toilet paper for the older child.

Infant Constipation

Constipation is most commonly due to a low fiber diet, low fluid intake, an irregular bowel movement, abnormal motility of the bowel, an acute illness, etc. It is rarely associated with other medical conditions. Many times, there is no identifiable cause for constipation. The following are common causes of constipation:

- *Bottle-feeding*: Generally, constipation in bottle-fed babies is much more common than breastfed infants. Stools are infrequent, firmer and darker than breastfed baby stools (once solid foods begin, the stool becomes firmer and more frequent). Some breastfed babies have bowel movements once every few days with no difficulties. However, under-feeding (not getting enough milk), whether in a breastfed or bottle-fed baby, leads to a lack of fecal bulk, which may result in constipation and is associated with poor weight gain.

- *Formula composition*: According to some experts, iron-fortified formula does not cause constipation. However, some mothers believe that iron-fortified formula does cause constipation. Some soy formulas cause more constipation than cow's milk based formula.

- *Weaning from breast milk to formula*: In the early transition period, weaning or switching from formula to cow's milk sometimes causes constipation.

- *Foods*: Bananas, rice cereal, and other foods with decreased fiber content increase the risk of constipation (cereal and milk taken excessively from the bottle can cause worse constipation).

- *A change in the child's diet*: Starting new solid foods (e.g., low in fiber) may be associated with constipation.

- *Insufficient fluid intake*: When your baby does not receive enough fluids, his body responds to dehydration by absorbing more water from whatever he eats or drinks and from the waste in his bowel, leading to a hard stool.

- *Milk allergy*: Cow's milk, egg, wheat or soy allergy, and excessive milk products can cause constipation.

- *Genetics*: There can be a familial tendency for constipation.

- *Fissures:* These are small cracks in the anal area. They result from the passage of hard stools, causing pain and further complicating the situation (infants are afraid to pass bowel movements).

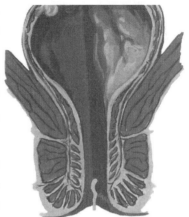

- *Tight anus/anal stenosis*: This may cause constipation; an examination by your doctor can simultaneously confirm and enlarge the anal canal.

- *Acute illness*: Fever and other symptoms can lead to constipation for a few days, as the infant is eating less and has no waste products (losing fluids from sweating, vomiting, etc.).

Toddler Constipation

- Toddlers can experience a negative phase or emotional upset that may lead to constipation.

- Changes in stools may be due to moving to new foods, a low fiber diet, a low intake of fluids, or a diet which is high in dairy products, bananas, and rice.

- The toddler who is potty training may be holding his stool in, which promotes constipation. The longer the stool is retained, the more fluid is absorbed from the stool and it becomes harder. Also, the intestine muscle weakens the longer your child is constipated, further worsening the situation.

- Toddlers may become involved in power struggles with their parents. Many toddlers will intentionally hold their bowel movements in, as they learn to assert their independence.

- Children may be "too busy" to go to the washroom if they are having too much fun playing a game or involved in something they do not want to leave.

- A lack of exercise (physical activity) may cause constipation, as exercise helps move the digested food through the intestine.

Tip: Constipation and Medical Conditions

Hirschprung's disease is a disease of large bowels with faulty nerve development that affects bowel motility. The chief sign of this disease is if your new baby delays or fails to pass the first stools (meconium) within first few days after birth. It can present in the newborn as a large bowel obstruction or, later, as chronic constipation.

Some other medical conditions that may be associated with constipation may include neurological (cerebral palsy), endocrine (diabetes, low calcium), obstructive (anal stenosis), etc.

Encopresis: Soiling From Constipation

- Encopresis is the repeated passage of stool or feces into inappropriate places such as underwear or floors.

- The problem usually begins with children passing very large stools or having pain while passing stools. Over time, the young child becomes reluctant to pass bowel movements and "holds" it in to avoid the pain. As more and more stool collects in the child's lower intestine (colon), the colon slowly stretches and the child loses the natural urge to pass a bowel movement. Often in the beginning, only small amounts of stool leaks out, producing streaks in the child's underwear. Parents often mistake this for not wiping very well. Eventually, more and more stool leaks until the child passes entire bowel movements into the underwear.

- In the majority of cases, Encopresis develops as a result of chronic constipation. Other causes include:
  - ❖ A diet high in milk.
  - ❖ Genetic predisposition.
  - ❖ Stool holding as a way of resisting toilet training.

- Encopresis is very upsetting for many parents as they have to frequently bathe their dirty child and discard soiled underwear. Many parents assume that the child is being lazy or soiling intentionally. In most cases, Encopresis is involuntary.

- Treatment for Encopresis is the same as that for constipation, rather than diarrhea.

Symptoms of Constipation

General Symptoms

- Many children experience symptoms differently. The child with chronic disease may present with no symptoms or just some irritability (evidence of discomfort). Children in which constipation is due to other medical issues may show related symptoms. The following are symptoms that your child may be constipated:

❖ Abdominal pain, cramping, and bloating.

❖ Decreased appetite.

❖ Gas and moodiness.

❖ Hard and dry stools.

❖ Getting red-faced.

❖ Legs drawn up onto the abdomen.

❖ Streaks of blood along the outside of the stool.

❖ Hard, round, or pellet shaped bowel movements.

❖ Less frequent bowel movements.

❖ Small liquid or soft stools that soil the child's underwear.

Breastfeeding & Constipation

• With breastfeeding, the newborn may have a soft, watery stool that is mustard color and is frequent throughout the day (with almost every feeding).

• Breastfed infants have an active "gastrocolic reflex" in the first one to two months of life, causing bowel movements every time the stomach is full.

• By the age of six weeks, some breastfed babies only have one soft bowel movement per week (considered normal). Generally, stools remain high in frequency until about two months of age.

• As long as the stools are soft and mushy and the baby is happy and comfortable, abrupt changes in the frequency of bowel movements (from several per day to one every several days) are not a problem since breast milk produces less waste than formula. These infrequent stools are not signs of constipation and are considered normal.

• When breastfed babies start with added formula or solid foods, stools become less frequent or they can become constipated.

• If you need to start cereal and your baby is already constipated, start with oatmeal as a first cereal food, since starting with rice cereal may worsen the constipation.

- If the baby is growing healthily, he may have anywhere from one to twelve stools per day in the first month or one stool every seven days or more until about three months of age.
- True constipation is not common in breastfed infants. If your baby has constipation, stools will be hard, round, or pellet shaped, even if your baby is healthy and gaining weight well.

Diagnosis

History
- The parent's observations, medical history and feeding patterns help a doctor diagnose constipation. Depending on your child's age, your doctor may ask the following questions:
- Is your child breast or bottle-fed?
- How often does your child have a bowel movement?
- How old was your child when he passed his first stool?
- What does your child's diet include?
- Is there visible pain or complaints made by your toddler during bowel movement?
- Is your toddler in the process of being toilet trained?
- Have any emotional or stressful events occurred to your child lately (e.g., toilet training)?
- Does your child have any blood in his stool?
- Is the stool your child passes hard? Any pain (abdominal)?
- Has your child been on any medication or in surgery lately?
- Are there any symptoms other than constipation noticed recently?
- Any recent illnesses or vomiting before becoming constipated?

Physical Examination & X-rays
- The doctor will assess your child's abdomen for masses of stool, etc.
- In a rectal examination the doctor will insert a finger into the rectum to look for stool abnormalities (e.g., hard stool, blood in the stool, tightness in anal area, etc).
- Sometimes, the doctor may order the following tests or refer your child to a specialist for further assessment:

❖ *Abdominal X-ray*: Examines stool amount in your child's intestine.

❖ *Barium Enema*: Examines the intestine for any abnormalities.

❖ *Anorectal Manometer*: Examines the muscle, reflexes, and coordination during the defecation process.

❖ *Rectal Biopsy*: Samples tissue from the rectum and looks for any abnormalities.

Prevention

The following are suggestions to help prevent constipation in your infant/toddler:

- Do not use mineral oil, enemas, or herbal supplements without first consulting your doctor.

- In hot environments, add water in-between your child's feedings depending on age as per your doctor's instructions (see *Water, Fluids & Drinks*).

- Do not offer an excessive amount of rice, banana, or rice cereal. Serve acidic foods (e.g., tomatoes, oranges, etc.) to the age-appropriate child.

- Increase your child's intake of high fiber fruits and vegetables such as peas, beans, broccoli, prunes, apricots, plums, strawberries, melon, whole grain cereal, etc.

- Do not offer excess dairy products or, unless your child is older than one year of age and able to tolerate it (see *Cow's Milk*).

- Do not frequently switch formulas before discussing it with your doctor.

- Ensure adequate daily fluid intake and increase fiber intake after one year of age. Fiber is proven to be of considerable benefit in regulating motility of the digestive tract. Ways to increase fiber in your child's diet include the following:

  ❖ Young infants between the ages of six to twenty-four months should work up to 5 grams of fiber per day. Children aged two to eighteen years should receive about 5-10 grams per day, while adults should take in 25-35 grams of fiber per day.

  ❖ Add one or more servings of fruits or vegetables per day. Fruits high in fiber include apples, berries, oranges, prunes, pears, raisins, etc.

Vegetables high in fiber include broccoli, Brussels sprouts, carrots, potatoes, cauliflower, lettuce, etc., and legumes high in fiber include kidney beans, hummus, lentil, peas, etc.

❖ Replace white bread with whole grain breads and cereals; offer brown instead of white rice. Offer 100% bran cereal for breakfast such as All-Bran, Bran Buds, etc.

❖ Always increase fluid intake when you increase your child's fiber intake: while increased water intake is recommended in cases of constipation, it is important to remember that the problem is too little water in the stool (not in the body). You should use increased fiber in the diet or substances such as sugar (Karo, Lactulose) to retain the water in the stool (otherwise, excess water will simply wind up in the urine).

- Encourage your child to be active every day.
- When your toddler is potty training, do not make it a source of tension and do not force him to sit for a long period of time (and don't hurry him, either). Try to make him sit on the toilet after meals and before bedtime.

Treatment

Treating constipation typically involves modifications in your child's diet and medications are sometimes required. Parents make mistakes with a constipated child in stopping all treatment as soon as the child has normal bowel movements. If the child has a tendency to constipation, it will likely reoccur. Also, the longer the constipation, the worse the motility of the bowel. You need to continuously clean the bowel until bowel motility is restored. Treatment for chronic constipation usually takes a long time and you need to keep your child's bowel content soft until it returns to normal. The following are some suggestions and treatment methods for the constipated child, according to age:

Birth to 6 Months
- Increase your baby's fluid intake (extra plain water, 1-2 oz/30-60 ml per day).
- If your baby is breastfeeding, then breastfeed more often, since breast milk produces softer stools.
- Feed more frequently if your baby is bottle-fed and add boiled water to his diet.

- You can add 10-20 g of sucrose or Dextrose/Lactulose per 4 cups/1 liter of formula or fluids.

- Add 1 teaspoon of dark sugary syrup or malt extract with every four bottles given per day for two to four days.

- Offer juices such as grape, prune, and apple twice a day. Prunes contain isatin, sorbitol, and soluble fiber. All of these have laxative effects and help prevent and relieve constipation.

- Sometimes, placing one tablespoon of Karo corn syrup in your child's formula (in 4 oz/120 ml of water) helps reduce constipation during the first few months of life.

- Decrease the use of bananas, rice cereals, and apple sauce (if started before six months of age).

- If constipation continues to be persistent, consider changing formulas after a discussion with your doctor.

6-12 Months

- Offer water in-between meals (1-2 oz/30-60 ml) to your baby's diet when starting solid foods.

- Offer more breast milk or formula.

- Add prune, pear, or apple juice in your baby's diet (1-2 oz/30-60 ml by bottle or spoon).

- Do not offer bananas, rice cereal, and apple sauce for a while. Use another grain such as barley or oatmeal.

- Offer fruits and vegetables that are high in fiber (see previous tip).

- Glycerin suppositories may be used. They melt in the heat of the rectum and lubricate it. These are helpful when the stool does not come out easily (it helps to initiate the defecation reflex). It is completely safe but do not use these for more than a few days.

- Glycerin enema (Baby lax) works well. It is a pre-lubricated tube with a squeeze bulb of pre-melted glycerin that is gently inserted into the anus about 1/2-3/4 inches/1.5-2 cm (squirted into the anus). You can lubricate the tip of the bulb syringe with olive oil.

- You may use a baby enema as a last resort and lubricate the tip of the syringe with olive oil. Insert the tip of the bulb containing one to three tablespoons of lukewarm water into the baby's rectum. Gently squeeze water into the colon and repeat if necessary.

1-5 Years

- Offer water and juices every day (2-4 oz/60-120 ml per day). Limit whole milk to 16 oz/500 ml per day. The colon is your body's fluid regulator. If your baby is not drinking enough, the colon steals water from the waste material and gives it to the body. This causes stools to be dry and hard.

- Offer fruits and vegetables that are high in fiber. Certain fruits and juice such as prunes, apple juice, apricots, etc., are rich in sorbitol. It is a non-digestible sugar that passes through the body into the colon and causes water to be retained or drawn into the stool mass.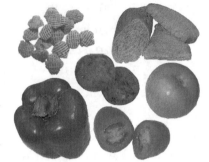

- Offer Lactulose, a non-absorbable sugar product that is processed by colon bacteria to produce an inflow of water into the stool mass. The dose is adjusted according to your child's response. Side effects include cramps and diarrhea, so it is better to start with a small dose and give one or more increased doses, as necessary (1-3 ml per kg per day). It is safe and well tolerated.

- Physical exercise is helpful in moving stools.

- Glycerin suppositories are helpful in the treatment of constipation, along with Baby lax.

- Mineral oil is a lubricant laxative that is a mixture of hydrocarbons dried from petroleum products (1-3 ml per kg per day). The oil can interfere with vitamin absorption. It is dangerous if it is aspirated to the lungs, so do not use it for children with neurological and swallowing difficulties. It is not recommended before the age of one year.

- Flax oil has omega three fatty acids that facilitate vitamin absorption. It is an alternative to mineral oil. One teaspoon per day can be taken orally with breast milk or water.

- Proper bowel habits help ease stool movements. Get your child in the habit of sitting on the toilet twice a day about 10 minutes after a meal.

- To ease your child's bowel movements, massage his stomach. Start at the bottom of the abdomen with circular movements and gently rub towards the top right of the stomach. Repeat this action about 5-10 times in each quadrant of the abdomen.

- When fissures exist, it is important to use stool softeners at all times (until they heal) to reduce additional trauma. You may apply aloe vera lotion to the area and medical cream, as recommended by your doctor.

Parent Concerns

Does constipation lead to stomach pain and decreased appetite?

- It is unclear whether constipation leads to stomach pain and decreased appetite.
- It is possible that acute constipation will cause abdominal pain, but less so with chronic constipation (at least until a certain point). Parents should not blame abdominal pain on constipation, as it is not always the case.

Are there certain formulas, which cause hard stool and constipation?

- Some babies develop constipation on soy formula.
- On the other hand, casein hydrolysate formula (e.g., Nutramigen) will cause looser stool than those seen with standard formula use (see *Stool Characteristics of Babies & Toddlers*).

Does iron-fortified formula cause constipation?

- Iron-fortified formula does not cause more constipation than formula with no iron.
- On the other hand, scientific research and a mother's observations may sometimes clash.
- Some mothers will argue that iron-fortified formula absolutely does cause constipation.
- You can try alternating formula with and without iron to see if the situation worsens or gets better.

I started my child on solid foods and now he has constipation/hard stool.

- The baby's stool consistency changes with dietary changes (transition to solids) or when cow's milk is started. Starting solids could be a contributing factor to constipation, among other factors such as not enough fluids and fiber intake, etc., that affect stool and bowel movement.
- Consistency may range from a firm to loose stool when starting solids.

- If you start rice cereal or other foods that are more constipating, you may want to hold off on these for a while and/or replace it with other cereals (e.g., oatmeal, etc.).
- Sometimes, the stool is initially hard when changing the diet; it may gradually become normal with no treatment. It could possibly indicate that your baby is not yet ready for the foods being given and needs some time for adjustment.

Is constipation only due to dietary habits & nutrition?
- Although the diet plays an important role in bowel movements and constipation, it is not the sole factor (see causes in this chapter). For example, decreased activity levels and eating styles in obese children may be a factor in constipation, along with emotion, psychological, neurological diseases, drugs, thyroid problems, etc.
- There is a significantly high prevalence of obesity in children with constipation by four to eighteen years of age. It may be the result of dietary factors, activity levels, and hormonal influence; however, this needs further clarification.

Is constipation commonly seen in vegetarian babies?
- Usually, vegetarians have less constipation due to their increased fiber, vegetable, and fruit use. However, some soy formulas given to vegetarian infants may cause a firm stool. You still need to ensure that your baby receives enough fluid, etc., and, after discussion with your doctor, you can try other formulas.

My child has diarrhea and has now developed constipation. Is this normal?
- This is normal since constipation usually occurs after diarrhea or the stomach flu, because the child lost fluids and did not eat much while sick; he may also have had excessive amounts of constipating foods. Also, the colon will initially reabsorb any fluid from foods to re-stabilize the amount of water the body needs. Continue offering fluids to your child and stop the excessive use of constipating foods (rice, banana, etc.).

Does incorrect formula preparation play a role in constipation?
- It is not clear whether the suggested ratio of water to powder in formula may cause constipation, as each baby is unique and some mothers with constipated babies add extra water in-between feedings while the baby is still gaining weight well.

- When preparing powder formula, you need to follow the instructions. If there is excess powder relative to the amount of water added, the baby may develop hard stools.

Can constipation be associated with Irritable Bowel Syndrome (IBS)?

- IBS can occur in the early childhood years and includes episodes of diarrhea and constipation accompanied by pain, bloating, and gas.
- IBS attacks usually occur in stressful situations and it does run in families.
- Treatment of IBS includes increased fiber intake and behavioral approaches to decrease anxiety.

Does massaging my baby's stomach help with bowel movements?

- Massaging your baby's stomach may help with digestion, relieves stress and colic, regulates breathing, etc. You can help your baby's bowel movements by gently massaging in circular movements the bottom right of your baby's abdomen up to the top right. If it does not help with bowel movements, it at least provides comfort and love.

What about botulism and constipation?

- Honey may contain bacteria that cause botulism. One of the first manifestations of botulism is constipation. It is the reason why honey is not recommended in the first year.

Should I worry about my son's umbilical hernia when he pushes for bowel movements and the hernia swells?

- Some premature, full term, and small for gestational age babies develop small umbilical hernias.
- Anything that causes an increase in intra-abdominal pressure makes it more bulging and prominent. However, it is not associated with pain or any problems.
- In most cases, the hernia usually resolves as the baby grows older.
- The baby's stomach is relatively small to the amount of food (breast milk or formula) he is fed. Do not overfeed while bottle-feeding.

Can my baby/toddler get addicted to laxatives if I offer them for too long?

- There usually is no addiction to laxatives, however the longer it is used, the higher the dose of medication needed.

- When glycerin suppositories are used, they are not recommended for use longer than two to four days. You do not want the rectum to lose the sense of stool that stimulates defecation.

Conclusion

- Constipation is a very common and frequent concern. It is important to understand its definition so that you can know when your baby has true constipation.
- While there are many non-organic causes (nutritional, emotional, etc.), there are also organic causes/diseases that your doctor will evaluate and test for, when necessary.
- It is important to treat constipation early and continue treatment until the problem has resolved, otherwise it can lead to a vicious cycle of worsening constipation.
- Treatment of constipation should be tailored to each individual child and his age. This is especially true for the young infant, in which case you will need to discuss treatment measures with your doctor.
- Good bowel habits early in life are important for bowel functions and the prevention of constipation.
- While constipation usually has no long-term complications, this depends on the cause (i.e. nutritional and/or medical).
- Consult your doctor when:
  - ❖ Your child cries when they are passing hard bowel movements.
  - ❖ Blood is present in the stool.
  - ❖ The stool is hard or passes after several days.
  - ❖ Pushing is not strong enough to expel the stool.
  - ❖ Soft stools leak from the anus and painful tears appear in the skin around the anus.
  - ❖ Your child has hemorrhoids or is constipated and vomiting.
  - ❖ Your child has a distended abdomen.
  - ❖ You have concerns about your child's growth and weight gain.
  - ❖ Your child has had constipation since birth.

❖ Leaky stool in the underwear (Encopresis).

❖ Constipation lasts longer than 3 weeks.

Tip: Anal Fissures

When your child's defecation is painful with no associated bleeding, it is important not to blame the problem solely on constipation. The anal area should be examined for fissures and other problems, which can sometimes be difficult to notice.

Crying & Fussing In Relation to Feeding & Nutrition

General

Crying may be described as an unpleasant sound. Typically, babies cry because they need to communicate to adults that something is not right.

The first few weeks of your baby's life will give you a "sneak peak" at your baby's personality (demanding or easygoing). Some babies have more persistent and recurrent crying than others. In time, you will learn to recognize the various causes of your baby's crying, whether it is due to hunger, pain, or another reason. It must be admitted that much of infants' crying occurs without any discoverable cause. However, simply trying to respond to your baby's needs will help him feel secure and comfortable. When you cannot console your baby, and if there are any other associated symptoms, then consult your doctor.

Causes

General (Non-Organic) Causes

- Often times, you will not know why your baby is crying or why he has stopped. There may be many times when he is crying for absolutely no clear reason at all. The following are possible causes of crying:

  ❖ *Colic* is fairly common until about three months of age.

  ❖ *Pain & medication:* Your baby may cry if he is in any type of pain such as that caused by teething, diaper rash, or if he is taking medications, etc.

  ❖ *Growth spurts:* Many babies seem to be fussy when they are experiencing a growth spurt, usually around seven to ten days, two to six weeks, three to nine months, etc (see *Growth Charts & Assessment of Growth Patterns*).

  ❖ *Environment:* It may be too cold or too hot (your baby's room should be at 71 F/22 C). Do not over clothe your child, as he may cry because he is hot and sweaty. Your baby may also have a desire to see his surroundings. Many babies (after the age of 6 weeks) are not content lying down with nothing to see. They quiet down when they are propped up so that they can see the fascinating activities going on around them.

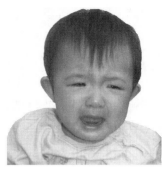

❖ *Activities and personality:* Your child cries to voice what he dislikes (e.g., in dressing or undressing, bathing, etc.). Your child may also feel lonely and want to be picked up and comforted. In young children, excessive crying may be due to insecurity.

❖ *Your own mood and anxiety:* The baby reacts to your own emotions. Some babies seem to sense their mother's anxiety and tenseness, and may cry as a result.

❖ *Independence and control* is especially seen after the age of two years, when your child wants his own way. Ignore the tantrums and do not frustrate him unnecessarily. The amount of crying by a baby commonly represents an interaction between his personality, his developing mind, and the personality of his parents (especially the mother).

❖ *Frustration,* especially when he is trying to do something beyond his capabilities.

❖ *Over-tiredness* (crying is usual): Some babies' cry whenever they are put to sleep. The baby discovers that when he cries, he is picked up and taken to his parents' bed. This usually forms into a habit of crying every night.

❖ *Weaning:* In this stage, much crying is due to efforts to force the child to take food, especially foods that he does not like. He may also cry if he is unable or not allowed to feed himself when he wants to.

Abnormal Causes (Not Related to Nutrition)
The following are some abnormal or organic causes for acute, recurrent, or persistent crying:
- *Infection:* Viral illness, urinary tract infection (UTI), ear infection, Roseola, etc.

- *Trauma:* Fractured bones, child abuse, etc.

- *CNS (Central Nervous System) Abnormality*: Malformation, infections, prenatal asphyxia, increased intracranial pressure, etc.

- *Eyes*: Corneal abrasion, foreign bodies, etc.

- *Cardiac*: Coronary artery defect, rhythm disturbance, heart failure, atypical Kawasaki disease (irritability can be prominent), etc.

- *Digestive*: Appendicitis, abdominal pain, anal fissure, stomach flu, etc.

- *Renal*: UTI, renal disease, etc.

- *Psychosocial*: Parent-infant interaction difficulties, maternal fatigue or depression, etc.

- *Metabolic*: Low sugar, calcium, sodium, etc.

- *Autism*: This is an occasional cause of persistent inconsolable cries.

- *Leukemia*: Bone pain in leukemia is an early cause of irritability and crying.

- *Hernia*

- *Strangulated digit by hair*: Hair is wrapped around your baby's finger or toe.

- *Unrecognized deafness*

- *Skin*: Eczema, hives, etc.

> **Tip: Your child has a hernia and is awaiting surgery**
>
> If he starts to cry suddenly, is vomiting, and swelling is noticed in the herniated area, then see your doctor immediately to ensure there is no strangulation of the hernia content.

Causes Related to Feeding & Nutrition
General Causes

- Causes for crying related to feeding and nutrition can be associated with bottle or breastfeeding (e.g., overabundant milk supply, insufficient milk intake, etc.). General causes may also include hunger and thirst, underfeeding or overfeeding, allergy (e.g., cow's milk, peanuts, etc.), force-feeding, malnutrition, low sugar (hypoglycemia), early solid food introduction, etc.

- Various vitamin and mineral deficiencies may be a cause for crying in your baby including iron, zinc, vitamin A or B6 deficiency, low or high sodium or calcium intake, etc.

- In addition, metabolic (e.g., phenylketonuria), Celiac disease (crying can persist until gluten is excluded), intoxication (e.g., herbal tea, etc.) and water intoxication (e.g., inappropriate preparation of formula, etc.) may cause crying.

Colic & Formula
- Colic usually appears in 25% of all newborns and causes may vary, but it usually disappears around the age of three months.

- In babies fed milk-based formulas, colic may be due to sensitivity to cow's milk protein or sugar. This will cause a build up of gas in your baby's intestine.

- Try the following suggestions, in accordance with consultation of your doctor, to reduce colic when formula feeding:

  ❖ Talk to your doctor about a trial of changing the type of formula your baby is feeding. Try soy-based, extensively hydrolyzed or hypoallergenic formulas (e.g., Nutramigen, etc.).

  ❖ Burp your baby often during feedings.

  ❖ Use a bottle and teat with less risks of air swallowing, since many babies swallow a lot of air during a feeding.

  ❖ Do not overfeed your baby by placing a bottle in his mouth every time he cries.

Colic & Gastroesophageal Reflux
- Gastroesophageal Reflux (GER) is when stomach acids are regurgitated into the esophagus, causing inflammation (esophagitis) and pain in your baby.

- GER is one of the most common medical causes of colic.

- About 1/3 – 1/2 of all babies experience some form of reflux during the first three months of life, however most babies outgrow reflux by seven to nine months of age.

- Try the following suggestions to ease your baby's discomfort:

  ❖ Keep your baby sitting upright for about a half-hour after a feeding.

  ❖ Feed your baby frequently and in small amounts.

  ❖ Do not overfeed or underfeed.

  ❖ Positioning your baby (see chapter on *GER*).

- In the absence of frequent vomiting, GER is an unlikely cause of infant irritability (see *Gastroesophageal Reflux*).

Breast & Bottle-feeding Related Causes

There are many reasons why babies cry in relation to feedings. Ensure that your baby is gaining weight at an adequate rate. If your child is not gaining weight well, then he may cry because he is still hungry (maybe you are not producing enough milk). Speak to your doctor about these concerns.

- *Milk flow is too slow or too fast*: The baby may gulp and choke with a fast milk flow, or he may want a faster milk flow during a slow let-down.

- *Too much air:* Your baby may swallow too much air during a feeding, causing him discomfort and gassiness. A large flow of milk with a nipple that has a large hole may cause the ingestion of air.

- *Mother's diet:* Your baby is sensitive to your diet (when breastfeeding) and possibly, to a particular food in the diet. As a result, he may spit up, vomit, or have colic, diarrhea, rash, nasal congestion, etc.

- *Other foods in the baby's diet:* These are foods other than breast milk or formula such as herbs, teas, solids, juice, drugs, vitamins, etc.

- *Feedings:* The baby may cry if he is not satisfied with a feeding (e.g., wants more). He may also cry after a feeding session to indicate that he may need to burp.

- *Switching breasts too quickly* may cause your baby to receive more lactose in the milk, leading to fussiness.

- *Gastroesophageal reflux, teething, and stuffy nose* are all contributing causes to crying.

Tip: *Support for the Tired Parent*

Ask for help from family and friends with your crying or fussy baby.

Try to rest at least once per day when your baby is asleep or being taken care of.

Know when the most difficult time is for your baby, and plan ahead to take care of him.

Do not feel bad about yourself as a parent and do not be discouraged if your efforts seem to have no effect. With time and patience, things will change.

Arrange home delivery of food and other necessary items.

Suspecting a Cause

- In the early months of life and with time, you will learn to suspect or know the possible causes of your baby's crying. The following are some examples of various types of cries and their meaning:

    ❖ *Hunger Cry:* This cry usually starts off slowly and builds up to a loud cry. Hunger cries are usually seen about two hours after the last feeding, so feed your baby when he is hungry (on demand, rather than on a schedule). There are warning cues, so feed him before he starts to cry.

    ❖ *Pain Cry:* This cry begins almost like a scream and then is suddenly followed by short gasps. Pain cries require immediate attention, since your child is most likely in some sort of pain. Consult your doctor if it seems persistent.

    ❖ *Upset Cry:* This cry sounds like a fussy, irritable, and mild cry meaning that your baby is upset about something such as tiredness, comfort ability, wants the pacifier, is upset by his environment, soiled diapers, gas or burping, etc. Try to soothe your baby by holding and rocking him.

- When determining the cause of a baby's crying, a doctor has to assess the relationship the baby has with the mother. Attachment, anxiety, family stress or breakdown, poor partner support, child abuse or tiredness, etc., are all related. This is important, since studies have proven that crying tends to diminish when parents hold or carry their babies more often and/or breastfeed on demand.

- Crying and irritability should be taken more seriously when comforting and consoling methods fail to remedy the situation.

- Other aspects to consider that may help in determining the problem include:
    ❖ When the baby is fussy (during or after feeding session, day or night).

    ❖ Age of baby (e.g., during the first three months, colic or a growth spurt may cause crying, etc. In a toddler it can be for independence and control, frustration, etc.).

    ❖ New formula or new solid foods.

- ❖ Any symptoms of illness/disease (rashes, fever, vomiting, allergy, etc.).

- ❖ Related feeding issues (e.g., breastfeeding: fast milk flow, slow milk flow, low milk supply; nose blocked, difficulty breathing, gastroesophageal reflux, etc.).

- ❖ Nature of parent and child bonding.

Measures to Control the Fussy Baby

The following are suggestions to help you ease your baby's crying and discomfort:

- Nurse your baby on demand, rather than on schedule.

- Burp your baby frequently to avoid a build-up of gas.

- Change his diaper.

- Cuddle your baby for comfort, and if this fails, then your baby could be hungry or thirsty.

- Carry your baby in a sling, if possible.

- Give your baby a stomach or back rub to relieve possible gas or pain.

- Reduce the amount of noise surrounding your baby, since this may cause your baby to be upset.

- Play some music to see what your baby prefers to listen to, or sing to your baby to calm him.

- Give your baby a bath.

- Rock or hold and gently bounce your baby to provide security while playing with him.

- Soothe your baby with a pacifier or your finger.

- If your baby wants to be carried all the time, simply minimize separations from his mother and stay in sight. This ensures that your baby knows you are there for him without having to always carry him.

- Take your baby for a walk outside for fresh air.

- Do not give your child any herbal remedies, since they will likely cause more gassiness or problems in your baby (many herbs are toxic to infants).

- Know when your child is tired and put him to sleep. Signs of tiredness may include frowning, arms and legs flailing, crying, clenched hands, etc.

Tip: Simethicone Drops

These medications (mylicon, ovol) are sometimes given to gassy babies, since they break down gas bubbles trapped in your baby's stomach and intestines. These are proven to be safe for babies; however they have not yet been proven to be truly effective in reducing the amount of gas passed by your baby.

Parent Concerns

Is it possible for me to know the problem according to the type of cry that occurs?

- In time, you will be able to learn your baby's reasons for various types of cries.

- Many times, there are no clear reasons for a baby's crying and you may not be able to identify the cause, especially when the baby is still a young infant.

- Also, infants and toddlers sometimes have episodes of persistent crying with no symptoms of illness. When the baby is taken to the doctor to be examined, no medical reason is found. In such cases, the reason is unclear and since, the baby calms down after a few hours, there is no need to do anything.

- Cries that occur after a feeding session with no other clear symptoms might be related to feeding, whether it be formula or breast milk.

How do I know if my baby is crying because he is sick?

- This type of cry is often, but not always, accompanied by other symptoms of illness. It is sometimes difficult for parents to know, so speak to your doctor anytime your baby's cry seems different than usual (especially if it is persistent).

My baby is neurologically impaired and has a strange cry. Is this normal?

- Babies with cerebral irritabilities, asphyxia, meningitis, etc., have a shrill, high-pitched cry.

- Some neurologically impaired infants may be feeble, whiny, intermittent, or sharp and piercing in their cries.

- Infants with hypothyroidism may have a weak, low-pitched cry.

- Infants with congenital heart disease or muscular weakness disease, stridor/laryngitis, etc., have a weak or hoarse cry.

How do I know if my baby is allergic to milk, if he has no other symptoms other than crying?

- Allergy to milk is not easily diagnosed and symptoms may be mild and unnoticed. Some of the following may help in diagnosing a milk allergy:
  - ❖ Mucus and blood in the stool.
  - ❖ Family history of allergy.
  - ❖ Baby has any other allergies (e.g., eczema).
  - ❖ Occasional regurgitation/vomiting.
  - ❖ Recent change in formula (e.g., breast milk to formula).
  - ❖ Maternal diet when breastfeeding (mother consumes excessive dairy products).
- Your doctor will need to rule out possible causes of crying. Your doctor may recommend a weeklong trial of extensively hydrolyzed, hypoallergenic formula (e.g., Nutramigen, etc.) be tried to see your baby's response.

My baby was crying for a few hours until I removed a piece of hair that was tight around his finger.

- When a hair is tied around your baby's fingers or toes, it is called Tourniquet Syndrome.
- This leads to less blood circulation, irritability, redness, swelling in the area and, in rare situations, amputation of the affected area. It may be the reason your baby was crying.
- In such cases, remove the hair from the area gently and see your doctor immediately.

My baby cries when he has bowel movements and until recently, he has had hard stools.

- This is probably an anal fissure, which is a small tear that develops in the opening wall of the anus. It is usually associated with constipation; when hard stools pass through the opening, they cause a crack in the lining of the anal opening which leads to inflammation.

- Often, your baby will cry when he is passing bowel movements due to pain from the fissure, and blood may be seen covering the surface of his stool.

- When the child is older, he may hold off passing the stool due to pain, which leads to a vicious cycle of retention, cracking, and pain. Holding the stool can prevent healing.

- Treatment of an anal fissure is like that of constipation (see *Constipation*). Your doctor may add anti-inflammatory cream/pain relief medication to soften the stool and you will need to keep the area clean after bowel movements.

Tip: Crying Helps (according to some experts)

You need to allow your baby to let out his cries to relieve tension.

Tears and crying are one response to relieve the body's energy and stress hormones.

An examination of tears showed the elimination of stress hormones. It helps to stabilize chemicals in the brain after an upsetting episode.

If you accept your child's crying and support it, he will have high self esteem as he feels you accept him unconditionally.

How should I behave when my baby cries?

Help relieve your child's tension and do not block his cries since he may learn that crying is unacceptable (as an adult this may lead to self-destructive behavior such as smoking to prevent crying). The following suggestions are how you should behave when either your infant or toddler cries:

Infant

1) Assess his needs (e.g., thirst, hunger, gas, etc.).

2) Comfort your baby by holding him and looking him straight in the eyes (this lets him know you are there for him). If he turns away, ask him to look at you and to feel secure with you.

3) Take deep breaths and relax.

4) Talk to your baby and tell him that everything is okay and that it is okay to cry.

5) Continue holding your baby until he stops crying.

Toddler (words usually replace toddler's cries)

1) Assess his needs and why he is crying.

2) Stay near your child (it is not really necessary to hold him), but show him you are there.

3) Do not send him to his room for crying.

4) Passively listen to your toddler and discuss with him how he feels at that moment, so that you can try and help him.

- Comforting your baby is not spoiling him. Studies have shown that when parents respond to a baby quickly, he often cries less and feels more secure. A baby who is fussy or crying may just want more contact or love from his caregivers.

Case Description

Simon is a 25-day-old boy who was breastfed for his first 2 weeks. His mother then decided to completely stop breastfeeding and started Simon on cow's milk based formula.

Every time Simon's mother fed him, he began to cry, bent his legs towards his abdomen, and occasionally vomited and regurgitated.

His mother described his stool as "jello" with no blood noticed. She also stated that Simon seemed more gassy and cranky. On examination, Simon seemed to be gaining weight well with no abnormalities.

He was suspected to have cow's milk allergy (a cow's milk based formulas was used) and was switched to extensively hydrolyzed, hypoallergenic formula (Nutramigen). After making the switch to a different formula, Simon's symptoms disappeared and he continued to thrive well. When Simon reached 10 months of age, a skin allergy test confirmed his milk allergy.

Conclusion

- Crying is a common way of communication and a way of relieving tension and/or anxiety for your baby.

- While it may be due to simple environmental causes (e.g., diaper change, temperature, etc.) and comfort reasons, crying may also be due to organic or abnormal causes.

- It is important to know your baby's cries and his needs so that you can respond appropriately when he cries. However, when you notice an unusual cry, with or without other symptoms, you must seek medical advice. Some causes may require your doctor to run laboratory tests, x-rays, or other modes of diagnosis.

- Do not assume blame for cries, which seem to be unclear or have no reason.

- See the doctor when:

  ❖ Feeding and sleeping problems occur past three months of age.

  ❖ There is no response when parents attend to crying.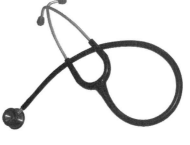

  ❖ He does not enjoy any type of play.

  ❖ The mother lacks sympathy for her child or makes crude comments.

  ❖ The mother does not bond with her baby or does not follow the doctor's advice.

  ❖ The mother experiences anxiety, depression, anger, etc.

  ❖ There are family troubles or breakdown, etc.

Section 6:
Food Allergy
& Food Safety

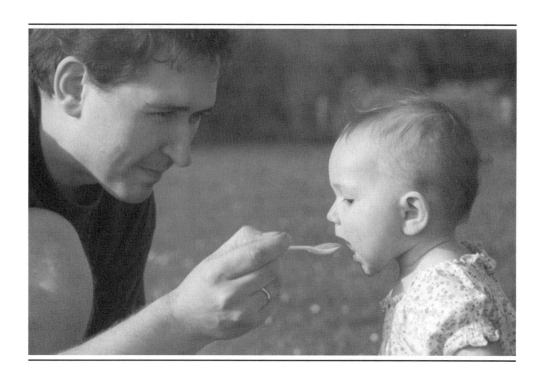

Feeding & Food Allergy

General

*F*ood allergies are a response by the body's immune system to food components that it identifies as foreign (e.g., milk protein). When a child has an allergy, the immune system overreacts by producing antibodies against the allergen. Once produced, these antibodies will react with special cells called mast cells (found in the lining of the nose, lungs, skin, and digestive tract). These release various chemicals, producing symptoms in different body parts. Most commonly, allergy symptoms can be tolerable while in some cases, symptoms may be severe (e.g., breathing problems, shock, etc.) and, rarely, life threatening.

About 80% of true food allergies manifest upon first exposure. For this reason, it is important to introduce new foods one at a time, so that you have a good idea of what your child is reacting to. There are also common non-food allergens that children can react to, which include pollen (tree, grass, weeds), molds, dust mites, animal products (e.g., dander), latex, drugs, etc.

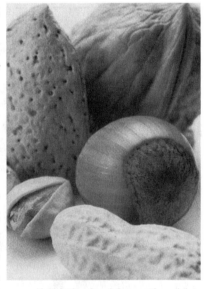

Food allergies are most common in the first few years of life and decline over the first decade. Within the first year, 2-3% of babies will have cow's milk allergy, 1.3% will be allergic to eggs, and 0.5% to peanuts. Infants have an 8% chance of having some sort of allergy, while the incidence in older children is 1-2%. By the age of one year, 50% will lose their allergy to milk; by the age of two years, 70% will lose their allergy, and, by the age of three years, 85%. "Transient" food allergy is typically seen with foods such as milk, soy, wheat, and eggs. When a food allergy does not disappear by five years of age, the chances are that it is a "persistent" food allergy. "Persistent" food allergies are typically seen with peanuts, tree nuts, fish, seafood, and sesame.

The types of foods that most commonly cause food allergy depend on the geographic area. For example, there is a higher incidence of allergy to soy in Japan, peanuts in the United States, fish in Scandinavia, etc. Within North

America, the following six foods account for 90% of food allergies in children: cow's milk, eggs, peanuts, wheat, soy, and tree nuts. With increased exposure to ethnic cultures, the spectrum of food allergy broadens.

Food intolerance is defined as the adverse reaction to food that results in symptoms that are not caused by the immune system (e.g., lactose intolerance). The digestive system is often involved, with resulting discomfort in the stomach and bowels. Food intolerance can be unpleasant, but it is rarely life threatening.

With food allergy, a child can react to a small amount of food (e.g., crumbs left on a fork) while food intolerance, unlike allergy, is dose specific (i.e. a child can tolerate small amounts of the particular food, but will have problems with larger amounts).

Common Food Allergies

Various foods may cause allergies in your child including fish, meat, corn, peas, tomatoes, strawberries, lentils, etc. The following are the most common food allergies noticed in children:

Eggs
- 80-90% of children with egg allergy will develop symptoms upon first exposure, while 76% of children will appear with symptoms after one hour.
- In a child with eczema, the prevalence of egg allergy is about 30%.
- About 44% of children will resolve their egg allergy by three to four years of age (see *Eggs*).

Wheat
- Wheat allergy is due to the protein in wheat (grain allergy is uncommon).
- Anything containing wheat flour (e.g., bread, pasta, cake, meat, etc.) should be avoided and replaced with rye, corn, rice, etc. (watch for labels containing hidden ingredients such as wheat flour).
- When you introduce cereals and breads to your child, you also introduce wheat for the first time, which is a potential allergen (especially when there is family history of wheat allergy).
- Wheat allergy usually resolves within the first few years.

Peanuts
- Peanuts contain about 28% proteins, 50% oil, 18% carbohydrates, and 4% ash.
- It is the most risky allergy, as it may cause anaphylactic shock.
- Most children (about 50%) will react to peanuts upon first exposure or contact.
- 90% of children with peanut allergy will have skin symptoms and 40% will have respiratory symptoms.
- Nuts and peanuts are not in the same family, but those with peanut allergy should avoid tree nuts, due to cross contamination. Tree nuts are also a common food allergy; these include almonds, Brazil nuts, pecans, pine nuts, pistachios, and walnuts.
- Pure peanut oil should be avoided.
- Touching peanuts and kissing someone who has consumed peanuts may trigger an allergic reaction.
- 25% or more of children outgrow peanut allergies by the age of six years (those with low allergic reactions).
- Medically retest for peanut allergy after two years, to see if it has been outgrown.

Cow's Milk & Formula
- Some formulas contain cow's milk or soy proteins to which your baby may be allergic.
- Your child may develop allergic symptoms upon exposure to products containing milk (e.g., milk based formula, cereal, etc.).

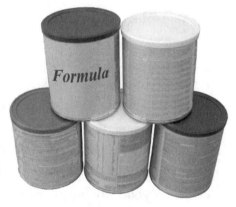

- Exclude milk and its products from your child's diet and from the mother's diet (if the mother is breastfeeding).
- Use substitute formulas such as soy bean formula (if not allergic to soy) or hypoallergenic extensively hydrolyzed formula.
- Do not use goat's milk, because of its similarity to cow's milk (see *Cow's Milk*).

- The American Academy of Pediatrics and the Canadian Pediatrics Society do not recommend the use of soy formula as a measure to prevent future allergies.

Cereal
- A number of cereals are reported to cause allergic reactions in sensitive children.
- Your child may be allergic to any type of cereal including wheat, rye, barley, oats, corn, and rice cereal.
- Sometimes, a child can react to more than one type of cereal.
- Some cereals contain additional cow's milk based formula, so if your infant is allergic to milk, then she may react to the cereal.

Causes
- Allergies may occur at any age. The cause is still unknown, but genetics play a major role in the development of an allergy.
- Some children are more likely to develop allergies due to strong hereditary links. Thus, when the parent has an allergic condition, the child is more likely to have an allergy problem.
- Allergic conditions that seem to run in families include hay fever, asthma, eczema, and food allergies.
- The following are the chances (out of 100%) that your baby will have a food allergy in relation to family history:
  - ❖ Up to 72%, if both parents have the same type of allergy.
  - ❖ Up to 43%, if both parents have different types of allergy.
  - ❖ Up to 32%, if one sibling is allergic.
  - ❖ Up to 20%, if one parent is allergic.
  - ❖ Up to 12%, if no parents are allergic.

Adverse Reactions to Food

Adverse reactions may occur after eating particular foods, including:

- Food Poisoning
  - ❖ This occurs when you eat contaminated food. You can develop vomiting, diarrhea, and abdominal pain soon after exposure to these contaminated foods.

- Enteropathy
  - ❖ This occurs particularly after the ingestion of milk (e.g., cow's milk, formula, or cereal with cow's milk) or soy in the diet.
  - ❖ It usually manifests with vomiting, diarrhea, and abdominal pain. It is not an allergic response (milk allergy tests are usually negative).
  - ❖ Treatment includes the elimination of any milk based products or soy products (if sensitive to any of these) in the diet. Most children recover spontaneously within two years.

- Food Intolerance
  - ❖ Food intolerance mostly involves the digestive system. It does not involve the immune system and it is not an immunologic type of reaction.
  - ❖ Symptoms include vomiting, diarrhea, bloating, and stomach pain. These symptoms develop after the ingestion of a large amount of the same food.
  - ❖ The patient may be able to tolerate smaller amounts of the food without experiencing any symptoms whatsoever (e.g., lactose intolerance).
  - ❖ Food intolerance is more of a delayed reaction and is not usually life threatening.

- Food Allergy/Food Hypersensitivity
  - ❖ This is when the immune system responds to specific foods ingested (usually, more than one system is involved such as skin, respiratory, digestive, etc.).
  - ❖ Reactions can be life threatening and immediate (right after eating the particular food).

- Oral Allergy Syndrome/Fresh Fruit Syndrome/Food Pollen Allergy Syndrome
  - ❖ Some reactions to fruits, vegetables, and nuts occur more often among individuals with pollen sensitivity and those allergic to grass and ragweed. The allergens (the substances causing the allergy) contained in fruits and vegetables are sensitive to heat, thus symptoms occur only with raw foods.
  - ❖ Symptoms appear after a few minutes of eating fresh fruits, raw vegetables, or nuts and include itchiness of the mouth, throat, roof of the mouth, and, sometimes, abdominal discomfort.

❖ Symptoms last 20-30 minutes and then disappear spontaneously. If this happens, spit the food out and rinse the mouth immediately (1-2% of patients respond with a life threatening reaction such as anaphylaxis).

❖ Common fruits that cause fresh fruit syndrome include peaches, apricots, bananas, apples, and cherries. It also occurs after the ingestion of almonds, hazelnuts, kiwi, carrots, celery, parsnips, tomatoes, etc.

❖ If the fruit is heated or frozen, symptoms do not usually occur.

❖ Cooked, canned, and microwaved fruits and vegetables are usually well tolerated, except for cooked celery, which can sometimes cause a severe allergic reaction.

❖ The oral allergy syndrome tends to occur in older children and is almost always preceded by pollen allergies (grass, trees, ragweed).

❖ It is common for patients to have seasonal allergies due to the cross reaction between the protein in the food and the pollen.

❖ An allergy test must be done with fresh fruits, vegetables, or nuts to confirm the allergy.

Allergy Symptoms

- Usually, an allergy occurs within 20-60 minutes of ingestion or exposure to food. However, the reaction may also occur two hours after ingestion and sometimes longer (rarely).

- The onset of symptoms with allergy is rapid and will usually disappear within four hours (and no more than six hours). Delayed development of symptoms of the digestive system develop several hours to a few days after food has been ingested and may be due to a non-immunologic reaction or food intolerance.

- Symptoms include one or more of the following: hives around the mouth and other areas of the body (face, eyelids, lips), swelling (in lips, tongue, eyelids), wheezing, hoarse voice (stridor), vomiting, diarrhea, and shock. A complete collapse (fainting, losing consciousness, and risk of death) may occur in severe reactions (anaphylactic reaction).

- *Anaphylaxis* is an extreme response to allergy that usually occurs immediately after exposure (sometimes, it happens up to two hours after ingestion). In severe situations (besides hives), the following may occur: swelling in the face and lip, vomiting, difficulty breathing, shock (decreased blood pressure, lethargy, etc.) that may lead to death. If an Epipen is available, it may help control this reaction (see following treatment suggestions).

- It is important to remember that food allergies may not include hives and that not all symptoms occur in the same individual in the same order of appearance. It may vary from person to person, type of food ingested, and the specific episode.

- Food allergies can manifest in various organs of the body and in different forms. There may only be one symptom (e.g., rash) or a combination of symptoms. Sometimes, it can be manifested by crankiness alone.

- Organ specific symptoms of food allergy include the following:

  ❖ *Respiratory* symptoms include a runny and congested nose, shortness of breath, and wheezing.

  ❖ *Skin* related symptoms include a rash, hives, redness, itching, and swelling.

  ❖ *Digestive* system symptoms may include vomiting, diarrhea, abdominal pain, swelling of the lips, and tingling of the mouth.

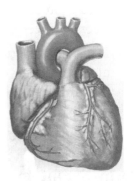

Tip: Hives or Urticaria

Hives are a rash of smooth, raised, pale welts surrounded by an inflamed (red and itchy) area of the skin. They come in various sizes and in various parts of the body, disappearing from one spot to occur in other spots quickly. By the time the child is brought in to see the health professional, the rash can disappear and reoccur later, usually lasting a few days. On rare occasions, the rapid onset of hives may signal an upcoming severe reaction (e.g., anaphylactic shock).

There are two main types of hives:
- Acute is the most common and lasts days to weeks (usually less than six weeks). Triggers may include a virus (e.g., cold), drugs, foods, insect stings, etc.
- Chronic hives last longer than six weeks and may occur almost daily for months to years. In 95% of cases, the cause is not identified and allergic testing is usually not helpful in identifying the cause.
- Seek medical treatment if your child has swelling of the face and mouth, makes noise, or has trouble breathing and difficulties swallowing.

Diagnosis

- The information (e.g., symptoms, history, etc.) you provide your doctor leads him to suspect allergy (or something else).

- Allergy testing reveals which foods cause allergic reactions in your child.

- If your child is taking medication and needs to do an allergy test, then talk to your doctor first, as your child may need to stop the medication for a period of time prior to the test (medications such as antihistamines may affect the test results).

- There are various allergy tests that can be done and these include the following:

  ❖ A *Prick Test* is the most common, simple, and inexpensive test. A small amount of allergen (the extract of a substance that is suspected to cause the allergy) is introduced by pricking the skin with a small needle to discover whether there is local redness or swelling. If the test is negative, then most patients will be able to tolerate the particular food without a reaction. The procedure is fairly painless, reliable, and sensitive. This test can be done at any age; however, reactions may be less pronounced in small children.

  ❖ *RAST (Radioallergosorbent)* measures the level of allergy antibodies (IgE) produced when your blood is mixed with a series of allergens in the laboratory. It is a blood test that is done when the skin test cannot be done. Blood tests can be used if you have eczema or if you are on a medication that cannot be stopped and may interfere with the test results (e.g., antihistamines). They can also be used if you have a history of anaphylaxis or if you just prefer not to have the skin test done. This testing is expensive.

  ❖ The *Immunocap* is a newer version of the RAST and it is used under the same circumstances. Depending on the level of allergen antibodies obtained by the test, your doctor will decide if your child can safely undergo the oral food challenge. The Immunocap is not routinely recommended, as the benefits of this test are still being studied and it is less sensitive than skin testing.

  ❖ *Elimination Diet:* Eliminate the suspected food for two weeks and then, slowly reintroduce it to identify which foods are causing the symptoms. This is only done under medical supervision. Be careful not to eliminate food types for long periods of time without medical advice, as there may be nutritional problems. This method is used when the answer is still unclear after a skin test and RAST results. It is not done with a true allergy. Discuss this method with your doctor.

❖ *Oral Food Challenge Test:* This is done by your allergist only after the blood test is negative and the likelihood of a reaction is negligible. You will be given a small amount (e.g., milk, etc.) to swallow and then, if there is no reaction, you will be given gradual and increased amounts of the same substance. These is done only in hospitals or in appropriate medical settings and performed only when it is absolutely necessary (due to the anaphylaxis risk) to confirm or to disprove allergy.

- Do not self diagnose a food allergy but, rather, talk to your child's doctor.

Treatment

General

- Treatment of food allergy involves three key aspects:

    1) *Avoidance* of the allergen and all foods that contain it, as well as foods with similar allergens that can cause similar allergic reactions (e.g., children allergic to peanuts react to soybeans, peas, or other beans in 5% of cases). Be sure to read labels carefully if you have an allergic child.

    2) *Antihistamines* for mild reactions such as hives, abdominal pain, itchiness, etc.

    3) *Epipen* (epinephrine) and steroid use for severe allergic reactions.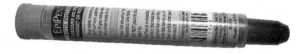

- You may need to consult a dietitian or nutritionist to maintain a nutritionally balanced diet for your child, and dietary supplements may be required along with changes in the breastfeeding mother's diet (e.g., a cow's milk allergy in the breastfed infant means that the mother stops or reduces drinking milk, using cream in coffee, butter on toast, etc.).

- Additional aspects for parents to consider and be better prepared to treat the allergic child are:

    ❖ *Medical*: Anticipate accidental exposure, recognize early symptoms and ensure the availability of treatment.

    ❖ *School*: Provision of a safe environment and training of the supervising staff.

❖ *Social*: Balance vigilance with normalization of activities (do not isolate your child, etc.).

- In addition, parents should watch for imported foods that may not include all the details of what is contained in them, shared utensils and equipment, risk of contaminated products, etc.

Tip: *Medical Alert Bracelet*

Providing your child with a Medic Alert bracelet is also a good way of alerting the ambulance immediately after an allergic reaction.

Epipen
- Epinephrine (or adrenaline) is a hormone produced by the body's adrenal glands in response to stressful situations. The Epipen is the first line of medication used to treat anaphylaxis. The Epipen comes in a self-injectable device, it is available in the junior and adult size (your doctor will decide according to your child's weight, etc.).

- There are also preloaded syringes that contain two doses of Epinephrine (TwinJect). A certain number of patients require a second dose to treat the allergic episode. Also, you may not use the first dose correctly or there may be a defect (in the Epipen; e.g., the auto injector). You may carry the TwinJect which contains two doses of Epinephrine or two Epipens. There are differences in cost, size, and ease of use, so discuss with your doctor what is best for your child.

- Children at risk for anaphylaxis reactions and who may require the use of an Epipen include those who have experienced a severe attack, children with allergies to peanuts, nuts, and shellfish, and children with asthma.

- The use of the Epipen will save your child's life, so be sure to always have it available wherever your child may be (47% of parents with a severely allergic child do not carry the Epipen with them at all times).

- Also, a child who is more than 20 minutes away from the emergency room must always have an extra Epipen. Do not dismiss its importance, as many allergic patients have died because an Epipen was not available to control the reaction.

- If your child goes to any activities that are supervised by another adult (e.g., school, day care, soccer practice, swimming, etc.) where you will not be present, you must be certain that the teacher, baby sitter, etc., knows exactly where the Epipen is, what the symptoms of exposure are, and what to do. Make up an instruction sheet to go over with them. Also, ensure that your child is well educated about her allergy (according to age, of course).

- *Use the Epipen when you begin to see the first signs of a reaction* as symptoms can worsen quickly. The Epipen must be administered immediately (as soon as a reaction occurs). In the case of previous severe reactions, it is recommended to be given immediately after contact with the triggered food, even before any reaction occurs. Once given, medical help should be called for (call 911), even if you see your child getting better (rebound or relapses can occur).

- Inject the Epipen when you see one or more of the following signs:
  - ❖ Rapidly spreading hives and swelling.
  - ❖ Difficulty breathing and tightness of the throat.
  - ❖ Dizziness and feeling faint.
  - ❖ Loss of consciousness.
  - ❖ Gagging or vomiting.

- Repeat use of the Epipen 10-15 minutes after the initial administration if the anaphylactic reaction continues or worsens.

- Side effects of the Epipen include paleness or flushing, dizziness, tremors, weakness, and a rapid heart rate.

- Practice the use of an Epipen with your child in case of an emergency, especially since 60% of those with an Epipen do not know how to use it correctly. Assistance is crucial.

- Watch the expiry date on the Epipen.

- *Three Key Points*:
  1) Epinephrine is the first line medication to be used in emergency treatment of severe life-threatening reactions.
  2) All individuals who receive Epinephrine must be transported immediately to the hospital.
  3) No person(s) should be expected to be fully responsible for self-administration.

> ### Tip: Common Mistakes with Epipen Use
>
> Epipen is not always available and carried everywhere with your child.
>
> Not teaching your child (when age appropriate) and caregiver(s) to use the Epipen.
>
> Injecting the wrong end of the Epipen.
>
> Pressing the Epipen too softly or not pressing it hard enough.
>
> Inappropriate handling and holding each end of the Epipen.

Prevention

There is no proven method to prevent allergy. However, the following may help, especially when there is family history of allergy (causing a higher risk in babies):

- Maternal lactation diet should probably not include peanuts and tree nuts. Also, consider eliminating eggs, cow's milk, and fish.

- Breastfeed as long as possible in the first year, since cow's milk causes more allergies. If you are not breastfeeding exclusively, use extensively hydrolyzed hypoallergenic formula.

- Introduce cow's milk as late as possible. If an allergy still occurs, use hypoallergenic or extensively hydrolyzed formula, as soy formulas may still cause an allergy.

- Delay the introduction of solid foods—begin after the age of six months.

- Wait a longer time (about a week) after introducing other new foods.

- Use less allergenic food first, such as the following:

  - ❖ Rice cereal first, then oats and barley.

  - ❖ Most vegetables and fruits do not cause a problem, but wait with tomatoes, berries, beans, and peas.

  - ❖ Wait longer to introduce shellfish.

  - ❖ Other foods that may cause allergies, such as nuts, peanuts, spices, and chocolate, are best introduced after the age of three years.

  - ❖ Delay introducing highly allergenic foods such as milk, peanuts, tree nuts, fish, eggs, etc.

Case Description

Ely was a five month old baby who was fed Isomil formula since birth. His mother brought him to the office because of sudden vomiting, blue lips, and lethargy, but no rash or swelling was present. This reaction occurred after Ely was fed oatmeal cereal.

After examining Ely, there seemed to be no source of infection. He did not look well, but the vomiting stopped after three hours and color returned to his face. Ely seemed normal several hours after eating the oatmeal cereal.

The mother was told that Ely probably had a milk allergy and that it was best not to use milk until he reached the age of one year. Ely continued on his usual Isomil formula and his parents were told that when he begins solid foods, they must read each label to ensure his food did not contain any milk products.

One month later, the mother tried giving Ely a cow's milk based formula and organic rice cereal. After one hour, the same symptoms occurred. Ely was rushed to the emergency room and discharged after a few hours. This second episode confirmed that Ely did, in fact, react to milk, as both the oatmeal cereal and the cow's milk based formula had milk products in them. A specialist then did a milk allergy test, but it did not confirm a milk allergy.

There is a condition called milk enteropathy, whereby the skin test is negative and only digestive symptoms appear with no rash. As a result, it is recommended that Ely not be fed milk or any other milk products until he can be reassessed in a year.

Conclusion: The diagnosis for Ely's symptoms is milk enteropathy. The skin test for this type of response is always negative. Ely was on soy formula, which means that he has an intolerance to milk, but not to soy (as 25% of those intolerant of milk are also intolerant of soy). The mother could have caused a severe reaction in Ely because she did not read the label properly and note that it contained milk products. Many cereals contain an added cow's milk based formula, which may result in a reaction. Another, but very remote, possibility is that Ely has lactose intolerance.

Parent Concerns

Does an allergy risk decrease if the pregnant mother avoids certain allergenic foods such as eggs, soy, or milk?

- Studies on children over their first five years show that a mother's allergen free diet has no influence on whether the child develops allergies.

- If there is family history of allergy to a particular food (e.g., nuts), pregnant mothers may want to avoid this allergen, as the baby has a 1-2% chance of developing the allergy.

- If there is no family history of allergy, it is not advisable to eliminate possible allergenic foods from the mother's diet.

- Speak to your doctor about allergen foods, as it is important for the pregnant mother to maintain a healthy and well balanced diet. Avoiding certain foods may decrease the intake of nutrients needed by the mother.

- Also, when you are breastfeeding and your baby has a specific food allergy, you should avoid eating the allergen during lactation. Trace amounts of the allergen can be transferred to your baby through breast milk.

Is there an ideal age for introducing peanut butter for the first time?
- There is no specific age for introducing peanut butter for the first time, unless there is family history of allergy, atopy, eczema, etc.

- Peanuts are a highly allergenic food and care should be taken when first introducing it to your child.

- The usual recommendation is to wait until your child is old enough to verbalize any arising symptoms, or later than three years of age, especially if there is family history of peanut allergy.

Does it matter when new foods are introduced in respect to allergy risk?
- Many books state that parents should wait three to seven days between new food introductions, however, in most cases, it is probably overkill. An allergic reaction is, usually, immediate upon first exposure; in a small number of cases, it can be delayed by a few hours or days (e.g., cow's milk allergy). About two days is sufficient, but consult your doctor in respect to your own unique child.

- The delay in introducing new foods should be considered along with these two aspects; the family history of allergy and high-risk allergen foods such as milk, soy, wheat, eggs, fish, and peanut butter.

What about Celiac disease and sensitivity to gluten?
- Gluten is a protein found in wheat, rye, barley, and oats.

- Children with Celiac disease are usually sensitive to gluten. It causes damage to the internal lining of the intestine, which leads to difficulties absorbing nutrients.

- The child may experience diarrhea, green stool, irritability, poor weight gain, etc.
- A gluten free diet usually works very well for the child with Celiac disease.
- Celiac disease is called an "occult" (or hidden) disease, which means that the child may grow poorly without showing any symptoms, except slow growth or slow weight gain. This is the reason why it may be detected at an older age.

Is there a link between allergy and hyperactivity?
- There is no clear link established between a specific food and hyperactivity. If you believe that consuming a specific food clearly shows any visual symptoms or behavior changes, avoid it and discuss your observations with your doctor.

I think my child has outgrown her allergy. Can I offer the allergenic food without talking to my doctor?
- No, you can never give your child the allergenic food at home without first discussing it with your doctor. If your child has outgrown it, a skin allergy test will be done to confirm this and, when re-offering allergenic food, it must be done under supervision (e.g., hospital, doctor's office, etc.).

Can nasal congestion be a sign of allergy?
- There are various symptoms associated with allergy, as stated in this chapter.
- Nasal congestion can be among these symptoms. However, there are many other reasons for nasal congestion beside an allergy (most often, the common cold).
- In persistent or severe cases of nasal obstruction/congestion, talk to your doctor about the possibility of an allergy and assess other associated symptoms.

Can stomach pain be associated with allergy?
- Young children have many reasons for stomach pain.
- Recurrent abdominal pain is common and, most of the time, its cause is non-organic and can be associated with pallor, umbilical pain, etc. Usually, this pain does not wake up the child at night and has no other associated symptoms.
- Pain in the stomach after eating may be due to reflux, ulcer, stomach inflammation, etc.

- Food intolerance may be associated with abdominal pain (e.g., lactose intolerance).

- Your doctor will consider allergy symptoms or evidence of food allergy. He will decide, according to the physical examination and family history, whether to do an allergy test.

Do dark circles under the eyes indicate the possibility of an allergy?

- Dark circles under the eyes can be part of an allergic reaction known as allergic rhinitis. Other symptoms are usually present with an allergic reaction. Dark circles can also occur because of nasal infections, as with the common cold.

Should we use hypoallergenic formula if there is a strong family history of allergy?

- Although some suggest this, it is usually not recommended to start directly with hypoallergenic formula, even if there is a family history of allergy especially since most do well with the standard starter formulas (cow's or soy milk based).

Tip: Assumption of Food Allergies and Formula Change

Symptoms like mild eczema, regurgitation (spitting up), nasal discharge (congestion), constipation or loose stool, colic, vomiting, dry skin, and redness in the cheeks, etc., are common and can be due to various illnesses. Thus, do not automatically assume that these are due to food allergies and change formulas on your own without consulting your doctor.

Can sleep patterns indicate or be affected by allergy?

- Restless sleep may be due to various reasons, depending on your child's age.

- Older children with allergies may have disruptive sleep patterns, while young babies may also sleep poorly due to skin itchiness, abdominal cramps, or other unclear causes and effects of an allergy.

Can a baby be allergic to breast milk?

- Usually, it is not the mother's breast milk that the child is allergic to, but rather the food ingested by the mother (e.g., dairy products, peanuts, etc.).

How long does it take for the food ingested to get to my breast milk?

- While it usually takes four to six hours from the time of ingestion, it may vary from an hour to a day. It depends on many variables such as what food was ingested, how often you nurse, your individual metabolism, etc.

- Some experts suggest that your baby's digestive system is more mature after the age of six months, so that food allergens cannot get through as easily as before.

- Rather than worrying about the food you eat, talk to your doctor if you believe there is a problem.

If my baby has eczema, is she at a higher risk for food allergy?

- People with eczema have a higher incidence of food allergy (1 out of 5). 35% of children with severe eczema have food allergies.

- However, there are foods that can trigger or aggravate the eczema, and avoiding these foods seems to improve the condition.

- At this time, there is not enough evidence that eczema is caused by allergy. 80% of patients with eczema end up with asthma or hay fever.

- Food allergy alone is not as common a cause of eczema as many people think. Even if there is a positive skin test to a food, it does not always mean that a food allergy is the cause of eczema. Proving the relationship may require a food challenge test supervised by your doctor. As such, very restrictive diets are not recommended for the treatment of eczema.

  Comment: A study was done to investigate the effects of breastfeeding on eczema and allergy with 4089 children, up until four years of age. It concluded that breastfeeding for longer than four months may reduce the risk of eczema and allergy for children up to the age of four years (*Allergy & Clinical Immunology*, 116: 657-61, 2005).

How can I differentiate between a cold and real allergy?

- Some children have repeated/frequent colds that prompt parents to ask whether their child has a cold or an allergy, as the child's nose is always running. With colds, the nasal discharge can vary from clear and running to yellow/green and thick. In allergies, it is clear and runny. In colds, sneezing occurs at the start of the cold and is sporadic, while in allergies, it is frequent and usually when in close contact with the allergen (e.g., dust, cat, etc.). In allergies, the eye, nose, and throat are itchy but are less itchy in the cold than in the allergy. Symptom duration is longer with an allergy than with colds (but it can be confusing when a child has frequent colds).

What foods should I watch for if my child has corn allergy?

- Starch, food starch, modified food starch (can be corn starch), vegetable starch, Maize, maltodextrins.
- Corn (fresh, canned, frozen, dried), corn oil, corn syrup.
- Dextrin, fructose, sorbitol, mannitol.
- Caramel colored foods.
- Corn starch is common in baking powder.
- Corn meal is usually used in corn bread, corn muffins, and corn chips.

My child had a rash around the mouth when he came in contact with citrus fruits. Is this an allergic reaction?

- Reactions to citrus fruits can cause contact dermatitis (rash around the mouth upon contact with fruit). This is not considered a food allergy, but develops due to the citrus fruit acidity level. Hold off on citrus fruits until later in infancy when the digestive system is more mature (see *Juices*).

Tip: Food Allergies Website

Check the website www.foodallergy.org as it provides good information about allergies for parents with allergic children.

Water, Fluids, & Drinks

General

Water and fluids are essential for the health of babies and toddlers. Water is the original health drink. It plays a vital role in how the body functions, regulates the body's temperature, moves nutrients throughout the body, and carries waste away in the urine. Water also dilutes the more concentrated waste products of solid foods.

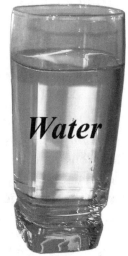

Young babies and toddlers have a greater need for water than anyone else, since they are more susceptible to fluid alterations and electrolyte imbalance. Newborns have greater water content than infants and young children. The surface skin area of newborns and premature babies is 3-5 times as great than that of the older child or adult. This surface area allows larger quantities of fluid to be lost in perspiration from the skin (fluids are usually lost through urine, feces, sweat, and breathing). The infant's metabolism is significantly higher than adults. They are less able to handle quantities of solute free water than older children, due to a relatively immature kidney function at birth. Babies are also more apt to become dehydrated when given concentrated formula. It is important to remember that the younger your baby is, the quicker she can become dehydrated and ill. This is the reason why babies require constant fluids.

Thirst & Recognizing Thirst

- Thirst is defined as a physiological need to drink. It may also be defined as dryness in the mouth and throat leading to the desire to drink. It is regulated by the brain, which sends signals throughout the body that fluid is required. When there is not enough fluid in the body, dehydration may then occur.

- A classic sign of thirst is a dry mouth.

- Children often do not recognize or express their thirst or need to drink. This is further intensified in the young infant where thirst is difficult to recognize. Older children may let you know by requesting "more milk or juice, please."

- After 6 months of age, you may offer water to ensure that your child is receiving enough fluids, particularly in situations where extra fluids may be needed (e.g., hot weather, etc.).

- Even when young children are thirsty, they may ignore the sensation.

- While there are various signs of hunger in infants and children, there is little research on how infants and children express signs of thirst. This is why this matter is confusing for both parents and doctors.

- It is the parents' responsibility to teach their child about the difference between thirst and hunger and how to express each feeling.

- Help them learn the required words and expressions that will allow them to express thirst or hunger (e.g., is your tummy growling or does your tongue feel sticky, etc.).

Sources of Water

- Water comes from breast milk, formula, and juicy foods.

- Until solid foods are started, all water is derived from formula or breast milk.

- The body, through metabolizing carbohydrates, protein, and fat, also produces water.

- A baby who is fed appropriate amounts of calories from breast milk or formula will get enough liquid (in regular conditions, and even in hot weather).

- For the breastfeeding infant or toddler, the mother has to make sure that she drinks appropriate amounts of water. This is to ensure that your breast milk contains enough water content.

- Formula-fed babies obtain water from formula, so be sure to mix the correct amount of water with the formula.

- There is a high concentration of salt and protein in cow's milk, which requires extra water to help get rid of the harmful by-products in the urine (it is another reason why cow's milk is not recommended before the age of one year).

- In the first five to six months, all fluids come from breast milk or formula. After that, it is derived from other sources such as juices, fruits, vegetables, etc. As the total quantity of formula or breast milk decreases, it is important to ensure that the total fluid intake does not decrease.

> ### Tip: *Contaminants in Water*
>
> Do not use water that has been sitting out for a long time (e.g., kitchen counter) and make sure that when using tap water, you let it run for two minutes before giving it to your child to drink, as contaminants accumulate overnight in the pipes. You may boil water for a full two to four minutes to sterilize it. Do not boil for a longer period of time since minerals may become concentrated and dangerous to your baby.

Types of Water

There are various types of water available:

- *Natural Mineral Water*: This is the purest form of water as it is bottled directly from a natural spring, without being pumped or forced. However, it contains high levels of minerals, some of which may be dangerous to your infant (making it unsuitable for infant feedings and formula preparation).

- *Tap Water*: This is the municipal drinking water and can be used for regular drinking water or when preparing formula (needs boiling). For the preparation of infant formulas or infant foods, or for drinking by infants, water from the cold water tap should be used. Water from the hot water tap may contain more lead and other non-biological contaminants because hot water can dissolve or leach them more readily.

- *Well Water*: This type of water comes from a hole that is bored, drilled, or otherwise constructed in the ground, tapping the water of an aquifer. Be cautious with the use of well water, as it may contain high concentrations of various elements (nitrates, fluorides, etc.) and bacteria.

- *Commercially Bottled Non-Carbonated Water*: The only commercially bottled non-carbonated water that is suitable for use by infants is natural spring water, drawn from underground springs (these are unpolluted). However, some spring water undergoes treatment and as such, this water has low mineral content and may be less suitable. Carbonated drinks are best avoided due to their high sugar and acid content, which can erode tooth enamel and lead to tooth decay.

- *Sparkling Water*: This is water that has been naturally carbonated (not suitable for infants).

- *Purified Water*: Purified water is water from which the contaminants have been filtered; it still needs to be boiled. It is also known as demineralized water.

- *Distilled Water*: This water has been completely purified of minerals. For this reason, it is not good to drink it.

- *Home Water Treatment*: Some water treatments increase sodium content and chemical filters can increase silver content or may contaminate water with bacteria. These are not recommended for infant feedings.

- *Bottled Water*: Most of this is not natural mineral water at all, but comes from processed local tap water. This is especially true if the bottle label reads "spring fresh" or "spring pure," etc.

- The best type of drinking water is that bottled directly from a local spring. It will normally read "Natural spring water bottled directly from the source."

- Whatever type of water you use, whether bottled or tap, should be boiled and cooled prior to formula preparation or serving as a drink to babies under the age of six months. Boiling the water kills the bacteria (boil for 5-10 minutes) and you may store it in a sterile container in the refrigerator (no longer than two days).

Tip: Purifying Water

Boiling is the most effective method of purifying water.

Other Beverages & Sweet Drinks

General

- Water contains no calories. This is the best and most recommended drink to quench your child's thirst.

- Other beverages and sweet drinks mainly supply sugar. Besides the calories these drinks provide, they have no special nutritional importance. However, beverages and sweet drinks other than water do provide your child with the satisfaction of a tasty beverage.

- Of course, most children prefer sweet and "fun" or very concentrated juices to plain, boring water.

- Encourage your older child to drink 8-10 glasses of water and other fluids per day.

Fluids Not Recommended

- Beverages with caffeine and theobromine such as coffee, colas, and hot chocolate are not recommended for infants, because they are stimulants.

- Fruit drinks, punch, soda, and sport drinks are also not recommended for your child as they contain high sugar, carbohydrate, inappropriate salt levels, and less of other important nutrients.

- Beverages with artificial sweeteners such as Aspartame are not recommended for infants and small children, since they interfere with other food intakes.

Fruit Juice as a Water Source

- When providing your child with fruit juices (if at all), be sure to use an amount which does not interfere with formula intake or breast milk intake.

- Excessive juice intake contributes to low nutrient and energy intake, causes diarrhea, and either inadequate weight gain or obesity (see *Juices*).

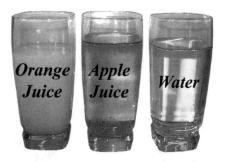

- Certain types of juices are more likely to increase the risk of diarrhea, especially if they contain high contents of sorbitol and/or fructose types of sugars. Dilute the juice when given as a water source (e.g., one part pure fruit juice with the other part cooled, boiled water).

- Also, note that juices are associated with nursing bottle syndrome and cavities.

- To satisfy your child's thirst or anticipated thirst, water is recommended.

Sweet Drinks

- In general, it is not recommended to add sugar or sweetener to drinking water in order to stimulate the baby to drink. Sweeteners are not recommended for young children, since their brains are more sensitive to it than adults. It is also better for the breastfeeding mother not to use any sweeteners for safety reasons (which are currently unclear, pending more research).

- Babies who have been used to sweet drinks will prefer sweet drinks. Those who use unsweetened water prefer the unsweetened water.

- For those children who refuse to drink or in situations of fluid loss, you may sweeten the drink to stimulate the baby to drink (known as "gentle" sweetening).

- It is preferable to combine juices and sweetened drinks in a cup and give these in-between meals, so that they interfere less with healthier nutrient intake.

When to Introduce

General

- Although there are some recommendations as to when water should be introduced, each baby is unique. Due to various factors (e.g., feeding method, weight gain or loss, illness, fluid intake, etc.), this should be discussed with your doctor.
- To complicate matters further, there is not enough research to indicate when infants are thirsty and how thirst should be quenched (e.g., formula, breast milk, water, etc.).

Breast & Bottle-feeding

- Water is added after six months of age, since there is no need to begin giving water before starting solid foods.
- Providing water in the first few days of life has been found to increase the risk and severity of newborn jaundice. Also, giving water in the first weeks of life may interfere with feedings since babies are full of water and drink less milk at feeding time.
- In normal situations, there is no need to add water in the first few months of a baby's life. Remember, formula or breast milk has enough water content. You may sabotage your milk production and cause your baby to fail to gain weight (the stomach does not yet differentiate between water and food; it considers volume), if you provide your child with too much water.
- Some recommend using plain boiled water, offered from time to time in the baby's third month of life, so as to accustom the child to a bottle.
- For the very young formula-fed baby, your doctor may suggest giving your child water in-between formula bottles.
- For older babies, you may offer water or diluted fruit juice in cups or in the bottle.
- Melons, peaches, tomatoes, or other juicy fruits may provide additional fluids.

Age	Introducing Water & Fluids
0-6 Months	There is no need to provide extra water. There is enough water content in breast milk and/or formula.
6-7 Months	Bigger and varied meals are provided at this stage. Your child may want to start drinking. Depends on the environment (how warm or cold is the house, etc.). Warmer environments will cause your child to be thirsty. You may provide extra water supplements and diluted juice (if at all) occasionally.
Sickness (fever, vomiting and diarrhea)	It is especially important to provide your child vomiting with water and food when they are sick. Provide more frequent drinks in small amounts, as suggested by your doctor.

Tip: Basic Point on Starting Fluids

It is suggested starting your child with water and extra fluids around the age of seven months, when she is sitting up well and has begun eating solid foods.

How Much Fluid Your Child Needs

How Much

- When deciding upon how much fluid your child actually needs, various factors must be considered, including her age, size, where she lives, what she eats, and how active your child is.

- There is no exact amount recommended for young babies.

- It is recommended to provide your baby with no more than 2-3 oz/60-90 ml of water at a time and offer it only after the baby has eaten.

- The amount of water that can be used each time increases with age. For example, children between the ages of one and three should have 5 oz/ 150 ml of water each time. Children who are ten years of age can take 9 oz/ 270 ml of water per drink.

- Normal fluid requirements can be estimated per body weight/per day as such:

  ❖ 3.5 oz per 2.2 lb/100 ml per kg for first 22 lb/10 kg of body weight.

  ❖ 1.75 oz per 2.2 lb/50 ml per kg from 22-44 lb/10-20 kg of body weight (in addition to above).

  ❖ 0.7 oz per 2.2 lb/20 ml per kg from about 44 lb/20 kg of body weight (in addition to above).

Excess Water

- Too much water can lead to a serious condition known as oral water intoxication.

- Excess water may cause seizures, low body temperature, bloating, or loss of consciousness, since too much water can dilute the sodium in the baby's bloodstream.

Dehydration

- Dehydration may be defined as a loss of body fluids, which are composed of water and salt. In this condition, your body does not have as much fluids as it should.

- It may be caused by not drinking enough fluids, losing too much fluids, or both (e.g., by vomiting, diarrhea, etc.).

- The most common cause of dehydration in babies and toddlers is the loss of fluids through diarrhea and vomiting, due to infection of the intestine.

- Symptoms of dehydration include decreased urination, dry skin, mouth and tongue, sunken eyes, and a "soft spot" on your baby's head (fontanel) with severe dehydration, elastic-looking skin, and dark, yellow urine.

- It is important to replace lost body fluids immediately when your child is dehydrated.

- If your infant is six months of age or younger and is losing fluids, then give her an oral rehydration solution (e.g., Pedialyte) in small, frequent amounts (1 tablespoon/15 ml every 15-20 minutes). However, if your child is six months of age to a year old, then increase the amount to 1 tablespoon/15 ml every 15-20 minutes (after discussion with your doctor).

- When your child is older than one year and is dehydrated, you may offer small, frequent amounts of clear fluids and/or an oral rehydration solution. Avoid offering any fruit juices or sugary drinks.

Hot Weather & Additional Water

- In hot weather, you may give 1-2 oz/30-60 ml of water between feedings to compensate for water lost in sweating. Most of the time, there is no need for this.

- Until six months of age, nursing more often or adding a little water on very hot days may offer additional fluid.
- Provide your baby with more fluids and water should she be sick (vomiting, diarrhea, fever, etc.) to prevent dehydration, as per your doctor's recommendations.

Developing Water Habits

- Many children prefer to drink fruit juices instead of plain water.
- These drinks supply a lot of calories (up to 35% of their requirement daily), and causes children to have a decrease of appetite for other, healthier foods. This can also contribute to tooth decay. The child will have added dental benefits by drinking fluoridated water.
- Therefore, offer your child water whenever she is thirsty or in-between meals, and have it available regularly throughout the day. This way, your child will not develop a fruit juice habit.
- Limit the use of fruit juice, powders, or granules when preparing drinks for infants.
- Keep bottled water available so that your child can easily use one.
- Set a good example and drink water yourself instead of soda.

Salts

General

- Salts used for cooking are made of sodium and chloride.
- Salt is important for the maintenance of bodily fluids, acidity, and normal nerve functions.
- Salt replacement is needed, since it is lost through sweat and the kidneys. It is also lost through various diseases such as Cystic Fibrosis, where salt can be excessively lost by sweating glands (especially in hot weather), so ensure that your child is taking enough fluids.
- Salt may be retained in the case of kidney disease, where the kidneys are unable to excrete it. The baby's kidneys cannot handle large amounts of sodium (salt).
- Too much salt may be a predisposing factor for later onset of high blood pressure.

- Do not use excessive salt in family foods, to prevent your infant from developing a liking for saltier tastes.

Salt Requirements

Age	Salt Requirements
0-6 Months	No need to add salt; enough is already provided in breast milk or formula.
6-12 Months	Between 250-750 mg/day of sodium. Serve foods that do not exceed this daily amount.
1-3 Years	One gram per day (less than 1/2 spoonful).
4-9 Years	1/2 spoon per day. Remember that many foods contain salt; you do not need to give an actual 1/2 spoonful of salt to your child!

- Requirements are modified depending on the state of your baby and if she presents with illnesses.
- Dairy foods and vegetables contain enough salt for your baby's requirements.

Decreasing Salt Intake
- 75% of salt intake is from processed foods and 10-15% is from natural foods with 5% of salt added during home preparation.
- You may decrease salt intake by doing the following:
  - ❖ Do not add salt when preparing foods.
  - ❖ Do not assume your baby needs extra salt simply because you enjoy it.
  - ❖ Purchase foods with less sodium content (read the label).
  - ❖ Feed your child fewer processed foods.
  - ❖ Use fresh spices with no added salts, as ready made spices have higher sodium content.
  - ❖ Powdered soups should contain no MSG or extra salt.
  - ❖ Low sodium tastes may be acquired gradually by slowly reducing the amount of salt used in foods.
  - ❖ Do not give your child snacks with high sodium or salt content.

- High levels of salt can be found in the following:
  - ❖ Milk products, cereals, legumes, nuts, and seeds.
  - ❖ Bread, cakes, cookies, salty cheese, hot dogs, sausage, hummus, and tuna with oil.
  - ❖ Kosherized meat contains large amounts of salt.
  - ❖ Processed foods can be high in sodium due to high salt content.
  - ❖ MSG is added to some foods (e.g., powdered soup, etc.).
- Small amounts of salt are found in fresh fruits and vegetables.

Other Fluid Issues
Caffeine Effects on Children
- 68% of boys and 62% of girls aged twelve to seventeen years consume one or more caffeinated drink per day.
- 21% of boys and 22% of girls aged twelve to seventeen years drink coffee or tea everyday.
- 26% of children between three to ten years of age drink at least one caffeinated beverage (usually as soda pop) each day.
- Caffeine effects include increased heart rate, high blood pressure, irritability, stomach pain, and interference with fine motor coordination.
- It causes behavior similar to ADHD (attention deficit hyperactivity disorder), frustration, and restlessness. Sleeping difficulties also arise, such as sleeping less over a week (3 1/2 hours less than those not drinking caffeine), and difficulty in falling asleep.
- Caffeine is a diuretic (it makes you urinate more often, potentially causing dehydration).
- In adults, it decreases calcium absorption and is probably has the same effect in children.
- Health Canada recommends a daily limit of 45 mg for four to six year old children, and 62.5 mg for children aged seven to nine and, lastly, 85 mg for children aged ten to twelve years.

Herbal Teas as a Source of Water
Many parents use herbal substitutes for various reasons.
- Herbal teas can contain stimulants, psychoactive molecules, and other active, naturally occurring chemicals, which can have harmful

consequences to a baby. Just because it's natural doesn't mean it's healthy (after all, arsenic and hemlock are both perfectly natural!).

- Herbal tea use is associated with toxic effects in babies and mothers; probably more so for those who drink large amounts of herbal mixtures while breastfeeding.

- At this point, there is not enough research regarding herbal tea safety for babies, pregnant mothers, and the breastfeeding mother.

Water Intoxication
- Excessive amounts of water given over a relatively short period of time may lead to water intoxication. This is manifested by confusion, dizziness, seizures, brain damage, coma, and possibly death.

- Young infants and children are most susceptible to water intoxication.

- It usually occurs in babies given tap water in the form of supplemental feedings or overly diluted formula. Less implicated liquids include juices, sodas, and tea.

- Talk to your doctor about the appropriate use of water in your child's diet.

Tip: Swimming and Swallowing Water

Infants and children who swim may swallow the water in the pool, and this may lead to blurred vision, nausea, vomiting, weakness, seizure, etc. Supervise your child when she is swimming and teach her to close her mouth in the pool.

Parent Concerns

What type of water should I offer my baby when traveling to a country with less sanitary conditions?

- Bottled water is a good choice for your baby when traveling to a country with less sanitary conditions.

- If your baby is bottle-fed, then you should take ready made formula with you. Make sure you wash your hands before handling any formula or equipment (especially after using the washroom). Consider bringing a good supply of sanitizing hand gel.

- Breastfed infants are less of a problem when traveling since the breast will provide the extra water your baby needs, especially in hot weather (as long as the mother is drinking enough fluids).

My 9-month-old baby has diarrhea. Should I dilute her formula?

- During an episode of the stomach flu, your doctor may recommend diluting the formula to provide more fluids to your baby. Diluting the formula decreases the amount of calories and sugar offered.

- You may dilute the formula about 1/2-1/3, but do not do this for more than two to three days, as it decreases the amount of calories your baby receives.

- You may also offer rice, banana, and apple sauce. Avoid offering any juices.

Tip: Diarrhea as a Manifestation of Urinary Disease

Diarrhea is not always a manifestation of the stomach flu; it can also be a manifestation of a urinary tract infection in children below the age of five years.

How do I know when my infant/toddler is thirsty and when she is getting enough fluids?

- As stated previously, a dry mouth is a late sign of thirst.

- Infants who are thirsty will cry, but it is difficult to know the "thirst cry," as there are many different cries.

- If your baby had a feeding session and began to cry, then rule out possible causes for her cry, and offer fluids in case she is thirsty.

- The following are some signs of how to know that your baby is receiving enough fluids:

  ❖ Frequent urination.

  ❖ Urine color (normal urine color is pale yellow; the darker the color, the more dehydrated your child is; the first urine of the morning is usually darker and more concentrated than normal).

- With infants and toddlers it is not possible to always know how frequently your baby urinates since she may urinate in her diaper and it can also be mixed with the stool.

- Also, a breastfed baby who is thirsty will probably regulate her fluid intake by feeding more often and taking in enough of the watery foremilk to satisfy her thirst.

Can I mix oral rehydration solution (e.g., Pedialyte) with formula?

- It is better to use water instead of oral rehydration solution with formula, since the use of oral rehydration solution alters the level of certain minerals.

Why is it important to increase my child's water intake during some illnesses?

- With many illnesses, children lose water due to fever, vomiting, diarrhea, rapid breathing, not drinking much because of pain, etc. It is important to provide extra fluids during this time to prevent dehydration.

My baby is healthy and breastfed. Does she need extra water?

- It is not recommended to offer your baby extra water when breastfeeding, since too much water may interfere with the feeding session (babies nurse less, thus leading to less growth). This may lead to decreased milk production and prevents the establishment of optimal milk supply since your baby is less interested in nursing and milk production depends on supply and demand. However, some studies have shown no effect on breastfeeding mothers and infants when a small amount of supplementary water is provided.

- Breast milk has the water the baby needs, and she is able to regulate her thirst.

- *Newborn Jaundice*: Some studies have shown that giving water to a breastfed infant may increase jaundice (bilirubin) by decreasing the urge to breastfeed, while some other studies have shown no significant differences in respect to jaundice levels and water.

- Infants and toddlers may require extra water when the weather is particularly hot and/or if your child has an illness like stomach flu, diarrhea, constipation, dehydration, etc. Also, the need for additional water increases as your child is being introduced to foods with less water (e.g., meats, etc.) and more fiber.

- Giving a few sips of water to your baby when she is less than six months old will not hurt her. However, if you provide too much water (do not give more than 4 oz/120 ml per day in the first six months), it may interfere with nutrient absorption and, in rare cases, cause water intoxication.

- When giving your baby water, always offer it lukewarm (whether breastfed or formula-fed). Also, use cold tap water and boil and then cool the water prior to giving it to your baby.

Safe Feeding & Food Safety

General

One of the major problems facing parents today is safe feeding and food safety for infants and young children. This chapter focuses on food safety measures and discusses the risks of food poisoning and choking and how to minimize these dangers.

Food Poisoning

General

- Infants and young children are among those most at risk for developing infections or a serious illness from food poisoning, because of their immature immune and digestive systems.

- Hygienic habits, particularly in older infants and children, are not yet developed and increase the risk of infections, as children will have the tendency to touch everything and put it into their mouths.

- Children may develop food poisoning after eating foods that are contaminated by a bacterial toxin or bacteria, such as Salmonella, E. coli, Listeria, Yersinia, etc. Organisms which cause food poisoning are found everywhere (air, soil, water, etc.).

- Symptoms may appear as early as half an hour after eating a contaminated food or as late as several days or weeks after ingestion. Symptoms of food poisoning include diarrhea, stomach pain, vomiting, fever, headaches, drowsiness, decreased urine output, pallor, blood or pus in the stool, rash, etc.

- Food poisoning can lead to serious complications (dehydration, kidney failure, or even death). As such, you should practice strict food safety (e.g., handling, storing, etc.) to decrease the risk of infections.

- If you are uncertain about whether a particular food is safe to eat, throw it out. It is better to be safe than to eat unsafe foods that may cause food poisoning in your child.

Predisposing Factors

Food poisoning and infections may occur from the following situations:
- Food preparation, storage, and feeding techniques:
  - ❖ Foods that are not well cooked (mild heat will not destroy all the bacteria).

552

❖ Storage without refrigeration in a temperature that will allow bacteria to grow (a reason to prepare food prior to feeding, when possible).

❖ Infected and/or unboiled water used in the preparation of formula/food.

❖ Feeding directly from a jar, and then using it to feed from again after it has been left out for a few hours (there will be bacteria growing in the jar from airborne spores and also from your baby's saliva).

❖ Touching your child's diapers while preparing food.

❖ The use of infected utensils and foods such as uncooked chicken, raw eggs, honey, sugar syrup, chicken, fish, meat, and vegetables that are not well cleaned.

- The use of a microwave will not kill all the germs, since different areas of the bottle will warm differently.

- Contact with animals, sick people who have skin lesions, or who are coughing and sneezing places one at risk for bacteria or bacterial toxins.

- Insufficient hand washing technique after using the toilet (salmonella bacteria or streptococcus).

Tip: Salmonella Poisoning & Eggs

To prevent salmonella poisoning, cook all eggs well and do not use products containing raw eggs.

General Suggestions & Hygienic Aspects
- Wash all kitchen utensils, cutting boards, counters, and sinks that are used for raw meat, poultry, or fish (especially when preparing food). Hot water and soap is a great way of cleaning surfaces and you may also use bleach solution or commercial sanitizing products (be sure to dilute to the recommended amount and read the instructions). Only use clean working areas when preparing foods.
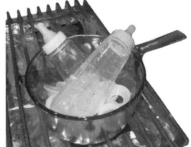
- Wash all fruits, vegetables, meat, and alternatives well under running tap water before and after peeling them to decrease pesticides.

- Prolong the cooking time for meat, chicken, and vegetables to ensure that it is well cooked. Serve foods soon after being cooked and, when that is not possible, store foods in the refrigerator until the next feeding.

- When heating foods after they have been stored, mix the food so that all parts reach a temperature of 70 degrees Celsius.

- Drinking water should be boiled for two minutes until your child reaches the age of one year (see *Water, Fluids & Drinks*).

- Do not store any foods in cabinets under the sink as insects and rodents can enter. Do not store food in painted ceramic or lead crystal containers since these can contain lead that may leach into the food (lead poisoning).

- Use a dishcloth instead of a sponge. Dishcloths can be washed regularly in hot water to kill germs. Sponges provide an environment for bacterial growth since they stay moist.

Hand Washing

- Hand washing is an important habit to learn for both parents and children.

- Always wash your hands before cooking, feeding your child, giving medications, after changing diapers, helping the child use the toilet, using the toilet yourself, handling pets or animals, wiping your child's nose and when taking care of a sick child.

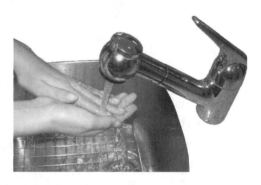

- Your child should always wash his hands (wash the hands for the infant) before eating or handling foods, after a diaper change, using the toilet, playing outdoors (especially in sand), and when playing with pets or animals.

  1) Make sure to use liquid soap from a container and mix it with water to cleanse properly.

  2) Rub your hands together while you are washing them for a count of 5. Wash in-between your fingers, the backs of your hands, etc.

  3) Dry your hands with towel paper and throw it into the garbage (one that opens with a foot pedal).

Refrigerating & Freezing Foods
- Refrigerating foods safely:
  - ❖ Keep the refrigerator at 41 F/5 C or lower.
  - ❖ Refrigerate hot foods immediately (within two hours after being cooked) or you may allow them to cool slightly before refrigerating. Refrigerate homemade baby food for no longer than 24 hours.
  - ❖ Leave eggs in their original carton and refrigerate them.
  - ❖ Store vegetables and fruits in refrigerator drawers.
  - ❖ After cutting meat and poultry into small pieces, place them in the refrigerator or freezer immediately.
  - ❖ When refrigerating raw meats and poultry, wrap them and place them in containers to keep their juices from contaminating other food.
  - ❖ Thaw baby food in the refrigerator.
  - ❖ Open the refrigerator doors only when necessary and close them immediately. Always keep the refrigerator doors tightly closed.
  - ❖ Clean away any spills in the refrigerator immediately.

- Freezing foods safely:
  - ❖ Keep the freezer temperature at 0 F/-18 C or lower.
  - ❖ Freeze homemade baby foods (pureed fruits, vegetables and meats) in clean ice cube trays then place the frozen cubes into smaller freezer bags for later use.
  - ❖ Cover anything placed in the freezer well with plastic wrap.
  - ❖ Label and date all freezer bags with masking tape.
  - ❖ Do not keep baby food in the freezer for longer than two to three weeks.
  - ❖ Avoid freezing commercially prepared baby food.
  - ❖ Baby food that has been thawed must never be refrozen.

Choking
General
- Choking may be defined as swallowing a foreign object that blocks the airways to the lungs.
- According to the Centers for the Disease Control and Prevention (CDC), the highest choking rates occur in babies under the age of one year.

Children have a natural tendency at this stage of life to explore things with their mouths.

- Symptoms of choking include the inability to breathe or cry, ineffective coughs, and if choking continues, your child's face can become blue, she may become limp, convulse, and then become unconscious.

- Choking is a major cause of fatal injury that may occur at anytime and in any location.

Common Foods that Cause Choking
- Common choking hazardous foods include foods that are firm, smooth, and slippery, or are round such as nuts, berries, grapes, and hard candies.

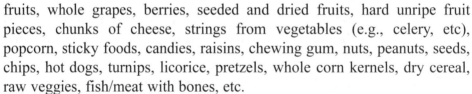

- Do not feed a child who is younger than four years any round, firm food unless it is completely chopped into fine, tiny pieces.

- Nuts should not be given at all to children who are under the age of six years.

- The following are foods that are common choking hazards, so keep them out of your children's reach: raw carrots, peas and fruits, whole grapes, berries, seeded and dried fruits, hard unripe fruit pieces, chunks of cheese, strings from vegetables (e.g., celery, etc), popcorn, sticky foods, candies, raisins, chewing gum, nuts, peanuts, seeds, chips, hot dogs, turnips, licorice, pretzels, whole corn kernels, dry cereal, raw veggies, fish/meat with bones, etc.

Feeding your Child Safely
- Whenever your baby is feeding, make sure she is sitting up. Do not allow any running, walking, or lying down while your child is still eating.

- Supervise your child at all times.

- Try to teach your child how to chew food well from an early age.

- Never hurry your child into finishing his meal quickly.

- Avoid round, firm, chunky, or raw foods (like those mentioned previously).

- Also, avoid stringy foods like celery and string beans.

- When offering your child food, offer only a few pieces at a time.

- Cut meat and poultry into pieces no larger than 1/2 inch/1.4 cm. If you are unsure of the size, cut the food into even tinier pieces.
- The following are suggestions for safe and healthy finger foods: well-cooked baby carrots, well-cooked apple chunks, tofu chunks, avocado dip, soft-cooked peas and beans, O-shaped cereals, whole-wheat toast without any crust, etc.

How to Prevent Choking
- Always observe your infant or child during a feeding. Ensure that they are sitting comfortably during feedings (solid foods should be eaten with your child sitting up with a straight back). Chewing should be encouraged.
- Remove any bones from fish, meat, or poultry.
- Remove grains and/or kernels from fruits such as prunes and apricots.
- Remove seeds from grapes and cut the grapes into small pieces.
- Cut all foods into bite-size pieces and serve in small portions. You may even moisten and soften dry foods.
- Avoid giving your baby round and firm foods such as carrots, celery sticks, grapes, hard candies, meat sticks, and hot dogs.
- Help and encourage your infant to eat food slowly and not be in a rush.
- Maintain a calm and warm meal atmosphere for your child.
- If your child is bottle-fed, make sure that the nipple holes are not too large.
- Only put water, breast milk, or infant formula into a child's bottle.
- Do not give your child solid foods before their time (see *Starting Solid Foods* and *Textured & Table Baby Foods*).
- Do not offer your child any foods when she is crying, laughing, lying down, walking, talking, or playing.
- Avoid feeding your child or allowing her to eat while you are in the car (it is harder to reach a choking child in the car).

Helping the Choking Baby
If your baby should ever choke, try not to panic. Stay as calm as possible and attempt to dislodge the foreign object to help re-open your baby's airway. The following are steps to help the choking baby:

1) Listen to your baby for breathing sounds by watching her chest rise and fall.

2) Do not spend more than 30 seconds listening and watching your baby, especially if you believe she is choking.

3) Have someone call 911 or, if you are alone, call 911 in the process of trying to dislodge whatever is stuck in your baby's throat.

4) Hold your baby on your forearm in a facedown position with her head pointed down to the ground (the baby's body should be firm against your forearm).

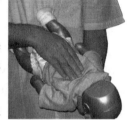

5) Using the palm of your other hand, deliver five firm blows to the back just in-between the baby's shoulder blades.

6) Your baby should begin to cry if the foreign object is no longer blocking her airway.

7) If however, the baby does not begin to cry after the back blows, lay her face up on your other arm. Be sure to support your baby's head with your hands and keep it lower than the trunk.

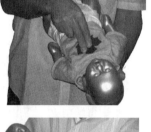

8) Place two to three fingers in the center of your baby's chest and deliver five thrusts (to the middle of the breast bone) in-between the nipples.

9) Raise the middle finger off the chest and use the other two fingers to thrust.

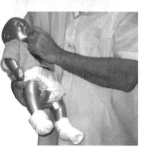

10) Repeat these steps until the object is expelled or the infant becomes unconscious.

11) IF YOUR CHILD BECOMES UNCONSCIOUS, then try the tongue-jaw lift:

   a) Place your thumb in the child's mouth over the tongue.
   b) Wrap your fingers around the jaw and lift her tongue and jaw forward.
   c) Use a hooking action with your finger to remove any visible objects (use one hooked finger to ensure that you will not further lodge the object).

12) If breathing does not resume, then attempt mouth-to-mouth resuscitation. If you look into your infant's mouth and see no sign of a foreign object, try to ventilate the baby with your mouth. Place your mouth over the baby's nose and mouth. Tightly seal your lips and blow

out. The baby's chest should move up and down. If it does not, then move the baby's head and neck into a slightly different position and try giving her one more breath.

13) If your child's airway is still blocked and you cannot get the foreign object out, continue with the back blows and chest thrusts until medical help arrives.

14) Hopefully, you will never be in this situation, but you can take one-day courses on Infant and Child Emergency First Aid through agencies such as the St. John's Ambulance Services.

Helping the Choking Toddler/Older Child

1) If your older child is coughing or is able to breathe and speak, then do nothing. However, if she is unable to do so, then call 911 or have someone else make the call while you are performing the Heimlich maneuver:

a) Stand behind your child and wrap your arms around her waist.

b) Place the side of your fist against your child's stomach (just above the navel and well below the lowest part of the breast bone).

c) Grab your fist with the other hand and press it into the child's stomach with a quick, upward thrust.

d) If necessary, repeat thrusts.

2) If your child becomes unconscious, place the child face up onto the floor and make sure that her head does not strike the floor. Do the tongue-jaw lift mentioned earlier and attempt mouth-to-mouth resuscitation. Give abdominal thrusts: Straddle the child's thigh and place the heel of one hand on the child's stomach (above the navel and well below the lowest part of the breast bone). Place the other hand on top of that hand with your fingers pointed towards your child's head. Give 6-10 quick, upward thrusts.

3) Repeat these steps until the object is dislodged and the child is breathing or until medical help arrive.

Feeding & Safety Tips

Food Safety Suggestions

- Serve food at room temperature, so that the tongue will not get burned.

- Try not to use the microwave but, if you must, be sure to thoroughly stir the food after and test its temperature before feeding the baby.

- Do not serve artificial sweeteners to your baby, since they are used for diet purposes only, which babies do not need.

- Your child should sit comfortably in a high chair when eating.

- To prevent botulism, do not feed honey to a child less than the age of one.

- Seal and store homemade foods properly. Ensure that safety seals have not been opened before. Remember to carefully cover and refrigerate all unused foods.

- When you travel with your baby, store bought baby foods may offer better safety than homemade foods (this prevents the chance of bacterial growth).

- Do not feed or use products with raw egg, and only give eggs after one year of age.

- As much as possible, keep away from processed foods with chemical additives.

- Delay serving your child peanuts until the age of four years.

- Make sure that all pot handles are turned in towards the back of the stove, as toddlers love to grab at things and this could lead to a nasty burn.

- Keep your child in a high chair or playpen when you are busy cooking.

- Do not put "a few drops" of alcohol, coffee, tea, cocoa, chocolate, or anything containing caffeine in your baby's food. This will cause your child irritability and alter calcium absorption.

- Do not use unpasteurized (raw) dairy products, juice, or cider.

- Do not serve smoked fish to your child since it may be infected with Listeria and may contain nitrates.

- It is unclear whether or not to serve your child tuna, since there is a small amount of mercury in it. It is probably safer not to give tuna until there is clearer evidence one way or another.

- Raw fish and smoked meat should not be served to your baby as they may contain various parasites and will not be chewed well.

- Foods with an increased amount of nitrates should not be given to your child.
  - ❖ Some vegetables such as beets, turnips, carrots, spinach, and collard greens may contain a chemical (nitrate) that can cause anemia in young infants (see *Vegetables*).
  - ❖ The amount of nitrates may increase if these vegetables are stored, so do not store these foods.
  - ❖ If you use these foods to prepare meals at home, serve them fresh, and use fresh water to puree then with, not the cooking water.

Foods to Avoid
- You should avoid giving your baby foods that are nutritionally poor or unhealthy, such as foods with high salt content and low fat foods (the child needs energy and fat is essential to central nervous system development in a child below two years of age; between two to four years, discuss any fat reduction with your doctor as it is dependent upon your child's nutritional status, etc).
- Do not give your child canned adult foods or canned vegetables and fish, since they contain too much salt and can contain too much fat, sugar, or salt.
- Avoid serving your child allergenic foods, since your baby may react adversely to foods given too early. The most common allergenic foods include wheat, eggs, sesame seeds, shellfish, soy products, nuts, peanut butter, and cow's milk.
- Avoid shellfish (regular fish may be given around nine to twelve months of age) and nuts until your child is at least three years of age and only offer whole cow's milk after the age of one year.
- Do not serve foods containing caffeine such as tea, coffee, cola drinks, and chocolate.
- Avoid foods that pose a choking risk or food poisoning danger.

Tip: Fat is Important for Brain Development

Fat is an important source of energy for your baby's development, at least until the age of two years. You may gradually introduce low-fat foods into your baby's diet after the age of two years, according to your child's nutritional status and upon discussion with your doctor.

Microwave Safety

- Foods are heated unevenly in the microwave, so stir or rotate the food midway through heating. If you do not do this, you will have cold spots where harmful bacteria may survive.

- Only use microwave safe containers and lids when heating foods.

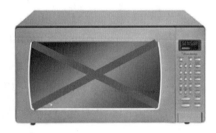

- Microwave safe plastic wraps should be loosely placed over foods for steam to escape. The plastic should not directly touch your food.

- Moist heat will help destroy bacteria.

- Other materials safe to use for covering food in the microwave include cooking bags, wax paper, and white, microwave-safe paper towels.

- Styrofoam or plastic containers should not be used in the microwave as they may emit harmful chemicals into the food.

- Do not use any metal or aluminum foils. They may get too hot and burn.

Juice Safety

- There is a difference between pasteurized and unpasteurized juice. Pasteurization is the act or process of destroying most harmful bacteria in certain foods.

- Most juices are pasteurized to kill harmful bacteria. Unpasteurized juices may contain harmful bacteria, which could be dangerous for your child.

- Children may get food poisoning from drinking unpasteurized juice since their immune systems are still developing.

- Most juice labels state whether or not the juice is pasteurized. If you are unsure about the status, do not buy or use the product. If you would like to use the product, simply boil it to kill any possibly harmful bacteria (see *Fruit Juices*).

Mercury & Shellfish

- A well balanced diet that includes a variety of fish and shellfish contributes to children's proper growth and a healthy heart.

- Almost all fish and shellfish contain small traces of mercury while others contain larger amounts of it, which may be harmful to your baby's developing nervous system. For this reason, it is recommended that young children eat fish and shellfish that are low in mercury to reduce exposure to mercury effects.

- Do not serve shark, swordfish, king mackerel, or tilefish since they contain high levels of mercury.

- The 5 most commonly eaten fish are shrimp, canned light tuna, salmon, pollock, and catfish, all of which are low in mercury content.

- Albacore "white" tuna contains more mercury than canned light tuna.

- Be sure that you wait till your children are the appropriate age for fish and shellfish and feed them these foods in small portions.

Outdoor Food Safety & Road Trip Feedings
- Keep the following suggestions and tips in mind when you are eating outdoors with your child or taking a road trip:
  - ❖ Keep cold food in a cooler with ice or frozen packs at or below 40 F/4 C.
  - ❖ Keep raw meat, poultry, and seafood securely wrapped so that the juices will not contaminate other foods.
  - ❖ Packaged fruits and vegetables should be labeled as to whether or not they are washed and ready to eat.
  - ❖ Place the cooler in the air-conditioned compartment of your vehicle (not in the trunk).
  - ❖ Limit the amount of times the cooler is opened.
  - ❖ Avoid introducing new foods (especially high-allergenic foods) right before or during a road trip.
  - ❖ When your child has food allergies, remember to bring along any medications (e.g., Epipen, etc.). You may need a letter from your doctor, especially if you are flying.
  - ❖ Avoid offering your child snacks in the process of driving a vehicle.
  - ❖ Carry a bottle warmer with you (if you warm your child's bottle) and make sure you have something to plug it into (e.g., cigarette lighter, adapter, etc.).

❖ Do not offer your child any perishable items (e.g., mayonnaise, etc.) to reduce the risk of infection.

❖ Carry extra nipples, bottles, ready-to-use commercially sterile formula, and feeding equipment with you.

Phytoestrogens & Soy Formula

- Phytoestrogens are substances that are found in soy beans. Infants that are fed with soy formula have higher levels of phytoestrogens than other babies. High levels of phytoestrogens have been a concern in that they may create hormonal imbalances, endocrine problems, and affect gonadal sex organs and their functions. No conclusive evidence has yet been reached regarding the risks of phytoestrogens in soy formulas; however, these risks have been reported in studies.

- Use formula including nucleotides (helps the immune system and assists in fat digestion) and DHA & ARA containing formula (important nutrients for brain and vision development). Do not use homemade formulas and goat's milk, as they do not contain the nutrient balance necessary for your baby's health.

E. Coli in Foods

E. Coli has been found in under-cooked beef, unpasteurized cider, and other foods (fruit juice, green salad, etc.); it may cause a serious condition known as hemolytic uremic syndrome (HUS). This condition may lead to kidney failure, neurological problems, seizure, and even death.

Section 7:
Growth Characteristics
& Assessment

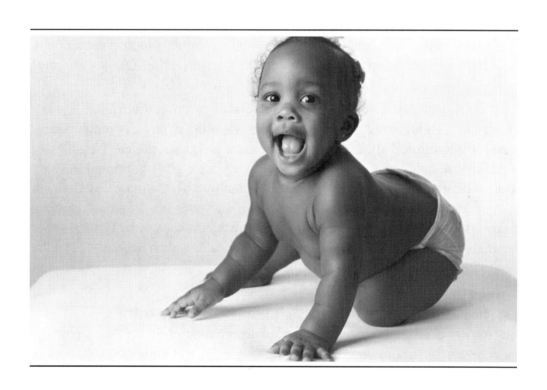

Growth Charts & Assessment of Growth Patterns

General

Each child is different and grows at different rates. Your child's physical growth refers to height and weight, as well as head circumference, in the first two years of life. The growth of a child is not constant. It tends to happen in growth spurts, which are defined as a period of rapid increases in height and weight. Growth spurts occur around ages 7-10 days, 2-3 weeks, 4-6 weeks, and at three, four, six and nine months (more or less); they generally last for 2-7 days. Studies show that children grow more rapidly in spring and summer than in the autumn and winter. Children also tend to grow more at night due to increased levels of growth hormone (another reason why it is important for your child to get enough sleep). During the growth spurt period, babies generally need to feed more and tend to be fussier.

It is evident that there is a strong relationship between nutrition and the growth of a child. Growth is often affected when the child has problems with health or nutrition. Failure to gain appropriate weight in the early months or years of life may have a negative impact on your child's brain and nervous system development. Moreover, nutritional quality affects your child's growth (e.g., excess calories will cause weight gain and obesity). Vitamins, protein, minerals, carbohydrates, and fat all affect growth, amongst other factors. Other normal growth factors include genetic heritage, diet and environment, and the absence of major, chronic disease.

Assessment of Growth, Growth Charts & Percentiles

- Growth charts allow your doctor to track your child's growth patterns over time. The process of graphing began in the early 1970's and has become the accepted method by which doctors monitor a child's growth and nutritional status.

> ### Tip: Growth Charts
>
> The following examples of Growth Charts are used in conjunction with many factors. Your doctor will include all factors influencing your child's growth (these charts are meant to be used as a general guideline); if you have concerns, discuss them with your doctor.

CDC Growth Charts

- Two sets of charts are used:

  1) Infants from birth to 36 months are measured for weight, length, and head circumference.

  2) Children between the ages of 2-20 years are measured for stature (height) and weight.

- When a child is being measured, it is important to select the appropriate growth chart; it must be selected based on both the age and gender of the child. The following table describes what measurements need to be taken and plotted onto the chart at two different ages:

Birth-36 Months of Age (same measurements taken for both boys and girls, but plotted on different gender charts)	Length-for-age Weight-for-age Head circumference-for-age Weight-for-length
2-20 Years of Age (same measurements taken for both boys and girls, but plotted on different gender charts)	Stature-for-age Weight-for-age BMI (Body Mass Index)-for-age

- The Center for Disease Control (CDC) published updated growth charts in 2000. These growth charts, used around the world, are based on the growth patterns of a limited group; primarily U.S. children, most of whom were formula-fed as babies.

- When breastfed babies are assessed using these older, standard charts, they appear to grow faster than the average during the initial three months, but then grow more slowly.

- Breastfed babies also tended to be taller and thinner when compared to babies in the mostly formula-fed group.

- The CDC collected data that included:

  ❖ An age range from birth to twenty years.

  ❖ Children who were breast and formula-fed.

  ❖ Children who represented an ethnic cross section of U.S. population.

  ❖ BMI (body mass index) data for children aged two to twenty years.

- The following are CDC Growth Charts examples:

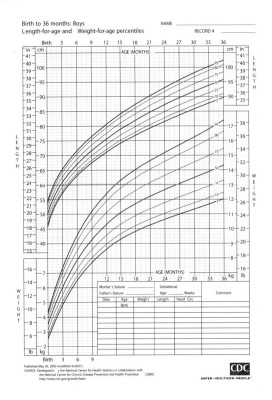

Birth to 36 months: Boys
Length-for-age and Weight-for-age percentiles

NAME _____
RECORD # _____

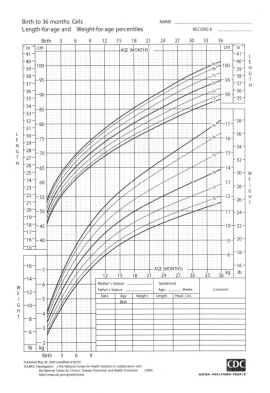

Birth to 36 months: Girls
Length-for-age and Weight-for-age percentiles

NAME _____
RECORD # _____

Published May 30, 2000 (modified 4/20/01).
SOURCE: Developed by the National Center for Health Statistics in collaboration with
the National Center for Chronic Disease Prevention and Health Promotion (2000).
http://www.cdc.gov/growthcharts

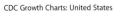

CDC Growth Charts: United States

CDC Growth Charts: United States

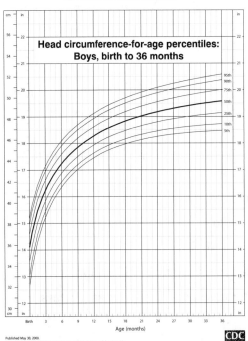

Head circumference-for-age percentiles:
Boys, birth to 36 months

Published May 30, 2000.
SOURCE: Developed by the National Center for Health Statistics in collaboration with
the National Center for Chronic Disease Prevention and Health Promotion (2000).

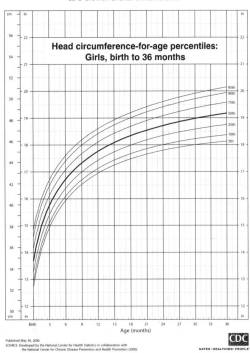

Head circumference-for-age percentiles:
Girls, birth to 36 months

Published May 30, 2000.
SOURCE: Developed by the National Center for Health Statistics in collaboration with
the National Center for Chronic Disease Prevention and Health Promotion (2000).

Printed with permission

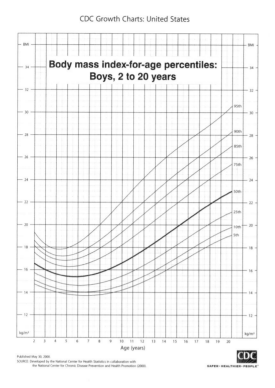

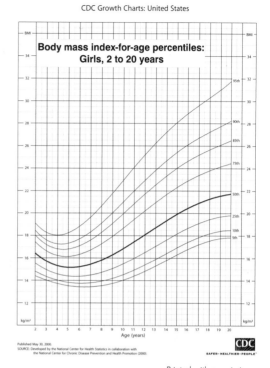

Printed with permission

WHO Charts

- In 2006, the World Health Organization (WHO) issued new growth charts based on data collected from children of several nations. The children studied were deemed to have optimal conditions for growth; the factors included exclusive breastfeeding for the first four to six months of life, good medical care, and smoke free households.

- It is assumed that from birth to age five years, children's growth is much more influenced by breastfeeding (considered the norm), good nutrition, access to health care, and other environmental factors rather than by genetics, ethnicity, where the child lives, etc.

- The WHO evaluated data that included:

  ❖ An age range from birth to five years.

  ❖ Only breastfed infants.

  ❖ Multiple ethnicity; data was collected from Brazil, Ghana, Norway, India, Oman, and the U.S.

  ❖ BMI data for children from birth to five years. (Allows for earlier diagnosis of excessive weight gain)

- In practice, the only major differences between the WHO and CDC charts are the weight patterns for the ages 6-20 months, with exclusively breastfed children appearing to fall off the CDC percentiles. Some doctors suggest cross-plotting these patients on the WHO growth charts.

- The actual recommendation to use the CDC growth chart (by the CDC) and the Canadian Pediatrics Society (CPS) predates the availability of the WHO Charts.

- Your doctor will use growth charts, preferably using WHO charts in the first few years of life and then switching to CDC growth charts thereafter.

- The following are WHO Growth Charts examples:

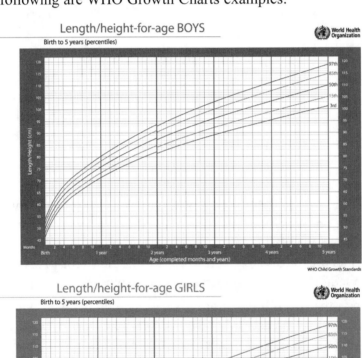

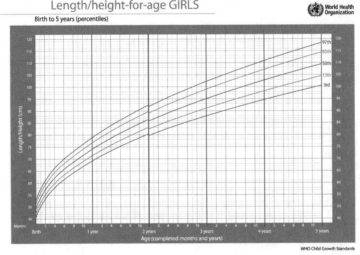

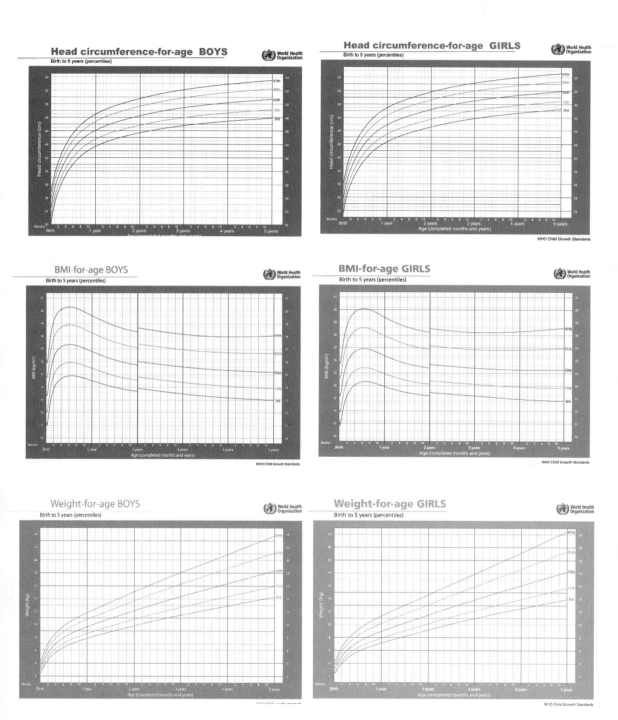

Printed with permission

Other Growth Charts and Percentile

- There are also growth charts specific to the premature or low birth weight infant and children with special health needs (disease specific growth charts such as Down's Syndrome, etc).

- Percentiles are used on growth charts as clinical indicators of growth assessment. They rank the position of a child compared to other children of the same age and gender group.

- There are 7 curves that follow the same pattern on a standard growth chart: 5th, 10th, 25th, 50th, 75th, 90th, and 95th percentile.

- The middle or 50th percentile represents the average growth for a specific age group. If your baby is in the 50th percentile, it means that half of the babies of that age group are heavier and half are lighter.

- Another example would be if your baby is in the 10th percentile for height. This means that 90% of babies the same age as your child are taller and 10 % are shorter.

- A baby in the 3rd percentile can be just as healthy as a baby in the 95th percentile.

- Children should have their height and growth measured on a regular basis so that doctors and parents are able to see how the child grows over time (as compared to the chart percentiles).

- Parents should not focus on one particular number on the growth chart. It is a matter of growth patterns over a period of time.

Additional Assesstment

- Growth assessment is determined through the use of growth charts, body mass index charts (BMI), ideal body weight, and skin folds.

Body Mass Index (BMI)

BMI for age (weight in kg/height in m2) is used to screen children 0-20 years of age (CDC, WHO). It shows whether the child's height and weight are proportional. With children, the BMI is based on gender and age to allow for change in the body's composition, as the child gets older. It is calculated by dividing body weight (kg) by the square of the height (kg/m2). It is then plotted on a curve to obtain a percentile value. Your child will be ranked in percentiles compared to other children his age and gender.

Ideal Body Weight (IBW)

At any given height, a child can have the ideal weight, which is called the ideal body weight (IBW). This is used as a method of calculating whether your child (at any age) is at a normal weight, underweight, or over-weight. To calculate the percentage of IBW, plot the length or height on a growth chart for age percentile. Locate the IBW as the weight at the same percentile as the height

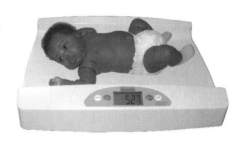

for the same age and sex. Divide the actual weight by the ideal body weight and multiply it by 100. The following chart is a basic overview of the percentage of IBW and its normal or abnormal meaning:

Percentage of IBW	Normal/Abnormal Meaning
Greater than 120%	Obese
110-120	Overweight
90-110	Normal
85-90	Mildly underweight
75-85	Moderately underweight
Less than 75%	Severely underweight

Skin Folds Measurement

Some nutritional doctors use the skin fold caliper measurement to determine if your child is carrying too much fat. This method measures body fat directly so that frame size and muscle mass do not interfere with the accuracy of the measurement. Further factors the doctor considers are the child's overall health, parent's height and weight, etc.

Normal Growth Patterns

- Although the child's growth rate is very rapid during the first year of his life, it slows down considerably in the second year. The following are normal growth patterns in children:

  ❖ The birth weight of a newborn correlates to the size, nutritional state, and general health of the mother.

  ❖ In the first 5 days after birth, the infant loses 30 grams of weight per day. The infant's weight returns to its original birth weight by day 10.

After day 10, growth occurs at a rate of about 7 oz/200 g per week in the first month of life.

❖ If the baby's weight is about 6.6 lb/3 kg at birth, this weight will double at 4 months of age and triple at 1 year of age.

- My experience has shown me that most large weight babies (greater than 8.8 lb/4 kg) gain weight more slowly in the first month than babies born at 6.5-7lb/3-3.5 kg.

- Growth rate slows down towards the end of the first year. In the second year of life, the baby will gain 5.5-6.5 lb/2.5-3 kg and in the third year, the baby will gain 4.5-6.5 lb/2-3 kg.

- During a period of decreased appetite or disease, growth may be stunted. The compensation growth period will help the child recover and return to his normal percentile growth curve.

- In the absence of appropriate nutrition, the compensation period will not fully occur; therefore it is important to ensure good nutrition during these vulnerable periods.

- After the first six months of life, genetic factors ultimately influence height. The growth percentile can shift (either increasing or decreasing) in the first four to six months to eighteen months of life.

- An infant who is smaller for his gestational age and has genetic predisposition to larger stature, usually experiences accelerated growth in the first six months. By eighteen months, a relatively stable growth percentile is established.

- The downward shift that is seen in large infants who have genetic tendencies for short stature and a decrease in weight may be confused with failure to thrive. Normally however, a stable percentile is achieved by eighteen months of age.

- The *head circumference* of a baby at birth is usually 14 inches/35 cm and 18.5 inches/47 cm by one year. This slowly reaches the average of 21.5 inches/55 cm by the age of six years. Head growth is the last thing to suffer from energy and food loss.

- The normal rate of growth in *height* is the following:
  1) Rapid in the first year (10 inches/25 cm in first year, 5 inches/12.5 cm in second year, etc.).

2) During mid-childhood, both boys and girls grow at a steady rate of about 2-2.5 inches/5-6 cm per year.

3) This amount decreases to 2 inches/5 cm per year just before puberty, with boys a little taller than girls.

4) During puberty, growth spurts occur in both males and females at about 12-18 inches/30-45 cm to reach mature height by age sixteen in girls and eighteen years of age in boys.

- The following table outlines normal growth in weight gain from birth to three years of age (any deviation from this chart is dependent upon your child and, if you are concerned, it may be discussed with your doctor):

Age Increase	Median Daily Increase	Median Monthly Weight
0-3 Months	0.9-1.1 oz/26-31 grams	2.2 lb/1 kg/month
3-6 Months	0.6-0.66 oz/17-18 grams	1.1 lb/0.5 kg/month
6-9 Months	0.4-0.5 oz/12-13 grams	0.73 lb/0.33 kg/month
9-12 Months	0.3 oz/9 grams	0.55 lb/0.25 kg/month
1-3 Years	0.25-0.3 oz/7-9 grams	

- Growth patterns of *breastfed* infants (WHO growth chart) are different from those of formula-fed infants. As such, there are growth charts to represent the different growth patterns of breastfed infants.

- These differences should be taken into consideration when assessing the growth of an exclusively breastfed infant so as to avoid unnecessary investigations, supplemental formula, or a too early introduction of solids.

- It is important to be familiar with the weight growth patterns of breastfed babies, so as not to wrongly conclude that the baby is not gaining sufficient weight.

- Breastfed babies tend to grow faster than formula-fed infants in the first six months of life and less rapidly from six to twelve months, although rates of growth in length and head circumference are similar.

Abnormal Growth Patterns

- Take your child for regular checkups at your doctor's office so that his measurements can be plotted on a growth chart.

- During regular checkups, your doctor will take measurements of your baby's length, weight, and head circumference and will record it in the baby's medical chart.

- When your child gets a little older (2-20 years of age), your doctor will record measurements *as needed* including height-for-age, weight-for-age, weight-for-height, and BMI (body mass index). Body mass index is an indicator of a child's body fat.

- An interpretation of growth parameters can help the doctor detect any medical or developmental problems.

- It is important to remember that kids do not grow at a constant rate, therefore taking your child's weight very often (e.g., very short periods of time between checkups) can sometimes show "jumps" in weight. Do not worry if this is the case. Also, do not worry if your child becomes slightly thinner around two to three years of age, as it is normal for growth to slow down.

- If you compare two points or more (eg. for weight) on the growth chart, you can see:
  - ❖ A *slow increasing line* represents the child is growing well.
  - ❖ A *straight line* indicates that the child is not gaining weight.
  - ❖ A line with a *sharp increasing (upwards) curve* shows that the child is gaining weight faster than usual and may need closer follow-up.
  - ❖ A line that is *slowly decreasing* indicates that the child is losing weight and needs a follow-up and/or assessment to rule out disease, nutritional deficiencies, etc.

- Follow-ups allow your doctor to identify early health problems. It will also permit assessment of how a dietary treatment program may help the child in either gaining weight (compensative growth) or continue losing weight (continuous loss or no weight gain, which may indicate persistence of a problem or inappropriate management of dietary program).

- Follow-up growth and nutritional counseling should be done for each child, especially children close to the extreme percentile, and more so for children with chronic diseases, frequent illnesses, etc.

- In the first month of life, it is important for the baby to be seen by a doctor a few times to check for any issues such as feeding difficulties, bottle/breast and first child concerns, proper weight gain, dehydration, etc. I normally see newborns a few times in the first month; however this varies in different pediatric offices.

- In the first year of a baby's life, taking his height and weight is frequently required.

- In the child's second year of life, the child's growth rate decreases to 28-57 grams per week. Therefore, growth parameters are assessed less frequently as growth changes are small.

Tip: Excess Food Intake

Excess in food intake will lead to increases in weight but fewer gains in height.

Parent Concerns

What does my child's growth monitoring tell me about his nutrition?

- Your child's growth lets you know whether or not he has any problems with his nutrition, which affects his growth patterns. It can help rule out diseases or various conditions, which secondarily affect nutrition.

Are boys and girls different in growth and what else affects my child's growth?

- Growth is gradual in both girls and boys during toddler and young ages.

- It is generally known that girls mature earlier than boys, so they gain more fat tissue in their breasts, hips, and thighs while boys gain muscle tissue.

- The following affects a child's growth:

  ❖ *Genetic:* Ethnic background, family and parent growth history, size, and shape.

  ❖ *General health*: Drugs, acute illnesses, and chronic conditions.

  ❖ *Gender:* Differences in male and female growth patterns.

  ❖ *Age*: Peak growth periods occur in infancy and puberty, with slower growth during childhood.

  ❖ *Activity level:* Amount and type.

  ❖ *Food intake and eating habits:* Type, amount, and how often.

My toddler is not gaining weight and does not care to eat so much. What can cause decreased appetite?

- Natural appetite, where some children will eat like wolves and others like birds.

- Interest in their surrounding environment (it is more exciting than eating).

- Growing independence, where the child enjoys feeding himself.
- Wide taste swings, where he will like a food one week and then reject it the next.
- Diseases.

Why does my newborn baby lose weight before he gains any?
- Newborns are born with extra fluid in their bodies. This allows them to do well on their own for the first 48-72 hours, until their mother is able to supply them with milk.

How do I know if my baby is feeding appropriate amounts of breast milk or formula?
- Your baby should have at least 4-5 bowel movements per day when he returns home from the hospital (normally one after every feeding). The stool should be a green transitional stool (different from the black stool he had at birth), to a yellowish stool. To be able to tell if your baby is feeding well, consult your doctor (weight assessment on the scale is most important).

What are some external indicators of good growth?
- Normal growth patterns (charted).
- Good appetite.
- Good bowel movements.
- Good sleep patterns.
- Skin is moist and soft, and hair is shiny.
- Good face color.
- Good gums that are not swollen.
- Good teeth with no cavities.
- Strong nails with good pink base color below.
- Good muscle tone.
- Concentration, listening, and behavior is good.
- Resistance to disease.

Why is it important to follow head circumference growth?
- Head circumference is assessed with each doctor's visit for the first two years of life.

- It is important to follow head growth as it reflects normal brain growth.
- If there is a sudden increase in head growth circumference, your doctor will investigate to rule out any brain disorders.
- For example, a small head (microcephaly) is when head circumference is at or below the 3rd percentile. This means that fewer than 3 children out of 100 in that age group and sex will have a head circumference that is smaller. A large head (macrocephaly) is when head measurement is placed at or above the 97th percentile.

My baby/child is not gaining weight. How often should I visit the doctor?
- The recommended frequency of visits to the doctor depends on the following:
  - ❖ The age of your child; during the first few weeks after birth, he requires visits every one to two weeks. Once your child is older, a visit every one to two months should suffice.
  - ❖ How poorly he is growing (in mild cases, visits may be less frequent; it depends on each case).
  - ❖ The reliability of the parents (nutrition intake etc.).
  - ❖ The doctor's experience and level of concern.
  - ❖ Associated chronic diseases (e.g., congenital heart disease, child with cleft palate, etc.).
  - ❖ If your baby is premature, frequent visits are required to assess appropriate weight gain.
  - ❖ If your child is obese, the frequency depends on the degree of obesity and the parents or doctor's wishes for a close follow-up and diet monitoring.

How often should my child be weighed or measured?
- Your child should be weighed and measured in the first 48-72 hours after being discharged from the hospital (if there are no problems and your baby is discharged after 24 hours).
- In the first month of life, your doctor will assess and dictate follow-up visits according to the mother's comfort, feeding difficulties and/or ensuring good weight gain.

- After the first month of life, babies should be measured again at two months, three to four months, six months, eight to nine months, one year, two years, and once a year after that. However, this may vary according to the doctor's office.

- Normal newborns with low birth weight or pre-term babies may require more frequent follow-ups for parameters of height and weight than normal newborns with normal birth weight.

What is failure to thrive and what causes it?

- Failure to thrive is failure to gain weight appropriately.

- Many times, a medical reason is not identified; it may be due to a variety of factors such as inadequate nutrition, an infant's temperament, inappropriate formula preparation, a feeding technique, poor socioeconomic status, inappropriate diet for age, parental or family stress, etc. (see *Failure to Thrive*).

Conclusion

- Growth charts should not become an anxiety for parents, as it is easy to be misled by or misinterpret them.

- They help the doctor to know when to investigate changes from normal growth. They help to identify early deficiencies and assess how treatment is helping (e.g., to increase weight, continued weight drop, problem is solved, etc.).

- When the doctor assesses the child's growth, he considers more than the curve of the growth chart. He is looking at factors such as other parameters of child development, activity, family history (genetic), etc.

- Regular height and weight growth follow-ups are good, sensitive indicators of nutritional and health status, which can be affected by various diseases.

- If an infant fails to gain weight on formula that is quantitatively and qualitatively correct, then something is wrong with the infant or the feeding situation, and not with the formula.

- Significant differences in activity among children account for variability in food requirements (basal metabolic rate, rapidity of growth, amount of non-utilized food lost in stool, and specific food action).

- The infant who is more active, tense, and kicking will require more calories than a placid baby. Crying may raise the metabolic requirement.

The Food Groups: Making Sense of Portion Size & Activity Level

General

The food groups provide parents with an overall idea of the type of nutritious and balanced diet necessary for their child. To plan a healthy diet that is appropriate for your child's age, it is not necessary to calculate the exact required calories, vitamins, and minerals. A simple and easy way to plan your child's menu is by using the food groups and serving units needed from each group for a specific age.

Within this chapter, both the American (*My Pyramid*) and Canada's Food Guide to Healthy Eating include the food groups, portion and serving size according to age group, etc. These aspects may change over time, so ensure that you are constantly updated. An updated food guide pyramid for the United States was released in 2005 by the USDA (US Department of Agriculture Center for Nutrition, Policy and Promotion) to help parents make daily food choices that adequately meet nutritional standards for their children (the food guide pyramid is now called *My Pyramid* in the U.S). The Canadian food guide from the Minister of Public Works and Government Services (2007) is also attached.

Both the American and Canadian food guide (February, 2007) recommend eating patterns for different genders and depending on levels of physical activity. The new Canadian food guide of 2007 now provides information on the recommended number of food guide servings per day by age and gender, what one food serving includes (examples of each food group are provided), and provides you with the option of completing *My Food Guide* for your child, according to your child's age, gender, and level of physical activity. This also provides you with further examples of food servings. The websites for all this information is www.healthcanada.gc.ca/foodguide or MyPryamid.gov.

Tip: Food Groups and Activity

If your child is very active and needs more food, choose exta servings from the various food groups, using age appropriate portions.

While there are five food groups, they are sometimes referred to as four food groups in this chapter (amongst others) because the separate food groups of vegetables and fruits are sometimes considered as a single food group.

Health   Santé
Canada   Canada

Your health and
safety... our priority.

Votre santé et votre
sécurité... notre priorité.

Eating
Well with
Canada's
Food Guide

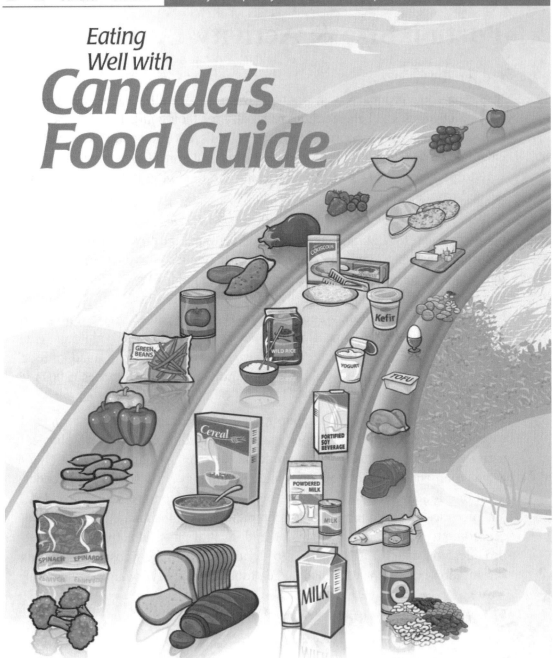

Canada

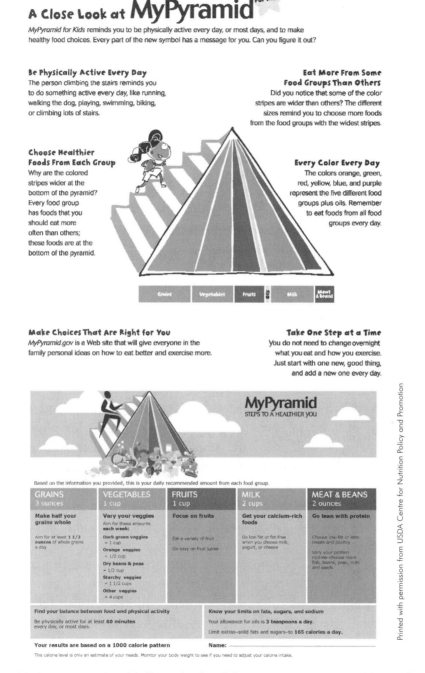

This is a general guideline obtained from www.MyPyramid.gov for an average two year old child. Please refer to the website for your specific child's age, height and activity level under the section entitled "My Pyramid Plan".

The Food Groups of the Pyramid

Grains	Rich in carbohydrates, fiber (if whole grain is used), B vitamins, and minerals. Examples: whole grain, breads, rice, pasta, cereals, etc.
Vegetables	Provide vitamins (A, C), minerals (potassium, iron), antioxidants, fiber, and carbohydrates. Choose brightly colored green and orange vegetables for more nutrient packed choices. Examples: carrots, tomatoes, potatoes, broccoli, etc.
Fruit	Rich in carbohydrates and vitamins, especially A and C, but they also provide potassium Examples: apples, pears, peaches, plums, clementines, bananas, etc.
Milk & Milk Products	Main source of dietary calcium and vitamin D, also high in vitamin A. A good source of protein. Examples: milk, yogurt, cheese, etc.
Meat & Alternatives	These are rich in proteins and include meat, poultry, fish, beans, eggs, soy based products, nuts, and seeds.

- In each group, there are components with special contributions to energy and body development. You cannot omit them when you are planning the daily menu.

- You still need to reach the best nutritional balance for your child and offer the right amount of food in each food group according to his physical activity. Remember, your role is to offer a healthy balanced diet in the right amounts, but it is your child's job to choose how much they want to eat. Always allow your child to self-regulate his food intake—children are born with strong self-regulating instincts.

A Word about Juice
- Sweets and soft drinks are not considered a food group, since they mainly contain sugar and very few other nutrients (too much juice can cause poor weight gain and chronic diarrhea in young children; it also reduces the child's appetite, etc.). They have no specific nutritional importance (other than empty calories), but they give satisfaction and act as a source of energy.

- Sweets and soft drinks need to be limited when given to small children. It is best to teach and encourage your child to drink water for thirst and use milk for beverage needs.

- Water and other liquid-containing foods help replenish body fluids as needed, especially during periods of activity or hot weather.

Grain Products

- Infant cereals may be offered until the age of two years. The Canadian Pediatric Society (CPS) recommends them (rather than regular cereals) to prevent iron deficiency.

- Crackers, bread, noodles, sticky rice, cereal, toast, etc., make for great finger foods, as children often enjoy the simplicity of these foods more than combination foods. But do offer cubed vegetables, fruits, pieces of meat and/or cheese along with grain snacks, so as to balance the food groups (make sure that the foods are age appropriate).

- Do not add sugar or syrups to grain foods.

Tip: Whole Wheat Bread Versus White Bread

Whole wheat bread offers a nutritional advantage over white bread, even though both are made of wheat flour. Whole wheat bread contains fibers that are rich in the outer bran layers and the nutritious inner germ of the wheat kernel. Whole wheat bread has more vitamins and minerals than bread made from refined wheat flour, from which the bran and germ have been removed. Look for "100% whole wheat" instead of "Wheat" and/or "Multigrain."

Meat & Alternatives

- Meat and meat alternatives are important to maintain iron store in the body; however, pay attention to the required serving sizes for young children—they don't require very much to meet their needs (1-2 oz/30-60 g per meal twice a day is all they need).

- Serve your child chopped meat, poultry, cooked egg, cheese, yogurt, beans, or peas. The texture of the meats offered should be appropriate for your child's stage of development and chewing ability—avoid hard/stringy meats, and give meats and proteins that are soft and cut into small pieces or served in a sauce for easy chewing.

- Be sure to serve meats and alternatives in moderation and limit the use of fried meats, gravy, and other sauces. Avoid processed meats such as bacon, sausage, luncheon meats, and hot dogs (high in fat, nitrates, and salt).

Fruits & Vegetables

- Serve soft and plain fruits and vegetables. If fruits are too hard, steam or poach them before serving.

- Do not add salt after cooking. Avoid excess sugar, oils, or butter.

- Remove all seeds and pits when serving fruits and vegetables. Cut grapes into quarters to avoid choking hazards.

Milk & Milk Products

- It is not recommended to start cow's milk until after one year of age (see *Cow's Milk*).

- Reduced fat and skim milk should not be used for children under two years of age, because milk is a key source of fat (needed for brain development and energy).

- Limit your baby's milk intake to about 16 oz/500 ml per day, as excessive amounts of milk will lead to increased calories and a decreased appetite for other foods.

- Offer your child milk products such as yogurt, cheese strings, slices of cheese, etc., for snacks, breakfast, or as part of a healthy lunch.

Fat

- Oils and fats are not a food group and are the least understood of all food types, but your child does need some for good health (see *Dairy Products for Infants & Toddlers* for comments on age and fat requirements).

- While it is suggested that adults limit foods rich in fats and oils, the young child (at least until two to four years of age) may be malnourished if he does not receive these (do NOT put children on a low fat diet).

- Until age four, children require more fat for brain development, with the following fat/energy requirements:

  - ❖ 30-40% energy from fat between 1-3 years of age.
  - ❖ 25-35% energy from fat between 4-8 years of age.
  - ❖ 20-25% energy from fat for ages 9-adult.

- Children can receive fats and oils from fatty fish (salmon), nuts, seeds, and liquid oils such as corn, olive, soybean, and canola oil. Vegetable oils are put through a process of hydrogenation that makes them firm and resistant to spoilage. Hydrogenated or "trans" fat have some of the same undesirable effects as saturated fats and interfere with the removal of cholesterol (can contribute to heart disease and certain cancers). As such, avoid trans fat.

- Healthy type margarines such as 55% polyunsaturated are also a good source of fat and vitamin E. Moderate amounts of butter also provide fat and vitamin E, as well as being a source of calories required for growth.

Tip: Types of Fat

The terms saturated, unsaturated, non-saturated, and polyunsaturated refer to the number of hydrogen atoms in each fat molecule.

- Omega 3 and Omega 6 are essential fatty acids found in corns and other oils made from sunflower, nuts, flax seeds, green leafy vegetables, etc. Omega fatty acids are important for brain and eye development.

- Once your child is four years of age, reduce fat caloric intake if excessive dietary fat is used with the following suggestions (see *Dairy Products for Infants & Toddlers* for further comments on fat):

  ❖ Switch from whole milk to 1-2% milk.

  ❖ Serve fish 2-3 times per week and avoid frying and bread coatings (also, avoid frequent servings of the following fish due to higher mercury levels: fresh tuna, shark, swordfish, and tile fish).

  ❖ Trim fat from meat and remove skin from poultry.

  ❖ Reduce butter use.

  ❖ Use low fat cooking methods—baking, broiling, poaching, steaming, and grilling.

Tip: Additions to the Food Groups

For preschoolers, foods outside of the 5 food groups are also part of healthy eating and contribute to the taste and enjoyment of eating. Thus, it is important to include other foods in healthy eating patterns, in amounts that do not displace food from other food groups. Use moderate amounts of food such as margarine, butter, and salad dressings and allow your child to enjoy the natural flavors of food (adding salt, seasonings, etc., in moderation and only after your child learns to like the natural taste of a food).

Activity Level & Calories

- The food groups in *My Pyramid* and Canada's Health Food Guide are a general guide to daily food requirements for children above the ages of two years.

- Daily food requirements are given according to age, gender and activity level (*My Pyramid and Canada Food Guide*).

- Physical activity is an important part of the pyramid since the level of activity affects how much a child needs to eat (the more active, the more food and calories he requires).

> ### Tip: Food Portions and Caloric Intake
>
> Kids naturally adjust their intake when they require more calories for growth and activity. Parents should not worry about making sure that their kids get all the required portions every day or focus on calorie counting, as this may create feelings of anxiety and feeding disturbances in the child.

- If you are concerned that your toddler is not eating enough of the various food groups, consult your doctor or dietitian. If poor weight gain is an issue, try to increase calories with such foods as peanut butter, gravy, added fats and oils, cheese, pudding, macaroni and cheese, etc., and talk to your doctor/dietitian about additional nutritional supplements.

Making Sense of Portion Size (Instead of Servings)

- The food guide shows you how to take foods in moderation and proportion (how much food a person should choose from each group).

- Variety is important for good health (it requires food from each food group).

- The food in each food group is divided into portions with similar caloric and nutrient components (e.g., carbohydrates, protein, fat, vitamins, minerals, fiber, etc.).

- Remember, a serving is not how much you eat at one meal. Rather, it is a reasonable amount of the food required to meet nutrient recommendations for a specific age/activity group.

- Servings in the food pyramid are now described more specifically in ounces, grams, and cups.

- Children do not need to eat food from all food groups everyday—they simply need a balanced diet over the course of two to four weeks.

- The following table shows common food items and what a toddler portion size is (1 toddler/young child portion size = 1serving) as a general guideline:

Milk, yogurt (2 servings)	1 cup/250 g (yogurt 3/4 cup)
Cheese (2 servings)	1 1/2 oz/50 g
Cereal (dry or cooked), rice, pasta, grains (3 servings)	1/2 cup/125 mL (1 baseball); 1 oz/30 g of cereal is about an adult hand or the size of a tennis ball
Fruits & vegetables (whole) (4 servings)	1/4-1/2 small piece
Chopped and cooked vegetables & fruits (4 servings)	1/2 cup/125 g (1 baseball); 1/2 cup/125 g of cooked vegetables = 1 baseball
Meat, poultry, fish, beans & peas (1 serving)	2.5 oz/70 g of meat, fish or poultry is about the size of a deck of playing cards or of a woman's hand
Bread (1 slice)	1 oz/35 g

Tip: Measures & Metric Equivalents

Spoon

3 teaspoons = 1 tablespoon

4 tablespoons = 1/4 cup; 8 tablespoons = 1/2 cup

1 teaspoon = 5 ml = 5 g

1 tablespoon = 15 ml = 15 g

Cup

1/4 cup = 60 ml

1/3 cup = 80 ml

1/2 cup = 120 ml

3/4 cup = 180 ml

1 cup = 240 ml

Weight

1 oz = 30 grams

1 pound = 454 grams

- There is no need to become obsessed with the use of a scientifically accurate scale to weigh each serving. Simply eyeball the servings and they should be around the approximate amount recommended.

- The amount of food required depends on the child's age, body size, activity level, growth rate, and appetite.

- The food guide gives a lower and higher number of servings for each food group. These ranges make the food guide flexible to use with family members with different energy and nutrient needs.

- There is a wide variation in portions of food consumed by preschoolers. That is why a child size portion is anywhere from 1/2 to the full size for food in each food group. Generally, the size of a portion increases with age (e.g., a two year old may eat 1/2 slice of bread whereas a four year old is more likely to eat a whole slice—both of these are counted as one child size serving).

Food Group Age Requirements: Servings & Portions

0-4 Months
Breast milk on demand and/or formula only (baby's digestive system can't handle solid foods at this age).

Age	Servings/Day	Oz/Ml Per Serving
0-1 Months	6-8	2-5 oz/60-150 ml
1-2 Months	5-7	3-6 oz/90-180 ml
2-3 Months	4-7	4-7 oz/120-210 ml
3-4 Months	4-6	6-8 oz/180-240 ml

4-6 Months
Breast milk on demand, or 4-6 servings of iron enriched formula of 6-8 oz/180-240 ml each.
Grain (iron-fortified baby cereal): 2 servings of 1-2 tablespoons per serving.

6-8 Months
Breast milk: on demand, or 3-4 feedings a day.
Formula: 3-5 servings of 6-8 oz/180-240 ml each.
Grains (iron-fortified baby cereal): 2 servings of 2-4 tablespoons per serving.
Grains (bread or crackers): offer 1-2 servings of 1/2 slice of bread or 2 crackers or 1 small baby cookie per serving.
Fruits: offer 2 servings of 2-3 tablespoons per serving.
Vegetables: offer 2 servings with 2-3 tablespoons per serving.

8-12 Months

Breast milk: on demand or 3-4 feedings per day.

Formula: 3-4 servings or 16-24 oz/ 240-320 ml per day.

Dairy: cheese, plain yogurt, or cottage cheese (no cow's milk); offer 1/2 oz/ 15 g to 1/2 cup/120 ml.

Grain (iron-fortified baby cereal/pasta): 2-4 servings of 2-4 tablespoons each.

Grain (bread or crackers): 2-3 servings of 1/2 slice or 2 crackers per serving.

Fruit: 2 servings of 3-4 tablespoons per serving or 2 oz/60 g per day.

Fruit juice: 1 serving of 3 oz/90 ml from a cup (if at all).

Vegetables:1 to 3 servings of 3-4 tablespoons.

Meat and alternatives (chicken, beef, pork, egg yolk, dried or cooked beans): 1 to 2 servings of 1-2 oz/30-60 g each, or 1/4-1/2 cup/60-120 ml per day, or 3-4 tablespoons per serving.

2 years and above

The following charts are the recommended number of servings per day and one food guide serving (Canadian recommendation):

Recommended Number of Food Guide Servings per Day

	Children			Teens		Adults			
Age in Years	2-3	4-8	9-13	14-18		19-50		51+	
Sex	Girls and Boys			Females	Males	Females	Males	Females	Males
Vegetables and Fruit	4	5	6	7	8	7-8	8-10	7	7
Grain Products	3	4	6	6	7	6-7	8	6	7
Milk and Alternatives	2	2	3-4	3-4	3-4	2	2	3	3
Meat and Alternatives	1	1	1-2	2	3	2	3	2	3

What is One Food Guide Serving?
Look at the examples below.

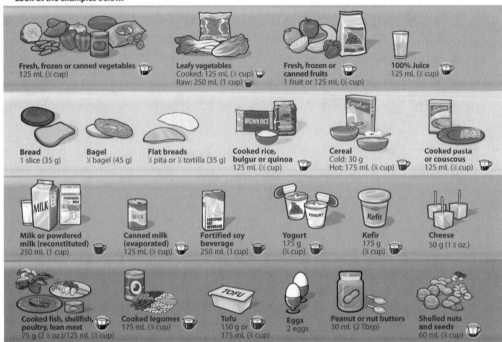

Rreproduced with permission of the Minister of Public Works and Government Services Canada,2oo7.

Tip: Food Guide Referrals

Please refer to the website www.healthcanada.gc.ca/foodguide for specific serving amounts for Canada and www.nal.usda.gov/fnic for the American food guide(s).

Refer also to the table of examples of the recommended number of food guide servings per day for Canada, *What Is One Food Guide Serving* and *My Pyramid* for the American food guide.

Practicality

- I have tried to make the food guide as practical as possible by providing parents with the guidelines, age requirements table, appropriate food groups, and using portions equivalent to a serving.

- Always discuss any concerns you may have about the food guide with your doctor, including any updated or new recommendations regarding serving size and number of servings per day.

- When problems/concerns arise, consult your health professional, a dietitian, or nutrition specialist to help you plan the appropriate menu for your child.

- Children do not need to eat food from all 5 food groups everyday—they simply need a balanced diet over the course of one to three weeks. Between the ages of one to three years, most toddlers need about 900-1400 calories a day, though counting calories is not necessary. Simply offer a variety of healthy options.

- Remember, that the amount per day required may change depending on your child's activity level, actual weight-for-age, premature birth, and children with special needs or diseases.

Parent Concerns

How much does my toddler need to eat per day?

- Most toddlers do well with 3 small meals and 2 snacks per day.

- An average toddler needs 1000 calories per day, however appetite varies among children by the day and by their activity level.

Does each meal have to contain all food groups?

- No, each meal does not have to contain all food groups. Base your toddler's meals on the food guide pyramid in a way that it all balances out over the course of one to two weeks.

Does the young child need fat?

- Fat is important for brain and eye development. It is also required for calories and growth, especially in the first two to four years.

- Fat is also important for healthy skin, hair, and wound healing.

- It adds flavor and helps with the absorption of fat soluble vitamins.

- After the age of two, children should receive 1/3 of calories from fat, and low fat milk and products may be introduced into their diet.

What is the difference between simple, complex carbohydrates and starches?

- Simple carbohydrates (sugars) are digested easily and quickly by the body, as they have simple structure molecules.

- Complex carbohydrates (also called starches) have a long chain of thousands of simple sugar molecules which are broken down and released into the blood stream slowly and steadily. After feeding complex carbohydrates, a feeling of fullness/satiety exists for several hours. These are found in foods such as grains, legumes, nuts, seeds, and the products made from breads and pastas, etc.

Is there a simple way to understand portion sizes and servings?

Practical Examples Of Food Amount and Servings*

Vegetable & Fruits

Vegetables

*1/2 cup (125mL) cooked, canned, or frozen vegetables (1 serving)

Light bulb

Fruits

*1 medium fruit (apple/ banana). (1 serving)

Baseball

Milk and Dairy

*1 glass of milk (250mL) (1 serving)

glass

*1 slice of cheese (1 serving)

disk

*1 1/2 oz. of cheese (50g) (1 serving)

dice (6)

*3/4 cup of yogurt *1/2 cup of ice cream (1 serving)

tennis ball

Grain Products

*1 slice of bread (35g) (1 serving)

cd case

*1 bagel (2 servings)

hockey puck

*1 pancake/waffle (1 serving)

cd

*1 cup of cold cereal (1 serving) rice or mashed potatoes (250mL) (2 servings)

baseball

*1 cup of cooked pasta

tennis ball

Meat & Alternatives

*2 eggs (1 serving)

*3 oz. (90g) of meat/fish/ poultry (1 serving)

*cooked fish, poultry, lean meat = 1/2 cup = 125mL = 75g=21/2 oz. (1 serving)

eggs (2)

deck of cards

*cooked legumes 3/4 cup=175mL (1 serving)

*1/4 cup (60mL) of shelled nuts & seeds *2 tblsp. (30mL) of peanut butter (1 serving)

*= fits Canadian recommendations for serving sizes

Nutritional Assessment

General

T he first few years of your child's life are an important time to develop healthy eating habits. Nutrients and calories are required for his growth and development. Appetites vary in young children as they grow, and it is your job to promote healthy eating habits that will serve your child well through his life.

What you teach him today could prevent a heart attack or diabetic amputation forty years from now. Keeping the long picture in mind can make it a bit easier to weather the temper tantrums that may arise when you offer your child water, instead of sweet juice or pop.

It is important for parents to provide their doctor with regular information about their child's eating habits, nutritional needs, religious dietary preferences, and overall health.

If any problems seem to arise or if you have concerns, your doctor can work with you (along with nutritional specialists and dietitians) to help you meet your child's needs.

How to Determine if Your Child is Growing Well

Steps of Nutritional Assessment

- Parents often bring their child to the doctor's office and casually state that their child is not eating well or is a picky eater and needs vitamin supplements. Do not start your child on any supplements without first consulting your doctor.

- Your doctor knows your child and will be able to tell you if he is growing appropriately (including height and weight on growth chart).

- When your doctor suspects that your child is not growing well (this decision is made after your doctor has considered several different points, not just weight gain), has failure to thrive, or possibly has a nutritional deficiency, he may do a nutritional assessment with the help of a nutritionist/dietitian.

- The following sections outline the steps which may be performed when there is the possibility of a problem.

- A nutritional assessment should include the following:

  1) History questioning by the doctor, including medical and food history.

  ❖ Medical examination and investigating signs of possible deficiencies if problems are suspected; measurement of height, weight and head circumference, body mass index, ideal body weight, etc.

  ❖ Dietary history table that parents can fill out to assess food intake.

  ❖ Lab tests may also be ordered, if required.

  2) The general medical history required by the doctor includes immunization history and status, medications previously or currently taken, diseases, illnesses or injuries, and medical or surgical procedures (unless your child is a regular patient).

  3) *A physical exam* is done when your child visits the doctor. Sometimes, a child's physical appearance may provide the doctor with signs of possible poor nutritional health.

  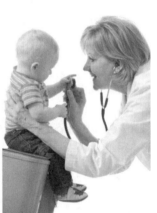

  ❖ Typically, a healthy child is strong, energetic, and has a "glow."

  ❖ Dental exams are also important, since teeth are greatly affected by nutrition. For example, a child with nutritional inadequacies may have redness, bleeding, swelling of the gums, and cavities (it is important to take your child for regular physical and dental exams).

  ❖ The measurement of height, weight, head circumference, and body mass index (BMI) helps to assess the child's growth and nutrition. It will be compared to his previous growth charts.

  4) Lab tests can be done if there is a suspected problem or your doctor notes a finding during a physical examination.

  ❖ Lab tests are sometimes done to relieve parental anxiety.

  ❖ The lab tests that will be ordered normally provide the doctor with nutritional data and include tests for ferritin, iron, calcium, phosphorus, vitamin levels, and, if appropriate, a thyroid test.

Dietary & Nutritional History

- Dietary history assesses your child's food intake and feeding schedule (*Table 1* following). These indicate how much and from which food groups your child is eating.

- Dietary history is important in assessing your child's nutritional health.

- Health care providers and dietitians can help you ensure that your child receives nutritious meals.

- Qualified physicians or pediatricians (MD), and Registered Dietitians (RD) conduct nutritional histories and assessments. If there seems to be a concern, then a dietary chart can be filled out and shown to your doctor. If there seems to be a problem after the chart assessment, a dietitian or nutritionist can help.

- Nutritional assessment looks at your child's usual nutrient intake (including calories), feeding interactions that may create feeding resistance, level of feeding skill (through feeding observation), etc.

- Some parents worry about the amount of food their child eats and may put extra pressure on their child to eat or finish a meal. Tactics such as force feeding, bribing/tricking, or distracting a child to eat will almost always cause feeding resistance and can negatively impact growth. Let your doctor know if you are using these tactics, so that he can properly understand your child's feeding patterns and behaviors (see *Picky Eaters*).

- Other includes the following questions about parent and child behavior interactions:

  ❖ Do you run after your child to feed him?

  ❖ Does he sit at the table with the family?

  ❖ Do you need to distract him to feed him, or are there any other distractions such as the TV, etc?

  ❖ Do you need to force, bribe, or coax him to eat?

  ❖ Do you push him to finish a meal?

  ❖ Were there any traumatic events (e.g., choking) that occurred previously, leading to food resistance?

  ❖ Are there any difficulties with certain textures?

❖ Is there a family history of picky eaters?

❖ Does he throw temper tantrums?

❖ What is his behavior at the table, and are there any rewards offered for food for eating, or favorite food as a reward for good behaviour?

Table 1: Dietary History Chart Parents Provide for the Doctor

Foods	How Much/Day	How Much/Week	How Much/Month
Breastfeeding			
Formula			
Milk, Cheese, Yogurt			
Cereal			
Vegetables			
Fruit			
Meat and Alternatives			

Parent Concerns

How do I provide my child with good nutrition?

- Offer a well balanced diet and set a positive calm, environment during meal times. Be sure you allow your child to choose the amount and what he wishes to eat from the foods you offer him. Your job is to ensure that the meal is balanced and that you provide positive feeding interactions, avoiding use of distractions, force feeding, or anxiety at meals. A child who is allowed to choose the amount of food he wishes and is left to self-regulate will, ultimately, eat optimally.

How do I know my child is growing properly?

- Usually, a growth chart will indicate to you and your doctor whether or not your child is growing at a normal, steady rate (see *Growth Charts & Assessment of Growth Patterns*). You may also keep track of everything your child eats and how much he eats of each food (dietary history) to see if he is receiving a proper nutritional diet. If he is, he should be growing properly, unless other factors are involved.

Failure to Thrive

General

Medically, a child is "failing to thrive" when he does not grow at the expected rate. His weight is disproportionate when compared to height and head circumference (among other factors). Failure to thrive may be associated with slow mental, physical, and emotional development. Poor nutrition during the infant and toddler stages may have permanent, negative effects on a child's mental development.

Your doctor uses a growth chart to see how your child compares to statistical norms. Your child does not have to be in the highest percentile of the growth chart to be considered healthy. While the growth chart is helpful for the doctor, it may be a source of anxiety for parents. It is easy to misread or misinterpret the chart, since it is dependent on various factors such as the genetic makeup of the parents, general health, nutritional status, period of growth arrest, diseases, changes over certain periods of growth, birth weight, gestational age at birth and weight, etc. (see *Growth Charts & Assessment of Growth Patterns*). Sometimes, a healthy baby may gain weight slowly, simply because of his unique growth patterns. Other times, a particular cause for slow weight gain may be found when visiting the doctor for regular visits. It is therefore important to have regular checkups with your doctor to assess appropriate weight gain or weight loss, and work on solutions if there are any problems.

Normal Growth Patterns

- Growth is very noticeable and rapid during the beginning stages of a baby's life.
- An infant usually drops less than 10 % in weight in the first few days of life as a result of loss of excess fluid. However, the weight is usually regained within about 10 days after birth.
- The following are normal growth patterns for the full term baby:
  - ❖ The baby who is developing and growing well usually doubles his birth weight by 4 months and triples it at the age of one year.
  - ❖ Typically, a baby eats 8-12 times in a 24 hour period in the first few weeks after birth.

❖ By the time the baby is two to three months old, the number of feedings has dropped but the amount taken at each feeding has increased because the baby's stomach is larger.

❖ By about four months, most bottle-fed infants will find sufficient nutrition from about 30 oz/900 ml per day of formula.

- In premature infants, normal growth can be calculated by subtracting the number of weeks of prematurity from the post-natal age. Normal growth charts may be used after "catch-up" growth has been attained (e.g., about 18 months for head circumference, etc.—see *Growth Charts & Assessment of Growth Patterns*).

Causes of Poor Weight Gain

General Causes

There are many causes associated with failure to grow at a normal rate, including:

- *Genetics*: If you and your spouse are relatively thin, your child may also be thin. While weight and development may appear to be slow, his nutritional and health status are good.

- *Activities and Calorie Requirements:* The very active child may be thinner than the inactive ones. Also, some children may require more calories due to their body build and level of activity (e.g., a tall baby will require more calories than an overweight baby—same weight but the height differs—as a tall baby's long muscles are more active, and hence use more energy).

- *Underfeeding*: Some babies do not receive or absorb enough formula or the appropriate solid foods for their age group or activity level, and will simply not gain weight. Sometimes, caregivers dilute the formula too much, so that the baby does not receive adequate nutrients.

- *Intentional Underfeeding:* Some parents intentionally underfeed their infants/toddlers to prevent them from being obese in the future. They limit their fat, sugar, and caloric intake. This can be dangerous to your baby. Infants and young children need calories and nutrients, which are appropriate for their normal growth and development (fats, for example, are necessary for normal brain development).

- *Regurgitation/Vomiting*: Frequent regurgitation and/or vomiting can also affect growth, even if the baby takes in appropriate amounts of food or milk. Most babies will gain weight appropriately (see *Gastroesophageal Reflux*).

- *Various Diseases*: Diseases such as infections, chronic diarrhea, liver disease, congenital heart disease, metabolic disorders, Cystic Fibrosis, diseases of the bowel, etc., or a chronic illness or medical condition (e.g., cleft lip and palate) can be associated with inappropriate weight gain.

- *Psychosocial Causes*: Parental inexperience or lack of education on appropriate feeding (e.g., rigid feeding schedule, diluted formula), poverty and malnutrition, neglect or abuse, mental illness in parents (e.g., postpartum depression, etc.), and substance abuse by a parent may all lead to a baby's slow weight gain.

Causes Associated with Breastfeeding
A breastfed infant may have additional causes for poor weight gain. Sometimes, the cause is evident (e.g., babies born with cleft lip/palate, vegetarianism, etc.) while in other cases, it is unclear and evaluation may be required along with follow-up weight gain, observation of breastfeeding, assessment of breastfeeding technique, etc. Other times, the baby is simply falling asleep before receiving enough milk. The problem is compounded if the baby has a passive temperament, or if a pattern of infrequent feeding that fails to meet nutritional needs is established. If the mother has chosen to feed the baby according to a schedule (not one determined by the baby), the child's growth can slow down or cease. Various factors associated with failure to thrive in the breastfed infant and related to the baby or mother are discussed below:

- *Limited Breastfeeding Sessions*
    - ❖ Inadequate frequency and duration of feeding is a major factor that can lead to failure to thrive in breastfed babies. It is important to know how long the feeding sessions usually last and whether it is the mother or baby that stops the session.

    - ❖ The volume of milk received depends on the length of the feeding and the effectiveness of the infant's suckling.

    - ❖ Limiting the amount of time your baby spends at the breast may cause your baby to receive more of the lower calorie foremilk and less of the higher fat content hind milk.

    - ❖ Mothers usually require feeding on demand by the baby for full stimulation of milk production in the breasts. Once the milk supply has been established through breastfeeding and no time limit is arbitrarily set, your baby will most likely seem satisfied after nursing only on one breast for a few minutes (this is normal for later stages of breastfeeding). Be aware of your baby's hunger cues.

- *Insufficient (infrequent) Feeding Sessions*
  - ❖ Some babies are "content to starve" and willing to wait long periods of time between feedings. Mothers may interpret this lack of interest as an indication that the baby is full.
  - ❖ Poor weight gain can be due to infrequent feedings and an inadequate let-down reflex (e.g., depressed mother, psychological factors, etc.).
  - ❖ Some babies are quite placid and need to be awakened to feed (see *How to Awaken a Sleep Baby*).
  - ❖ Moreover, inappropriate formula supplements or pacifier use may decrease your milk supply, since babies nurse less often and/or meet their sucking needs with a pacifier instead of the breast.

- *Disorganized Suckling*
  - ❖ Disorganized suckling affects the amount and type of milk your baby receives (foremilk, hind milk). It is a temporary condition, usually seen in babies less than 1-month-old and in mothers who receive obstetrical and various anesthetics medications.
  - ❖ The mother may report that:
  - 1) The baby's suck does not feel very strong, has pain with nursing or that the baby is not doing anything when put on the breast.
  - 2) The baby may suck and swallow 1-3 times at the beginning of a feeding (the chin can be observed to move rapidly in a brief manner).
  - 3) The mother is unable to identify a swallow for a short time or the baby falls asleep (a sleepy or ill baby may not suck vigorously).
  - ❖ Breastfeeding positions that are sub-optimal often contribute to poor breastfeeding, as they do not provide the baby with an opportunity to suckle properly. Although older babies can suckle in a wide variety of positions as a result of well-developed musculature and maturity, an infant is unable to control his body as easily.

Tip: Sucking Problems

Persistent poor sucking, particularly when associated with a delay in developmental milestones may suggest neurological dysfunction.

continued

In some cases, the neurological problem is transitory and is caused by the immaturity of the central nervous system (CNS). As the infant matures, feeding problems disappear.

- *Maternal Diet*: Failure to thrive can occur if a breastfeeding mother is severely restricting her own dietary intake, as she herself is not well nourished and her milk will not contain the needed nutrients.

- *Vegetarian Mothers Vegetarian Toddlers:* Care must be taken to ensure that specific proteins and amino acids, along with certain vitamins and minerals that are usually derived from animal sourced foods are provided (see *Vegetarian Babies & Toddlers*).

- *Low Milk Supply*: Although it is rare, some mothers do not produce enough milk to meet their infant's needs. In such cases, the doctor may suggest formula supplementation, along with consultation with a lactation specialist to encourage milk production (see *Insufficient (Low) Milk Supply*).

- *Tongue Tie:* A small piece of skin under the tongue (the frenulum) may be too tight to allow your baby to suckle effectively (see *Tongue Tie & Breastfeeding*).

Indicators of Poor Weight Gain

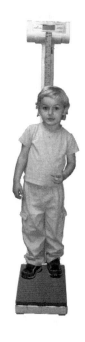

- The following are what parents should look for when you suspect or are told about poor weight gain in your infant/child:

  ❖ It is important to consider whether your infant is formula-fed or breastfed since growth patterns are different in each. Refer to the growth charts, have an idea of whether your child is losing or gaining weight, consider your child's stature, and discuss this with your doctor (see *Growth Chart*).

  ❖ Babies who have not regained their birth weight by 2-3 weeks of life, or the baby who is gaining less than 4 oz per week, require further consideration by your doctor.

❖ Genetics play a role in weight gain. For example, if both parents are slim, then the baby may not gain weight quickly. However, weight should increase at a steady pace, so follow up with your doctor to evaluate weight gain on a regular basis.

❖ Be alert to the following risks for poor weight gain: premature babies, the child with chronic disease, a child with irregular meals, a child with stress/poverty, a child with behavioral difficulties, picky eaters, major changes in the child's appetite, symptoms of vomiting, abnormal stools (e.g., malabsorption syndrome), etc.

• Discuss with your doctor any of the above concerns. If children have their weight and height measured regularly, their growth over time may be assessed and compared with other children of the same age and sex in the growth chart.

Tip: Indicators of Poor Weight Gain in the Breastfed Infant

First, consider the normal growth patterns of breastfed infants. Secondly, it is important to distinguish between the natural slow gainer from a slow weight gain issue. The naturally slow infant gains weight slowly but steadily. This child maintains a particular growth curve and increases in length and head circumference.

The following are indicators of poor weight gain in the breastfed infant:

Does not regain birth weight by 2-3 weeks after birth.

Does not gain at least 1 lb/450 g per month for the first 4 months.

Serious drop in growth rate, including length and head circumference.

Feeding on smaller amounts and less often than the recommendation for your baby's age group.

Fewer wet diapers.

Baby looks thinner and skin is wrinkled.

Baby wakes up quickly in-between feeds, or stays awake most of the time to show the mother that he is hungry.

Baby cries after a feeding session (see *Insufficient (Low) Milk Supply*)

Diagnosis

• The doctor caring for your baby will perform a physical examination that includes growth parameters (plotted and compared), as well as a medical history.

- Remember, that the younger your baby is, the more checkups he requires to detect any growth or developmental problems. Also, in the case of the breastfed infant, observation of breastfeeding is necessary by your doctor or lactation specialist.

- *Medical history* questions may include the following:
    - ❖ Was the child growing normally and then growth slowed down?
    - ❖ Does the child eat well (food type and feeding history)?
    - ❖ What type of feeding schedule do you use?
    - ❖ Is the infant breast or bottle-fed?
    - ❖ What kind of foods is the toddler eating?
    - ❖ What medications does the child take?
    - ❖ Is the child developing normal social and physical skills?
    - ❖ Questions about parent-child relations and social interaction.
    - ❖ Is the child vomiting or does he have diarrhea?
    - ❖ How are the child's stool types and patterns?
    - ❖ Are there any stress or health issues in the family?

- *Laboratory tests* are not always necessary, however if the cause for poor weight gain is not clear or there are suspected complications (e.g., iron or vitamin deficiencies), lab tests may be considered. Common tests include blood tests, hormonal studies, stool studies, and x-rays.

- In some cases, treatment may include an entire team of health professionals; it may be composed of the child's primary doctor, a nutritionist or dietitian (assess the child's dietary intake), an occupational or speech therapist (assess sucking or swallowing problems), a social worker (if failure to thrive is caused by the parents), a psychologist (problems in the home), etc.

Treatment of Poor Weight Gain

General Treatment

In most cases, treatment is given outside of the hospital with follow-up visits to your child's doctor as needed. There are several things a parent may do to increase the baby's weight:

- When feeding your baby, it should be a relaxed experience, whether you are breastfeeding or bottle-feeding.

- If your baby is regurgitating or vomiting, your doctor may consider thickening the food or providing medications.

- Ensure your technique of feeding and preparing formula is appropriate, including the amount of foods given. Your doctor may recommend starting to feed cereal at an earlier age.

- When your baby falls asleep during a feeding, wake him up and feed him at night to increase caloric intake.

- If the baby is feeding only on small amounts every time, feed him more frequently (as tolerated).

- Burping during feedings may sometimes help your baby continue to feed.

- Formula high in calorie content or high calorie foods may be required if the problem still does not resolve itself.

- Consultation with a dietitian may be required to increase the calories in your child's diet. A pediatric occupational therapist may be needed to improve oral-motor feeding skills, if the infant develops severe feeding problems.

- Any nutritional deficiencies are to be corrected with the help and advice of your health professional (e.g., iron deficiency if the child has developed anemia).

- Ensure optimal treatment if your child has a chronic condition, and treat specific conditions or causes for poor weight gain.

- Follow-up closely with your specialist with regular measurements of height and weight until growth has improved.

Tip: More Severe Failure to Thrive

A child with severe failure to thrive needs to be hospitalized so that he can be nourished properly. At the same time, possible causes are assessed, including parent and child interaction during feedings, etc.

Treatment for the Breastfed Infant
- The breastfeeding mother should be eating a healthy, well balanced diet with a good amount of fluid intake and as much rest as possible.

- Increase the frequency and length of feeding sessions and, upon consultation with your doctor or lactation specialist, you may also need to add formula or start solids earlier than normally recommended.

- Do not limit the amount your baby can feed on one breast, but rather, switch gradually to the other (remember that fat content is received at the end of the breast so do not switch breasts too quickly). Make sure that your child empties the breast before switching to the other breast. Always offer the second breast after your baby has completely emptied the first one. Do not worry if your baby seems full after the first breast.

Tip: Achieving Proper Lactation

Observation by a lactation specialist to assess breastfeeding technique can help to more appropriately position the baby for breastfeeding and quickly change the dynamic between mother and baby; this can help improve the situation.

Parent Concerns

My four and a half month old baby is breastfeeding and he seems hungry all the time. Why is he not gaining weight? Should I start him on solid foods or formula?

- You must first consult your doctor to assess your child's weight gain. If your doctor says that your child is gaining weight well, then there is nothing for you to do.

- However, if your infant is not gaining weight properly, then it would be preferable to add solids given with a spoon, rather than to serve formula in a bottle. If you give your infant cereal, you may add pumped breast milk to increase both caloric content and your milk production.

- Talk to your doctor or lactation specialist about assessing your breastfeeding technique and ruling out low milk supply (see *Insufficient (Low) Milk Supply*).

Sometimes, it feels as though my milk production is suddenly less, or "dried up." Is this normal?

- Some experts believe that sudden, "dried up" milk is rare.

- Many mothers will switch to formula on their own initiative when they believe their milk has "dried up." Talk to your doctor or lactation specialist before starting on formula supplements.

- Remember that there can be a variation in the amount of breast milk from day-to-day and sometimes, even morning to night.

- Also, if your breast feels soft or less full after a couple weeks of breastfeeding, it is normal, since breast engorgement is no longer present.

Are there any conditions that may present in failure to thrive without noticing any evident symptoms in the child?

- There are conditions, called *occult* (hidden) conditions, which may not show any clear signs except for failure to grow. These conditions may be suspected by your doctor and appropriately evaluated. The following examples of conditions include:

  ❖ Chronic gastroesophageal reflux.

  ❖ Mal-absorption (primarily Celiac disease).

  ❖ Infections (e.g.,perinatal, renal, etc.).

  ❖ Subtle oral motor difficulties in children with neurological conditions.

  ❖ Multiple cavities may make eating and chewing difficult, contributing to failure to thrive.

  ❖ Large tonsils and adenoids (feeding difficulties and hypoxia = shortage of oxygen to the body).

How should I keep track of my child's growth?

- Each measurement of height, weight and head circumference is put into a growth chart that looks like a graph. As new height and weight measurements are added, we can see if your child is following a natural growth pattern (see *Growth Charts*). Frequency of measurements is up to your doctor and your concerns.

Practical Tips & Conclusion

- The main cause of failure to gain weight in infancy is that the baby is not feeding enough, whether he is breast or bottle-fed.

- Generally, you do not have to worry about slow weight gain if your baby is happy, active, and his weight gain is proportionate to his height.

- Various factors are responsible for growth and one should consider genetics, physical activity, breast or bottle-fed, additional solid foods taken, social and environmental factors, etc.

- The most important thing to consider when your baby is not gaining weight well is your baby's welfare. You need to consult with your doctor regularly and watch your child's weight closely.

- If you are part of a small group of women who cannot produce enough milk, you can always combine breastfeeding with bottle-feeding. See lactation specialist.

- See other chapters for more causes and treatment options, such as the picky eater, how to know if my child is growing, prolonged food refusal, etc.

Sample Menus for 6-12 Months

For older children, the number of food servings for each food group is discussed in various chapters.

6-8 Months
Breakfast & Mid-Morning Snack
Breast milk or iron-fortified formula
3-4 tablespoons of infant cereal
2-3 tablespoons of strained fruit

Lunch & Mid-Afternoon Snack
Breast milk or formula
4-6 tablespoons of vegetables
2-5 tablespoons of strained meat

Dinner & Before Bed Snack
Breast milk or formula
3-5 tablespoons of vegetable/meat combination
2-3 tablespoons of strained fruit
Breast milk or formula or 3-4 tablespoons of infant cereal

8-12 Months
Breakfast & Mid-Morning Snack
Breast milk or formula
Grain cereal (oatmeal, rice, or various mixed cereals)
Fruits or vegetables (apples, pears, peaches, apple sauce, bananas, etc.)
Cheese, yogurt, or eggs*

Lunch & Mid-Afternoon Snack
Breast milk or formula
Meat and alternatives with cereal (chicken and rice, turkey and rice, beef and barley, tofu and wheat germ, peas or lentil, etc.)
Fruits and/or vegetables (squash and pears, bananas and sweet potatoes, avocado and/or apple sauce, etc.)
Yogurt and cheese*

Dinner & Before Bed Snack
Breast milk or formula
Protein and/or cereal* (cereal and yogurt and turkey, chicken and vegetables, lentil soup)
Fruits and/or vegetables (mixed vegetables, pear sauce and/or baked squash, avocado and mashed tofu)
Dairy* (cream cheese and apple sauce, teething biscuits, yogurt and fruits)

---

*These are optional foods and depend on your baby's age and ability to eat all of the above.

Eggs: Egg yolk is given at 9-10 months of age, while egg whites are added at one year of age or later (especially when there is family history of egg allergy).

Remember to use more textured, lumpier, and finger foods at this age.

Infant Obesity: Prevention & Treatment

General

Defining infant obesity is a difficult and controversial issue, because there is no clear definition of "overweight" in the first year of a baby's life. Possible definitions of infant obesity may include the following:

(1) The state of being overweight according to the standard growth charts.

(2) Weight exceeds growth percentiles in height.

(3) Both height and weight exceed the 97th percentile on a growth chart.

There is a misconception among parents that a fat baby is a healthy baby. The fact is that a fat baby is not necessarily a healthy baby (obesity is a risk factor for the development of type 2 diabetes and future complications). The concern with an overweight infant is that if the baby is larger than "normal" weight, then he is at a higher risk of being an overweight child. Not all obese infants become obese children, and not all obese children become obese adults. However, there is a greater likelihood that obesity, beginning even in early infancy, will persist throughout the life span. A study conducted of 1650 babies concluded that babies who gain weight quickly or faster than normal during the first 6 months of life, are likely to be overweight at the age of two years. It may foreshadow obesity during childhood and adulthood (*British Medical Journal* 331: October 2005).

Causes

There are various contributing factors to infant obesity that may include the following:

- Exposure to *excessive calories* during the infancy stage may lead the infant's metabolism to increase the number of fat cells in the body.

- *Bottle-feeding* (either in the amount given or the frequency of feedings): Although breastfed infants are thought to be less overweight than bottle-fed babies, I see breastfed babies who are very chubby and a small number who are largely overweight (when checked against the breastfed baby growth chart). Whether this is due to *"too frequent breastfeeding"* (feeding by schedule rather than on demand, etc.) or other factors (e.g.,mother's breast milk composition – i.e., leptin hormone in breast milk, genetics, baby grazing on the breast, etc.) is not clear.

- *Overabundant breast milk supply* can result in a more rapid than normal weight gain.

- *Starting solid foods, particularly cereal, earlier than recommended* and in excessive amounts or offered in a bottle, may lead to an obese or overweight baby.

- *Genetic factors or a family history* of obesity play a role, as overweight mothers may have large babies. They may tend to feed their infants larger food portions, laying the foundation for childhood obesity.

- *Diseases and syndromes* may be a cause of infant obesity (e.g., hypothyroidism, Pradder Willi Syndrome, Beckwith Wideman syndrome, etc.).

  ❖ Physical activity, at least in the early months of life, is probably not a significant contributing factor to infant obesity.

Prevention & Treatment

- Overfeeding your infant is a very common problem, however it is even more harmful to underfeed your baby. Parent should always consult their doctor before modifying their infant's diet. Parents are not advised to place their overweight baby on a diet, but to rather, re-examine feeding patterns upon discussion with the doctor. Treatment for the overweight or obese infant means slowing down the excessive weight gain. Prevention and treatment measures include the following:

- Do not feed your baby an *excess amount of formula*, because this may lead to a chubby baby, spitting up, abdominal pain, and excess weight gain. Consult your doctor about any overfeeding issues or concerns you may have and periodically assess his weight gain (see *Feeding By Schedule or On Demand: Amount & Frequency*).

- With the breastfed infant, *feed on demand* and respond to your baby's hunger cues. Do not feed for every cry, comfort, etc.

- If you are breastfeeding and your baby grazes at the breast, he will learn to eat when he is upset or distressed and use food to relieve this stress. Consider offering your baby a pacifier, since some babies crave sucking.

- *Do not introduce solid foods earlier than suggested* (e.g., to help your baby sleep through the night, etc.), since this has been found to increase the chance of childhood obesity. The suggested age for solid food introduction is six months (depending on your baby's weight gain, etc).

- Do not add *cereal*, as it is rich in calories, to your baby's diet (and especially earlier than recommended) if he is developing appropriately for his height and weight (watch other food intake, especially iron).

- Do not introduce juices before the age of nine months, if at all. Use water instead.

- Do not allow your child to keep his bottle as a companion day and night, since he will learn to feed whenever he is bored or upset.

- Feed by hunger cues. Stop feeding when your baby seems to be full (turning his head or no longer opening his mouth, etc.). Do not make him finish every bottle, finish a jar of baby food, or finish off everything on the plate.

- Do not hurry or rush your child's feedings—take your time and allow him to feed slowly.

- Avoid sweets until your child is at least one year of age.

- Avoid serving your child foods to keep him occupied during free time. Instead, give your child something to play with.

- Increase the level of physical activity in your baby by playing with him. Babies who gain weight quickly during the infancy stage begin to slow their weight gain once they become more physically active (crawling, running, walking, rolling, etc.).

Tip: Research on Feeding and Obesity

The type of feeding (breast milk or formula) your baby is given has been greatly debated in terms of its role in infant obesity. Research seems to indicate that breastfed babies are less likely to become obese children or adults than formula-fed babies. However, new research contradicts this statement.

Comments & Conclusion

- Feeding on demand is feeding your baby when he is hungry by responding to your baby's hunger cues. This technique seems to develop healthy, appropriate eating habits. Frequent feedings on schedule may lead to obesity (e.g., a four month old infant being fed on two hour intervals).

- Factors that may increase the chances of obesity are genetics, parental obesity, the obesity hormone in breast milk (studies on this are, to date, inconclusive), etc.

- It is important not to restrict your child's diet in the early years of life. Instead, provide adequate calories and a healthy, well balanced diet. Offer healthy food choices rather than unhealthy ones (e.g., "junk" food).

- While studies show some correlation of obesity in infant and the early years of life to obesity in adulthood, it is practically impossible to predict adult obesity based only on this criterion. In any case, obesity should be addressed as early as possible.

The Overweight & Obese Child

General

Obesity is a condition of excess body weight in the form of fat. The incidence of obesity is very high in North America and its prevalence is increasing, due to unhealthy eating patterns and lack of physical activity.

Obesity is an important health issue and one of today's major medical problems. It can lead to hypertension, heart disease, diabetes, pain in the hip joint, breathing difficulty while sleeping, and lower life expectancy.

The most traumatizing and widespread complications of childhood obesity are psychosocial issues. Obesity is the least socially acceptable condition among children today. Overweight children may suffer from low self-esteem, psychological and social adjustment issues, depression, feelings of low self-worth, and so forth.

It is very important to teach your child good eating habits from an early age, as the first 3 years of life lay the foundation for obesity. The probability of childhood obesity persisting into adulthood is estimated to increase from about 20% at 4 years of age to approximately 80% by adolescence. The first three years of life are a critical period, so as soon as you see that your child has a tendency to become obese, it is important to make changes as early as possible.

Tip: Drastic Weight Change

Children who experience a drastic weight change (gain or loss) should see a doctor. It is also important to find out how your child perceives his weight and whether he wants to do something about it. A weight management problem is doomed from the start if it is only the parents who perceive the problem, and not the child.

Causes & Risk Factors

Genetics & Familial

- Obesity tends to run in families, suggesting a genetic cause.

- When both parents are obese, there is an 80% chance that the child will become obese as well. When both parents are slim, the child has a 20% chance of becoming obese.

- At any age of childhood, having an obese parent increases the child's risk of being overweight as an adult. Obese parents more than double the risk of adult obesity in both obese and non-obese children younger than the age of 10 years.

- Some genetic diseases have obesity as a part of other symptoms (e.g., syndromes such as Pradder Willi or Cohen Syndrome, etc.).

- Along with genetics, environmental factors also influence the likelihood of obesity. For example, a high birth weight, maternal diabetes, and obesity in family members are all factors which increase the risk of your child becoming overweight.

Lifestyle & Parental Dynamics

- The family lifestyle affects obesity in children. Families share lifestyle and diet habits that sometimes contribute to excess weight.

- Typically, obese parents are less active and consume high calorie foods, and then pass these habits to their children.

- Events such as separation, divorce, moving, etc., can be stressful for the young child and he may respond to this stress by overeating, exercising too little, or both. You need to find out what the problem is and try to change the situation to help your child to feel better (you can help an older child cope with stress by teaching him to talk about the problem, write it down, draw, cry, punch a pillow, etc.).

- It is important to examine family and parental dynamics such as low income and socioeconomic status, as these may contribute to a lack of consistency in healthy food choices and safe places for activities.

- Over-controlling parental behavior affects the child's eating patterns, and parental food choices influence the child's food preferences.

Physical Activity

- There is a decline in physical activity that has worsened with technological advancement. For example, watching television or playing video games results in decreased physical activity and increased food consumption.

- Children today are 40% less active than they were 30 years ago. The average child in Canada watches three to five hours of television per day while snacking.

Other Risk Factors

- *Extent and duration of breastfeeding*: This is inversely associated with the risk of obesity in childhood. However, recent studies do not confirm the positive effects of breastfeeding and obesity in children.

- *Timing of complementary food introduction*: Some experts believe that the timing of when complementary foods are introduced to the child plays a role in obesity. However, studies have not shown any consistent links between the timing of food introduction to childhood obesity.

- The *early period of life* may increase the risk of childhood obesity. As such, early intervention will help optimize growth and development in your child while promoting healthy eating and activity patterns from a young age.

- *Adolescence* is a critical time period to develop obesity that persists into adulthood. Adolescents are also at risk of poor diet and exercise habits.

- *Medication and medical illness* (e.g., hormonal imbalances, metabolic diseases, etc.) can cause obesity, but it is uncommon.

Tip: Medical Complications of Obesity

Cardiovascular health (increased blood pressure, hypercholesterolemia, etc.).

Endocrine system (insulin resistance, impaired glucose tolerance, type 2 diabetes mellitus, etc.).

Fatty liver; polycystic ovary syndrome (in adolescent girls).

Lungs (asthma, obstructive sleep apnea, etc.).

Orthopedic (slipped capital femoral epiphysis).

Psychological and social consequences (less likable, difficulties making friends, poor self-esteem, teasing, risk of early disorders, depression, etc.).

Decreased quality of life is associated with obesity in school aged children.

Diagnosis

- While diagnosis is evident when seeing an obese child, it is possible to detect signs of upward weight gain at an early stage. The percentile growth line on the graph going from the usual linear growth to the line above, indicates the start of obesity. This is the time to intervene, before your child develops a life-long weight problem.

- Your doctor may ask you questions related to obesity risk factors to rule out any other medical causes, as most of the time, extra weight is functional obesity (from diet and lifestyle, rather than medical causes) as well as, psychological implications. Some of these questions may include:

  - ❖ The family history of obesity.

  - ❖ Diet and eating patterns, including the number of meals and snacks, types of meals and snacks offered (food groups offered, foods high in fat and calories, sugar in beverages, etc.), and portion size (food limits, overeating, large portions, etc.).

- Hunger and fullness sense: Does your child like to eat? Is he always hungry or asking for food? Does he get full? Does he know when he gets full (e.g., tummy hurts, going to burst, blowing up, etc.).

  - ❖ Restricted access and food limits: Studies show that children are more likely to over-eat when placed on food restrictions and/or limits.

  - ❖ Eating for stress or anger: Parents sometimes quiet their child by giving him food every time he is upset or stressed. This teaches the child to get into the habit of eating every time he is angry or stressed (emotional eating).

  - ❖ Physical activity: Is your child active? Is he playing video games or watching television all day long? Is there any involvement in household chores or sports activities? Are there any activities done as a family?

> ### Tip: Regular Meals, Food Control
>
> According to a recent study, overweight children skip the breakfast meal more often than children of normal weight. Studies also show that there is decreased consumption in fruits and vegetables and an increased consumption in such foods as French fries, potato chips, candy, chocolate bars, etc.

- A physical examination by your doctor will usually show normal findings, except for growth parameters. Lab tests are mostly unnecessary and depend on any abnormal findings (they may include thyroid and liver function tests, and a glucose screen).

- Physical examinations assess the degree of obesity and muscularity, body type, height and weight measurements, etc. The doctor will measure the following:

Body Mass Index (BMI)

❖ Your child's height and weight will be plotted on a growth chart. These growth charts consider the child's body mass index (BMI), which shows whether the child's height and weight are proportionate. With children, the BMI is based on gender and age to allow for change in the body's composition, as the child gets older.

❖ BMI is widely used to define overweight and obesity as it correlates well with more accurate measures of body fat, and is derived from easily available data on height and weight. It is calculated by dividing body weight by the square of the height. It is then plotted on a curve to obtain a percentile value.

❖ Your child will be ranked in percentiles compared to other children his age and gender. If, for example, your child were in the 85th percentile (meaning that his weight is higher than 85% of children his age and gender), he would then be considered overweight. If your child were in the 95th percentile and above, he would be considered obese.

Ideal Body Weight (IBW)

❖ Obesity is also defined medically, based on the child's weight relative to height. At any given height, a child should have the ideal weight, which is called ideal body weight (IBW). The child whose weight is 20% above his IBW is considered obese.

Skin Fold Measurement

❖ In addition, some doctors use skin fold caliper measurement to determine if your child is carrying too much fat. This method measures body fat directly, so that bone size and muscle mass do not interfere with the accuracy of the measurement.

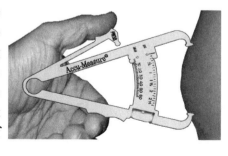

❖ Further factors the doctor considers are the child's overall health, and the parents' height and weight, etc.

Tip: High BMI and Weight Management

A child who is older than two years of age and whose BMI is above the 95th percentile should be evaluated in a pediatric center before a weight management program is considered.

Prevention & Treatment Measures

- In order not to compromise child growth and development, the treatment of the obese child is different than that of the obese adult.

- Restricting a child's diet when he is under the age of two years may affect growth and development of the body and brain, so follow up with your doctor on your child's height and weight gain and get suggestions for healthy eating habits. Consult a dietitian to help you plan a balanced diet for your child.

- The key to success in the prevention and treatment of the overweight or obese child is changes in lifestyle, exercise, healthy eating habits, encouragement, close and supportive follow-up, family behavior modifications, decreasing sedentary behavior and motivation (parent/child). Motivation to make a change by the parents is a key factor. Many parents do not acknowledge how important their role is in developing and maintaining a child's eating habits at a young age, as they may predispose and/or perpetuate the problem.

- Treatment of the obese young child should focus on weight maintenance rather than weight loss. Regular follow-ups are needed every 1 to 2 months for close monitoring of prevention effectiveness and to provide positive reinforcement. As treatment progresses, less frequent visits are required.

- Depending on the patient, your doctor may refer you to a center with multidisciplinary team that may include a pediatrician, dietitian, endocrinologist, cardiologist, respirologist, gastroenterologist, social worker, and psychologist.

Family Behavior Modification

- Young children are especially dependent on adults for nourishment, activity planning, and attitudes towards health (among other things).

- Behavioral changes in the family are needed, as parents are considered to be the primary agents of change in the young child (e.g., in an active household, children are more likely to be active).

- Short-term diets that seek quick and drastic weight loss are unrealistic and unhealthy for young children. Incorporate small, gradual changes into the family's daily routine.

- The first step for parents is to take the position of being a role model (i.e. encouraging healthy behavior). These attitudes and behaviors directly affect children's actions.

- A balanced parental approach (without being too rigid and controlling) is important in maintaining good nutritional standards in your home. Do not show too much concern about weight, but rather focus on health, good exercise, and eating habits as a family. If you restrict access to snacks and foods, your child is more likely to eat when he is hungry.

- Studies show that children who sit at the table with the family are more likely to eat a healthy, well balanced diet. Provide a positive and encouraging environment at the table when eating that may include:

  ❖ Always eat at the table.

  ❖ Allow no distractions during the family dinner.

  ❖ Offer support and reinforce healthy eating habits.

  ❖ Offer balanced and nutritional foods.

  ❖ Teach normal and healthy eating habits from an early age.

Healthy Eating
- Encourage three balanced meals and two small snacks per day (breakfast is especially important).

  ❖ Breakfast is an especially important meal and is proven to increase academic performance in children. Children who tend to skip breakfast have poor attention, less concentration, and are more at risk of developing nutritional deficiencies. Offer your child breakfast every morning, with foods such as fresh fruits, whole wheat pita with cottage cheese or peanut butter, bagel with cream cheese or eggs, grilled cheese sandwich, etc.

❖ There should be at least three food groups offered in at least one meal every day (see *The Food Groups: Making Sense of Portion Size & Acitivity Level*).

- Encourage fiber-rich foods (e.g., cereals that are low in sugar, vegetables, fruits—keep the skin on fruits and potatoes, etc.). Fiber is naturally filling and can help manage weight (fiber also helps normal bowel function and is rich in vitamins and minerals).

- You can start a meal with a soup or a salad. Offer at least two vegetables at dinner and use vegetables in sandwiches or as snacks (great finger foods). Give fruits each day as a snack or with breakfast and/or lunch.

- Serve tasty and healthy snacks in-between mealtimes (e.g., fruits, cheese, whole grain crackers with low fat cheese, rice cakes, low fat milk, homemade fruit smoothies, low fat yogurt, sliced apples, bananas, cooked and diced potatoes, well cooked carrots, whole grain crackers, dry cereal, strawberries, etc.) that do not contain much sugar. Keep healthy, low fat snacks in the house, and limit junk food servings to one or none per day. Cut down on snacks and sweet drinks between meals.

- Choose lower fat and high calorie foods.
  - ❖ Decrease consumption of fast foods such as French fries, potato chips, chocolate, etc.

  - ❖ Take the skin off poultry, serve lean meats, trim fats off meats, and use lower fat dairy products. Avoid fried foods (e.g., onion rings, fried chicken and fish, French fries, etc.)—grill, bake, or microwave instead. Limit the amount of oils in cooking (two tablespoons per family meal). Limit vinaigrette style dressings to two tablespoons per serving and avoid creamy dressings and sauces. Offer fruits for desserts.

  - ❖ Avoid saturated and trans fats (they worsen insulin resistance) and use unsaturated fats such as olive oil, canola oil, almonds, walnuts, fish oil, etc.

  - ❖ Make healthy choices such as offering grilled chicken sandwiches with baked potato instead of fries and a cheeseburger; offer thin crust veggie pizza with a sprinkle of cheese instead of pan crust pepperoni with extra cheese, etc.

- Select water rather than juice or soft drinks (see *Juices*). Your child needs to learn to drink water when he is thirsty.

- Offer your child a variety of healthy foods at mealtime and allow him to decide what he would like to eat.

- Offer portions that are suitable for your child, with options for second servings. This allows him to serve himself when possible.

- Healthy lunch bag suggestions may include the following:

  ❖ Bake a chicken and shred it or slice it to use for lunches all week.

  ❖ Add chopped vegetables like tomatoes, cucumbers, spinach, carrots, celery, etc., to your child's lunch. You may even add a light dressing for extra flavor.

  ❖ Create a cold rice salad by chopping up various vegetables, and meat or chicken.

  ❖ Pretzels are a much better snack than potato chips.

  ❖ Pack 100% pure juice boxes as beverages.

  ❖ Include fat-free strawberry or oatmeal bars, graham crackers, and raisin cookies instead of chocolate chip cookies, brownies, etc.

- A study from the Canadian Institute for Health Research found that kids who purchased lunch at school were 47% more likely to be overweight than those who brought lunch from home.

- Do not just take out everything unhealthy in your child's diet. Simply add healthy foods to the diet, and slowly phase out unhealthy choices. Make simple dietary substitutions, such as serving low-fat milk to children two years and older.

- If you do not succeed in offering certain healthy foods, try again. Studies have shown that a new food often has to be served 8-15 times before a child will accept it. Relying on the same few foods that your child always accepts may seem easier, but it makes a balanced diet less likely.

- How and where dinner is eaten makes a difference, as well. Children who eat dinner with their families at least three times a week are less likely to be overweight or obese, because they eat healthier foods. Eat meals with your child at the family table with no distractions, since it can interfere with hunger and satiety cues.

- Try to make healthy food choices and do not place any pressure on your child to eat or follow a strict diet.

- Set a daily mealtime schedule so that meals and snacks are not rushed and your child is not pressured to eat.

- Watch foods eaten at restaurants, as they usually contain a higher sugar and fat content than foods eaten at home (also watch the portion size).

Physical Activity/Exercise

- Physical activity and exercise is very important for good health for the family as a whole. Do not focus or "single" out one child as he may feel punished.

- The key to promoting physical activity in the young child is to incorporate these activities into daily life. Although your child may have opportunities to be physically active in school, sports and/or on the playground, they may not provide sufficient exercise.

- Create and maintain an environment that is conducive to active play. It may include using the stairs whenever possible, walking to the store, taking daily trips to the park, walking the dog, playing games, bicycling, dancing, swimming, basketball, etc.

- Parents can designate an area in the house for free play, so that even in bad weather your child will have a place to play active games. Also, parents can be involved in these physical activities.

- Find an affordable activity that your child enjoys, and makes active living a part of the daily routine.

- *For children who are between the ages of 12-18 months:*
  - ❖ Pull toys to encourage children to pull themselves up or walk.
  - ❖ Soft balls or beanbags may be safely thrown to help children develop throwing patterns and sports activities.
  - ❖ Allow children to carry various fun objects from one place to another (inside or outside).

- *For children who are between the ages of 18-24 months:*
  - ❖ Play games that encourage children to move about at various speeds and directions.
  - ❖ Kick balls with your child so he learns how to balance.

❖ Help the child walk on his own, up and down stairs.

❖ Play "Simon Says" to provide movement flexibility development such as touching the nose, twisting, nodding heads, etc.

❖ Play music, and sing and dance with your child

- Parents can decrease sedentary time by removing the television from their child's bedroom, limiting "screen" time (less than two hours per day), setting a good example by involving the whole family in physical activity, encouraging the child to walk to school whenever possible, etc. The Canadian Pediatric Society suggests no more than an hour of television per day for preschoolers.

Tip: Decreasing Sedentary Time

Reinforcing decreased sedentary time is more successful than reinforcing increased physical activity.

How to Handle Overeating & Teaching Fullness

- Children do not stay full for a very long time. They have small stomachs, high energy levels, and rapid growth, so they are probably hungry most of the time.

- Do not deny your child food because he is overweight or obese. Simply offer healthy food choices when he is hungry.

- The following are ways to help teach your child fullness:

❖ Encourage the whole family to eat slowly and eat together.

❖ Teach your child that "full" means content, no longer hungry, and comfortable, but with no sensations of a heavy stomach after a meal.

❖ Let your child self-regulate his own portion size.

❖ Play the tummy talk game: Let your child feel what a tummy full is like before starting to eat by placing his hand on the tummy and then asking, what "full" feels like. While eating, ask your child if he is getting full and explain that full means light but that hunger is no longer there and, at end of the meal, again ask what his tummy is saying.

Tip: Nutrition & Eating Out

Limit outside eating to less than once a week.

Do not "upsize" foods.

Avoid ordering foods with words such as fried, buttery, cheesy, crispy, gravy, creamed, marinated in oil, etc.

When ordering, use low fat dressings and sauces, ketchup or BBQ sauce, low fat milk or water, baked/broiled/poached foods, split large portions or take home leftovers, and watch bread intake with the meal.

Section 8:
Specific Feeding
& Nutrition Issues

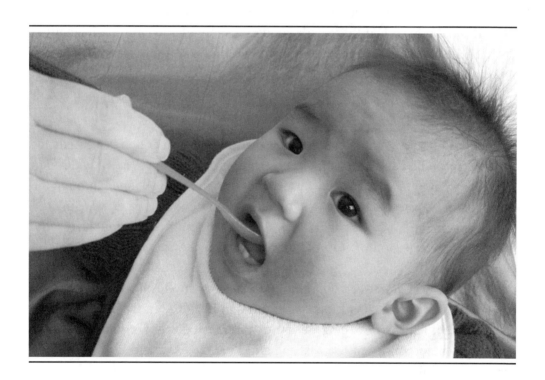

Iron & Iron Deficiency

General

Iron is a necessary mineral for body function and good health. It is important to enzyme systems, which are responsible for the smooth functioning of the body. These systems do not function properly in iron deficient children, resulting in tiredness, weakness, sleepiness, etc. Iron helps the body resist colds and infections while, at the same time, promoting a stronger immune system. It is also required for brain function, as neurotransmitters (chemicals in the brain that carry messages from one nerve to another) require iron to function properly. In addition, iron is an essential component of the hemoglobin molecule in red blood cells that carry oxygen through the body. When there isn't enough iron available (iron deficiency), a child's body cannot produce enough hemoglobin, leading to anemia.

Iron deficiency is the most common single nutrient deficiency worldwide, mainly affecting older infants, young children, adolescents, and women of childbearing age.

Babies are born with a small amount of iron in the liver and bone marrow, which is received from the mother. This store of iron supplies the baby through the first 4-6 months of life. After this period, iron must be obtained through the diet. Young children between 6-24 months of age are at greater risk for iron deficiency anemia, because their rapid growth requires more iron. Typically, the danger time period of iron deficiency anemia is when children transition from iron-fortified foods (e.g., formula and infant cereals) to solids, which contain less iron. Moreover, children often start on cow's milk around the age of one, which may cause a loss of iron through bleeding in the digestive tract (tiny amounts, but over a long period of time, this becomes significant). As such, it is important to ensure that the child receives enough iron in the first two years of life (by this age, one in fifteen American babies are low in iron).

Types & Sources of Iron

Types of Iron & Its Absorption

- There are two types of iron found in foods:
  - ❖ *Heme iron* is found in animal foods (e.g., red meat, chicken, pork, fish, and lamb) and is the best absorbed (10-20%) type of iron.

❖ *Non-heme iron* is found in vegetables, cereals, fruits, eggs, and fortified food products and is less absorbable (about 7%).

- The amount of iron in a specific food is not important. What is important is the amount of iron which your body absorbs. For example, a grown woman can get half of her daily iron needs from 5 oz/150 g of lean steak; to absorb the same amount of iron from spinach, she would need to eat nearly 4 lb/1.8 kg of it.

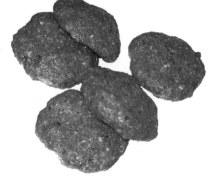

- Overall, iron absorption is affected by the type of iron in the food, other foods eaten at the same meal, and the body's need for iron.

- The amount of iron that can be absorbed from a variety of foods range from 1-20%; undigested iron goes directly to the stool. The percentage of iron absorbed from the following sources are:

  ❖ Breast milk: approximately 50-70% (lactoferrin and vitamin C contribute to efficient absorption).

  ❖ Iron-fortified cow's milk formula: Approximately 3-12%.

  ❖ Iron-fortified soy formula: Approximately less than 1-7% (soy contains phytates, which interfere with iron absorption).

  ❖ Cow's milk: Approximately 10 % or 0.5 mg of iron per liter (increased calcium levels interfere with iron absorption).

- The amount of iron can vary according to its formula type and manufacturer. Consult your doctor and check the formula before serving it to your baby.

- Children who are iron deficient will absorb the available iron more efficiently than those with normal iron levels.

- To increase iron absorption, try the following after consultation with your doctor:

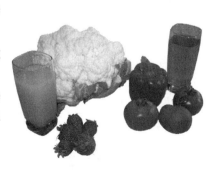

  ❖ Use a variety of vitamin C rich vegetable sourced foods to increase iron absorption (e.g., squash, legumes, hummus, etc.).

❖ Iron absorption may be increased by eating vitamin A and the amino acid cysteine containing foods such as eggs, wheat, and cheese.

❖ Sugars in fruits will help iron absorption.

• Factors that decrease iron absorption include:

❖ Phytic acid found in bran, wheat, soy, and bread can interfere with iron absorption. Thus, do not serve them at or near the time you serve iron-rich foods to your child.

❖ Phosphates (in milk and eggs), vegetable fiber, and other minerals (calcium, zinc) interfere with iron absorption.

❖ Cow's milk and medications (e.g., antacids) can interfere with iron absorption and should not be taken at the same time as iron supplements.

Sources of Iron

While introducing solid foods, parents should pay attention to foods that contain good sources of iron. For example, about two tablespoons twice per day of iron-fortified cereal will supply the iron needs of a baby or toddler, especially if you add vitamin C rich fruits or vegetables (these enhance iron absorption). The following list contains foods that are good sources of iron (in no particular order), not including breast milk or iron-fortified formula (already discussed above):

Cereals (iron-fortified): 1 oz/30 ml = 4-8 mg iron	Bagel: 1 oz/30 g = 1.8 mg iron
Tomato Paste: 4 oz/120 ml = 3.9 mg iron	Sweet Potatoes: 4 oz/120 g = 1.7 mg iron
Lentils: 4 oz/120 g = 3 mg iron	Tuna: 3 oz/90 g = 1 mg iron
Chicken: 4 oz/120 g = 1 mg iron	Liver: 4 oz /120 g= 6.5 mg iron
Hot Dog: 1 = 0.5 mg iron	Beef: 4 oz/120 g = 3.5 mg iron
Artichokes: 4 oz/120 g = 2.5 mg iron	Dried Fruits (peaches, raisins, apricots, figs): 1/2 cup = 2-3 mg iron
Tofu: 3 oz/90 g = 2-7 mg iron	Egg Yolk (white has no iron): 3.5 mg iron per 100 g
Pumpkin & Sunflower Seeds*: 1 oz/30 g = iron	Black-Strap Molasses*: 1 tbsp = 3.5 mg 2-4 mg iron

* Pumpkin, sunflower seeds, and blackstrap molasses (unless pasteurized) should not be given to a child younger than two years of age.

- Other good sources of iron include legumes, watermelon, wheat germ, turkey, beets, collard greens, mushrooms, spinach, brown rice, parsley, carrots, chickpeas, winter squash, peanut butter (when age appropriate), etc.

How Much Iron is Required?

- Most babies are born with iron stores. Babies get the iron they need from these stores, combined with breast milk and/or iron-fortified formula.
- Iron needs increase around six months of age when babies' iron stores are reduced. Infants will require the *absorption* of 0.4-0.6 mg per day of iron to maintain adequate stores.
- The recommended iron intake is as follows:

Age	Iron Intake Per Day
7-12 Months	11 mg a day
1-3 Years	7 mg a day
4-8 Years	10 mg a day
9-13 Years	8 mg a day

- *Premature babies* require extra iron, since they are not in the womb long enough to develop sufficient iron stores.
- Most *full-term babies* are born with large stores of iron, designed to get them through the first four to six months, but they still need iron every day, especially since these stores often are reduced after a period of time.
- This is the reason why, beginning at birth, formula-fed babies should receive iron-fortified formula until the baby is one year old, or even later if the baby prefers formula to whole cow's milk.
- Also, there is an increased demand for iron during growth spurts (e.g., birth to two years, toddler age and adolescence) since there is increased red blood cell production when the body is experiencing these changes.

Risk Factors & Causes for Iron Deficiency

The causes of iron deficiency are too little iron in the diet, poor absorption by the body and blood loss (from the intestinal tract; e.g., milk protein allergy, inflammatory bowel disease, etc.). The most common reason for iron deficiency in infants and children is the inadequate supply of iron. The following are risk factors that might lead to develop iron deficiency:

- Premature or low birth weight babies who begin life with less iron stores.

- Formula-fed babies who are given low iron formula.

- The infant (if started before one year) or toddler who is receiving a high amount of cow's milk (more than 20 oz/600 ml per day) may have blood loss in the digestive system and decreased appetite.

- The child who is a poor or picky eater may have low iron intake.

- The child on a vegetarian diet or with a mother who is breastfeeding and is on a vegetarian diet, because the combination of low iron foods and high fiber in the diet leads to decreased iron absorption.

- Mothers with significant iron deficiency or on low iron diets, causing reduced iron content in breast milk.

- The mother who exclusively breastfeeds her baby past the age of six months. At this stage, the baby requires additional iron from other food sources.

- Some low income social groups that switch early in infancy to cow's milk because it is less expensive than formula or those children who consume large amounts of tea (tea blocks iron absorption).

> ### Tip: Bottle Versus Cup Use and Iron Deficiency
>
> In one study of 12-38-month-old children, it was found that children who were drinking milk from a bottle were almost three times as likely to be iron deficient as children drinking cow's milk from a cup. This is because bottle-fed children are more likely to keep the bottle throughout the day and drink large amounts of milk, compared to when using a cup to drink.

Diagnosis of Iron Deficiency

- Iron deficiency develops slowly in most infants and children, so that they are usually asymptomatic (in contrast to acute anemia).

- Routine anemia screening is not considered absolutely necessary, as anemia is uncommon in well-fed babies. At the same time, babies with mild to moderate anemia may not display any symptoms (asymptomatic) and the only way to know if they are anemic is through a blood-screening test.

- Since each child is unique, screening should be considered at various ages according to risk factors and/or presence of symptoms.

- If you believe that your child is anemic, look at the following list of symptoms caused by iron deficiency and anemia (signs and symptoms vary with severity of the deficiency) and the time it takes for anemia to develop:

  ❖ Paleness in the face.

  ❖ Weakness, fatigue, shortness of breath.

  ❖ Irritability (fussiness), hyperactivity, short attention span (difficulty concentrating).

  ❖ Constipation, decreased appetite, and poor weight gain.

  ❖ Brittle, flat and thin fingernails; sore and swollen tongue.

  ❖ Intolerance of cold temperatures.

  ❖ Children whose iron deficiency are partly due to cow's milk may be fat and flabby with poor muscle tone.

  ❖ In some cases, children exhibit pica symptoms (craving to eat things that are not foods such as ice, sand, dirt, starch, etc.).

  ❖ When your child has iron deficiency and anemia, there can be psychomotor delay, and intellectual, emotional, and immune system impairment.

- Research has proven that there is a close association between iron deficiency anemia and reduced mental, motor, and behavioral functioning. These effects seem to be long lasting.

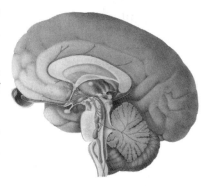

- It is unclear whether iron deficiency is the sole cause of impaired development in behavior, cognition, and psychomotor skills. It is concluded that iron deficiency anemia is a major cause in the impairment of these skills.

- In anemic children, studies provide evidence that increasing their iron levels improve school performance, concentration, efficiency, short-term memory, and I.Q.

- Even if hemoglobin and blood levels are normal, iron stores may still be deficient as it takes a few months for the hemoglobin circulating in the blood to show decreasing levels.

- Anemia screening should be considered in infants and toddlers, especially in high-risk infants such as those born with low birth weight, premature babies, and mothers who are anemic or vegetarian mothers, etc. Anemia is also noticed more at the toddler age, a period requiring parents to pay attention to the food their child eats (screening may be necessary). This is because the chances of anemia are decreased in the first year of life due to iron-fortified cereals and formula.

- Your child's doctor will order simple blood tests to assess whether the anemia is due to iron deficiency. The doctor may add other tests to look for possible contributing factors (e.g., a stool test to assess iron loss in the stool, etc.).

- Iron deficiency anemia is suggested by:
  - ❖ Low hemoglobin value.
  - ❖ Red cell size, color, and number.
  - ❖ Low serum ferritin (measures iron stores).

How to Prevent & Treat Iron Deficiency

Prevention

- It is important to prevent iron deficiency anemia since there are various consequences associated, such as psychomotor delay, cognitive and developmental skills impairment, etc.

- Premature babies and very low birth weight infants have sub-optimal iron stores at hospital discharge (blood is also lost through blood tests) and will require iron supplementation before or by the time they reach eight weeks old until twelve months of corrected age.

- Making wise food choices for you and your baby may prevent iron deficiency anemia:
  - ❖ If your baby is bottle-fed, use an iron-fortified formula starting at birth. Do not use low iron formulas, as they do not contain enough iron for the growing baby's needs.
  - ❖ If you exclusively breastfeed your baby, after six months add iron-fortified cereals and iron rich solid foods to her diet.
  - ❖ Try to use iron-fortified cereal until your baby is 18 months of age to make sure your baby is getting enough iron.
  - ❖ Cow's milk should be introduced only after one year of age and limit its intake for toddlers. This is because cow's milk is low in iron in the first

place, and it may cause bleeding in the intestines with a resulting loss of iron. Limit your toddler's milk intake to no more than 16 oz/500 ml a day.

❖ Combine foods that are high in iron with foods that are rich in vitamin C, such as meat and potatoes, fruit, iron-fortified cereal and raisins, etc.

❖ Some professionals suggest preventing iron deficiency anemia during the second year of a baby's life by daily iron supplements (iron drops, iron-fortified vitamins, iron-fortified nutritional drinks). Discuss the matter with your doctor if you have any concerns.

Treatment

- Your doctor may choose to treat your child with iron supplement medication to build up iron reserves, usually for about four months or longer (depending on the degree of anemia, causes, etc.).

- Taking iron drops may be limited due to a combination of an unpleasant metallic after-taste, the dark staining on the child's teeth, and abdominal discomfort.

- When offering iron medication to your child, offer it between meals with juice or vitamin C rich fruits to increase iron absorption. Do not give it simultaneously with cow's milk, since this decreases iron absorption.

- The following are dietary measures to provide enough iron in your child's diet:

  ❖ Use baby and toddler jar foods that are good sources of iron. Baby jar foods include beef, veal, turkey, combined foods such as chicken with vegetables, beef with vegetables, turkey with vegetables, etc. Use meat and poultry with combinations of vegetables rich in iron and use infant iron-fortified cereals. Toddler jar foods include beef, vegetable and pasta casserole, toddler turkey rice and vegetables, chicken cacciatore, beef stroganoff and toddler cereals enriched with iron (do NOT use adult cereals since iron absorption is less; use baby brand cereals).

  ❖ Compare labels on the jars and buy such foods as "chicken and vegetables" since these will contain more iron rich meat or chicken than a jar that reads "vegetables and chicken."

  ❖ Plain meat provides more protein and iron than mixed dinners such as chicken and rice.

❖ Avoid giving tea, too many bran muffins, or too much cereal, as it decreases iron absorption.

❖ "Sprinkles," which contain iron and other micronutrients, can be sprinkled onto any compatible foods that are prepared at home. These help improve compliance, acceptability, and ease of use, especially in the area of difficulty accessing iron-fortified foods.

❖ When preparing homemade foods, iron rich foods should be given in combination with foods that are rich in vitamin C, as the baby will be able to absorb the iron better (e.g., combine eggs & juice, etc.). Good sources of vitamin C include oranges, mango, kiwi, cauliflower, broccoli, watermelon, strawberries, red and green peppers, and juices with added vitamin C.

❖ Use as little cooking water as possible when preparing foods, since iron leaks into the water. Using less cooking water will increase the iron content in foods.

• The following table provides general guidelines to follow when preparing certain homemade foods:

Food Category	Guidelines
Grains & Cereals	If grains and cereals are the only source of iron, especially when you exclusively breastfeed, talk to your doctor, since homemade cereals are not enriched with iron.
Meat, Poultry, Fish, Liver & Eggs	Be sure to use boneless, skinless chicken breast. Use liver, pork, chicken, beef (3.5 oz/100 grams of pureed beef supplies about 1.5 mg of iron), veal, ground beef, chopped liver, liver and meat combinations, meatballs or chicken balls, chicken fingers, tuna balls or salad, meat with spaghetti. Example of including iron in a chicken meal: Cook chicken liver with chicken stock for ten minutes on low heat. Place it in a blender with cooked vegetables. Add iron-fortified formula and blend until desired consistency is reached.
Vegetables	You may include vegetables in your child's diet alone or in combination. For example, beef and chick peas, spinach, artichokes, mixed vegetables with tuna, soybean puree with chicken, chicken and broccoli, turkey and peas, wheat germs, lentils, etc. When your child is of an appropriate age, you may add collard greens and

Food Category	Guidelines
Vegetables	leafy vegetables like chard or kale, etc. You may puree vegetables, as 3.5 oz/100 grams of pureed vegetables provide 0.3 mg of iron.
Fruits & Juices	Serving fruit juice during mealtime increases iron absorption. Serve dried fruits such as apricots, peaches, figs, prunes, etc.

- It is important to understand that while meat and poultry products are a great source of iron, vegetables also play a role in keeping a well balanced diet.

Tip: Potato Skins Have Extra Iron

Potato skins have 5 times more iron than the rest of the potato. Feed the skin along with the potato. Do not remove the skin from the potato when preparing homemade French fries.

Case Descriptions

Case One:

Adrian, a fifteen-month-old boy, came for a regular checkup at his doctor's office. The doctor noticed that Adrian was pale. Questioning the parents revealed that Adrian had been pale for a few months. He had also been irritable, and seemed to be developmentally delayed, as he was not yet walking. He was drinking 35 oz/1050 ml of cow's milk a day, and ate very little in the way of meat (a bit of chicken, sometimes), vegetables, or solids, except for small amounts of rice cereal. There was no family history of anemia or bleeding.

On *examination*, Adrian was pale, irritable, weighed 18 lb/8 kg, and displayed a mild weakness of the limbs and trunk.

Laboratory tests showed Hemoglobin levels of 51 gram %, very low serum ferritin of 4 (the norm is 100-300 mic/L), abnormality in red blood cells in size, shape, and color, etc., and other evidence of an iron deficiency. A chest x-ray showed mild enlargement of the heart.

Treatment was started with iron supplement medication, and the child's diet was discussed. The clinical condition and its level had required several months of treatment. One year later, Adrian has gained weight, is less irritable, and his general motor skills have been improved—he looks well.

Case Two:

Sarah, a 20-month-old girl, had swollen eyelids for 5 days in a row. Her mother noticed this and brought her to the doctor. There were no other symptoms of infection, nor any family history of blood or kidney diseases. Sarah recently had ear infections and cold symptoms, which had passed.

Sarah's doctor confirmed swelling of the eyelids and also noted a possible mild swelling of the legs. Blood and urine tests were ordered and revealed low protein and albumin levels in the blood, normal urine analysis with no protein loss in the urine, and normal blood renal function.

Sarah's mother stated that Sarah drank more than 32 oz/1 liter of cow's milk per day, more juice than was recommended, and did not eat not many meat products.

The diagnosis was iron deficiency due to cow's milk enteropathy. Cow's milk caused a loss of iron and protein in the bowel (in this particular patient)—all reasons for Sarah's swollen eyelids.

Sarah was started on iron drop supplements, and was put on a cow's milk-free diet, with Nutramigen formula. Iron rich foods were also introduced into her diet.

In this case, the iron loss and blood in stool were due to excessive use of cow's milk, leading to anemia and protein loss, which are manifestations of enteropathy.

Parent Concerns

How do I know that my child is iron deficient if she already has a pale skin type?

- While your child's pale skin may be an indicator, you will not be able to definitely know that your child is iron deficient or has anemia unless the doctor runs tests. Often, anemia due to low iron is discovered in a routine test done for other reasons.

- You and your doctor can assess your child's diet and see if it is low in iron-containing foods. You will also be able to see if your child is consuming too much cow's milk.

- Even though the child has an already pale skin type, she may be paler than usual, she gets tired more easily, or has evidence of blood loss in the stool (due to cow's milk sensitivity).

- Skin color is not a reliable indicator of iron deficiency anemia.

How much cereal does my baby need after the age of 6 months?

- The answer depends on how much formula or breast milk your baby takes.

- At the age of 6 months and older, babies require 10 mg of iron per day and, if formula is used alone, this can be met with 27 oz/810 ml of fortified infant formula or three times as much low-iron formula (not practical, due to large volume—it's unlikely your baby will be willing drink that much!).

- In general, use *at least* 1/2 oz/15 g or 4 tablespoons per day of dry cereal with formula or cereals with fruit (you can prepare the cereal with formula instead of water).

- Basically, the required cereal intake depends on how much iron-fortified formula you use, other foods and types that are taken (remember that at six months of age, the baby's solids diet is vegetables and fruit, so she lacks a significant source of iron and needs cereal to be iron-fortified).

Does iron and formula cause constipation in my baby?

- Research studies do not support the fact that iron in formula causes constipation in infants and toddlers. However, research on the one hand and the "real" thing on the other can be different.

- It has also been noted that some iron drops or pills lead to constipation, according to parents.

- A little constipation is a small negative effect of iron-fortified formula, compared to its benefits (better to have a little constipation that can be dealt with than related iron deficiency difficulties).

- Sometimes, I ask parents to alternate between days with iron-fortified formula and days without (e.g., one day with, one day without). Re-assessment of the situation a few weeks later may show that the infant is able to tolerate iron-fortified formula "when the baby's bowel improves."

Can my baby get enough iron if I prepare home cereals?

- If you feed your baby homemade cereals instead of commercial iron-fortified cereals, your baby may not get enough iron.

- Use brown rice and/or millet, which contain iron. However, you should speak to your doctor about further iron supplementation, since these grains do not contain enough iron for the growing baby.

My baby is taking supplemental iron and I notice she has staining on her teeth. Is this due to iron, and what can be done?

- Some infants or toddlers develop staining of the teeth if they take iron with vitamins in liquid form. It is harmless and usually disappears once the child stops taking the vitamins.

- To prevent this happening, use chewable forms of vitamins whenever possible, and brush or clean the spots with a towel.

- Take your child to the dentist to ensure that these spots on the teeth are not due to other causes.

Is there such a thing as iron poisoning?

- Yes, there is. Iron overdose is a leading cause of poison-related diseases and deaths in young infants and children.

- Iron overdose may cause liver damage, low blood sugar, and shock. It may sometimes cause intestinal bleeding, abdominal pain, and vomiting.

- Parents usually feel that they should be providing great amounts of iron when additional iron is recommended, but, to prevent toxicity, you must only give the amount recommended by your doctor.

- NEVER give your child any type of vitamins and minerals (including iron) without first discussing it with your doctor.

- Be sure to keep iron supplements out of reach of children. They can mistake them for candy.

Tip: Hemochromatosis—Too Much Iron

Some people are born with a rare condition called Hemochromatosis, where too much iron is absorbed and stored in various organs. People with this condition are at a higher risk for iron poisoning.

Is there a difference between the iron stores in full-term babies and premature babies?

- Yes, there is a difference in iron stores. Full-term infants are born with four to six months' worth of iron supply in the body. After that, they will require iron supplements for their diet.

- Premature and underweight babies may only have enough iron stores for two months. They require iron supplementation (as recommended by your doctor) much earlier than full-term infants.

Does iron affect my baby's stool color?

- Iron may cause a black stool.

- In some children, the reaction between the normal bacteria of the digestive system and the iron sulfate causes the stool to turn dark brown, green, or black.

- There is no need to be concerned or alarmed about this when it occurs after iron supplements are started.

- If the baby has black stool and is not on any iron supplements, see your doctor immediately, especially if your child looks sick.

What about vegetarians and iron?

- Vegan diets that do not include any animal foods can result in iron deficiency anemia, as there is decreased nutrient and caloric consumption.

- Less iron is absorbed from vegetables than from animal food sources, so the vegetarian infant should have foods enriched with iron from vegetables, fruits, and foods rich in vitamin C to increase iron absorption.

Tip: Spinach is Not a Very Valuable Source of Iron

Spinach is not as valuable of an iron source as it is often thought to be due to its phytates content. Phytates—and tannins which occur in tea and coffee as well— decrease iron absorption.

My child has anemia with low iron. How long is treatment needed?

- It usually takes two to four months for the iron supplements to improve hemoglobin levels in the blood and refill the body's iron stores.

- Various factors such as treatment compliance, severity of anemia, causes of anemia, etc., can affect the length of treatment.

- Your doctor will be able to suggest the duration of treatment and follow-ups.

Can I keep my child on iron-fortified formula after the age of one instead of starting her on cow's milk, since she does not like cow's milk too much?

- Some experts recommend keeping your toddler on iron-fortified formula for as long as she wants, since it is considered to be better for your child than cow's milk. Formula ensures the provision of iron and other good nutrients.

- Cow's milk has low iron content and low absorbable iron. It is known to cause a decrease in appetite, iron loss, and anemia (especially if it is ingested in excessive amounts).

- For very sensitive babies, you may try soy formula, hypoallergenic formula, or extensively hydrolyzed cow's milk formula, where proteins are broken down into smaller and more tolerable pieces (less allergy risk). You may use these formulas for infants and toddlers with cow's milk allergy.

My child's hemoglobin level was in the normal range, but the doctor suggested that we give her iron. Why?

- A normal hemoglobin level does not necessarily mean that your child is not anemic.

- It only means that her blood is not low in iron; however, her iron stores may be low.

- To be certain, the doctor measures the serum ferritin, which is the level of iron in the blood that accurately reflects body iron stores. This test detects iron deficiency in the early stages.

- Abnormal hemoglobin levels may take a few months to detect, because the body uses stored iron first.

Conclusion

- Iron deficiency anemia in the first two years of life can have lifelong developmental consequences. It has been shown to be just as dangerous during the second year of life as it is during the first year. Great efforts should be made to prevent it through appropriate nutrition, prevention, and, when needed, medication. Additional information for parents can be found at Paediatr Child Health, vol. 12, page 333-334, April 2007.

- Often, a routine blood test done for other purposes provides evidence of anemia. This leads to appropriate treatment and assessment of possible causes (mostly dietary habits).

- Once treatment has started, follow-up is important to ensure compliance with medication and ensure that your child is improving. This is also to ensure that there are no other ongoing causes of iron loss (e.g., medical causes).

- With the use of iron-fortified formula and cereal, the incidence of iron deficiency anemia has decreased in infancy. It can still remain a problem in the second year of life, so ensure that your child is not drinking too much cow's milk, and feed her an appropriate, nutritious diet.

- Watch your toddler for such things as decreased appetite, increased intake of juices (leads to decreased appetite), picky eating, etc.

- Because iron is associated with long-term cognitive and motor development, parents should watch that their child is receiving the appropriate amount of iron and discuss concerns with their doctor.

Picky Eaters

General

Picky or selective eaters are usually children under the age of three or four years, who have strong food preferences, accept only a limited number of foods, and are unwilling to try a new food. Picky eaters are usually defined by their parents' perception, since there is no scientific definition. It is a common problem among toddlers and children, causing tremendous concern and issues for parents, some of which often include:

- ❖ Eating too little or too much.
- ❖ Prolonged mealtimes and inappropriate mealtime behavior.
- ❖ Failure to advance to table foods.
- ❖ Lack of self-feeding.
- ❖ Poor food acceptance and nutritional balance.

It is estimated that 25-35% of parents report that their toddlers are picky eaters. Pickiness usually declines as the child grows older, but those who do not outgrow it by the age of nine or ten years may remain picky eaters.

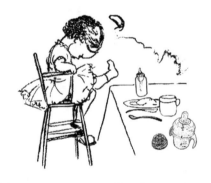

Complications from feeding problems may result in nutritional deficiencies of vitamins and minerals (especially iron and zinc), malnutrition, teeth problems, and the risk of eating disorders (anorexia and bulimia at older ages). Severe feeding problems are rare, affecting only 1-2% of children. These young children refuse to eat (hunger strike), have growth problems, and most (up to 70%) of these children will continue to have feeding difficulties between ages of four to seven years.

For successful feeding, it is important to remember the concept of *division of responsibilities,* popularized by feeding therapist Ellyn Satter. Parents are responsible for providing what, where and when children eat and, in turn, the child is responsible for how much, when to eat or not, according to hunger mechanisms. Through understanding why your child is a picky eater, and understanding the basics of toddler nutrition, you may be able to improve your child's eating behaviors.

Causes of Picky Eaters & Feeding Difficulties

General

Picky eaters are toddlers and young children with behavioral feeding disorders. They present poor food acceptance or resistance due to altered behaviors and/or child-parent interaction around food. *Picky eating is not considered to be a disease.* The question is whether or not these children are "born" to be picky eaters or if the environment (e.g., parental behavior, feeding habits, etc.) influences their feeding behavior. It is probably a combination of both. Many times, parents misinterpret their child's eating behaviors as a problem, when, in fact, it is a developmentally appropriate response on the child's part.

Picky Eaters with No Nutritional Deficiencies

Picky eating does not usually lead to nutritional deficiencies. The following are causes or reasons why children (with no nutritional deficiencies) are picky eaters or display food refusal:

- The child's growth and weight do not always increase smoothly or gradually, as their appetite may be inconsistent.

- Toddlers do not grow as rapidly in the second year of life as they did in the first year (a period of slower growth). This sometimes results in a decreased appetite and decreased food consumption.

- Some toddlers are not necessarily hungry at mealtime, while others do not enjoy their meals, and some have strong food preferences.

- *Super tasters* (those with more taste buds than the norm) tend to be picky eaters and have stronger food dislikes. They are more sensitive to spicy or bitter food tastes.

- Some foods are more likely to be refused, since they have limited toddler appeal (looks or smells different, too much on the plate, etc.).

- The toddler stage is recognized as a time for the child to gain some control, developmental individuality and rebelliousness (e.g., forced to do something she does not want to do). The child may want to test the limits of control on the parents, especially at mealtimes (gets what she wants if she refuses food, a determination to self-feed).

Picky Eaters with Nutritional Deficiencies

- Studies show that a small number of picky eaters may have nutritional deficits (e.g., iron, zinc, vitamins, etc.). These children are difficult to recognize, because they seem healthy.

- A food intake assessment and lab tests may reveal nutritional deficiencies in your child, as it is difficult to know which children have nutritional deficiencies and which do not when both groups are healthy looking.

- Also, the picky eater with a prolonged food jag (consuming a particular food for a long period of time) may be at greater risk for a nutritional deficiency.

Parental Behavior

Parental behavior mismanagement may play an important role in developing feeding problems in early childhood and may include one or more of the following issues:

1) Parental force-feeding.

2) Purposeful distraction.

3) Mealtime environment.

4) Nutritional issues.

Parental Force-Feeding

- Force-feeding includes a variety of tactics by parents to get their child to eat against her will. These tactics may include restraining the child's arms, forcing the spoon or food into the child's lips or mouth, feeding while the child is asleep, etc.

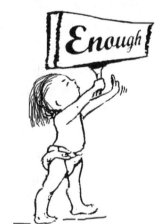

- Parents often force the child to eat (where the quantity is often excessive), possibly because of:

  ❖ Inappropriate knowledge of portion size.

  ❖ Simply wanting their child to eat more if they have more on the plate.

  ❖ Anxious over parental skills and weight loss.

  ❖ Learned from their childhood to "push" foods.

  ❖ Lack of understanding of a toddler's appetite.

  ❖ Not understanding the need for independence in their children.

  ❖ Comparing their child to obese children and feeling that their child is too "thin."

❖ Cultural reinforcements.

❖ Pressure from other family members, etc.

- Young children who are force-fed will often refuse to eat, even when they are hungry. The child who is force-fed or forced to finish everything on the plate is not permitted to allow her sensory feeling of fullness to determine when to stop eating, but is rather dictated to from external sources (parents). This frequently leads to food refusal or overeating and the development of an inaccurate definition of fullness.

- It is important to let your child decide how much to eat, while the parents decide what food is offered. Allow your child to self-feed (if developmentally ready) and provide her with her own spoon or fork to increase her sense of feeding control.

- Remember that appetites constantly change and thus, the amount eaten is quite variable.

Mealtime Environment

- Parents will often provide large snacks or additional snacks in-between "supposed" regular mealtimes to compensate for non-consumed calories in the previous meal or in general. Snacks are usually comprised of low calories and low nutritional value. This is why it is important to provide your child with *structured* daily meals and small snacks.

- Some parents will prolong feeding times (length of meals) in the hopes of encouraging more food intake. Follow your child's hunger cues and allow her to decide if she would like more food.

- Many times, parents worry about the cleanliness of the eating area, stopping the meal or not allowing the child to make a mess. Parents will frequently and immediately wipe their child's hand and mouth. Interrupting the flow of eating during mealtime in this manner may not allow your child to learn fullness and hunger and may suppress her appetite.

- Concerned parents may also give extra attention to their child's intake during mealtimes, for eating adequately or inadequately. This can lead to reinforcement for poor eating behavior.

Tip: Discipline at the Appropriate Time

There are better times than mealtime to make discipline an issue.

Purposeful Distraction
- Distraction at mealtimes should be avoided, as it may lead the child to lose focus in the hunger and fullness cues.
- It teaches your child that mealtime is about playing and entertainment rather than eating.
- Moreover, purposeful distraction takes away the pleasure of eating and the understanding of nutrition, hunger, and fullness.

Sometimes, parents use diversions to persuade a child to eat such as a toy, book, television, game, candy bribe, etc. Instead, teach your child about food and nutrition and be creative with food games, etc.

Nutritional Issues
- Parents often provide children with excessive amounts (e.g., 30 oz/900 ml) of milk, juices, or sugary drinks. This will lead to decreased appetite and consumption of high-energy foods, low fiber intake, teething problems, risk of obesity, and diabetes. Juices and sugary drinks are not nutritious and should be given in minimal amounts, if at all. It is better to replace these with water.
- Some parents provide inappropriate food textures for their child's age and skill, because of a fear of choking, the convenience of faster feeding (pureed foods), or because of lack of knowledge about age appropriate textures. For example, a child may hold food in her mouth as it dissolves since she is not yet able to chew (rotary chewing develops at about eighteen months of age). Often times, parents misinterpret the child's inability to consume food properly as refusal or feeding problems (see *Textured & Table Baby Foods*).

Abnormal Behavior: Medical & Psychological Causes
- *Neurological*: Children with neurological problems may experience more gastroesophageal reflux, failure to thrive, regurgitation/vomiting, chronic constipation, oral, motor, and feeding difficulties.
- *Gastrointestinal Disorders*: These include gastroesophageal reflux, mal-absorption, Celiac disease, Cystic Fibrosis, chronic constipation (pain or cramping during or after meals, because the colon squeezes when the stomach begins to get full), and swallowing and oral motor difficulties.

- *Developmental Delay*: These children may have disorders in processing or properly perceiving smell and taste sensations (e.g., very sensitive to taste, smell, and texture). They may also experience oral motor difficulties and behavioral feeding issues.

- *Sensory related aversion:* These children (e.g., autistic, etc.) in particular have rigid food selections (specific pattern of preferred textures and flavors) and are sensitive to the sight and smell of certain foods and odors. These children have different perceptions and do not accept the variety of food groups very well. You may use various tastes, textures, and flavors (e.g., bland, salty, spicy, sweet, crunchy, etc.) for food acceptance. Usually, these children do not respond well to behavioral management.

- *Oral aversion*: These children have preferences for certain textures and food types. This usually resolves itself over time. However, in some cases, these preferences may be due to true oral aversion wherein exposure to a specific food may be associated with gagging or other symptoms. Speak to your doctor and/or dietitian. They may refer you to an occupational therapist to assess your child's oral motor function and swallowing abilities.

Post Traumatic Feeding Disorder: A child who has experienced an episode of choking may refuse some foods with variable textures, for fear of choking again. These children sometimes develop panic responses if they are offered food with "harder" textures (not soft foods). There is no specific treatment for this disorder. It usually resolves on its own. Allow your child to eat to her own ability during this period. Do not force solid foods, as this may prolong the problem and the anxiety your child feels. Talk to your doctor if the problem persists; a behavioral psychologist may help.

Anxiety Childhood Disorders & Psychological Anorexia: Children with these disorders usually have a low appetite and they may limit their food intake. Infants who receive poor emotional nurturing have little appetite and feed poorly (often in the lower percentile). On the other hand, these children may present with obese dietary patterns where they tend towards excessive food intake. They may be uncomfortable in the feeding situation and unsatisfied most of the time. In the preschool child, this disorder can represent a continuation of the feeding difficulties present during infancy. The child may have a history of delayed self-feeding or chewing, chewing but not swallowing foods, gagging and/or choking. Coaxing, bribing and family scenes may center on the child's refusal to eat. Moreover, anorexia may be the child's way of getting attention and manifestation of autonomy. It can also be a symptom of dysfunctional parent/child relations.

How to Manage the Picky Eater & Behavioral Feeding Problems

General Nutritional Aspects

- Optimal treatment of a child with a behavioral feeding disorder includes supportive counseling, parental consistency, and follow-ups with the doctor.

- Behavioral tactics should be discussed with the parents/caregiver to help reverse the feeding resistance and treat underlying reasons for picky eating and feeding problems. Feeding observations and history questioning will guide the health professional in offering suitable advice.

- Uncomplicated feeding disorders with no major psychological or parenting issues usually have a good response rate (two to three weeks). If parents seem to be struggling for longer than approximately two months (with no improvements), then the situation should be re-assessed, possibly with a behavioral feeding specialist or psychologist.

- The following are some general nutritional aspects to follow:

  ❖ A well balanced diet should include milk (either breast or formula), grain cereals rich in iron, vegetables, fruits, chicken, fish, milk products, eggs, water, etc. Toddlers do not have a sense of what constitutes a balanced diet and they need our guidance to help them determine what sort of things are best to eat and when.

  ❖ Divide the day's food into three principal meals with high caloric value and two to three intermediate small meals consisting of fruits, snacks, and yogurt. It is important that the child not skip intermediate meals as this may cause hunger, leading to nervousness, impatience, and tiredness.

  ❖ It is also important to give breakfast to your child. Having breakfast will prevent a drop in blood sugar (leading to nervousness, inability to concentrate, and tiredness). It will also lead to improvement of memory, learning, etc. You may use carbohydrates, protein, and fats such as bread, cheese, eggs, yellow cheese, and milk.

  ❖ Your child must eat a variety of foods over a period of time, over ten days, say, and not necessarily all varieties in one day. Your child's food preferences can change from time to time; this is normal for the growing toddler.

❖ The young child's diet should not be very high in fiber or too low in fat. Avoid sugary foods, as they are empty calories and replace more nutritious foods.

What Parents Need To Do

General

- Do not let your child eat randomly throughout the day, so that she is not hungry when it comes time for dinner, and do not allow free access to the refrigerator.

- Have regular family meals (at the same time) as often as possible and scheduled snacks, so that your child will not eat all day long (toddlers thrive on a consistent and predictable approach).

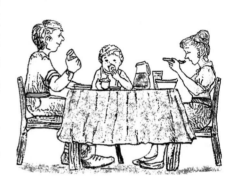

- Feed your child's curiosity by allowing her to try different tastes, learning what goes with what.

- Do not push/force your child to eat if she is not hungry, but at the same time, do not wait until mealtime to feed her if she is hungry. Adjust to your child's "hungry" clock, since she does not estimate mealtimes as adults do.

- Let your child choose her speed of eating and food satisfaction, but up to a certain limit, to complete a normal sized meal for their age (within 30 minutes for meals and 15 minutes for snacks).

- Do not compare your child to other children. Each child has her own unique characteristics.

- Do not insist on the logical order of dinner before dessert. Allow your child to have dessert before dinner, sometimes.

- Continue to introduce food which was previously refused at a later time.

- New foods should first be offered in small portions, and the amount should be increased gradually. Praise your child when she finishes her food.

- Offer appropriate textures for your child's age and skill.

Environment during Meal Time

- Feed your child in a quiet place, without the distractions of television or toys.

- The baby/toddler should be positioned comfortably, in a manner that is developmentally appropriate for her age (e.g. high chair).

- Parents or caregivers feeding the child should have a calm, positive attitude during meal times.

- Meal times should be pleasant, and children should be included in the conversation. Do not center the meal solely around your child, as it is family time.

- Tell stories about food and let her know that it is okay if she does not feel like eating a certain food today.

- A friendly and supportive environment always encourages the picky eater to eat.

- Parents who exhibit appropriate mealtime behavior should ensure that their child adheres to appropriate behavior as well. Both parents and children should follow the following mealtime rules. Mealtime rules should be explained before each meal until the child is complying consistently:

  - ❖ Do not allow toys at the table or the highchair; mealtime is not playtime. If your child is self-feeding and no eating is taking place (of course, some play is normal), pick up the spoon and take over feeding.

  - ❖ Do not immediately give your child napkins when she gets dirty, otherwise she will associate food with dirt.

  - ❖ Do not offer your child what she wants on the table, as this gives her a sense of control and leads to bad eating habits. Stick to the routine of providing two to three appealing foods at a sitting and let her decide how hungry she is (make an exception when she is acutely sick).

  - ❖ Remain seated while eating from the beginning to the end of the meal.

  - ❖ No throwing food (meal is ended if she throws food in anger).

  - ❖ Food should be removed from the child if she is playing with her food for longer than fifteen minutes.

  - ❖ When mealtime is finished, remove the plates from the table, regardless of whether or not your child has finished eating.

❖ If the child did not finish eating her foods, do not lecture or condemn her. Do not give your child any desserts or snacks until her next scheduled meal. It might be hard, but don't give in on this.

❖ If mealtime rules are broken, the child should practice correct behavior. If the rules are broken three times, discipline your child with a time out.

Enhance Interest & Motivation

- Give foods in various shapes, colors, and textures to stimulate your child's appetite.

- Let your child eat with her hands to encourage self-feeding and exploration (it may enhance her satisfaction). Don't be scared that she won't learn how to use utensils.

- When the child does use utensils, provide her with interesting and fun utensils.

- Let your child be involved in the preparation of the food and setting the table. This enhances her interest in eating.

- Encourage your child to eat by offering a new food 10-15 times before giving up on it. A recent study found that repeated exposures to a new food made acceptance of that food more likely.

- Show the child that you are enjoying the same foods you are offering her. Introduce one food at a time (but not in a pushy manner).

- Have finger foods that your child can feed herself with, while you are spoon-feeding her as well. This combination sometimes keeps the baby happy and occupied.

- For picky eaters, it may be a good idea to use few spices; also, they may prefer a new food if they see you eat it.

Food as a Reward or Punishment

- Do not use food as a reward or punishment, since she will learn to do the same back to you.

- Do not use food as a pacifier or a bribe. If you give sweets and snacks to keep your child quiet, you can dull her appetite for the next meal.

- On occasion, you may give your child favorite foods that are not nutritionally sound (about every two weeks).

Beverages

- Do not give your child large sweet or sugary drinks just before a meal, since this will fill her up and cause appetite loss. If your child is thirsty, offer water before the next scheduled meal or before and after a snack (it can be provided freely without restriction).

- Excessive juice intake and milk will decrease your child's appetite.

Overcoming Food Refusal in the Picky Eater

- When children refuse foods, it is the parent's responsibility to make foods more appealing to increase the chances of food acceptance.

- Portion size is important, but so are the color and contrast of foods. Provide your child with small portions, and give different foods on another plate. Allow your toddler to decide whether or not she wants to eat it; the bigger variation in color, the more appealing the food will be. The following are appealing foods and colors that your toddler may enjoy:

  ❖ *Red*: Tomato (raw or pureed), radish, beans, strawberries, red skinned apple, etc.

  ❖ *Green*: Cucumber, broccoli, kiwi, green skinned apple, cabbage, peas, etc.

  ❖ *Orange*: Carrots, baked beans, cheese, peaches, sweet potato, etc.

  ❖ *Yellow*: Cheese, egg yolk, sweet corn, pineapple, etc.

- You may also try changing the way foods are offered or add fun ways to dress up foods in order to enhance food acceptance such as the following:

  ❖ *Fun Dips*: Children like to eat foods they can dip into a sauce such as cream cheese, peanut butter (thinly spread), guacamole, pureed fruits or vegetables, yogurt, etc.

  ❖ *Nutritious Spreads*: Children enjoy spreading their foods, so show them how to spread food on bread, toasts, crackers, etc.

❖ *Top It:* Top foods with nutritious items like yogurt, apple sauce, tomato sauce, melted cheese, etc.

❖ *Slice It Up*: Cut foods that you serve into various shapes and sizes to make them more appealing and fun to your child.

❖ *Drink It Down*: Make foods that your child can drink, such as milkshakes and smoothies out of fruits and vegetables.

- With specific food refusal, try the following suggestions for each particular food group (see appropriate chapters in *Section 4: Starting Solid Foods & First Year Feedings* for further tips and tricks on overcoming refusal):

Specific Food Refusal	Tips & Tricks
Vegetables	Serve raw or grated vegetables, instead of cooked.
	Use different preparation methods at different temperatures.
	Mix vegetables with other food groups and make eating vegetables fun by taking your child grocery shopping with you.
	Soups are a good way to get your child to eat vegetables, or hide vegetables in a sauce.
Meat & Alternatives	Hide meat in soups, sauce, and casseroles. Keep offering small amounts of well cooked, cut up meat on a regular basis.
	Use meat alternatives such as fish and poultry (remove bones), eggs, hummus, tahini, tofu, and well-cooked mashed legumes (lentils, chick peas, and soy beans).
	Cook fish with sauce or colored vegetables.
Fruits	Let your kids pick the fruits they enjoy when they shop with you.
	You may puree fruits and use it as a homemade topping sauce.
	Mix fruits with Jell-o or with yogurt.
	Serve dried fruit, fruit smoothies, and milkshakes.
Eggs	Serve egg in different forms or add it to other cooked foods.
	Replace eggs with protein alternatives such as fish, meat, yogurt, cheese, etc.

Facts About Snacks

- As solids become the most significant part of a child's diet, snacks help improve their nutritional intake. Snacks are good if they are eaten in moderation and not so much that they affect the three usual main meals.

- Choose nutritious snacks that aren't normally eaten during meals.

- Snacks are also a great way of helping your child learn how to pick up food with her fingers and put it in her mouth.

- Give two to three snacks per day, so that they don't affect mealtime. However, sweets and snacks should not be made readily available. If the child sees a variety of nutritional foods, she will pick something to eat from there, if and when she is hungry. If snacks are refused, put them away and do not offer them until the next meal.

When To Be Concerned

When Not to Worry

- Parents usually come to see the doctor for other reasons and state that their child is not eating foods in a "by the way" manner.

- They may not realize that their child may be getting more foods than they know. Many times, when parents are asked to write all of what their child eats in a week, they notice that, in fact, the child is eating enough.

- There is usually no reason to worry if your doctor confirms that your child is growing and developing well for her age. If your child is progressing well, not only in weight gain but also developing well for her age (e.g., walking, talking, climbing), it means she is receiving proper nutrition.

- However, if your child is a picky eater, discuss ways to improve the picky eating habits with your doctor.

When To Be Concerned

- If you are concerned and anxious about your child's picky eating habits, speak to your doctor. Feeding observations will clarify contributing factors to feeding problems and confirm the diagnosis.

- Always see your doctor if your child experiences the following:
  - ❖ Your child continues to lose weight or is not gaining weight over a period of time.
  - ❖ Difficulty sucking, swallowing, and chewing, or she is vomiting.
  - ❖ Developmentally inappropriate acceptance of textures or the inability to graduate to textured foods.
  - ❖ Food jag—your child is eating the same food(s) for a long period of time.
  - ❖ Symptoms of vitamin/mineral deficiencies such as (see *Vitamins & Minerals*):
    - Tiredness, recurrent infections, depleted fat mass.
    - Growth arrest, edema, mental confusion, irritability.
    - Smooth tongue, soft and bleeding gums, teeth cavities.
    - Cracked lips and fissure in the corners of the mouth.
    - Protruding ribs, muscle weakness, bow legs/wrist.
    - Dry skin, easily bruised skin that is pale and wrinkled.
    - Hair loss, brittle nails.
    - Thin, round and curved nail ends.
    - Skin rash and eczema around the mouth and anus area.
- Observations of feeding may show:
  - ❖ Parents' actions, such as tricks to open the mouth and the child's response (angry, cry, distressed).
  - ❖ Excess cleaning of the child and surroundings (e.g., chair, face, and table) associated with feeding interruption and over-concern for messiness.
  - ❖ Offering what the child wants to settle her (e.g., giving a bottle).
  - ❖ Force-feeding.
  - ❖ Lack of control over feeding or restraining and lack of eye contact.
  - ❖ Use of distractions or tricks.
  - ❖ Prolonged feeding time.
  - ❖ Pockets foods in the mouth cheeks.
  - ❖ Eats only with distractions.
  - ❖ Self or no self-feeding, etc.

The Doctor's Office

- When consulting your doctor, you will probably be asked the following questions to help both of you understand why your child is a picky eater or has these eating habits. Your doctor will assess:
  - ❖ The environment at mealtimes.
  - ❖ What foods are developmentally appropriate for your child.
  - ❖ Who is responsible for the difficulties.
  - ❖ If there are medical causes.

The Doctor's Questions

Tell me which foods your child refuses to eat?

- Sometimes, there is a pattern of specific foods which the child refuses.

Tell me your child's diet history, such as what she ate yesterday?

- Diet histories allow parents (as well as the doctor) to discuss and review how the child is given food and what foods are rejected.

What do you do when your child refuses food?

- Understanding mealtime behavior of both the parents (punishment, force feeding, rewarding, trying to feed when upset, etc.) and the child allows the parents and the doctor to assess any inappropriate behavior which may add stress to you or your child (are you concerned about the mess at feeding time?).

Was anyone else (e.g., parents) in the family a picky eater?

- Almost always, the answer to this question is yes. This allows the family of the picky eater to see that having strong food preferences is a natural developmental stage.

Does your child snack or drink excessively before mealtime?

- Excessive use of juice, cow's milk, and snacks may be affecting your child's eating behavior at mealtime.

Are there or were there any additional symptoms, such as those of vitamin or mineral deficiencies (as discussed earlier), known neurological or developmental diseases or any possible psychological trauma?

- The next step is the physical examination by your doctor to ensure that there is normal growth in weight and height, and no physical signs of nutritional deficiencies. Although parents ask for lab tests to be done on their child, there is usually no need (especially when your child is growing well) unless the doctor is concerned. An observation of the mother while feeding her child may be necessary, showing some of the previously mentioned aspects.

- After questioning, history taking, and physical examination, the doctor may ask you to provide her with a detailed dietary record of your child's intake over the last week to 10 days. This will show the doctor whether or not your child is eating a well balanced diet (from all 5 food groups and in appropriate portions) over a period of time, and assists in the detection of any abnormal feeding behavior. At the same time, this dietary record will show you that your child is, in fact, eating an appropriate quantity of various foods when you look at the bigger picture.

Parent Concerns

My child is a picky eater. Is there something wrong with her?
- Parents should know that there is nothing wrong with their child and being a picky eater will not put your child in harm's way.

- The child is simply adjusting to her growing needs and will not starve herself as long as food is available.

- Watch your child's eating habits and know how to feed your child according to her picky food preferences (see previous suggestions). Discuss any concerns with your doctor and have regular checkups to ensure that your child is growing well.

I feel incompetent, guilty, and angry and I worry, since my child does not do what I say.
- Discipline is a completely different and separate issue from the picky eater.

- The worst time to try to discipline your child is at mealtimes, since excessive parental anxiety and forced feedings will lead to feeding problems in early childhood.

- Being a picky eater is usually considered a normal developmental stage that will disappear, so you do not have to feel this way.

- As a parent of a picky eater, you should educate yourself to know how to properly feed your child and follow recommendations on behavior and mealtimes.

- As children grow and change, so do their needs and preferences.

I am concerned about my child's food portion size.

- When your child is full and has eaten enough, there is no point to try and force the rest of the food on her, as it may predispose her to obesity.

- Typically, parents give their child far more than they are able to eat, and then they worry that that they have not finished their meal.

- It is better to give your child a small portion and have her ask for more food.

My child is eating "junk/bad" food and I'm concerned about her diet.

- It is important to remember that there is no such thing as "bad food."

- Junk food such as chips, chocolate, and sodas are not "wrong" to eat. They simply have to be given in moderation.

- Help your child make better food choices, rather than depriving her of junk food:

  ❖ Offer a range of nutritious snacks that she likes and keep junk food out of reach.

  ❖ Try offering fun food choices instead, such as pizza, granola bars, bagels and cream cheese, a peanut butter sandwich or a muffin, etc.

How can I tell if my child is getting enough to eat since she is a picky eater?

- If you are worried about your child's food intake because she is a picky eater, you may keep a dietary intake log to record your child's diet (to be discussed when you see your doctor for assessment and concerns). This will allow you and your doctor to see if your child is eating a healthy, well balanced diet from all 5 food groups (it may be evident that, over a period of time, she is eating healthily, even if her daily intake doesn't look like it).

- Also, your child's regular doctor will know your child and her past medical history; physical examinations will be able to compare her growth over time in growth curve charts to assess changes in weight and height.

My child does not want to eat much at dinner. Should I be concerned?

- If your toddler has had a good breakfast and lunch, then she may not want to eat much at dinner time, which is perfectly normal.

- Most young children will only eat one or two full meals each day. It is uncommon for a toddler to eat three good meals per day.

- The stomach of a toddler is usually as big as her fist, so a portion size is sometimes a tablespoon and it's enough to fill her. Also, limit your child's juice intake to none (use water instead), so she has room for solid foods and consumes less "empty" nutrients, which lead to decreased appetite.

My 2 1/2-year-old child prefers to eat only pizza, spaghetti, French fries, hamburgers, and a large volume of milk. She refuses almost all other foods. What should I do?

- This preference for a specific food and refusal of other solid foods is called a food jag.

- The child is "obsessed" with the type of food and its consistency, presentation, color, shape, etc., and refuses other types of food.

- Try some of the suggestions to deal with food refusal suggested in this chapter.

- Try offering various foods from all 5 food groups and offer them on a plate in small portions (2-3 types of food on one plate). Present these foods in different ways, and offer them in a relaxed manner that allows your child to feel in control of the situation.

- You may also try to gradually mix small amounts of other solid foods with her favorite foods. Slowly increase the amount of other food types and be patient. Learning to accept new food takes time and you may need to offer it many times before your child accepts it.

- If your baby cries and refuses to try the foods offered on the plate, do not bring her alternative foods. This teaches her that picky and fussy behavior works.

- As a prevention measure (beginning in the early months), do not ignore her food preferences, and do not force her to accept foods that are "good" for her. Allow her appetite mechanism to function normally. Offer a variety of foods, different in preparation and presentation, and offer them in small portions (don't overwhelm her).

My 15-month-old baby is a picky eater and looks underweight. Is it okay to give her more toddler formula since she does not take much other foods?
- Giving excessive amounts of formula may provide your baby with enough calories, but certainly not a well balanced diet.
- It is understandable that you are anxious about your child's food intake, however, the more formula you give, the less chance there is that she will take other foods.
- Toddler formula, if it replaces whole cow's milk, is okay and possibly better, but not in excessive amounts. Try offering your child other foods for a well balanced diet and good eating habits (see suggestions in this chapter).
- Compared to whole cow's milk, toddler formula has more appropriate levels of protein, vitamins, and minerals (vitamin E, C, niacin and iron).
- Speak to your doctor regarding growth concerns.

Should I force my child, who is a picky eater, to finish her dinner?
- You should never force your child to finish a meal.
- Mealtimes should be pleasant, enjoyable, and relaxing.
- As long as your child is growing normally and gaining weight well, allow her to establish her own independence during feedings.
- Remember that most children will only eat one or two full meals per day, even though they are provided with three well balanced meals.

My 22-month-old baby is a picky eater. She will take food I offer and keep it in her mouth for a long time before swallowing it. What do I do?
- This phenomenon is known as pouching. It occurs in toddlers and young children who do not like the taste/texture of a particular food, or have emotional stress related to parents trying to "push" the food in the mouth of the picky eater.
- The child keeps food she does not like in her mouth (pouches), and holds it to be chewed over a long time. However, this phase passes on its own.
- Sometimes, an unknown or large amount of food may trigger a fear of choking.
- It is risky to leave a poucher in bed or allow her to go to sleep with food in her mouth, as it can lead to choking when she falls asleep.

- You can try to persuade your child to swallow or spit up the food, clean the food out with your finger, offer a drink of water to rinse food remnants, etc. Sometimes, you can pinch her nostrils shut and the child will spray out the food.

Vitamins & Minerals

General

*V*itamins are organic substances that are essential for normal growth and development. They must be obtained through food sources, because the body cannot produce them (with a few exceptions including vitamin D, K, B-3, Biotin, and Niacin). Vitamins are involved in biochemical processes in the body that help release energy from digested foods and regulate the metabolism. They help with bone formation, connective tissue, fight diseases and infections, and heal injuries and wounds. Basically, vitamins are a vital part of our body's normal functioning, growth, and maintenance.

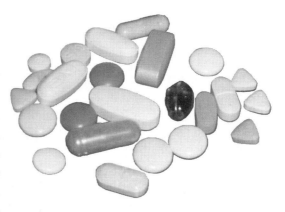

Minerals are substances (solids and crystalline) that are required for certain metabolic processes and cannot be synthesized by the body. They have structural roles within the body. Minerals are required for growth and development of the teeth, bones, and formation of red blood cells.

Both vitamins and minerals are vital for overall mental and physical well-being. Most people receive all the nutrients they need through eating a varied diet that includes all 5 major food groups. In some cases, vitamin and mineral supplements are required for people who cannot or do not eat a healthy diet, or for those who require more nutrients because of medical issues. A daily multivitamin is given to 25-50% of children in the United States, although it is usually not necessary for children eating an average diet. The question of adding or not adding vitamin and mineral supplements to your child's diet is a matter which confuses many doctors and parents. The decision should be made with your doctor and/or dietitian. Though, it is evident that the best and recommended way for a healthy child to obtain needed vitamins and minerals is to eat a well balanced diet. A daily diet of varied foods can provide the required vitamin and mineral nutrients for maintaining a healthy body. Vitamin and mineral supplements will not make your child's diet healthy.

Types of Vitamins & Minerals

Vitamins

- There are two groups of vitamins that are classified according to the material they dissolve in—water or fat:

Water-Soluble Vitamins

- Water-soluble vitamins are not stored in the body, as they are dissolved in water. They need constant, daily replacement because they are excreted with urine (they have a lower risk of accumulation in the body).

- These vitamins include the *vitamin B-complex group* and *vitamin C.* The vitamin B complex group includes B1 (thiamine), B2 (riboflavin), niacin, B6 (pyridoxine), folic acid, B12 (cyanocobalamin), Pantothenic acid, and biotin. It helps children's bodies produce energy, build brain cells, develops red blood cells, and helps fight against illness and infection. Vitamin C plays a key role in helping babies and children absorb iron.

- Many fruits and vegetables contain water-soluble vitamins.

Fat-Soluble Vitamins:

- Fat-soluble vitamins dissolve in fat and need fat for their absorption. They are stored in the fatty parts of the liver. You must eat some fats to absorb these types of vitamins.

- Sources of fat-soluble vitamins include animal fat, vegetables, liver, and oily fish.

- These vitamins include *vitamins A, D,* and *K,* which are stored in the liver and vitamin *E,* which is distributed throughout the body's fatty tissues.

- Vitamin A is important in the development of eyesight in a child, especially night vision. This vitamin is required for the development of healthy skin and the formation of bones and teeth.

- Vitamin D is known as the sunshine vitamin, since the body can provide this nutrient from sunshine on your skin by using cholesterol from your body. Vitamin D is important for children, because it increases the absorption of calcium into the bones and assists in a healthy heart and nervous system.

- Vitamin E is significant in developing the baby's metabolism and protects the body from pollution (especially the lungs). Breast milk contains four times as much vitamin E as cow's milk.

- Vitamin K is used in the child's body to control blood clotting and is important in bone formation.

Minerals
- Calcium, phosphorus, and magnesium account for 98% of the body's mineral content by weight.
- Calcium absorption increases in the presence of other nutrients such as milk, lactose, amino acids, and vitamin C. Calcium absorption decreases with increasing levels of phosphorus, oxalate, or phytates.
- Too much protein may increase the amount of calcium excreted in the urine.
- Iron is a major constituent of hemoglobin, which is the red blood pigment that carries oxygen to tissues in the body.
- Other minerals (e.g., zinc, fluoride, copper) are only required in miniscule amounts and are involved in multiple processes that takes place in the body's metabolism.

Who Is At Risk for Vitamin & Mineral Deficiency

There are various factors to be considered when determining who is at risk of nutritional deficiency. The following groups of children are at risk, and may require vitamin and mineral supplements:

Breastfed & Formula-fed Full Term Infants (First Year)
- Breast milk usually provides full nutrition for an infant and is enough to support their growth and development at this stage. It provides the nutrients your baby needs for at least the first 6 months of life, except for vitamin D. The American Academy of Pediatrics (AAP) and the Canadian Pediatric Society (CPS) recommend supplementing vitamin D to breastfed babies.
- Formulas fed infants do not need the additional vitamin D, as it is added to formula.
- Both the AAP and CPS state that vitamin supplements are probably not necessary for healthy children over one year who consume a varied diet.

Tip: Vitamin K injection at Birth

Vitamin K is given at birth, usually in the form of an injection.

Vitamin D Deficiency
These infants are at risk of a vitamin D deficiency:
- Babies who are breastfed (exclusively after six months of age).

- Babies who are not exposed to any sunlight, or live where there is little sunlight.

- Babies whose skin is dark.

- Babies who are born to a mother with vitamin D deficiency.

- Infants with increased consumption of non-fortified milk substitutes, such as soy and rice beverages.

Tip: Can the Sun Be Enough to Produce Vitamin D?

It is unclear how much sun is required to produce vitamin D in the body. 5-30 minutes in the sun twice a week on the face, arms, hands, or back should be enough for a young baby. They are not supposed to be in the sun for long. Using protective clothing or sunscreen stops natural vitamin D from being produced, so try to get 15 minutes of exposure before putting on sunscreen.

It is not recommended to use sunscreen on infants younger than six months of age, because of the risk of chemical absorption through their thin skin. Infants are sensitive to sunburn.

Another factor to consider is where you live; there may be winter periods that do not allow for sunlight and vitamin D to be formed.

For all of the above reasons, a vitamin D supplement is required in breastfed infants and when rickets are noted. Infant formulas and regular milk is fortified with vitamin D.

Premature Babies
- Premature babies who weigh less than 3.3 lb/1.5 kg will most likely require multiple vitamins and minerals.

- These vitamins are provided in the mother's milk.

- Supplemental iron is advised, either as iron-fortified formula or as a liquid medication in breastfed or low iron formula-fed premature babies (from two weeks of age to twelve to fifteen months).

- Vitamins D, E, K, and folic acid are especially important for premature and low birth weight infants. Vitamin D should be given to both premature and full term breastfed babies. If your premature baby is bottle-fed with standard formula, vitamin supplements are advised until the baby ingests appropriate amounts of formula. If a special formula is used, check its vitamin content to see if supplementation is required.

Vegetarians & High Fiber Diets

- Vegetarians are those who do not eat or feed their babies any animal foods (see *Vegetarians*).

- A vegetarian diet affects vitamins B12, D, calcium, iron, zinc, and other nutrients.

- Vegetarian diets are nutritionally sound if they include a variety of nutritious plant foods, especially vegetables, whole grains, nuts, beans, and products which are fortified with vitamins and minerals. Close attention to combinations of different types of plant protein is necessary.

- Vegetarian infants and toddlers may require vitamin and mineral supplements to make up for the food types they are not eating.

- High intake of fiber in a child's diet decreases the absorption of minerals and other nutrients. However, some studies show that there is no risk posed on these high-fiber diets, unless the child only eats a narrow variety of foods, and/or if there is malnutrition.

Picky Eaters

- Picky eaters usually seem to have a poor or restricted diet. Most, though, have no nutritional deficiencies.

- A small number of picky eaters who may be at risk are those who eat the same foods most of the time.

- Make sure that foods readily available in your house are nutritious and the foods your picky eater decides to eat are varied and full of nutritional value (see *Picky Eaters*).

- A very small number of picky eaters may require the assistance of vitamin and mineral supplements to prevent nutritional deficiencies.

Children with Diseases

- Mal-absorption diseases (e.g., cystic fibrosis), liver diseases.
- Chronic disease (e.g., Irritable Bowel Syndrome, etc.).
- Metabolic diseases.
- Feeding difficulties.
- Emotional or physical distress.

Other Risk Factors
- Children who need special consideration are those with:
  - ❖ Symptoms of vitamin/mineral deficiency.
  - ❖ Egg, milk, and dairy allergy.
  - ❖ Gluten-free diet.
  - ❖ Physical/emotional stress.
  - ❖ Children with failure to thrive.
  - ❖ Inappropriate family diet and cultural aspects.
  - ❖ Prolonged food refusal and lack of dietary variety.
  - ❖ High intake of sweets.
  - ❖ Early or inappropriate weaning diet and children on a diet for obesity.
  - ❖ Social aspects (low income, lack of knowledge, irregular family meals, poor parent-child interaction, etc.).
  - ❖ Eating disorders or inadequate appetite.

- There are children who show no obvious risk factors or clear symptoms, and yet have a vitamin/mineral deficiency.

Symptoms of Vitamin & Mineral Deficiency

Vitamin and mineral deficiencies are rarely seen these days; however, deficiencies may cause various illnesses and diseases. Many signs and symptoms are not only due to vitamin deficiency, so discuss any concerns with your doctor. The following is a list of some general symptoms to look for, alone or in combination:

- *General*: Tiredness, recurrent infection, growth arrest and weight loss, edema, mental confusion, seizures, and loss of appetite (lack of vitamin C, niacin, vitamin B6, Biotin, vitamin B1, vitamin A and D, iron, calcium, etc.).

- *Eyes*: Dark and dull circles under the eye, eyes sensitive to light and night blindness (insufficient vitamin B12 = riboflavin).

- *Nose:* Eczema around the nose (insufficient vitamin B12).

- *Throat:* Smooth tongue, soft and bleeding gums, cavities in the teeth, cracked lips, and fissures at the corners of the mouth (insufficient niacin).

- *Chest:* Protruding ribs (insufficient vitamin D, rickets).

- *Neuromusculoskeletal:* Bowed legs and/or wrist, muscle weakness, arthritis, and paresthesia (burning or prickling sensation); (insufficient vitamin C, B1, B6, B12, D).

- *Skin and hair:* Dry, easily bruised, pale, wrinkled, dry sparse hair, hair loss, eczema, skin rashes, and slow healing wounds (insufficient vitamin C, niacin, vitamin B6, A, and K).

- *Nails:* Brittle, thin, white bands across the nail, and round and curved nail ends (insufficient vitamin C, B2, Biotin, Vitamin A, iron).

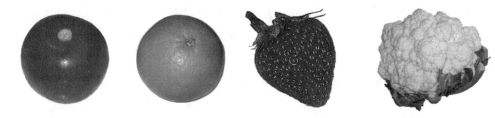

Vitamin C Rich Food Examples

Tip: Zinc Deficiency

Symptoms include a loss of appetite, skin inflammation around the mouth and anus, diarrhea, hair loss, failure to gain weight, increased susceptibility to infections, and white spots on nails (do a blood test for low alkaline phosphatase and zinc).

- Other minerals such as iron and calcium are discussed in appropriate chapters.

How to Keep Nutritional Value in Foods

- Nutrients are often lost from foods during cooking. However, foods must be cooked if they are being served to small babies. Use the following points to keep nutritional value in foods when preparing your child's meals:

  ❖ Ensure food quality vegetables by making sure they are fresh and clean from disease (no brown spots in leafy vegetables, etc.).

❖ Retain vitamin and mineral content by using the cooking water to puree vegetables and for other uses (the exception to using the cooking water is with high nitrate vegetables like carrots and beets).

❖ You may also maintain nutritional value by cutting vegetables into small pieces before cooking them, using the smallest amount of water possible, and adding water gradually when needed.

❖ Cook vegetables for as short a time as possible.

❖ Due to loss of nutritional content, it is generally suggested not to heat vegetables or fruits with vitamin C (when possible).

❖ Do not excessively heat foods in the microwave as this has an effect on the quality of proteins, vitamins B, and vitamin C.

❖ Vitamin C can easily be destroyed, and its nutritional value can be affected during prolonged heating and cooking or when prepared a long time before the actual feeding (prepare foods approximately one hour before a feeding).

Providing Vitamin/Mineral Supplements: Approach & Risks

General

Each child should be considered and approached individually for vitamin supplements. Giving vitamins and minerals will rapidly correct the deficiency, as long as they are child-appropriate. Once you and your doctor have decided that it is best to provide your child with multivitamins, there are things you should know about which ones to choose:

• Read the labels on all vitamin and mineral boxes before buying them.

• Follow the directions on the label closely so that you do not give high doses of vitamins and minerals, as they may be dangerous.

• Look for the "USP" (for U.S. Pharmacopeia) on the label, as this means the supplement meets strength, purity, disintegration, and dissolution standards set up by the testing organization (or the sister Canadian organization).

• Check expiration dates on supplement bottles and, if one is not shown, do not buy it.

• Choose any multivitamin bottle for children and make sure it is labeled for *children* and check that what you buy is suitable for your child's age.

• Unless your doctor prescribes iron supplements, make sure iron is not part of the multivitamins you give your child.

- Choose fun shaped vitamins to make it easier to give them to your child. Make sure, though, to keep the bottle out of reach so that your child does not take extra and risk harm.

- It is important to buy vitamins that your child will take, so consider taste as well.

- Usually, vitamins come in drops for very young children and chewable tablets for the older children.

- Give all vitamin and mineral supplements with meals so that they are better absorbed, and to avoid an upset stomach.

- Remember, that vitamin supplements are *not* meals, nor do they replace a meal.

- Store all supplements in a safe, out of reach, dry, cool place. Avoid hot or humid storage locations such as the bathroom.

Risks of Vitamin/Mineral Supplements
- It is important to realize that excess amounts of vitamins may cause ill effects and/or interfere with the functioning of other vitamins and minerals.

- More is *not* always better. It is wrong to assume that vitamins will not cause damage if taken in excess amounts. For example, taking excess vitamin B6 may cause nerve damage, difficulty walking, and numbness.

- Minerals, on the other hand, may interfere with your body's ability to absorb or use another mineral. An example of this is taking too much zinc, which interferes with copper absorption.

Nutritional Screening & Assessments
Nutritional Screening
- It is important to assess your child's dietary intake in reference to the 5 major food groups, in addition to related questions and examination of your child, along with a detailed nutritional analysis. This will help you and your doctor see if your child has developed a nutritional deficiency.

- Compare your child's weekly diet to the food groups and, if your child is greatly lacking in one of the food groups, discuss with your doctor about multivitamins for your child (see *The Food Groups*: *Making Sense of Portion Size & Activity Levels* for portions, serving size, etc.).

- In addition to dietary intake, assessment of your child's height and weight is a vital indicator of nutritional deficiency. Slow weight gain and stunted growth in height may reflect nutritional deficiency or other medical problems. Assess and compare past growth to actual growth.

- Nutritional screening is important since no single food can supply all the nutrients required. A healthy, well balanced diet will supply the nutrients your child needs for growth and development.

Lab Tests
- Lab tests do not always show deficiencies in vitamins and minerals. They simply cannot account for all vitamins and minerals required by our bodies.

- Also, blood concentration levels are not usually reflective of vitamin or mineral status, or an impending deficiency.

- Vitamin and mineral concentration is maintained in the blood, even when the body stores are depleted. For example, iron stores decrease before hemoglobin levels in the blood decrease.

- These aspects are further complicated by the fact that children differ in what foods they eat, their ability to absorb it, their individual needs, and so forth.

- Some vitamin and mineral levels can be measured in blood tests (e.g., vitamin D, zinc, iron, calcium, folic acid, vitamin B6, etc.). However, its usefulness is limited by the wide variation that is considered normal.

Case Description
Sundeep was born in June of 2000; he is of South Asian heritage. When a milk allergy was diagnosed, he was switched over to soy milk. His diet consisted of breads in the morning, apples, bananas, rice, vegetables, or some meat at lunch, and for dinner, he would have fruit, chappati bread or rice, and mango juice. According to his parents, Sundeep was not a "good eater."

His parents noted an abnormal shape to their 18-month-old boy's legs. On examination, Sundeep had bowing in his wrists, ankles, and legs. His chest also showed a prominent area of swelling in his rib cage. Laboratory tests confirmed that he had a low level of calcium and elevated alkaline phosphatase.

Sundeep was diagnosed with Rickets, secondary to low calcium (hypocalcemia and hypophosphatemia). Treatment included doses of 2000-6000 IU/day of vitamin D for a few months. Sundeep's parents were advised to reduce the amount of chappati bread in his diet, as it is high in phytates, which prevent absorption of calcium. After treatment, Sundeep was walking and running well and his legs seemed to be straightening.

Follow-up appointments include appropriate diet counseling, vitamin D supplements, lab tests, x-rays, and normal sun exposure throughout the summer. In most cases of bowing, treatment improves it by three years of age. If there is still an issue, an orthopedic referral is considered. Some cases may even require surgery.

Parent Concerns & Tips

How do I help my child meet her vitamin D requirements?

- Consume milk and dairy and encourage your baby to follow your guide for healthy eating.

- Look at the labels to make sure that foods are fortified with vitamin D (e.g., soy beverages or yogurt).

- Include fatty fish in the diet.

Is it true that early vitamin supplementation causes an increased risk for asthma?

- A study done on more than 8000 patients stated that providing your child with early vitamin supplementation may cause an increased risk for asthma (Pediatrics, July 2004).

My child is a good eater (eats everything). Does she need vitamins or minerals?

- Your child's diet has to be varied, balanced, and offered in appropriate amounts according to the 5 food groups, to avoid the risk of nutritional deficiencies.

- The appearance of your child cannot always tell us that her nutrition is well balanced.

- Some studies show that even in cases of good eaters, children do not consume enough calcium, iron, zinc, and vitamin E.

Should I give large doses of vitamin C to prevent my child from getting a cold or infection?

- No, do not give large doses of vitamin C. No studies have shown any differences in children taking vitamin C and those taking normal, whole fruits.

- Vitamin C in large doses can be associated with Vitamin C toxicity and is not recommended for children. Toxicity is associated with kidney stones, deposition of oxalate in the heart and other tissues, diarrhea, anemia, urinary tract infections, decreased absorption of vitamin B12, and copper deficiency.

- There is no conclusive evidence that infants or children should be given additional vitamin C to prevent or treat colds. A diet that is varied and includes fruits, tomatoes, peppers, spinach, broccoli, etc., will supply enough vitamin C so that no supplements are required.

Does my child need to eat every recommended serving in the food pyramid every day?

- It is not necessary to give these recommended servings every single day.

- It is more important to average out what is eaten over a two-week period to ensure a well-balanced healthy diet with all the essential nutrients. In fact, the body has a remarkable ability to regulate the balance of minerals, unless illness occurs.

Can vitamins and minerals improve my toddler's appetite?

- Despite some parents' beliefs that vitamins are needed to stimulate a child's appetite, this is simply not the general case.

- Very rarely, in some more severe cases of deficiencies, there may be an associated appetite loss and replenishing the missing vitamins and minerals may help improve your child's appetite. Appetite stimulants are not usually used in children, but discuss this with your doctor.

My 4-year-old daughter has whitening of nails parts—does she need vitamins?

- Whitening of the nails is called Leukonychia and can cover a part of or the entire nail. White bands on the nail are common and are usually of no major significance. These are probably the most common nail condition noted in children.

- Sometimes, parents worry about this problem, but it is usually benign and, frequently, the result of minor injury to the nail. In these cases, it disappears in about 8 months, the time necessary for the nail to completely re-grow.

- Rarely, whitening of the nails may be due to severe liver abnormality, heavy metal poisoning, and zinc deficiency.

- It is common in children who pick and bite their nails.

Conclusion

In a perfect world, your child's diet would include plenty of vegetables, fresh fruits, whole grains, and dairy and milk products. The reality is that many children eat a narrow range of healthy foods that do not meet the recommendations of the Canadian or American Food Guide.

In 2004, a Canadian community health survey on nutrition found that 7 out of 10 children between four to eight years do not eat the recommended daily 5 servings of vegetables and fruits. This is a habit that is likely to short change them of folic acid, vitamin A and C, and minerals (magnesium). Also, children in this survey do not receive enough vitamin D and calcium. More than one third of children between four to nine years do not receive the recommended daily intake of two servings of milk products (it's even worse with older children).

In a 2001 USDA study, the diets of most children aged two to nine years were found in need of substantial improvements to meet dietary recommendations. In addition, the percentage of children with good diets had fallen from 36% to 17%.

When you add additional obstacles (e.g., picky eaters, vegetarian diets, hectic schedules, etc.), it can be difficult to ensure balanced meals. The argument could be made to add vitamin and mineral supplements to your child's daily routine. Multivitamins and mineral supplementations do more than just ensure that your child receives the nutrients missing from her diet. Many studies indicate positive effects on intelligence, and the increased likelihood of good behavior in children. For example, picky eaters who do not eat at least one serving of meat and alternatives per day may take vitamins with iron; kids with an allergy may benefit from supplements, especially those allergic to milk or multiple foods (e.g., calcium, vitamin D and E, B2 and niacin), etc. Do not put a young child on a low fat diet, as they need fat to absorb vitamins and minerals used in brain and bone development.

Remember that there are risks with taking large or excessive amounts of vitamin and mineral supplements. They can be toxic, and they cannot make up for a child's consistently poor diet. Please refer to the new Canadian Food Serving Guide for Healthy Eating and the US MyPyramid for portion size and child age.

Vegetarian Babies & Toddlers

General

Vegetarianism means consuming foods that do not contain animal and/or animal byproducts. Parents decide to make their children vegetarians due to perceived health benefits and ethical, philosophical, religious, ecological and, occasionally, economic reasons. The decision to raise your child as a vegetarian should be carefully thought out. It is your duty as a parent to take the time to ensure that your child still receives essential nutrients which are more easily found in a diet containing animal products. You should have appropriate help from health professionals with solid nutritional knowledge.

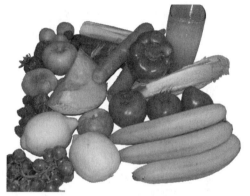

While vegetarian diets seem to be somewhat beneficial for adults, it may lead to growth and development problems in small children. Some studies have shown that some vegetarian children have slower growth and nutritional deficiencies, while other vegetarian children have been found to have growth rates which do not differ from non-vegetarian children of the same age. Vegetarianism is inappropriate for optimal growth in infants and young children. It may lead to nutritional complications in a child (different than those of an adult). A parent needs to have solid nutritional knowledge and continuous consultation to plan the vegetarian child's menu. There is a constant need for growth and nutrition follow-up with doctors, nutritionists, and dietitians. The following deficiencies may occur in a young child who eats no animal foods: calories, proteins, iron, minerals (calcium, zinc), vitamin D or B12 (necessary for growth and brain development) and riboflavin. The positive aspect of not consuming any meat is that your child will have less cholesterol and saturated fat nutrients. This may reduce the future risk of heart disease, gallstones, obesity, strokes, and certain types of cancers.

The American Academy of Pediatrics does not recommend a vegan diet for young children. Instead, they recommend using combinations of milk and its products with eggs, cereal, fruits, vegetables, legumes and nuts. If followed carefully, the right combination will provide the necessary food nutrients.

Types of Vegetarians & Nutrient Risk

Vegans
- These are "hard-core" vegetarians who do not consume any animal products, including red meat, fish, poultry, eggs, and dairy products.
- Vegans rely only on plant products such as vegetables (e.g., lentils, beans, soy products, etc.) and fruits.
- *Nutrients at risk* with the vegan diet include protein, iron, calcium, zinc, vitamin B12, vitamin D, and riboflavin.

Partial or Semi-Vegetarians
- Semi-vegetarians consume plant and dairy products, poultry, and seafood (only eating fowl and fish). They do not consume any beef, lamb, pork, goat, etc.
- *Nutrients at risk* with the partial vegetarian diet include iron, zinc, and calcium.

Lacto Vegetarians
- "Lacto" is the Latin word for milk.
- Lacto vegetarians consume plant and milk products, while avoiding all animal products (e.g., red meat, fish, poultry, and eggs), except for dairy.
- *Nutrients at risk* for the lacto vegetarian diet include vitamin D, iron, zinc, calcium, and protein.

Lacto-ovo Vegetarians
- "Ovo" comes from the Latin word for egg.
- These are the most common type of vegetarians.
- Lacto-ovo vegetarians eat plant products and vegetables, eggs, milk, and dairy products. They do not consume any animal flesh or byproducts including red meat, fish, seafood, and poultry.
- *Nutrients at risk* for the lacto-ovo vegetarian diet include iron, zinc, and calcium.

Ovo Vegetarians
- Ovo vegetarians only consume plant products and eggs and avoid all meat and milk products.
- *Nutrients at risk* for the ovo vegetarian include protein, minerals (especially iron, zinc, and riboflavin), and vitamins D and B12.

Nutrients of Special Concern

Protein

- Vegetable proteins have a limited amount of amino acids compared to animal proteins. This requires you to pay more attention to your protein needs, if you are only consuming plant proteins.

- Quality and quantity are important to consider when providing proteins.

- Vegans must eat a variety of plant proteins to get all the amino acids they need. *Vegan protein sources* include the following: cereals and grains (rice, corn, rye, wheat, pasta), green vegetables (Brussels sprouts, asparagus, broccoli, cabbage, spinach, squash, potato), legumes (beans, lentils, peas, soy, tofu, hummus, peanuts), nuts (almonds, walnuts, cashews), seeds (sesame, sunflower), and soy products (e.g., soy milk).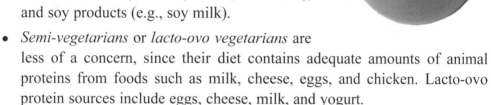

- *Semi-vegetarians* or *lacto-ovo vegetarians* are less of a concern, since their diet contains adequate amounts of animal proteins from foods such as milk, cheese, eggs, and chicken. Lacto-ovo protein sources include eggs, cheese, milk, and yogurt.

Fibers

- Vegetarian menus are rich in fiber and may interfere with the absorption of iron, calcium, and zinc.

- Fibers have low caloric value and provide a feeling of satiety and stop the feeling of being hungry.

- In order to decrease the risk of excess fiber, you may do the following:

  ❖ Use foods low in fiber with high caloric value such as tree nuts, avocado, hummus salad, and peanut butter.

  ❖ Replace some of the fruits you give your child with some fruit juices, refined grain products, and peeled vegetables.

  ❖ To decrease the feeling of satiety, feed small amounts more frequently during the day.

  ❖ Remove the skin of vegetables and fruits only after they are cooked to keep their nutritional value.

Vitamin D & B12
- Vitamin B12 is only found in animal products and it is important for cell division within the body.
- A vitamin B12 deficiency causes anemia and neurological damage (lacto-ovo vegetarians do not generally have vitamin B12 deficiency).
- All exclusively breastfed children with a vegan diet require additional vitamin D, beginning at two weeks of age. However, if the baby is formula-fed, vitamin D is provided in the formula. Vitamin D levels are found to be especially low in vegan diets.
- Food sources of vitamin B12 include fortified breakfast cereals, low-salt yeast extract, milk, and dairy products.

Minerals: Iron & Calcium
- Choose foods that are rich in iron, calcium, and zinc.
- Increase mineral absorption with fruits and vegetables rich in vitamin C.
- Children on a vegan diet should receive calcium supplements.
- The most common occurence of iron deficiency is found in semi-vegetarians, especially, in vegans.
  - ❖ Sources of iron: prune juice, pureed apricots, lentils, cereals, beans, and orange and dark green vegetables.
  - ❖ Sources of calcium: fortified soy milk, cheese, green vegetables, beans, lentils, ground almonds, sesame, tofu, etc.

Energy & Fats
- Babies and toddlers need calories and lots of nutrients to meet their growth needs and energy demands.
- Allowing some animal products, such as eggs and dairy products, into your child's diet provides energy and growth (when she gets older, she can become a vegan if she chooses).
- Provide foods that are high in fat and good sources of fatty acids.
- Use avocado, margarine, or oils liberally when preparing lentils and bean dishes, and use nuts and almond butter regularly.

Breastfeeding & the Vegetarian Mother
- A vegetarian diet in a breastfeeding mother affects her milk quality and the baby's nutrition. It is important to ensure that the mother delivers

appropriate amounts of vitamin B12, D, B2, calcium, and iron through her breast milk.

- Take the following precautions if you are breastfeeding and a vegetarian:

  ❖ Breastfeed your baby for at least one year, if possible. This will ensure that the necessary nutrients are completely supplied for the first six months of life and most of what is required will be supplied for the rest of the year. This is assuming that the mother is taking all the necessary nutrients, including supplements of vitamin B12 and folic acid. If you cannot breastfeed for the year, use soy formula; talk to your doctor.

  ❖ Add the following supplements when breastfeeding: vitamin B12, D, folic acid, minerals, and iron.

  ❖ Use whole grain cereals, bread, tofu, and other soy based products to provide added protein when the baby moves to solid foods.

  ❖ Watch your child's weight gain and caloric intake since growing babies need many calories (use high caloric foods such as avocado).

  ❖ Ensure your baby receives enough calcium by using fortified juices, calcium supplements, tofu prepared with calcium, broccoli, and vegetables with dark green leaves.

  ❖ For nursing vegan mothers, calcium and vitamin D supplements are usually recommended to reduce the baby's risk of developing rickets, and to maintain your own nutrient balance.

  ❖ Eat fatty foods, such as salmon and other fish or DHA rich eggs and omega-3 fatty acids (e.g., soy, canola, etc.). Vegans need to look at other resources for these elements.

  ❖ Near the end of the child's first year, you may use cooked brown rice, mashed chickpeas, and other legumes such as beans and peas.

Timing of Food Introduction in Vegetarian Babies

A vegetarian diet can provide all the nutrients required for growing babies, if done properly. You must ensure that your baby receives plenty of foods rich in calcium, vitamin B12, vitamin D, and protein. The timing of solid food introduction for vegetarian babies is similar to that of non-vegetarians:

0-4 Months

- Do not start introducing solid foods earlier than 4 months.
- If your baby is exclusively breastfed, then solid foods should not be given before the age of 6 months (this is a new recommendation; see *Starting Solid Foods*). Feed your child breast milk and/or soy formula.
- Talk with your doctor about when to start solid foods.

4-6 Months

- When weaning to first foods, you may introduce pureed fruits (e.g., banana, pear, apple, etc), rice mixed with breast milk or formula, mashed lentils with some added vegetable oil, or smooth purees with vegetables (e.g., potato, carrot).
- Do not give your baby wheat, oats, milk, nuts, or eggs.
- Iron-fortified cereal is a reasonable first food choice for vegan infants, since it provides energy and iron and is easily digested (it may be mixed with breast milk or formula).

6-8 Months

- Breast milk or soy formulas still provide important nutrients for your baby.
- Continue cereal and begin introducing other foods such as breads, crackers, toast, strained fruit, juice, vegetables, and pureed legumes.
- Good sources of protein such as well mashed, pureed or cooked tofu, soy yogurts, and beans should be introduced.

9-10 Months

- Breast milk or soy formula should be continued so as to provide important nutrients.
- As solid foods become a larger part of the child's diet and replace milk or formula, choose foods that are rich in calories and nutrients such as mashed tofu, bean spread, mashed avocado, and stewed, dried fruits.
- Provide your child with a variety of grains, fruits, and vegetables such as cereals and breads, pieces of soft cooked fruits and vegetables, pureed legumes, bananas, sweet potatoes, avocado, well cooked pasta, soy cheese, and yogurt.

11-12 Months

- Breast milk or soy formula (24-32 oz/750-1000 ml per day) may be continued.

- Provide a varied, well balanced diet for your child.

- Give your child foods such as rice, pasta, canned or cooked fruits, peeled raw fruits, cooked vegetables, bite-size pieces of soy burgers, etc. (you may start butter after one year of age).

Further Information

- Remember that a child between the ages of 6-12 months requires 700-1000 calories per day (see Vegetarian food guide, accessible on the Internet).

- Give your child small, frequent meals of concentrated energy foods (vegetable oil, lentils, avocado, cheese, or smooth nut butter) throughout the day. Regular meals and snacks can help ensure adequate energy intake (sugar is not a good source of energy).

- When introducing new foods to your baby, be sure to watch for allergic reactions. Leave three or more days in-between the introduction of new foods (see *Feeding & Food Allergy* for more details).

- Do not give your baby the following food items as they are choking hazards: candies, tofu dogs, popcorn, raisins, overly sticky foods, and make sure oatmeal is not too thick.

- An appropriately planned diet can meet the nutritional needs of vegetarian infants and toddlers for growth and development.

- Various nutritional deficiencies can occur in your baby, if they do not receive proper nutritional intake and that is why it is imperative to feed your child a variety of foods from all the major food groups.

Tip: Organic Foods

Use organic food whenever you can to ensure no pesticides or herbicides are in your baby's food. You can buy jarred organic food if you are not making your own foods. If you are not a vegan, organic milk and yogurt can be an easy way of providing daily protein. A big bowl of organic yogurt and granola requires hardly any preparation.

How to Raise the Vegetarian Child

Feeding Advice

It is important to know what to feed your child when raising a vegetarian. It is your responsibility to ensure that all the nutrients are received for optimal growth and development. The following are some things you must do in order to optimize your child's vegetarian diet:

- Give your child a varied diet with healthy, fresh foods.
- Introduce new foods to your child by pairing them with favorite foods.
- Provide your child with plenty of legumes, as they are full of protein and fiber.
- Prepare fun and tasty foods such as vegetable soups (be creative).
- Give your child soy milk (about 20 oz/600 ml per day) since it is high in protein.
- Add tofu to puddings, soups, shakes, sandwiches, desserts, etc., for that extra protein boost. Tofu is a great food for young children, since it is rich in protein and fat, but low in fiber.
- Serve whole-grain breads (full of fibers, vitamins, and nutrients).
- Give your child lots of green, leafy vegetables (sources of calcium) like broccoli—after one year of age—and add dips for fun.
- Serve soy cheese if you do not use dairy products.
- Avocados are great for children since they are full of fat, calories, and nutrients. Add avocado to dips, spreads, toppings, etc.
- Serve your child veggie versions of hot dogs and burgers, as they are high in protein (beans are also high in protein and fiber).
- Provide 3 meals per day, plus snacks in-between the meals.
- Limit your child's fluid intake immediately before meals, since fluids can be filling. Use water in-between and at the end of a meal.
- Add calories whenever you can with extra spreads on bread, oil when baking, adding soymilk powder to baked goods, etc.
- Speak to your doctor about giving your child multivitamins to ensure proper nutrient intake.

Vegetarian Toddler Food Guide (1-4 Years)

Food Group	Toddler Servings Needed/Day (the equivalent of 1 serving is in brackets)
Breads & Cereals	4-6 oz/120-180 ml of iron-fortified infant cereal + 1-2 toddler size servings of other breads and cereals per day (e.g., 1/2 slice of bread, 1/4 cup/60 ml of rice, cooked grain, cold cereal).
Vegetables	2-3 toddler size servings per day (1/2 cup/125 ml salad, 1/4 cup/60 ml cooked vegetables, etc.).
Fruits	2-3 toddler size servings per day (1/2-1 fresh fruit, 1/4 cup/60 ml cooked fruit, etc.).
Beans & Beans Alternatives	2 toddler size servings per day (1/4 cup/60 ml of cooked legumes, 2 oz/60 g. Tofu, etc.).
Grains	6 or more servings (1/4-1/2 cup/60-125 ml cooked cereal, grain. or pasta or 1/2-1 cup/125-250 ml of ready-to-eat cereal).
Fortified Soy Milk	3 servings (1 cup/250 ml each time of fortified soy milk, infant formula, or breast milk).
Fats	3 servings (1 tsp of margarine or oil).

Consult the vegetarian food guide on Canada's Health Food Guide on the internet for serving number and portion size as this may vary, and you should also consult your doctor.

Meal Options

Depending on your vegetarian type, you may use some of these combinations and options for the vegetarian toddler:

Breakfast Options
Scrambled eggs, whole-wheat toast, orange juice, grapefruit, fresh fruit, calcium fortified orange juice or soy milk, iron-fortified cereal, etc.

Breakfast Option 1:
2 small pancakes or 1 waffle, 1/2 banana, 1/2 cup/125 ml orange juice, and add fortified infant cereal.

Breakfast Option 2:
Hot or cold cereal with added fortified infant cereal (1/2 – 1 cup/125-250 ml), 1/2 cup/125 ml soy milk, 1/2 slice of toast, and 1 tsp of nut or seed butter.

Lunch Options
Green, lentil or tomato salad, peanut butter sandwich, fresh fruits, rice, yogurt, cottage cheese, calcium fortified soy milk, minestrone soup, apple sauce, etc.

Lunch Option 1:
Pasta with tomato sauce, 1 cup/250 ml veggie ground, veggies and dip and 1/2 cup/125 ml soy milk.

Lunch Option 2:
Tofu salad sandwich, bean and vegetable soup and 1/2 cup/125 ml soy milk.

Dinner Options
Chopped vegetables, salad, pasta, cheese, soy milk, potato soup, rice pudding and soy milk, lasagna with cheese, steamed broccoli, vegetarian burgers, tofu, red beans and rice, etc.

Dinner Option 1:
Veggie burger, oven fries, salad with oil-based dressing and 1/2 cup/125 ml soy milk.

Dinner Option 2:
2 pieces of pan-fried tofu, 1/4 cup/60 ml rice, squash and peas, and 1/2 cup/ 125 ml soy milk.

Snack Options
Toasted bagel, bran muffin, fresh fruits or vegetables, whole graham cracker, yogurt, soy milk, fresh fruit shake, calcium fortified juice, etc.

Snack Option 1:
1 cup/250 ml soy milk, 1/2 frozen banana, 3 strawberries and 2 tsp of soy milk powder.

Snack Option 2:
Crackers with a veggie plate or a muffin with nut butter.

Supplements
Supplements for your child (or a breastfeeding mother) should be based upon your doctor's recommendations.

Parent Concerns

What is the best way to assure growth in my vegetarian child?

- The best way to assure that your child achieves an optimal growth rate is to provide your child with a sufficient amount of calories for growth. However, some vegetarian children experience difficulties gaining weight well, due to dietary restrictions. Feed your child various fatty foods to increase her caloric intake through such foods as avocado, nuts, butters, dried fruits, seeds, and seed butters (be sure to brush your child's teeth to prevent decay).

- Remember, your child should not have any restriction on fat under the age of two, due to rapid growth and high needs for calories during this time.

- Between the ages of one to three years, your child's diet should contain approximately 30-40% of calories from fat.

Why is protein a concern, and what are adequate or inadequate types of protein?

- There are two types of protein, known as complete and incomplete proteins.

- The *complete protein* contains adequate amounts of essential amino acids for health and is found in products such as meat, milk, fish, and eggs. "Essential" simply means that the body cannot produce these amino acids and they must be obtained from outside sources.

- The *incomplete protein* does not contain all of the essential amino acids. Grains and beans are incomplete protein sources.

- To obtain all of the essential amino acids, you must combine different incomplete proteins to receive the appropriate necessary amino acids. Examples of combinations for complete proteins include the following: Legumes combined with seeds, nuts, dairy, or grain, grain and dairy, beans on toast, cereal with milk, rice with beans, peas, lentils, or with milk, veggie burgers, corns and beans, granola and yogurt, and hummus and pasta with beans or cheese.

Toddlers: Principles in Feeding & Related Aspects

General

The diet of a toddler is very different from the infant's diet. Most of the infant's nutrition is derived from breast milk and/or formula, while the toddler has a bigger need for a variety of foods. During the toddler stage, children are exposed to different foods and tastes. They learn to compare and choose and express what they think (sometimes to the parents' dismay).

This chapter discusses principles of feeding young children to ensure appropriate nutrition for normal growth and development as well as good eating habits.

Growth Requirements

- It is important to remember that growth slows by 1/2-1/3 in the second year of a child's life, proving the fact that children eat less after the first year. The baby is learning her environment, improving motor and social development, and is less focused on food. The toddler is becoming more independent and competent at feeding herself.

- Many toddlers will only eat between one to two full meals per day, so it is important to offer your child a well balanced diet (especially with snacks).

- The amount of food eaten varies from child to child, and from day to day. It is also influenced by growth and activity level. On average, a one year old child requires approximately 1000 calories per day (this varies with body size, activity level, etc.).

- It is important to provide children between one to three years of age with 16 grams of protein per day. Proteins are the building blocks and help provide new tissue for growth (1 oz/30 g of chicken or meatballs contains about 7 grams of protein; 1 chicken thigh contains about 6 grams of protein; 3.5 oz/100 grams of raw ground beef contains about 16 grams of protein; 1 large egg contains about 6 grams of protein, etc.).

Well-Balanced Diet

The Importance of a Well-Balanced Diet

- A well balanced diet from all major food groups is important in ensuring that your child receives all the necessary nutrients; it should include milk (formula, cow's milk, breast milk) and dairy, cereal and grains rich in iron, vegetables, fruits, meat/chicken/fish, legumes, eggs, and water.

- If you offer many different foods throughout the week, you can be reasonably sure that your child is getting the nutrients she requires. If a child is not eating enough variety (e.g., eating too much of the same food such as cakes, cookies, highly processed snacks, hot dogs, etc.), it is unhealthy.

- Regularly scheduled meals and snacks are important in the growth and development of your toddler for the following reasons:

    ❖ Spaced out meals encourage a varied intake of foods from each of the food groups. It is hard to achieve proper nutrition if snacking throughout the day is the norm.

    ❖ Regular meals promote regular bowel habits.

    ❖ With small children who have small appetites, regular "re-fuelling" is required.

    ❖ There is a lowered risk of dental decay when the child eats consistent and regular meals.

    ❖ Meal times allow for the opportunity to socialize with your children and set the example in respect to food choices and eating behavior.

- The following are important parts of a well-balanced diet in your child:

    ❖ Offer various foods from different food groups, paying attention to color, consistency, shape, smell, and taste.

    ❖ Offer the daily, required foods in appropriate amounts (servings and portions).

    ❖ Alternate between foods with high and low fat content.

    ❖ Offer nutritious snacks between meals (for nutritional completion).

    ❖ Small and frequent meals rather than large, less frequent meals (children have no patience for large meals, so the smaller meals must be of greater nutritional value and should be considered part of your child's overall nutrition for the day).

    ❖ Not too high in fiber or too low in fat.

    ❖ Avoid sugary foods.

    ❖ Limit juice intake to 2 oz/60 ml per day (if at all; offer water instead).

❖ Limit intake of fried foods and unhealthy snacks (e.g., French fries, chocolate, hot dogs, cookies, cakes, ice cream, highly processed snacks, etc.).

❖ Good vitamin and mineral intake (e.g., calcium, iron, etc.).

❖ Appropriate mealtime behavior.

> ### Tip: *Food Safety and Choking*
>
> Between the ages of one to three years, watch for safety aspects to prevent choking. The toddler may eat any foods, except those which pose a safety risk (see *Safe Feeding & Food Safety*).

Breakfast

- Get your child used to eating breakfast in order to break the night fast. If your child does not eat in the morning, the body will continue fasting and will break down proteins from the muscle and fat reserves. There may also be signs of physical/intellectual tiredness such as impatience, absence of listening, and possibly even a loss of appetite.

- It is important to include carbohydrates and some protein in your toddler's breakfast. However, it is more important to provide your child with carbohydrates than protein in the breakfast meal, since carbohydrates provide immediate sugar to the body. Your child will be less tired and will be able to concentrate better.

- Choose foods from grain products, milk products, vegetables, fruits, and alternatives to meat. Easy breakfast menu items include toast, fruits, cereal, yogurt, a peanut butter sandwich, cheese and crackers, pizza, grilled cheese sandwiches, scrambled eggs, apple sauce, cottage cheese with fruit, bran muffins, oatmeal pancakes, and French toast.

- The following breakfast options depend on your child's age, so do not worry if your child is not eating all of these (some have bigger appetites than others):

  ❖ Breakfast Option 1:
  1 cup/250 ml iron-fortified infant/toddler cereal mixed with whole milk, 1/2 pear or fruits.

  ❖ Breakfast Option 2:
  4 oz/120 ml of whole milk, 1/2 slice of toast with 1/2 teaspoon of butter, 2 pieces of cheese and 1/2 banana.

❖ Breakfast Option 3:

1/2 mashed banana (or other fruits like apples), 1 poached egg, 1/2-1 slice of toast and 1/2 cup/125 ml of milk.

Do not rush your child's time when eating breakfast, since it is an important meal in the day.

Lunch

• Lunch is an important time for children, as energy levels begin to decrease midday. Children need a range of nutrients to get them through the afternoon. If they do not have a good lunch, their learning can be affected.

• The following are some suggestions for healthy lunches:

❖ When making a lunch, follow and include a choice of each one of the food groups including grain products (whole grain bread, tortilla wraps, rice cakes, leftover pasta, etc.), fruits and vegetables (raw veggies, mixed green salad, unsweetened canned fruits, etc.), milk and milk products (plain yogurt, cheese strings, soy drinks fortified with calcium, cottage cheese, etc.), and meat and alternatives (hard-boiled eggs, tuna, salmon, etc.).

❖ Get creative and make lunches as appealing as possible by including a range of shapes (cut sandwiches into shapes, make melon balls, etc.) and colors (carrot sticks, grapes, etc.).

❖ Think variety: For example, alternate bread types if you usually make sandwiches with white bread; try whole wheat bread, raisin bread, or a bagel. Offer a variety of different fruits, and try new types of cheese and vegetables.

❖ Keep it simple with foods that are easy and quick to eat. For example, peel an orange ahead of time and slice it, or offer low fat, healthy pretzels.

❖ Use high fat spreads such as butter, mayonnaise, margarine, etc., sparingly.

❖ Avoid fried foods like potato chips.

❖ Pack long lasting energy foods, including ready-to-eat vegetables and whole grains (breads) that help kids feel the energy longer. Have a good source of lean protein such as cottage cheese, lean meat, eggs, etc., that helps them even out the energy to prevent fatigue.

❖ Make lunch healthy by trying not to rely on convenience foods and pre-packaged meals, which are high in salt, sugar, and calories, and low in vitamins and minerals.

❖ With drinks, pack bottles of flavored water or cold milk, and avoid soda pop.

❖ With older children, involve them in planning and preparing lunch.

❖ Lunch Option 1:
One boiled egg, 1/2-1 slice of bread, 1 teaspoon margarine, 1/2 grated apple, 1/2 cup/125 ml of milk, and add 1/4-1/2 cup/60-125 ml of vegetables.

❖ Lunch Option 2:
One fish finger or stick, 1-2 tablespoons of mashed potato, 1 canned pear, 1/4 cup/60 ml custard, 1/4 cup/60 ml of milk, and add 1/4-1/2 cup/ 60-125 ml of vegetables.

❖ Lunch Option 3:
Combination of cherries, tomatoes, carrots, cheese slices, crackers, and apples; OR a fresh fruit salad with melon, grapes, strawberries plus cheddar cheese slices, and a whole wheat bun and butter.

Dinner

• The dinner meal contributes to a good night's sleep, at a time when your child's body is growing. As such, it should include protein, carbohydrates, and fat.

• Examples of dinner items include pasta, homemade pizza, chicken fingers, vegetable soup, meat, bagels with avocado, vegetables, etc.

❖ Dinner Option 1:
1/2 oz/15 g of chopped chicken or 1 chicken nugget, 2 tablespoons of peas, 1/2 slice of whole wheat bread, 1/2 cup/125 ml of milk and 1 small banana.

❖ Dinner Option 2:
1 oz/30 g of cooked minced meat, 2 tablespoons of brown rice, 1 table-spoon of cooked butternut squash and 1/2 cup/125 ml of canned fruits.

Intermediate Meals & Snacks
- Young children may get a large part of their daily foods from snacks.
- You may provide your toddler with 2-3 snacks (mini meals) per day.
- Kids like snacks for various reasons, some of which include the following:
    - ❖ Kids enjoy the taste of snacks.
    - ❖ Many snacks come in different shapes and sizes, which children enjoy.
    - ❖ Children enjoy the fact that they can eat snacks while they are doing something else.
- Do not use the same food snacks all the time—offer your toddler a wide variety of grains, fruits, vegetables, etc., so that she may receive all the necessary nutrients she requires.
- Provide healthy, nutritious snacks and make sure that snacks are not too high in sugar. Fruits and vegetables are the most obvious nutritious snack foods and comprise most of the finger foods (see *Finger Foods for Babies & Toddlers*).
- Snacks enriched with protein, minerals, and vitamins are a great way of increasing nutritional value in your child's diet.
- Kids snack on whatever is handy. Having wholesome snacks available, whether store bought or homemade, is part of a parent's job. Junky snacks push the nutritious foods out of children's diets and contribute to tooth decay and obesity.
- The following are some suggestions for snack options:
    - ❖ Serve raw vegetables (when age appropriate to prevent choking), such as broccoli, cauliflower, carrots, celery sticks, green pepper slices, red pepper sticks, tomato wedges, and zucchini.
    - ❖ Offer your child various types of fruits such as berries, grapefruit slices, orange slices, grapes (cut in half), pineapple pieces, sliced kiwi, mango slices, peach slices, apple sauce, etc.
    - ❖ Raisins and other dried fruits have fallen from favor as snacks, because they consist of sugars (albeit natural) that stick between children's teeth and promote tooth decay. Consider moving dried fruits from snack time to the main mealtime.
    - ❖ Make milkshakes or smoothies by blending various fruits into a blender until they reach the desired consistency.

❖ Use cookie cutters to make fun-shaped sandwiches for your child.

❖ Cold cooked pasta (elbow macaroni) by itself or served with grated cheese makes a good snack food.

❖ Toast can be made more interesting by buttering it lightly or sprinkling it with a little cinnamon and sugar or Parmesan cheese before cutting it with a cookie cutter.

❖ Spread mashed banana (or other spreads) on mini rice cakes or small pita breads.

❖ Stuff celery sticks with cream cheese or peanut butter. Raisins may be added on top of the spread (remove the strands from the celery).

❖ *Snack Option 1:*
5 oz/15 grams of cheese, 1/2 slice of bread, and milk for a drink.

❖ *Snack Option 2:*
1/2 cup/125 ml of yogurt and 1/2 mashed ripe banana or 1 oat cookie.

❖ *Snack Option 3:*
2 tablespoons of peanut butter and 2 whole grain crackers.

❖ *Snack Option 4:*
1/2 cup/125 ml of milk and 1 tablespoon of dried fruit.

Tip: References to Other Food Guides

You may check www.nc-sc.gc.ca for Canada's Healthy Food Guide and the USDA Food Pyramid Guide (*My Pyramid*) for serving numbers and portion size for each age. You may also refer to *The Food Groups: Making Sense of Portion Size & Activity Levels*.

Nutrition Specifics

Cereals & Grains

• Cereal is a favorite family breakfast food. It provides good nutrients such as fiber, B vitamins, zinc, and iron.

• Grain products include bagels, croissants, pancakes, waffles, rice, tortilla, muffins, pitas, taco shells, pasta, crackers, crepe, noodles, buns, etc.

- It is better to buy pure grain cereals or fruit cereals. Parents should also buy grain cereals (whole wheat or wheat bran).
- Watch out for granola cereals, which may contain 4-9 grams of fat per serving and especially watch for hydrogenated oil.
- One cup of a nutritious cereal may supply as much as half the daily nutritional requirements for 15 of the top vitamins and minerals.
- Add milk or yogurt to cereals to boosts their nutritional content.
- Use brown rice, as it contains more than three times the amount of fiber of white rice (1/4 cup/60 ml of brown rice contains almost 1 gram of fiber).

Sweets, Sugars, & Alternatives
- You do not have to totally ban sweets; simply keep them to a minimum.
- Sweets provide few nutrients and are bad for the teeth. They also lead to less of an appetite for healthy food.
- If you offer sweets to your child, make sure to give them at the end of the day and not in-between meals.
- Choose sweets that can be eaten quickly, rather than sucked or chewed on for a long time. Provide fruits or unsweetened yogurt for dessert at meals (cheese is good, as it neutralizes cavity causing acids that form in the mouth).
- Offer milk and/or water more often (offer juice after the child has finished a meal).
- Do not use artificial sweeteners due to the risk of low caloric intake.
- Do not serve foods that are rich in sugar or have sugar as their biggest component. Choose foods that have lower sugar content than those that have a higher content.
- The following foods are high in sugar:
  - ❖ Sweet biscuits and cookies, cake, juice drinks or sweet drinks, chocolate, honey, sugar, jam, milkshakes, ice cream, candies, and chewy sweets.
- The following foods are low in sugar alternatives:
  - ❖ Plain or cheesy biscuits, low sugar cakes, bread sticks, banana loaf, water, fruit juice that is fresh or diluted with water, rice crispies, corn flakes, raisins, reduced sugar jam, cheese spread, milk or yogurt with fresh fruit, and small amounts of dried fruits.

- Do not use sweets to reward or punish your child. They will become intensely valuable to them, and this will make it harder to control the amount your child eats.

Salt, Spices & Food Spicing
- Highly salted foods are not recommended for children.
- There are no clear studies that show a relationship between salt and the development of high blood pressure in adult life.
- Infants do not like salt, so it is easy to get them used to food with no salt or only a small amount of salt.
- It is better to limit the use of salt, even in early childhood. Use salt in moderation and only use high sodium processed foods occasionally (One to three times per week).
- Sources of salt include breast milk or formula, table foods (especially hot dogs, powdered soups, and cheese), etc.
- Maintain a sort of "gentle" spicing that is not hot, acidic, or salty (see *Spices & Flavors*).
- Do not use MSG (monosodium glutamate).
- Use oils like canola, soy, and olive (alone or combined).

Fat & Cholesterol
- Do not limit fat and cholesterol intake if the child's growth is following a normal growth curve and do not restrict fat below the age of two years. After the second year of life, about 30% of calories should be from fat.
- Do not excessively serve foods with saturated fatty acids such as fatty milk, butter, margarine, yellow cheese, and white cheese with high fat content.
- Use a variety of vegetable and animal fats.
- There is no proven correlation between cholesterol levels at young ages and in adults.

Nutritional Fiber
- While fiber is important in adults, small children do not need quite as much.
- Fiber decreases the child's appetite by providing her with a feeling of fullness.
- This may interfere with growth and caloric intake, and decrease the absorption of calcium, zinc, and iron.
- Fibers are mostly found in breads, oatmeal, and rice.

- To calculate your child's daily fiber requirements, add 5 to her age (e.g., a 2 year old needs 7 grams of fiber per day).

Foods Not Recommended

The following foods do not offer your child adequate nutrition and encourages some unhealthy preferences. These foods contain added fat, sugar, or salt; fried foods such as French fries or home fries, iced cake or iced cookies, sugar coated cereals, flavored drinks or soft drinks, chocolate (see following), chips, and other salted snack foods.

- *Chocolate*: Moderation is the key to chocolate consumption without guilt, though it should not replace a well balanced diet. The general rule is the more cocoa, the better the chocolate is nutritionally. Dark chocolate contains the highest concentration of flavonoids (antioxidants). A square of dark chocolate may contain only about 50 calories, while most commercial candy has well above that amount. Chocolate is also a weak stimulant. It has the same amount of caffeine as 1 cup/250 ml of decaffeinated coffee. In addition, theobromine, which is an ingredient in chocolate, is more effective in stopping persistent coughing than codeine medication. Chocolate also seems to prevent blood clotting and the fat content in the cacao bean has components which cause good feelings in children. Furthermore, chocolate provides energy to the brain and magnesium, which causes relaxation.

- *Cola Consumption*: The caffeine added to cola as a flavoring agent is found to increase the risk of hyperactivity disorder (even just 3/4 of a can of coke). Please note that many of the clear and brightly colored soft drinks have caffeine added to them—sometimes in even larger amounts than the colas!

Behavior & Feeding

Reasons Your Child May Not Eat

Consistent meals and snacks for toddlers are important, as children like to have a routine. Between one to three years, parents are still able to interfere with their child's menu. However, taste preferences and the decision to eat particular foods will gradually develop in your toddler. The following are reasons why your child may not eat:

- Frequent snacking in-between meals, especially when snacking is close to mealtime.

- Juice or milk drinks decrease a child's appetite and produces a feeling of fullness.
- Acute illnesses or chronic diseases may be associated with appetite loss.
- Some children lose their appetite for a few weeks after a bout of stomach flu.
- In some periods of normal growth and development, the child does not eat much, as there is not much growth occurring (this is normal).
- For specific food refusal, refer to the appropriate chapters.

Messy Eaters & Learning to Feed Independently
- As toddlers begin to feed themselves, be prepared for the mess. This is the first real step your child makes towards independence. Showing independence is a normal developmental stage in your toddler. This includes food refusal to see how parents react, among other things (mealtime tantrums, etc.).
- Stay calm and have a relaxed, positive attitude during meal times.
- Usually, your child will make determined efforts around seven months of age to feed herself, but she does not have good enough coordination yet to get all the food into her mouth.
- At the beginning stages when the baby is hungry, start to feed her with a spoon and keep the bowl out of reach. If your child grabs the spoon, use two spoons at the same meal. Fill one and put it in the bowl so that she can pick it up. Fill the other one and keep it ready for when the spoon turns over on the way to her mouth. When this happens, pop your full spoon in and fill her mouth so that she can try again.
- The baby may put her finger into the bowl and push the food into her mouth. Once your child's hunger is satisfied, let her join you as you continue feeding her.
- Allow your child to learn by feeding her with plastic utensils that have curved handles that are easier for her to place in her mouth.
- Eating solid foods may make your child thirsty, so offer your baby formula or breast milk at meal times and tip the cup for her (since she cannot hold it on her own yet).
- Around 15 months of age, your child will make attempts to feed herself by spoon or fork, so cut the food into bite-sized pieces.

- Remember, your child is learning new things everyday, and now she is practicing how to eat. Everything is new to your child and she is using everything to learn (fingers, hands, and arms).
- Feed your child in a high chair or booster seat to decrease the chance of choking and messy spills everywhere.

Mealtime: A Happy Time
The following suggestions may make mealtimes more fun and less frustrating:
- Make mealtime a social, happy gathering.
- Present foods in different shapes, sizes, colors, and themes.
- Provide your child with small portions on her plate—do not overwhelm her with too much food. She will let you know if she is still hungry.
- Allow your child to feed herself as much as possible (even if she makes a mess).
- When your child refuses a certain food, do not stress or get upset over it. Simply offer it at the next meal or snack.
- Your child learns according to what you practice, as well. Serve your child the same foods that your family is eating.
- Be patient with your child and take your time during meal times. Keep the environment relaxed and calm.
- Do not force your child to finish all her food and do not use food as reward or punishment.
- Remove food from your child if she has not been eating for at least 20-30 minutes.
- Expect a mess when feeding your child and stay calm about it.
- Do not have distractions such as the television on during meal time.
- Supervise your child at all times, especially when she is eating.
- Encourage your child to always sit down when she is eating.
- Remember that your child's appetite varies all the time and she is not always hungry when adults are.
- Praise your child if she is trying new foods or shows appropriate behavior at the family dinner table.
- Discuss positive things at the table and, basically, have fun during meal times.

Helpful Tips

Vomiting & Food Rejection

- This type of vomiting must be distinguished from any underlying organic causes.

- The doctor will usually question the parents on the child's eating history.

- Vomiting is an effective means of manipulating or attracting the parents' attention.

- It can be associated with rejection of certain foods, while at the same time being used to manipulate parents on other issues (bedtime, child bonding, etc.).

- This type of vomiting on demand is rarely a cause for nutritional concern, but it needs to be assessed around the social and emotional family issues.

- Treatment for vomiting and food rejection may include the following:

  - ❖ Do not manipulate the diet in efforts to prevent vomiting.

  - ❖ Do not force feed and repeatedly present the rejected foods (in time, your toddler will accept new foods).

  - ❖ Do not give excessive attention—allow time for persistent cries or short cries before providing comfort.

  - ❖ Clean the vomit without any anger or emotions, since these emotions may give too much attention and reinforce the behavior. Simply ignore the behaviour.

Minerals

- It is important to use foods that are rich in iron, calcium, and zinc, such as the following:

  - ❖ Iron rich foods include enriched iron formula and cereal, meat, chicken, and soy.

  - ❖ Calcium rich foods include formula, milk enriched with calcium, most milk products, legumes, and soy based foods.

  - ❖ Zinc rich foods include formula, fortified cereal, meat, chicken, wheat, squash, fish, liver, dairy products, nuts, dried beans, and whole grain bread.

- Remember that toddlers are particularly prone to iron deficiency anemia (see *Iron & Iron Deficiency*), because they may have an increased intake of cow's milk, picky eating habits, are not on formula anymore, are using adult types of cereal, have a decreased appetite, etc. Because of this, parents need to make the effort to prevent iron and mineral deficiencies in their toddlers.

- Note that the most common deficiencies in toddlers are iron, calcium, zinc, vitamin B6 and vitamin A (see *Vitamins & Minerals*).

Milk & Calcium

- Milk source foods are the richest source of calcium.
- Do not offer too much cow's milk (more than 2 cups/500 ml a day), as this will affect your child's appetite. It may also increase the risk of iron deficiency anemia.
- If your child refuses milk, then calcium may be obtained from cheese, yogurt, sardines, fish, etc. (see *Dairy Products for Infants & Toddlers*).
- Milk is a major source of energy, so use whole fat milk and dairy products when your child is one to two. When your child is older than two years, you may then start to use reduced fat milk if you and your doctor have concerns about her fat intake.

Toddler Formula

- Toddler formula is good to use, especially in the picky eater. It will ensure that your child is receiving a more balanced diet.
- You may continue offering toddler formula after one year, as long as you do not give excessive amounts (which may lead to decreased consumption of other foods and nutrients).
  - ❖ Encourage your toddler to eat more solid foods, so that formula does not get in the way of other foods.
  - ❖ About 16 oz/500 ml of formula are acceptable to match the calcium and phosphorus levels your child needs. One benefit of toddler formula over whole milk is that it contains the omega-3 fatty acids that are found in breast milk.

Tip: Toddlers & Breastfeeding

Breastfeeding benefits toddlers nutritionally, immunologically, and psychologically. Breast milk continues to be a valued source of nutrition for toddlers. 15 oz/ 450 ml of breast milk provides a child between one to two years with these daily requirements; 29% energy, 43% protein, 36% calcium, 75% vitamin A, 76% folate, 94% vitamin B12, and 60% of vitamin C.

References

Periodicals and Bulletins

1. Alder, E.M., et al. 2004. "What influences the timing of the introduction of solid food to infants?" *British Journal of Nutrition* 92: 527-531.

2. Aldous, M.B. 1999. Nutritional issues for infants and toddlers. *Pediatric Annals* 28: 101-105.

3. Almnoth S., et al. 1990. No need for water supplementation for exclusively breastfed infants under hot and arid conditions. *Transactions of the Royal Society of Tropical Medicine and Hygiene* 84: 602-604.

4. American Academy of Pediatrics, committee on breastfeeding. 2005. Policy statement: Breastfeeding and the use of human milk. *Pediatrics* 115: 496-506.

5. American Academy of Pediatrics, committee on nutrition. 2001. Policy statement: The use and misuses of fruit juices in Pediatrics. *Pediatrics* 107: 1210-1213.

6. American Academy of Pediatrics. 2003. Policy statement. Prevention of pediatric overweight and obesity. *Pediatrics* 112: 424-430.

7. Anonymous. Patient Information. 2005. Eggs: a good source of nutrition for children. *Advance for Nurse Practitioners* 13: 19-20.

8. Arenz S., et al. 2004. Breastfeeding and childhood obesity—a systematic review. *International Journal of Obesity and Related Metabolic Disorders* 28: 1247-1256.

9. Ariza A.J., et al. 2004. Childhood overweight: management approach in young children. *Pediatric Annals* 1: 33-51.

10. Arts-Rodeas, D., et al. 1998. Feeding problems in infancy and early childhood: Identification and management. *Paediatric: Child Health* 3: 21-25.

11. Baker, R.D. 2002. Infant formula safety. (Commentaries). *Pediatrics* 110: 833-836.

12. Baker, S.S. 2000. Iron fortification of infant formula. *Pediatrics* 105: 1370-1371.

13. Baker, S.S., et al. 1989. American Academy of Pediatrics. Committee on nutrition. Calcium requirements of infants, children and adolescents. *Pediatrics* 104: 1152-1157.

14. Balbus, J.M., et al. 2001. Is the water safe for my baby? (Review). *The Pediatric Clinics of North America* 48: 1129-1152.

15. Ballard, J.L., et al. 2002. Ankyloglossia: assessment, incidence, and effect of frenuloplasty on the breastfeeding dyad. *Pediatrics* 110: 63-68.

16. Barchner, H. 2003. Cow's milk allergy is different from lactose intolerance. *Archives of Disease in Childhood* 88: 1029-1030.

17. Barton, D. Schmidt, et al. 1992. Encopresis 20 management mistakes. *Patient care* 26: 221-231.

18. Brown, K.H., et al.1986. Milk consumption and hydration status of exclusively breastfed infants in a warm climate. *Journal of Pediatrics* 108: 677-680.

19. Bruce, R. C., et al. 1997. Hyponatremic seizures secondary to oral water intoxication in infancy: Associated with commercial bottled drinking water (review). *Pediatrics* 100: (6) E4.

20. Buchan, I.E. et al. 2005. Early life risk factor for obesity in childhood: Early feeding is crucial target for preventing obesity in child. *British Medical Journal* 331: 453-454.

21. Canadian Pediatric Society. 2004. Weaning your child from breastfeeding. *Paediatrics & Child Health* 9: 254-255.

22. Canadian Pediatric Society 2004. Weaning from the breast (position statement). *Paediatrics & Child Health* 9: 249-252.

REFERENCES

23.   Caroccetti, M., et al. 2004. Parental belief and practices regarding early introduction of solid foods to their children. *Clinical Pediatrics* 43:541-547.

24.   Carruth, B.R., et al. 2004. Prevalence of picky eaters among infants and toddlers and their caregivers decision about offering a new food. *Journal of the American Dietetic Association* 104: 57-64.

25.   Carruth, B.R., et al. 2000. Revisiting the picky eater phenomenon neophobic behavior of young children. *Journal of the American College of Nutrition* 19: 771-780.

26.   Cathey, Mary, et al. 2004. Picky eating: a toddler approach to mealtime. *Pediatric Nursing* 30: 101-107.

27.   Chatoor, I. 2002. Feeding disorders in infants and toddlers: diagnosis and treatment. *Child & Adolescent Psychiatric Clinic of North America* 11: 163-83.

28.   Christofides A., et al.2005. Iron deficiency anemia among children. Addressing a global public health problem within a Canadian context. *Paediatrics & Child Health* 10: 579-601.

29.   Corrylos, Elizabeth, et al.2004. Breastfeeding: Best for baby and mother. Congenital Tongue Tie and its impact on breastfeeding. *American Academy of Pediatrics* Summer: 1-6.

30.   Danowski, L., et al.2002. Selection from current literature attitudes and practices regarding the introduction of solid foods to infant. *Family practice* 19: 698-702.

31.   Dennison, B.A. 1996. Fruit juices consumption by infants and children: a review. *Journal of the American College of Nutrition* 15: 45-115.

32.   Duffy, V.B., et al. 2000. Food acceptance & genetic variation in taste. *Journal of the American Dietetic Association* 100: 547-647-655.

33.   Edan, A.N. 2005. Iron supplementation for 1 to 2 years olds. *Pediatrics* 106 (5): 1166.

34.   Edmund, L.D. 2005. Parent's perception of health professional response when seeking help for their overweight children. *Family Practice* 22: 287-292.

35.   Ells, L.J., et al. 2005. Prevention of childhood obesity. Best practice & research. *Clinical Endocrinology and Metabolism* 19: 441-454.

36.   Emmett, P., et al. 2000. Types of drinks consumed by infants at 4 and 8 months of age: a discipline study. *The ALS PAC study team. Public health nutrition* 3: 211-217.

37.   Foote, K.D., et al. 2003. Weaning of infants (Review). *Archives of Diseases in Childhood* 88: 488-492.

38.   Garrison, M.M., et al. 2000. A systematic review of treatment for infant's colic. *Pediatrics* 106: 184-190.

39.   Garza, C. De Onis, et al. 2004. Rational for developing a new international growth reference. *Food and Nutrition Bulletin* 25: 5-14.

40.   Green, F.R. 2001. Do breastfed infants need supplementary vitamins? *The Pediatric Clinics of North America* 48: 415-423.

41.   Griffth, D.M., et al. 2004. A randomized, controlled trial of division of tongue-tie infants with feeding problems. *Archives of Disease in Childhood* 89: (S1) A2.

42.   Guffin, I.J., et al. 2001. Iron and breastfeeding. *The Pediatric Clinics of North America* 48: 401-413.

43.   Gundaker, Claudia, et al. 2002. Lead and mercury in breast milk. *Pediatrics* 110: 873-879.

44.   Halterman, J.S., et al. 2001. Iron deficiency and cognitive achievement among school-aged children and adolescents in the United States. *Pediatrics* 107: 1381-1386.

45.   Harder, T. et al. 2005. Duration of breastfeeding and risk of overweight: A meta-analysis. *American Journal of Epidemiology* 162: 397-403.

46.   Harrod-wild, K. 2002. When to introduce solids. *Journal of Family Health Care* 12: 4.

47.   Health Canada. 2004. *Vitamin D supplementation for breastfed infants: Health Canada recommendation 2004* http:// www. Healthcanada.ca/nutrition.

48.   Hiscock, H., et al. 2004. Problem crying in infancy: MJA practice essentials. *Pediatrics* 181: 507-512.

49. Hitchcock, N.E., et al. 1985. The growth of breastfed and artificially fed infants from birth to twelve months. *Acta Paediatrica Scandinavia* 74: 240-245.

50. Hoekstra, J.H., et al. 1995. Fluid intake and industrial processing in apple juice induced chronic non-specific diarrhea. *Archives of Disease in Childhood* 73: 126-130.

51. Howard, R. Cynthia, et al. 2003. Randomized clinical trial of pacifier use and bottle feeding vs. cup feeding and the effects on breastfeeding. *Pediatrics* 8: 511-518.

52. Kassing, D. 2002. Bottle feeding as a food to reinforce breastfeeding. *Journal of Human Lactation* 18: 56-60.

53. Keanne, V., et al. 1988. Do solids help baby sleep through the night? *American Journal of Diseases of Children* 142: 404-405.

54. Kelosa, K.M., et al. 1997. Nutrition during pregnancy. *American Family Physician* 56: 205-216.

55. Kelso, John K. 2005. The introduction of solid in relation to asthma and eczema. *Pediatrics* 116: 539.

56. Kelso, M. 2003. Nuts allergy in school children. *Pediatrics* 112: 459.

57. Kramer, M.S., et al. 2002. Optimal duration of exclusive breastfeeding (review). *Cochran database of systematic reviews.* (1) C D 003517.

58. Krebs, N.F. 2000. Dietary zinc and iron sources, physical growth and cognitive development of breastfed infants. *Journal of Nutrition* 130: 358-360.

59. Krebs, N.F., et al. 2002. Zinc and breastfed infants: If and when is there a risk of deficiency. *Advance in Experimental Medicine and Biology* 503: 69-75.

60. Kumor, K. 2001. Screening for anemia in children: AAP recommendation—A critique. Pediatrics 108: 56.

61. Lanigan, J.A., et al. 2001. Systematic review concerning the age of introduction of complementary foods to the healthy full term infant. *European Journal of Clinical Nutrition* 55: 309-320.

62. Lever, R., et al. 1998. Randomized controlled trial of advice on an egg exclusion diet in young children with atopic eczema and sensitivity to eggs. *Pediatric Allergy & Immunology* 9: 13-19.

63. Li, D.K., et al. 2006. Use of a dummy (pacifier) during sleep and risk of sudden infant death syndrome (SIDS): population base care control study. *British Medical Journal* 7:332: 18-21.

64. Lifshitz, F. 1996. Weaning foods: The role of fruit juice in the diet of infants and children. *Journal of the American College of Nutrition* 15: 1-3.

65. Lozoff, B., et al. 2000. Poorer behavioural and developmental outcome more than 10 years after treatment for iron deficiency in infancy. *Pediatrics* 105: 51.

66. Lumerg, J. 2005. Is the picky eater a cause for concern? *Contemporary Pediatrics* 22: 71-72, 75-76, 79-82.

67. MacDonald, A. 2003. Is breast best? Is early solid feeding harmful? *Journal of the Royal Society of Health* 123: 169-179.

68. Matthew, O.D. 1991. Science of Bottlefeeding. *Journal of Pediatrics* 119: 511-519.

69. Mayer, E.J., et al. 1998. Reduced use of IDDM (Diabetes) among breastfeed children. *Diabetes* 37: 1625-1632.

70. Mennella, J.A., et al. 1998. Early flavor experiences: research update. *Nutrition Review* 56: 205-211.

71. Michaelsen, K.F. 2000. Cow's milk in complementary feeding. *Pediatrics* 106: 1302-1303.

72. Migrath, S.M., et al. 2004. State of the science: feeding readiness in preterm infants. *The Journal of Perinatal & Neonatal Nursing* 18: 353-371.

73. Milner, J.D., et al. 2004. Early infant multi-vitamin supplement is associated with increased risk of food allergy and asthma. *Pediatrics* 114: 27-32.

74. Mocknin, M.L., et al. 1989. Infant sleep and bedtime cereal. *American Journal of Diseases of Children* 143: 1066-1068.

75. Morin, K. Solid, 2004. When and why. *MCN American Journal of Maternal Child Nursing* 29: 259.

REFERENCES

76. Morland-Schultz K., and P.D. Hill. 2005. Prevention of and therapies for nipple pain: A systematic review. *Journal of Obstetrics, Gynecology & Neonatal Nursing* 34: 428-437.

77. Morrill, J.F. 2005. Risk factors for mammary candidosis among lactating women. *Journal of Obstetrics, Gynecology & Neonatal Nursing* 34: 37-45.

78. Muraro, A., et al. 2004. Dietary prevention of allergic disease in infants and small children. *Pediatrics, Allergy & Immunology* 15: 291-307.

79. Neifert, M., et al. 1995. Nipple confusion: towards a formal definition. *Journal of Pediatrics* 126: 125-129.

80. Nichols, M.I., et al. 2002. Preventing pediatric obesity: assessment and management in the primary care setting (review). *Journal of the American Academy of Nurse Practitioners* 14: 55-62.

81. Owen, Christopher G., et al. 2005. Effect of infant feeding on the risk of obesity across the life course: A quantitative review of published evidence. *Pediatrics* 115: 1367-1377.

82. Reed, A., et al. 2001. Consideration in planning vegan diet. *Journal of the American Dietetic Association* 101: 670-676.

83. Romeo, S. 2001. Transitioning to table foods. The parent's offers and the child eat... sometimes. *Advance for Nurse Practitioners* 9: 63-64, 67-68.

84. Rosenberg, L. 2000. Bottle to cup: A formula for easy transition. *Contemporary Pediatrics* 17: 118.

85. Sachidev, H.P., et al. 1991. Water supplementation in exclusively breastfed infants during summer in the tropics. *Lancet* 337: 929-933.

86. Saloojee, H. 2001. Iron deficiency and impaired child development. *British Medical Journal* 323: 1377-1378.

87. Sanchez, J.E., et al. 2001. Methemoglobinemia and consumption of vegetables in infants. *Pediatrics* 107: 1024-1028.

88. Silmer, M.A., et al. 1984. Exclusive breastfeeding for 9 months. Risk of iron deficiency. *Journal of Pediatrics*: 104: 199-198.

89. Skinner, J.D., et al. 2001. A longitudal study of children's juice intake and growth: the juice controversy revisited. *Journal of the American Dietetic Association* 101: 432-437.

90. Skinner, J.D., et al. 1999. Fruit Juice intake is not related to children's growth. *Pediatrics* 103: 58-64.

91. Sicherer, S.H., et al. 2003. Symposium: Pediatric food allergy. *Pediatrics* 111: 1591-1594.

92. Smith, M.M., et al. 1994. Excess fruit juice consumption as a contributing factor in non-organic failure to thrive. *Pediatrics* 93: 438-443.

93. Victoria, Cesar G., et al. 1993. Use of pacifier and breastfeeding duration. *Lancet* 341: 404-407.

94. Welsh J.A., et al. 2005. Overweight among low-income preschool children associated with the consumption of sweet drinks: Missouri, 1999-2002. *Pediatrics* 115: 223-229.

95. Wharton, B.A., et al. 1999. Low plasma vitamin D in Asian toddlers in Britain. *British Medical Journal* 318: 2-3.

96. Wood, R.A. 2003. The natural history of food allergy. *Pediatrics* 111: 1631-1637.

97. Woolridge, M.W. 1986. The anatomy of infant sucking. *Midwifery* 2: 164-171.

98. Zeger, R.S., et al. 2002. Current issues with vaccination in egg allergy. *Journal of Allergy & Clinical Immunology* 110: 834-840.

99. Ziegher, A.G., et al. 2003. Early infant feeding and risk of developing type 1 diabetes-associated autoantibodies. *Journal of the American Medical Association* 290: 1721-1728.

Books

1. Briggs, B., Road Freeman and S. Yaffe. 2002. *Drugs in Pregnancy & Lactation: 6ᵗʰ Edition*. Philadelphia, London. Williams and Wilkins.

2. Deitz, W.H. and L. Stern. 1999. *The American Academy of Pediatrics. Guide to Your Child's Nutrition*. New York. Villard Books, Random House.

3. Kalnins, D. and J. Saab. 2001. *The Hospital for Sick Children. Better Baby Food*. Toronto. Robert Rose Books.

4. La Leche League International. 2004. *The Womanly Art of Breastfeeding: 7th Edition*. USA. Penguin Groups.

5. Linardakis, Connie. 2001. *Homemade Baby Foods: Pure & Simple*. New York. Three Rivers Press.

6. Murkof, Heidi and Arlene Eisenberg. 2003. *What to Expect the First Year.* New York. Workman Publishing.

7. Newman, Jack. 2003. *Dr. Jack Newman's Guide to Breastfeeding*. Toronto. Harper Collins Publishing.

8. Shelmov, Steven P. 1998. *Your Baby's First Year*. New York. *The American Academy of Pediatrics*, Bantam Books.

9. William, J. 2005. *Baby and Child Health. The essential guide from birth to 11 years:1ˢᵗ Canadian Edition*. Canadian Medical Association DK.

10. Yaron, Ruth. 2005. *Super Baby Food*. Brainerd, Minnesota. Bang Printing, F.J. Roberts Publishing.

11. Younger, Meek, and Sherill Tippins, eds. 2002. *American Academy of Pediatrics New Mother's Guide to Breastfeeding*. New York. Bantam Books.

Index

INDEX

INDEX

Pertussis, 106
Pesticides, 152, 268
Phenylketonuria, 144
Phototherapy, 99-102
Phytates, 375, 641
Phytic acids, 147, 630
Phytoestrogens, 147, 404, 564
Pica, 633
Picky eater, 644-663
    And specific food refusal, 655
    Causes, 645
    How to manage, 650
    Mealtime environment, 647
    Parental behavior, 646
Pincer grasp, 385
Pizza, 376
Plugged milk ducts, 50
Plums, 329
Poisoning, food, 523, 552
Polycarbonate bottles (see *Bottles*), 184
Polyunsaturated fats, 587
Popcorn, 240, 277
Portagen, 153
Potatoes, 313
    Mashed, 274
    Sweet, 313
    White, 313
Pouching, 662
Poultry, 286
Powder formula (see *Forms of Formula*), 171
Premature nipples (see *Nipples*), 164
Prick skin test, 400
Progesterone, 60
Prolactin, 6, 66
Prosobee, 483
Protein (complete & incomplete), 355
Public breastfeeding, 80
Pumpkin seeds, 630
Pumps, 122
    Techniques
    Types
    How to
Purified water, 540
Pyloric stenosis, 464
Pyramid, food, 583
Radioactive scanning, 107
Radioallergosorbent test (RAST), 527
Raisins, 277, 450, 484
Ready-to-feed formula (see *Forms of Formula*), 173
Recipes
    Banana puree with rice, 336
    Cheese omelet, 415
    Chicken & rice mix, 368
    For 4-6 months, 324

For older than 6-7 months, 325
Fruits & yogurt, 336
Fun with fish, 367
Great meatballs, 367
Homemade cereal, 309
Homemade vegetables, 324
Oatmeal & banana cereal, 309
Older than one year, 326
Puree with pears & apples, 337
Recreational drugs, 108
Reflex
    Extrusion, 249
    Gag, 235
    Gastrocolic, 480
    Rooting, 185, 235
    Tongue-thrust, 247
Reflux (see *GER*), 436-478
Reflux esophagitis, 466
Regurgitation, 428, 464
Relactation, 212
Rental pumps, 125
Replacing bottles (see *Bottles*), 162
Reusable bottles (see *Bottles*), 160
Rhinitis, 321, 535
Rhubarb, 278
Rice
    Brown versus white, 306
    Cereal, 232, 256
Rickets, 148, 673
Safe feeding & food safety, 552-564
    Choking, 555
    E. coli, 564
    Feeding safely, 556
    Food poisoning, 552
    Hand washing, 554
    Outdoor food safety, 563
    Refrigeration, 555
Salad
    Dressing, 235
    Vegetables for, 316
Salmonella, 335
    Egg cooking safety and, 414
Salt, 546
Sample menus
    4-6 months, 308
    8-12 months, 353
    10-12 months, 366
    One-year-old, 383
    6-12 months, 609
    6-8 months, 323, 336
    8-10 months, 366, 389
Sardines, 356
Scurvy, 328
Sequence of food introduction (by age), 232

About the Author

Dr. Maurice Levy

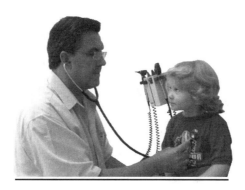

I am a Pediatrician practicing medicine and pediatrics for the last 30 years. I trained and worked in various hospitals around the globe including Belgium (1972-1973), France (1973-1977), Tel Aviv (1977-1980), finishing my medical degree at the University of Tel Aviv, Israel in 1980.

I have trained in Pediatrics from 1980 to 1986 at Edith Wolfson Hospital in Holon/Tel Aviv, Israel and developed a special interest in nutrition back in 1986 when I began working at St. Justine Hospital, Montreal, in the department of endocrine, metabolism and nutrition. Patients encountered included those with nutritional problems and Pradder-Willi Syndrome who were very obese due to a voracious and uncontrollable appetite.

I also began doing research at St. Justine Hospital, studying the effects of various diets on mice with similarly induced human liver diseases. This led me to obtain a research degree of Masters in Clinical Science.

Following that, I worked at the University of Montreal and began a PhD program on diabetes and cholesterol findings in the cell mitochondria. I then moved to the Hospital for Sick Children in Toronto and worked for about ten years there. Initially, I worked in the Mother Risk Clinic in the department of clinical pharmacology and toxicology and provided medical advice to parents and health professionals regarding the effects of breastfeeding, drugs, and infections on the pregnant mother and fetus/newborn.

Moreover, I trained in pediatric nephrology at the Hospital for Sick Children (HSC) and dealt with sick patients on dialysis and with renal diseases, requiring many dietary recommendations and adjustments (e.g. in patients with acute and chronic renal failure, in nephrotic syndrome patients, adjusting their minerals, vitamins and protein intakes, etc).

After leaving HSC, I worked as an active staff member at North York Branson Hospital, Toronto and became Chief of Pediatrics for about 5 years, for which I had multiple responsibilities. The latter were not only those extended to children in the hospital but also, in the nursery as well, where there were newborns and premature babies requiring medical knowledge in feeding and nutrition along with other associated medical problems.

At this time, I was also a member of the Medical Advisory Committee Board at the hospital. Along with these responsibilities, I was responsible for the pediatricians within the department. One of my duties was to support and teach pediatricians, students and other health professionals in various medical aspects including those related to feeding and nutrition. The teaching aspect had already begun in 1981, while working in the hospital in Israel. I taught students affiliated with the University of Tel-Aviv, Israel. That teaching has continued until now with students from the University of Toronto and doctors from there as well.

From the time at North York Branson Hospital (which is now North York General Hospital - NYGH) until now, I work at NYGH and in my office, dealing with extensive newborns, infants, toddlers and older children as a primary care and consultant. In my medical practice, I see many infants and children who are healthy and those with various diseases requiring specific needs such as those with cleft lip & palate, cystic fibrosis patients, vegetarians, those with congenital heart disease, etc.

While in previous years, I was a member of various committees in the hospital (including the Research Ethic Board Committee), in recent years, I am the Head of Research for the Pediatric department and an active staff member at NYGH. I am responsible for the assessment and permission of various research propositions with many research topics done by pediatricians of my department. Actually, I continue to have an extensive and active practice in pediatrics.

Furthermore, I have published many articles in important medical journals of various topics. In fact, I was a writer in a journal magazine (La-Isha) writing about pediatric topics and answering parental concerns and questions, already in 1982.

Despite the fact that feeding and nutrition of infants and children is extremely important, unfortunately it is not well-taught in schools and students or other health professionals bear much of the parents' guessing as well. They, like the parents, look for books or any other sources for further daily and practical information.

My past medical experiences and activities until present day, dealing with countless children and parents of infants and young children and dealing with health professionals, allows me to provide much advice & handouts regarding feeding and nutrition aspects of daily concerns. Careful research and observation over the last 30 years of experience have inspired me to write this book.